嚴 潔編著 尹鋼林譯

圖解中國針灸技法

SKILL
WITH ILLUSTRATIONS
OF CHINESE ACUPUNCTURE
AND MOXIBUSTION

湖南科技出版社
科學出版社

封面、扉頁題字：伍純道
協助編寫人員：丁果元
　　　　　　　胡志光
　　　　　　　曾淑芳
插　圖　繪　制：汪浣新

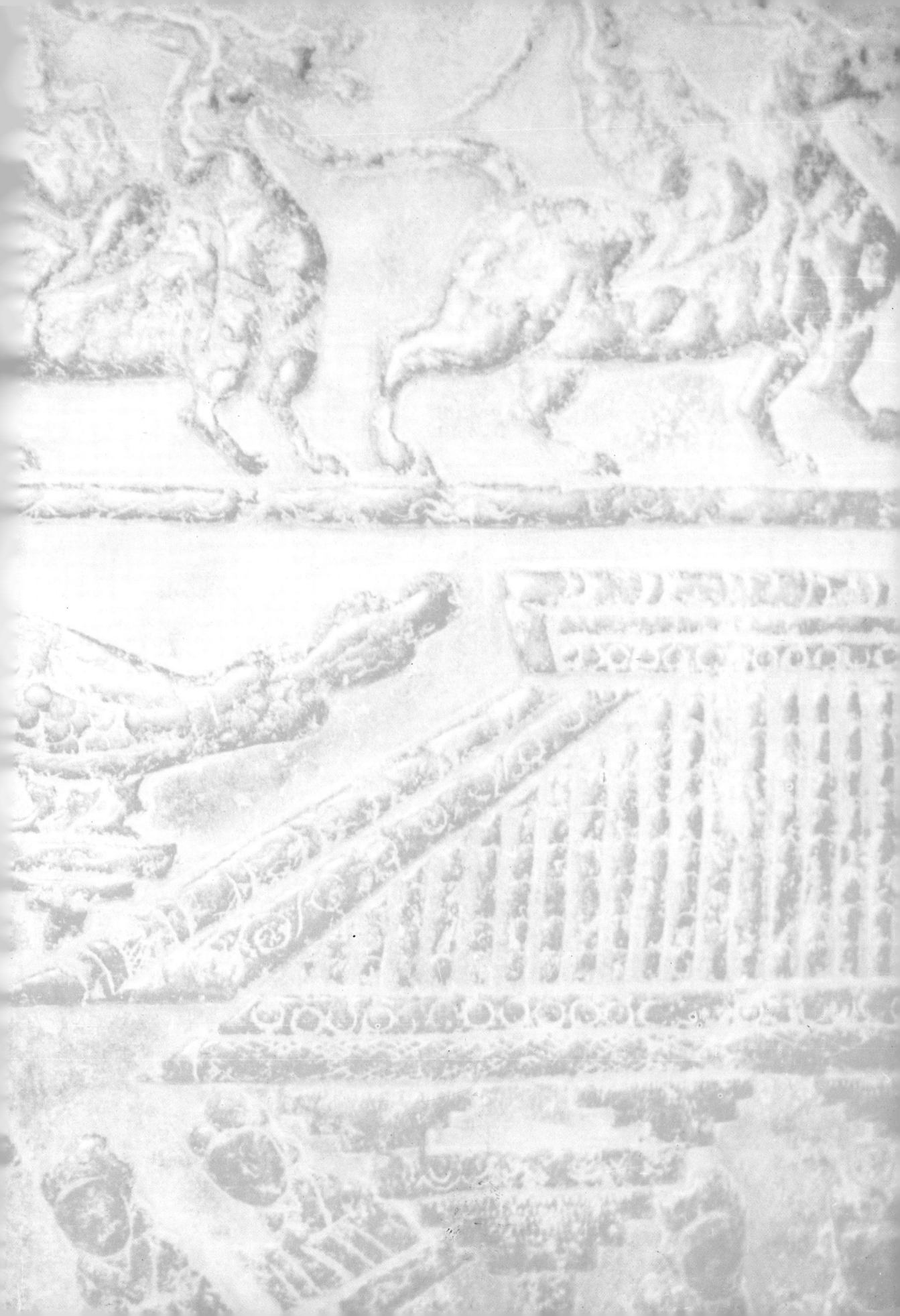

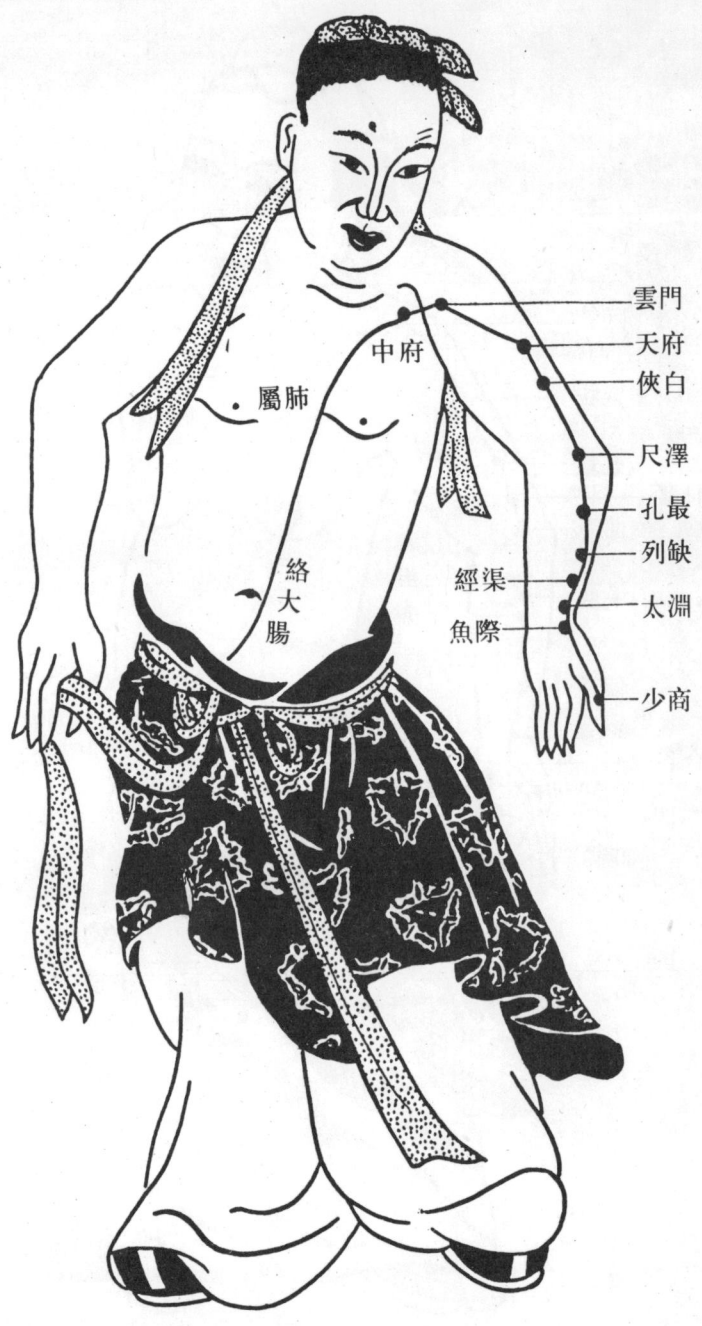

中國古代經絡圖——手太陰肺經
Ancient Chinese Meridian Picture – The Lung Meridian of Hand-Taiyin

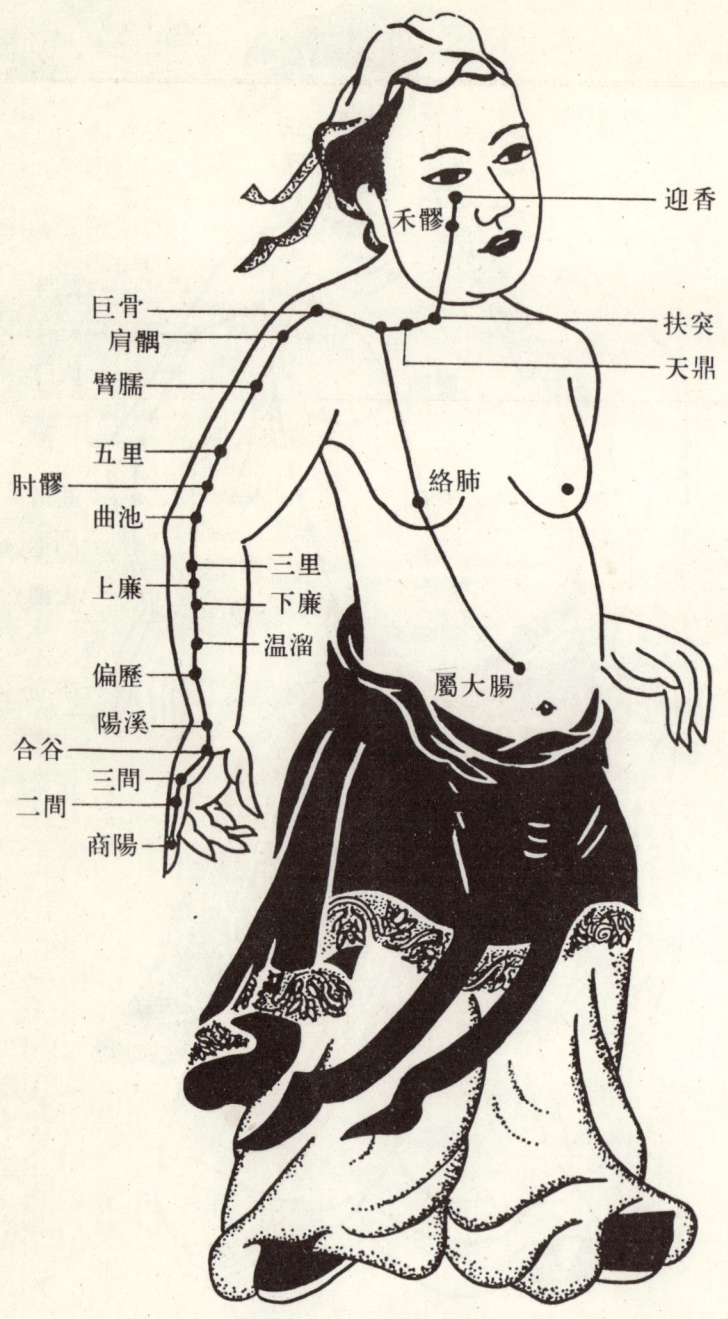

中國古代經絡圖——手陽明大腸經
Ancient Chinese Meridian Picture – The Large Intestine Meridian of Hand-Yangming

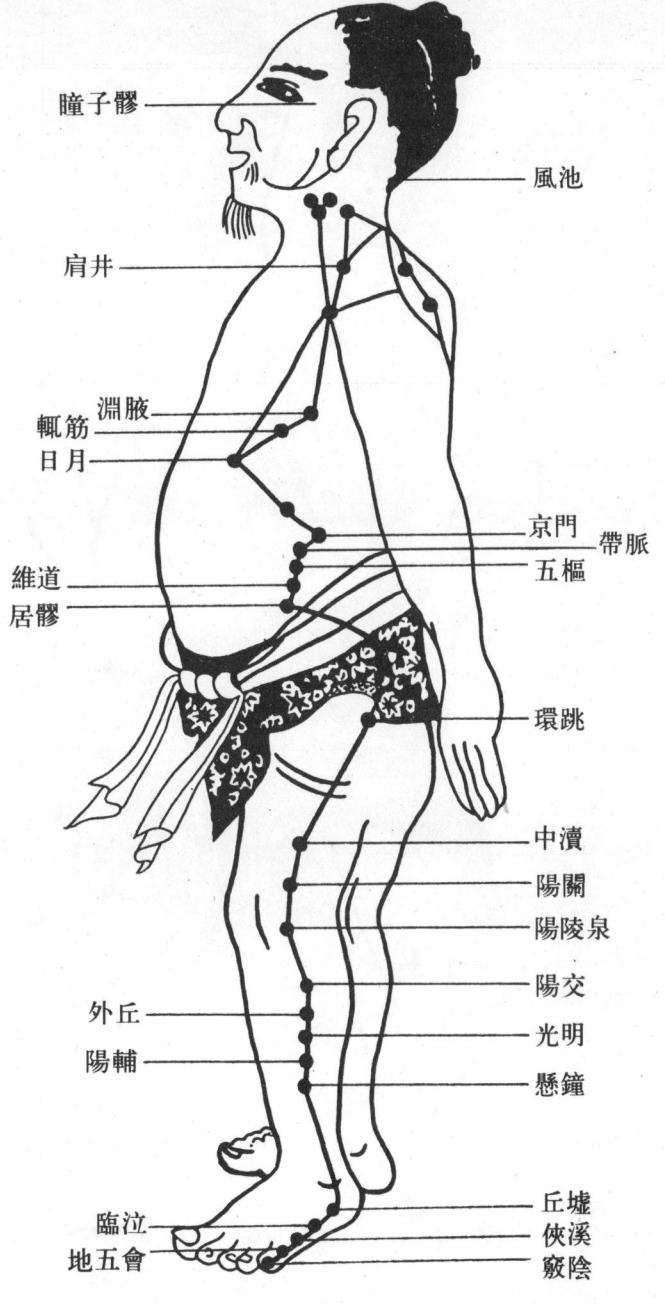

中國古代經絡圖──足少陽膽經
Ancient Chinese Meridian Picture – The Gallbladder Meridian of Foot-Shaoyang

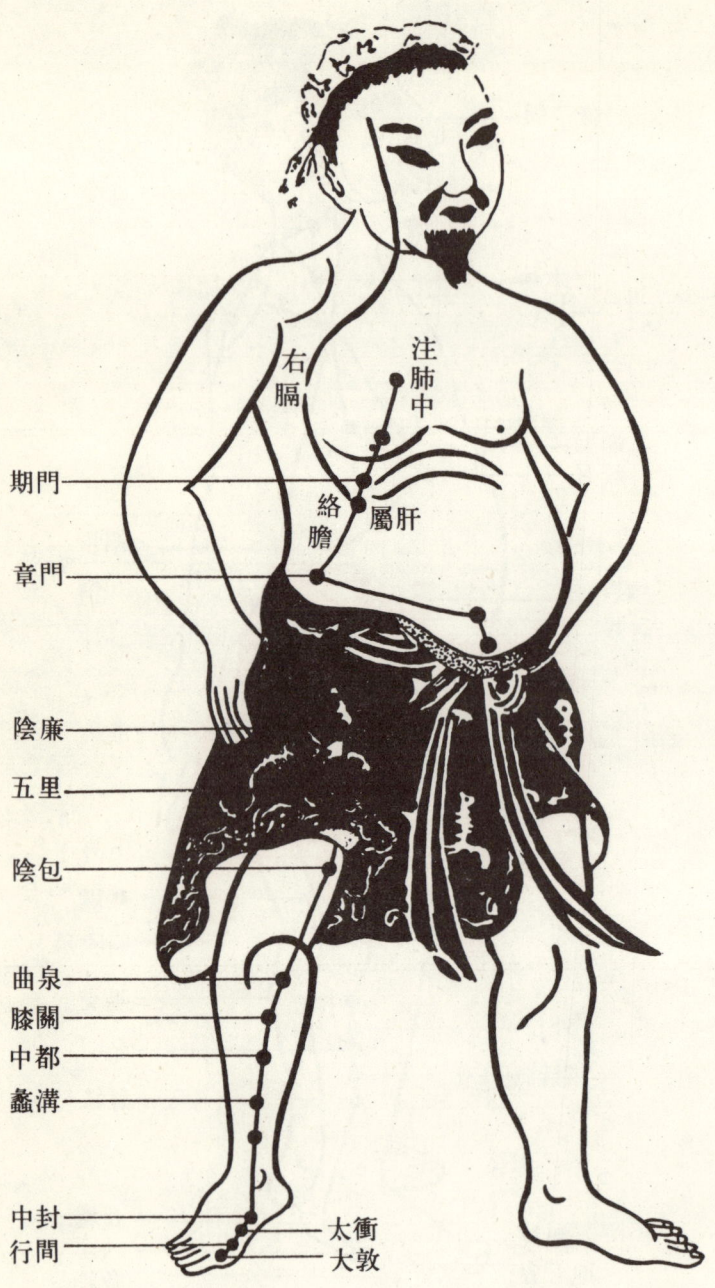

中國古代經絡圖──足厥陰肝經
Ancient Chinese Meridian Picture – The Liver Meridian of Foot-Jueyin

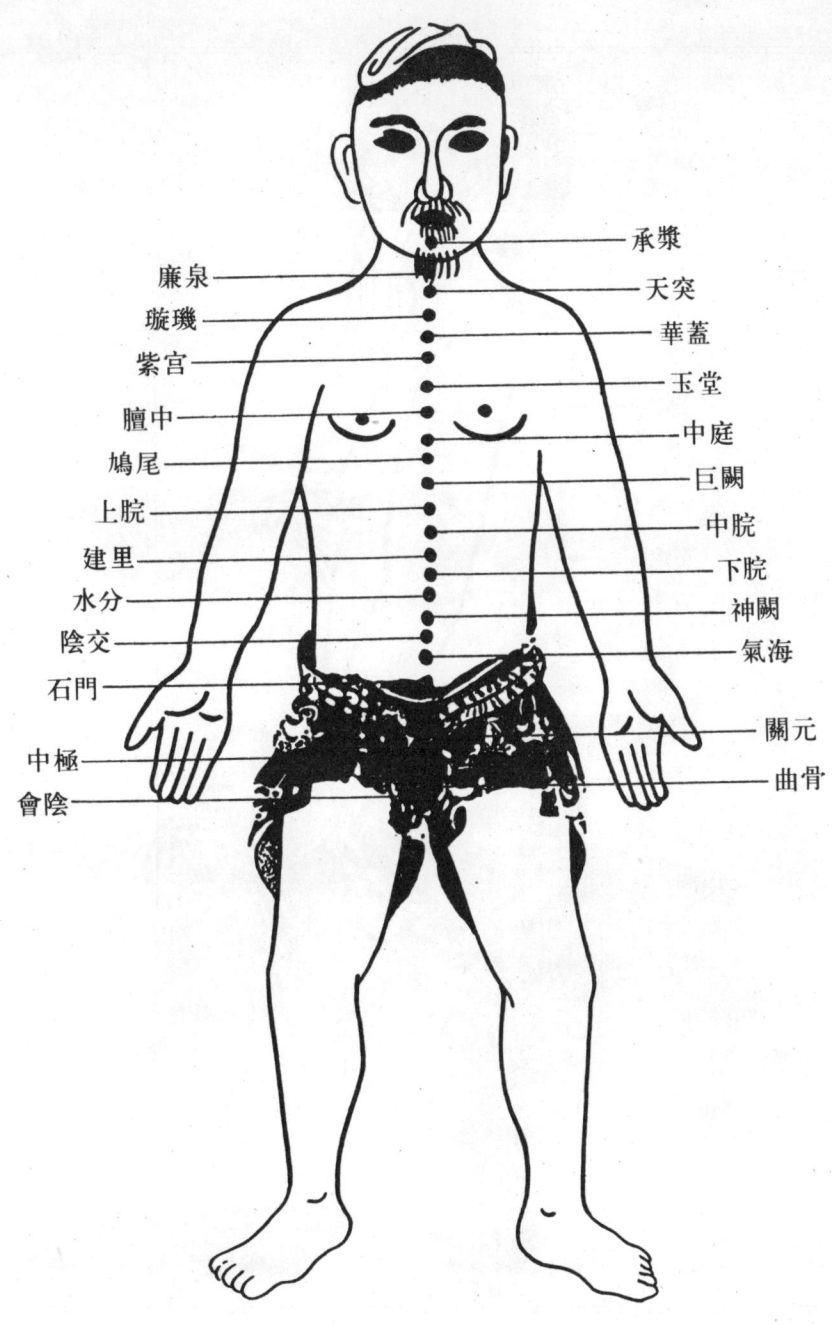

中國古代經絡圖──任脈
Ancient Chinese Meridian Picture – The Ren Meridian

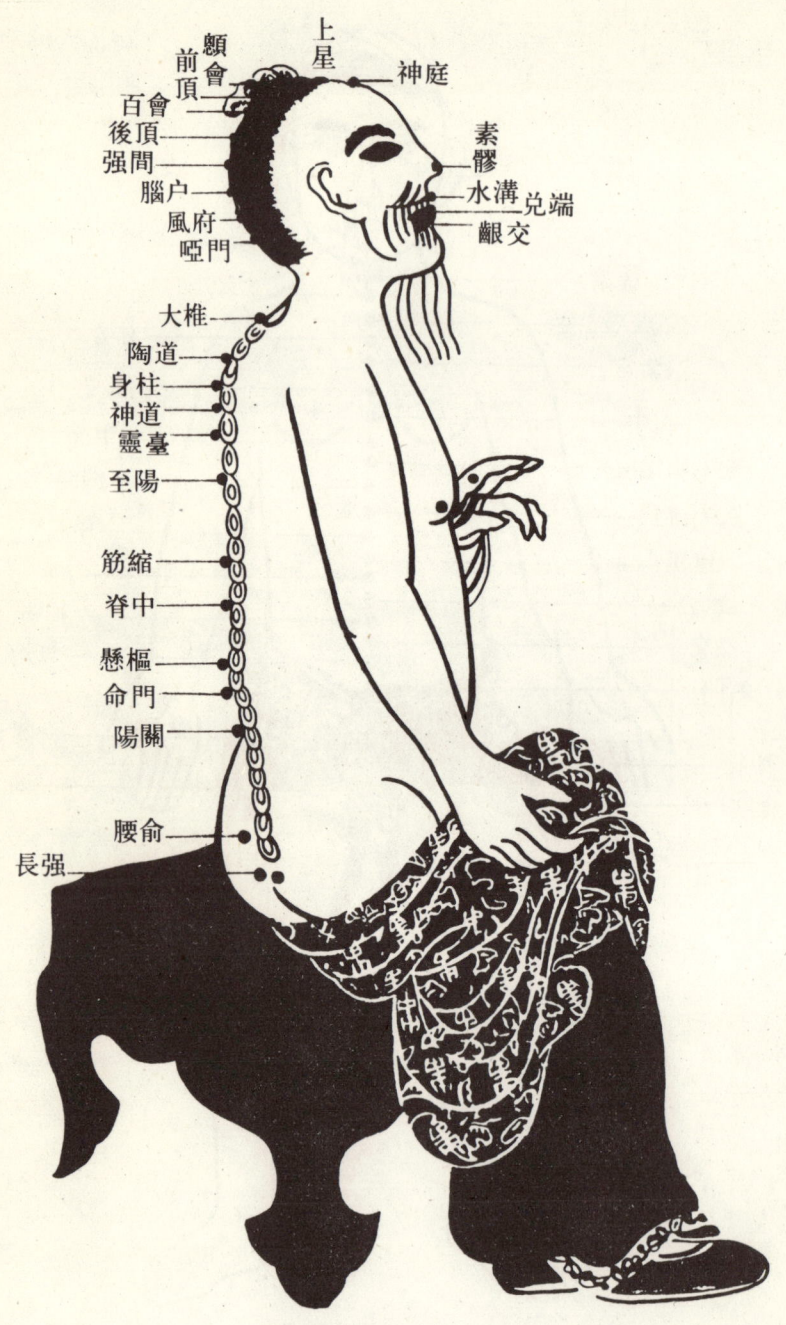

中國古代經絡圖──督脈
Ancient Chinese Meridian Picture – The Du Meridian

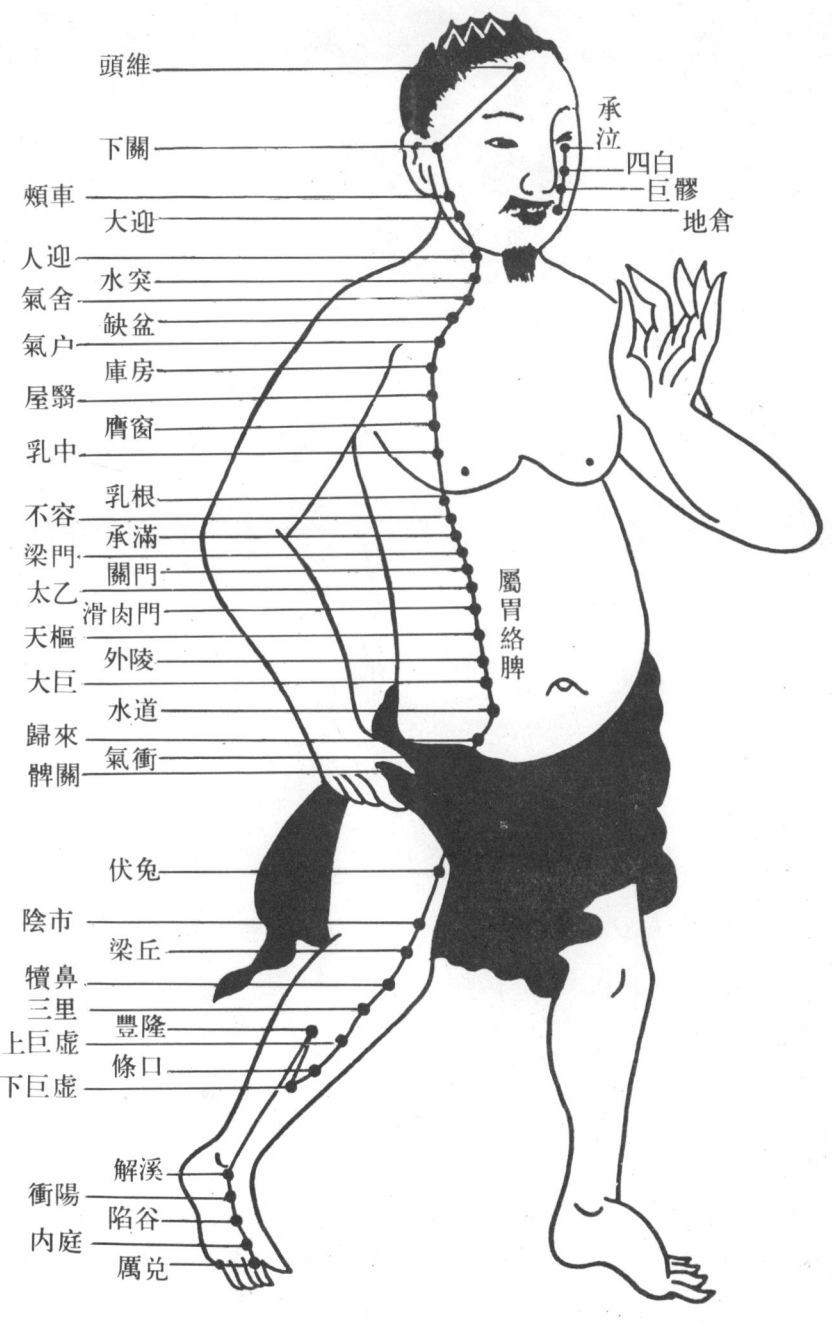

中國古代經絡圖──足陽明胃經
Ancient Chinese Meridian Picture – The Stomach Meridian of Foot-Yangming

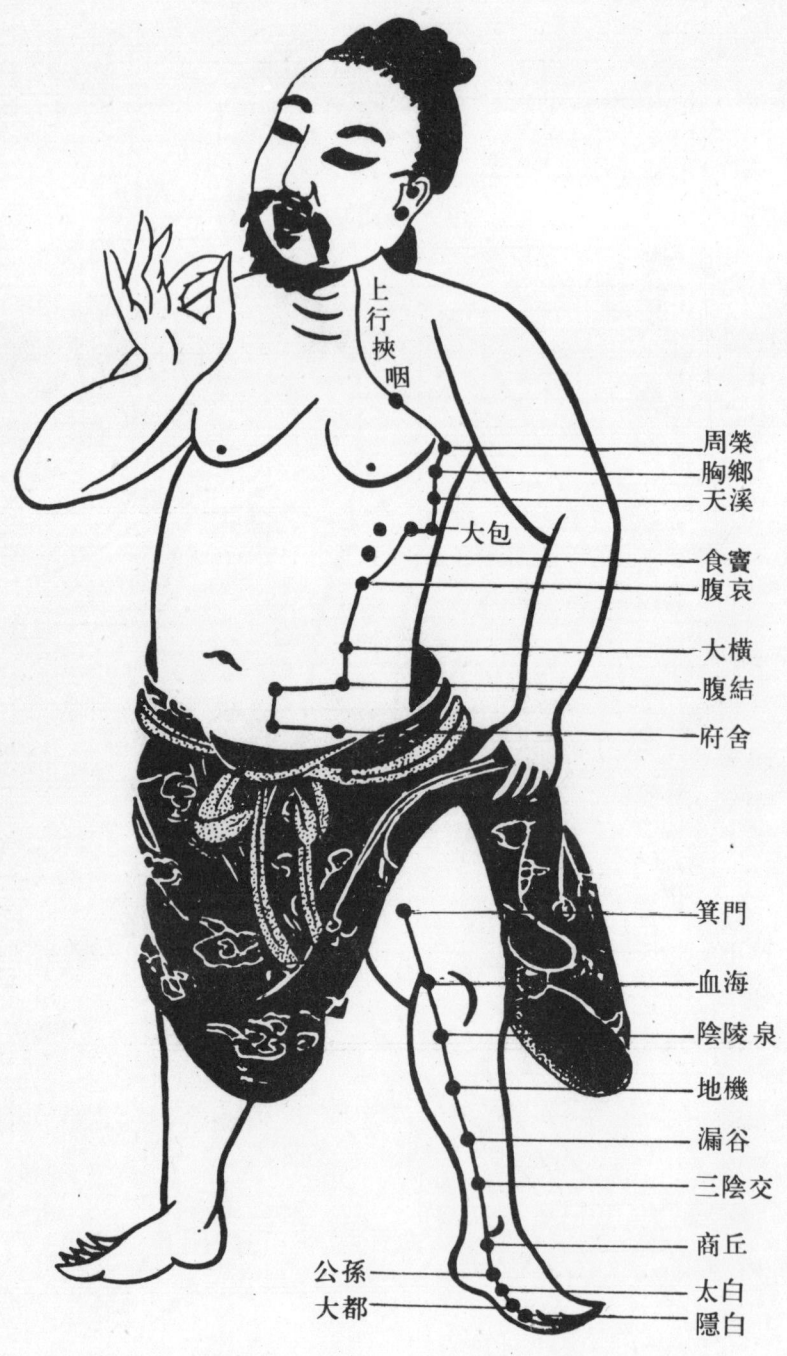

中國古代經絡圖──足太陰脾經
Ancient Chinese Meridian Picture – The Spleen Meridian of Foot-Taiyin

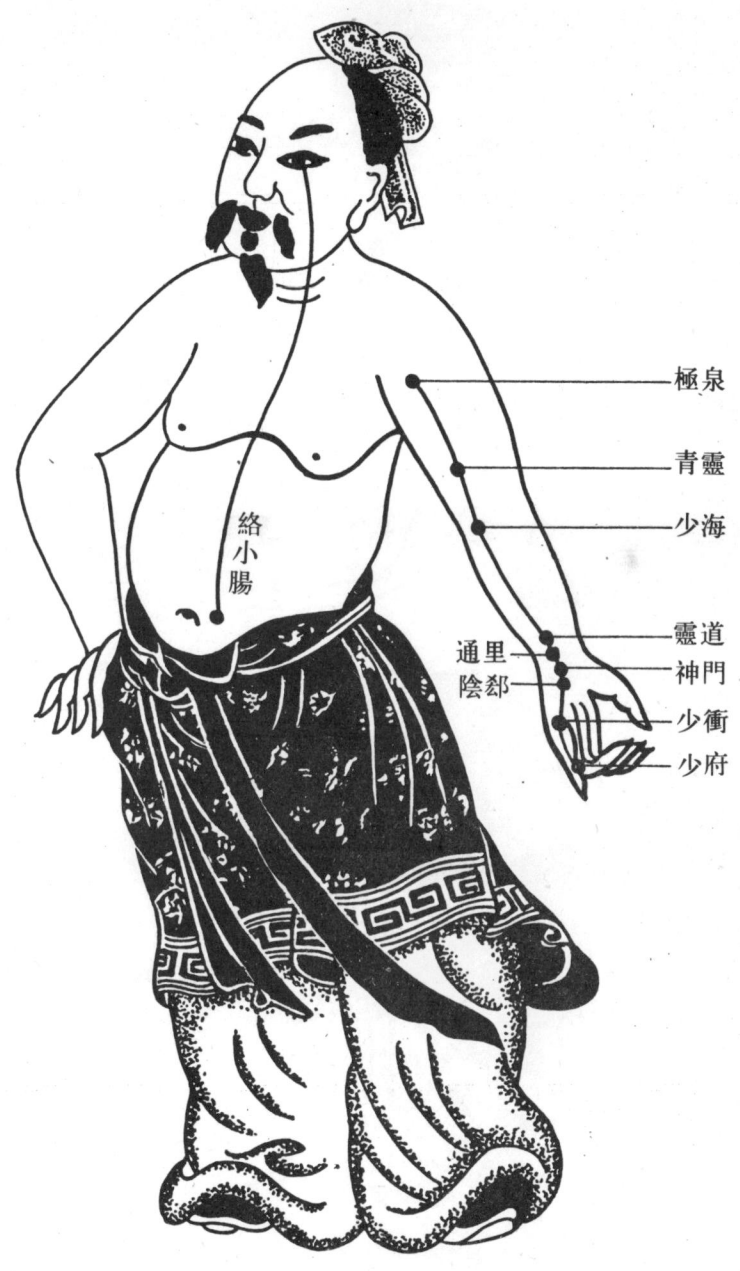

中國古代經絡圖──手少陰心經
Ancient Chinese Meridian Picture – The Heart Meridian of Hand-Shaoyin

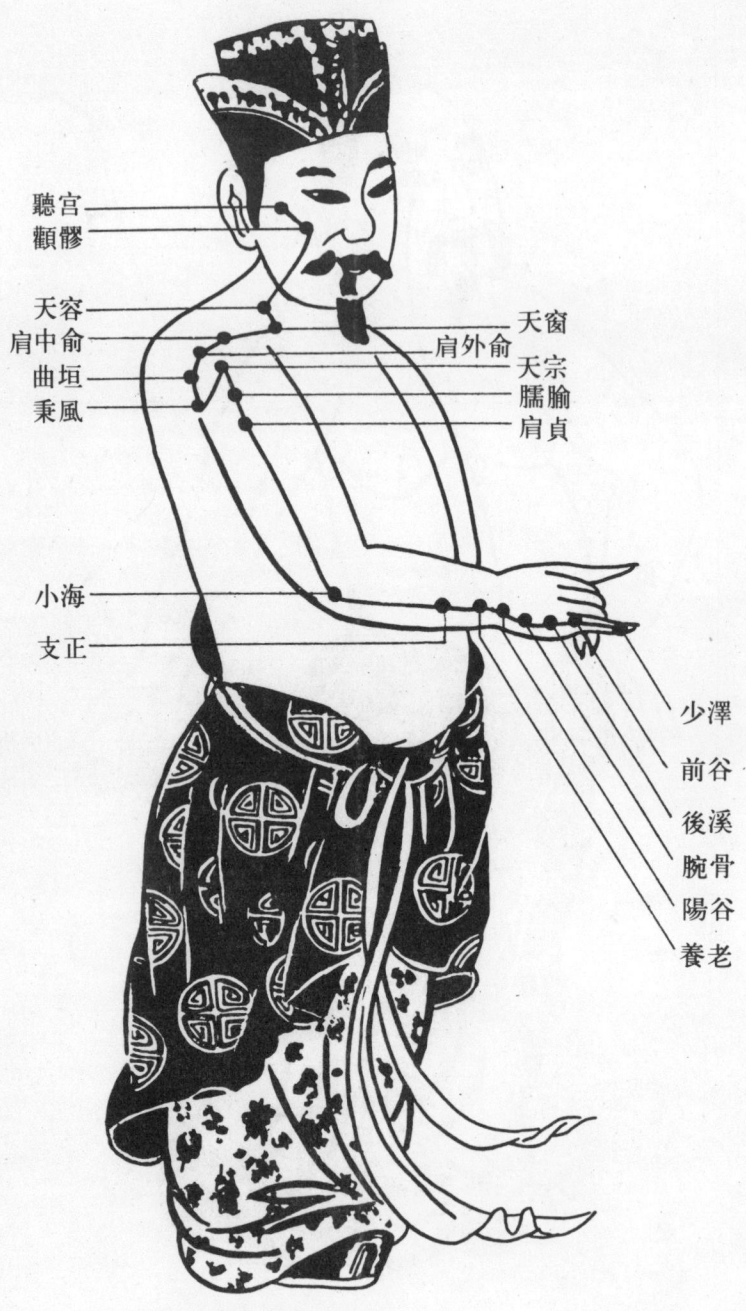

中國古代經絡圖──手太陽小腸經
Ancient Chinese Meridian Picture – The Small Intestine Meridian of Hand-Taiyang

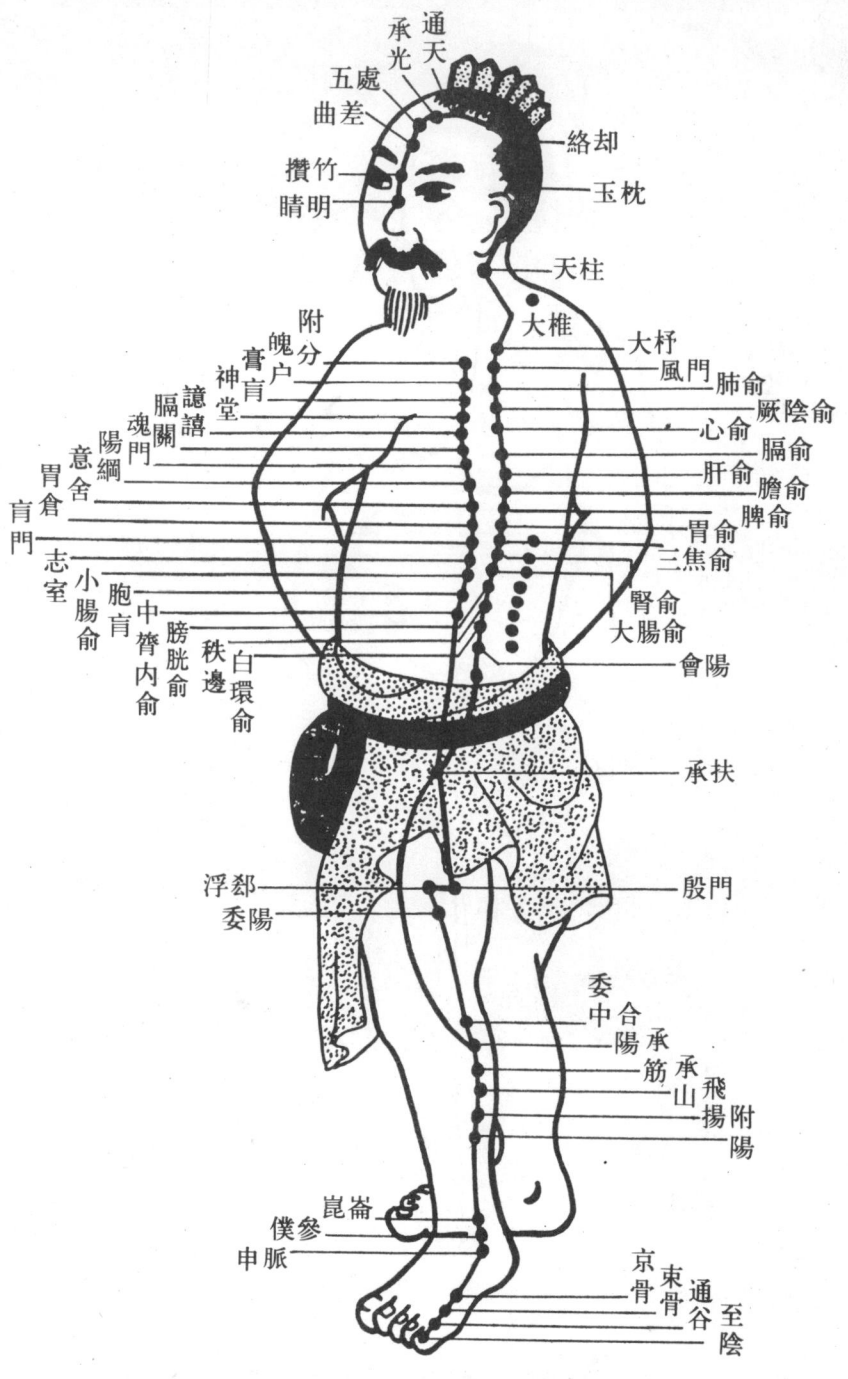

中國古代經絡圖──足太陽膀胱經
Ancient Chinese Meridian Picture – The Bladder Meridian of Foot-Taiyang

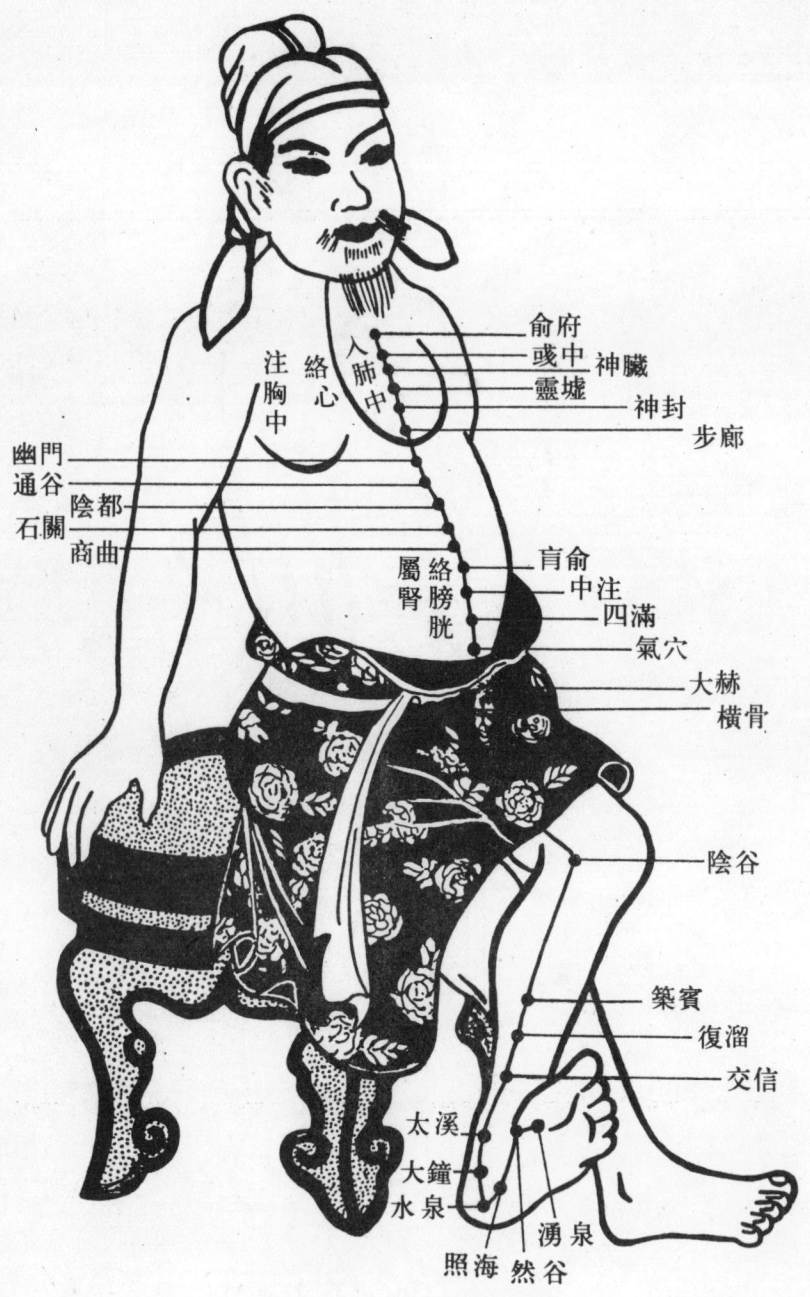

中國古代經絡圖──足少陰腎經
Ancient Chinese Meridian Picture – The Kidney Meridian of Foot-Shaoyin

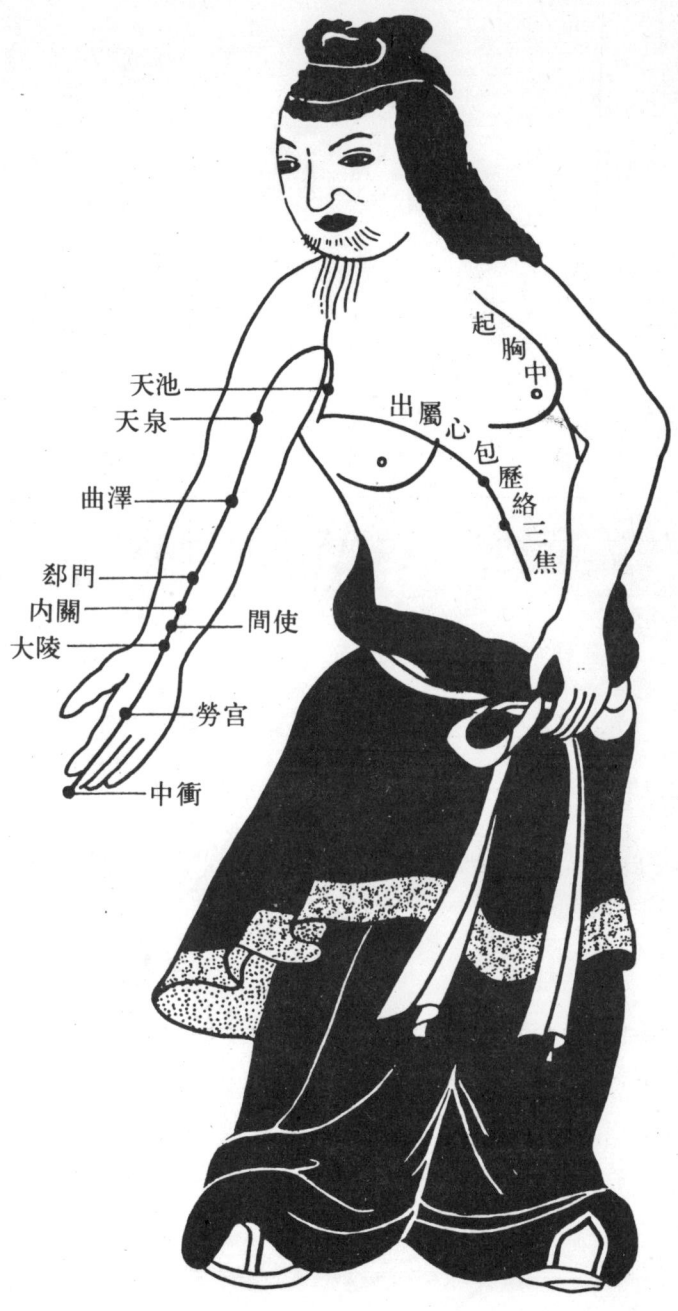

中國古代經絡圖——手厥陰心包經
Ancient Chinese Meridian Picture – The Pericardium Meridian of Hand-Jueyin

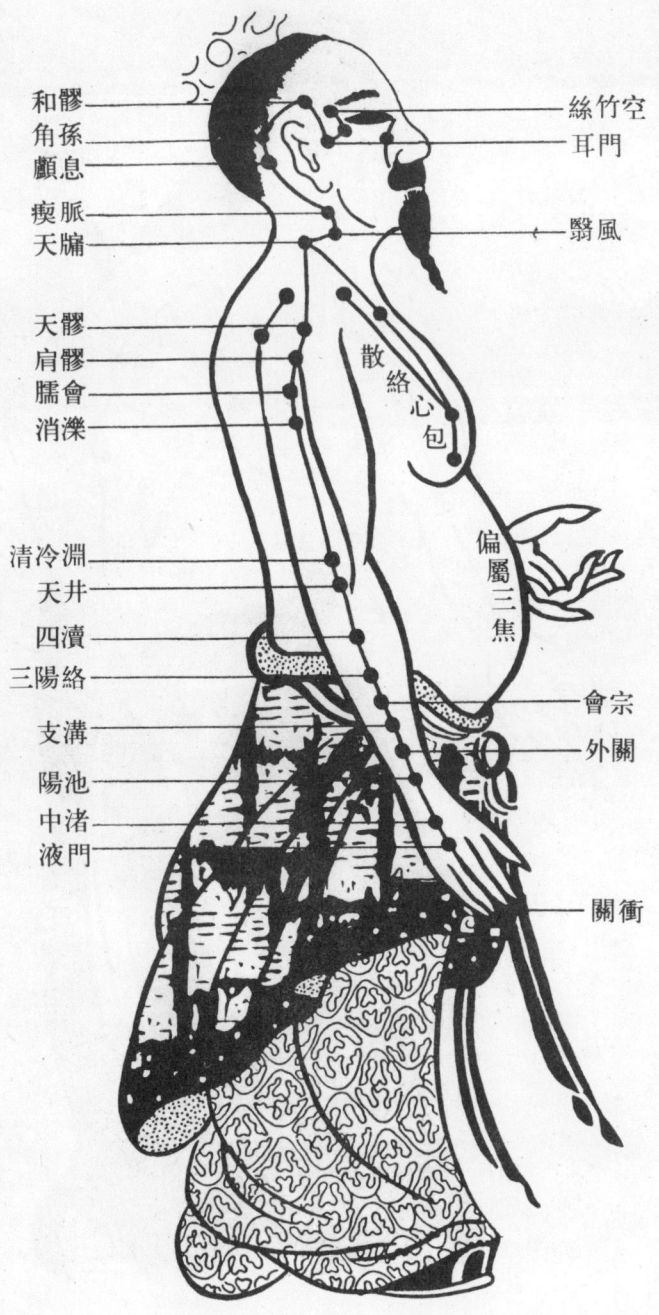

中國古代經絡圖——手少陽三焦經
Ancient Chinese Meridian Picture — The Sānjiao Meridian of Hand-Shaoyang

序

　　起源于中华大地的针灸医学,几千年来为中华民族的繁衍昌盛作出了巨大的贡献,当前已经传到世界上120多个国家和地区,成为世界医学的重要组成部分。

　　随着时代的前进,科学的衍化,传统针灸医学也在不断地发展,一方面深入发掘了古代针灸医学的学术宝库,另一方面运用现代科学理论、技术、手段对传统针灸医学体系作了全新的阐发与探索,从而大大地拓展了传统针灸医学的学术视野与临床范围。成为世界医学之林中独树一帜的医学体系。

　　针灸治病、器具虽简,但疗效神奇。其奥妙何在呢?行家们知道,除了取穴准确,配穴得当之外,操作技法是最活跃的因素,对针灸医师来说,它是一门需要长期体验、细心揣摩方可掌握的手法艺术,自然也是古今中外针灸学家极为关注的学术分支。早在《黄帝内经》里,就记载了五刺应五脏、九刺应九变、十二刺应十二经及几种重要的针刺补泻手法和灸法补泻要领。宋元以降,关于针灸技法的经验总结日臻活跃,有许多专门论著问世。不过,总的研究格局略显沉寂,本世纪50年代以后,随着针灸医学声誉雀起,针灸技法的专题研究逐渐步入系统,务实的轨道,成为针灸临床研究的热点。今有湖南中医学院严洁副教授等编纂的《图解中国针灸技法》一书即反映了这一领域研究的成果。该书不仅搜集了古今众多流派、专家的针灸操作技法,以图文并茂的形式加以介绍,是一本对针灸操作具有指导性的专著,同时,该书又对针灸技法这门应用技术的体系建构上作了探索,将其分为腧穴技法、分类技法、临床技法,这就使得该书在构思上颇具新意,当然,关于针灸技法体系的研究还需要不断地深化,希望作者在这一专题方面能有新建树。

　　此外,该书采用中英对照形式出版,不仅为国内学习、研究针灸技法提供了重要的参考书,同时有利于针灸学术的国际交流。这也反映作者的学术视野不同凡响。总之,该书的出版是一件可喜可贺的好事,故略书愚见,以向同道推荐。

世界针灸学会联合会主席
中国针灸学会副会长
中国民间中医医药研究　　王雪苔
开发协会理事长
1991年10月于北京

FOREWARD

Originating from China, acupuncture—moxibustion has made a great contribution to the thriving and prosperity of Chinese nation for several thousand years. Up to now, it has spread to more than 120 countries and regions all over the world and becomes an essential component of the world medicine.

With advance of the human society and development of the science, traditional Chinese acupuncture—moxibustion makes progress constantly. On the one hand, the academic treasure of ancient Chinese acupuncture—moxibustion has been deeply explored. On the other hand, theories, techniques and means of modern science have been employed for researching and expounding the traditional acupuncture and moxibustion in a new way. Thereby, the traditional acupuncture and moxibustion has broaden its field of academic vision and sphere of clinical application and becomes a unique medical system in the world medicine.

In the treatment of diseases by acupuncture and moxibustion, the equipment is simple, but the effect is miraculous. What is the mystery of this? It is well known by acupuncture—moxibustion connoisseurs that in addition to accurate selection of needed acupoints and appropriate combination of the acupoints, the manipulation skill is the most important factor in the attainment of the expected results. The acupuncture—moxibustion technique is a technical art which is indispensable to an acupuncture—moxibustion doctor, and it can be grasped only thorugh a long term of practice and elaborate study. As a result, its knowledge has become an academic branch of acupuncture and moxibustion, which has been concerned about by specialists of acupuncture and moxibustion in modern and ancient times, in China or elsewhere. As early as in 《Yellow Emperor's Internal Classic》 which was written in the period from the Spring and Autumn Period to Han Dynasty (770 BC—220 AD), it is recorded that the "five needling techniques" should be used in accordance with the pathological changes of the five zang-organs; the "nine needling techiques", with the differences of the nine types of syndromes; and the "twelve needling techniques", with the pathological changes of the twelve regular meridians; and some other important principles of reinforcement and reduction with acupuncture and with moxibustion are also introduced. After Song and Yuan Dynasties (960—1368), the activities of summarizing experiences of acupuncture—moxibustion techniques became more and more brisker, and many treatises on them were published. But, generally, no great academic breakthrough in the research of acupuncture—moxibustion techniques was seen in these periods. Since 1950's, the research of acupuncture—moxibustion techniques, with the advance of their reputation, has gradually become systematic and practical, having an ever—increasing appeal in clinical research. It should be pointed out that the book《Skills with Illustrations of Chinese Acupuncture & Moxibustion》compiled in Chinese and English by Prof. Yan Jie and her cooperator just reflects the achievements of the scientific rearch of this field. As a monograph of acupuncture—moxibustion techniques, it has gathered and collected the acupuncture—moxibustion manipulation skills and technics of diverse academic shools and doctors in modern and ancient times, and introduces and explains them with words and figures. So, it can give guidance and directions to acupuncture and moxibustion manipulation. Moreover, with some new ideas by dividing acupuncture—moxibustion techniques into skills relating to acupoints, abstract or basic skills, and clinical skills, it makes valuable exploration to the establishment of an applied science----acupuncture—moxibustion technique. Of course, constant and further efforts should be made in the research of acupuncture—moxibustion technique system and it is hoped that the authors of this book make some new progress in this field.

Additionally, published in Chinese and English, this book can be used as an important reference for study and research of acupuncture—moxibustion techniques by Chinese doctors and students, and meanwhile, as a textbook for acupuncture—moxibustion study by foreign learners and practitioners. Thus, it will play an active role in the promotion of academic exchange on medical science between China and other countries, and it also shows that the authors have high academic aspirations.

In a word, the publishment of the book deserves congratulations. Therefore, I write down this foreward with pleasure to recommend it to acupuncture—moxibustion learners and practitioners。

Prof. Wang Xuetai
Chairman of the World Federation of
Acupuncture and Moxibustion Societies
Oct. 30, 1991

前 言

在中国传统医学体系中,针灸学是最重视手法与技巧运用的科目之一。因此,在经验医学时代,针灸学更多地被称之为"针术""灸术"。相传作为中国古代神医化身的华佗,就是一位针术高超、灸法不凡的专家,他临床运针技法娴熟,炉火纯青。虽用穴极少,却能自如地控制针感的发放,随意调动经气,常常是手到病除。可惜他神奇的针灸之术仅传了其弟子樊阿一人。其实,象华佗这样的针灸高手代有人出,各怀绝技。不过,在古代针灸文献中却难窥历代名医神针妙术的风采。据古代针灸文献的宏观考察,我们发现晋唐以后针灸学术重心由经验走向理性,即由"术"转向"经",并逐渐形成一种重经轻术、重心法轻手法的学术倾向。关于这一特点,只要翻一翻现存针灸医籍目录就不难理解。而且许多冠以刺灸法术的文献也大多是未刊本,其内容详于心法,略于手法。这种文献缺乏的状况既是中国针灸技法整理、研究工作沉寂的表现,同时也是历代这方面研究、传播迟滞的原因。当然,限制针灸技法记述、整理、研究与传播更为重要的原因应该是其自身的经验性与灵活性。如同中国古代的舞蹈艺术,针灸手法技巧的习得是某一个体在临床中长期反复体验、揣摩、感悟的结果。它各具特点、富有创造性,且不易从操作者身上分离出来,成为超越时空的标准化程式。因此,它只能参师面授,而不异时异地旁通。同时,单纯的语言形式不易准确地把握与刻划出针灸手法技巧的奥妙,且针术越高超,技巧越神奇,语言则越显得苯拙、艰涩。难以超越"只可意会,不可言传"的表述障碍。所以,当确立本书编写意向时,除了感觉到文献参考资料不足之外,更强烈的感觉是必须改变传统的以文达意的记述与研究形式,代之以图文互参的形式,以充分表现中国针灸富有特色与个性的手法技巧。故此有了编写"图解本"的设想。当然,更理想的形式应该是有连续动感、细部特写的影像片资料,但目前尚有些技术上的困难,当然希望能在本书出版后,尽快摄出与该书配套使用的录像片。

编纂之初,除了编写形式的求新之外,另一个困扰编者的学术难题是中国针灸技法体系的逻辑建构。很显然,本书对中国针灸技法这一概念的理解和把握不只是一大堆经验层次的术式与方法,而是试图将它作为一门独立的应用技术学科来认识,来整理和研究。在这里,较一般意义上的技巧、手法而言,针灸技法的逻辑内涵大大地扩展了,成为伴行于针灸基础理论与针灸临床治疗学,既抽象、又具体的技术体系。经过深入地研究和探讨,我们将这一体系分为腧穴技法、分类技法、临床技法三大块。其中腧穴技法主要述及各个穴位的进针范围、针灸宜忌等,由于它与经穴知识交叉较多,且不是具体的操作过程中的主体内容,故未独立成章,而是与经穴知识一并归于"预备知识"。同在"预备知识"之中还介绍了针灸操作器械等内容。真正构成针灸技法体系主干的是相对成熟的,且颇具共性的分类技法和因病因人而异的临床技法,很显然,分类技法是在临床技法之中抽象、归纳出来的基本操作规程和要领。而临床技法又可视为是分类技法在临床过程中的运用。两者互为因果。但是,临床技法的内容更丰富,它不仅仅只是分类技法的演绎形式,实质上还包括很大一部分尚未被分类技法归纳的名医技法,这一部分内容是最富有活力和个性的临床技法,甚至许多已形成临床绝招,不过,尚有待进一步研究、定型、并作出充分的阐述,待其成熟后仍可归纳到分类技法之中去。本书力图较多地搜罗、介绍这些名医技法,以丰富分类技法与临床技法。其实,在针灸技法标准化、规程化研究尚不充分的时期,分类技法也带有较大的个性色彩,本书所介绍的分类技法亦有许多待商榷和补充之处。因此希望海内外同道能给予建设性的指导,以便共同建构更为完善、严谨的针灸技法体系。

其次,在本书策划之初,考虑到中国针灸正大步走向世界,为适应海内外读者学习、掌握中国针灸技法的需要,确定以中英对照形式编纂本书,但愿这一初衷能有助于海内外针灸界的学术交流。

值得指出,除了编、译者之外,对本书投入较多的还有本书的责任编辑,从选题策划到提纲的确立、结构的调整、文字的修润,以及插图的修改,做了大量默默无闻的工作,谨向他表示感谢。

本书的出版,还凝聚许多针灸界、出版界前辈的扶持与帮助,世界针联主席王雪苔教授欣然赐序、大百科全书出版社全如缄编审悉心审阅译稿,科学出版社赵世雄同志在技术设计方面的热情指导,都使该书增色不少。在此谨表示诚挚的谢意。

严 洁 尹钢林

1991 年 10 月 20 日

PREFACE

As being one of the subjects which attach the most importance to technics and skills in traditional Chinese medicine system, acupuncture—moxibustion was once termed as "needling skill" and "moxibustion skill" during the experiential medicine times. It is said that Hua Tuo, taken as the miracle—working doctor incarnate in Chinese ancient times, was a great master of acupuncture-moxibustion with highly skillful needling and moxibustion techniques, who attained perfection in applying needling craft in clinics, and, as being able to control a patient's needling sensation and move a patient's meridian—qi at his will even with a few points selected at each treatment time, he usually made diseases relieved at his touch. But it is a pity that his miraculous needling skills were passed on only to Fan A, one of his disciples. Actually, every dynasty of China had its own doctors with high skills of acupuncture—moxibustion like Hua Tuo in the history, each of them having his or her own unique mehtod of curing diseases. Unforturnately, there are few records on the miraculous needling mehtods of the outstanding doctors of various dynasties in Chinese ancient literature of acupuneture and moxibustion. If reviewing ancient literature about acupuncture and moxibustion, one can see that after Jing and Tang Dynasties (265—907), the academic focus of the research of acupuncture and moxibustion shifted from clinical experience to rational knowledge, namely, from research on the "skills in hand" to the " rules in mind ". Thereby, an acadcmic tendency of stressing the theory and ignoring clinical technics was gradually formed in acupuncture and moxibustion field. Moreover, not much literature about skills of acupuncture and moxibustion was formally published before and their contents are rich in the theory of acupuncture and moxibustion but sketchy in concrete manipulation methods. The condition lacking in literature about acupuncture—moxibustion manipulation skills is the sign indicating deficiency of sifting and research work of Chinese acupuncture and moxibustion skills before. Meanwhile, it is also the cause of their slow dissemination. But, the more important cause of limited record, collation, research and spread of Chinese acupuncture and moxibustion technique lies in its own nature of experience and flexibility. Mastering acupuncture—

moxibustion technics and skills, in most conditions, is the result that an individual clinically learns, practices, experiences, and tries to fathom them over and over again for a long term. This is just like ancient Chinese dancing art. As each manipulation method of acupuncture—moxibustion has its own character, rich in creation, and difficult to be seperated from its operator for the purpose of making it standardized beyond time and space. The most possible way of learnig and grasping it is face—to—face teaching and studying between a master and his or her students. Namely, in general, one can not learn and grasp acupuncture—moxibustion technics far from his teacher in time and distance. Additionally, the things behind acupuncture—moxibustion technics and skills can hardly be grasped and expressed only through speech or written language. In describing acupuncture—moxibustion techniques, the more skillful the needling method is and the more subtle the manipulation is, the more clumsy, and abstruse the language used looks like. This is described as "it can be only understood by the mind but can not be expressed by language." The obstacle of expression with language is very difficult to be overstepped. When planning to compile this book, we felt it necessary to compile a book to collect and systematize acupuncture—moxibustion skills because they are very important in the system of traditional Chinese medicine and there is not enough extant literature relating to them to meet the clinical needs. And what is more, we strongly felt that, in order to make full expression of the manipulation skills of Chinese acupuncture and moxibustion which are rich in distinctive features, it was necessary to change the traditional way of recording, describing and collating them only with language and we should replace it with a new way of using both language and illustrations. For this reason, we had a tentative idea to compile a book of skills with illustrations of acupuncture and moxibustion. Certainly, the more ideal form in expressing and studying acupuncture and moxibustion manipulation methods is video materials which can show continual motions of an acupuncture or moxibustion manipulation procedure and have a close—up shot of meticulous manipulation method. But in current time, there are some technical problems to be solved in producing a video tape like this. We hope a video tape used as conveyance of this book will be made out as soon as possible after this book being published.

  In addition to seeking for a new way———adding a lot of figures of acupuncture—moxibustion skills in the written language expression———a different method from the traditional way in researching and systematizing the acupuncture and moxibustion technique, we attached the importance to the establishment of a logical frame of Chinese acupuncture and moxibustion technique system, which was a big obstacle we had and should surmount at the beginning of compiling this book. With the establishment of the system, we plotted the construction of this book and tried to make it more logical and theoretical. Obviously, when researching and collating diverse manipulation methods of acupuncture and moxibustion for compiling this book, we took the Chinese acupuncture—moxibustion technique as an independent subject of applied science but not just as the simple manipulation method at the experiential level. In this book, therefore, the acupuncture—moxibustion technique has been greatly enlarged in its connotation as compared with other techniques, becoming an abstract and concrete technique system which is independent and closely related to the fundamental theory and clinical therapeutics of acupuncture—moxibustion, another two subjects of acupuncture-moxibustion science. After making a deep research, we divide the system into three parts: skills relating to acupuncture points, basic or abstract skills, and clinical skills. The "skill relating to acupoints" refers to the knowledge about the depth and angle of needling and remarks in needling at an acupoint. As being largely overlapped with the acupoint knowledge and only taken as a supplementary contents in concrete manipulation procedure, it, with acupoint introduction, is included in the "Preparatory Knowledge" but not listed as an independent chapter in this book. The "Preparatory Knowledge" is the first part of this book in which some other supplementary contents such as equipment of acupuncture and moxibustion are introduced additionally. The "basic or abstract skill" refers to a manipulation method of acupuncture—moxibustion which is comparatively mature and widely accepted, and the "clinical skill" refers to any method of acupuncture—moxibustion which is applied to treatment of a concrete disease in clinics according to the conditions of the disease and patient. The basic or abstract skill and the clinical skill constitute the main part of acupuncture—moxibustion technique system. Obviously, the abstract skill, which is about the basic manipulation rules and essentials, is abstracted and drawn from clinical skills, while the clinical skill can be considered as an abstract skill in clinical application. Although both of them have inter-causality of each other the clinical skill is richer in contents as compared with the abstract skill. In addition to being taken as a deductive form of the abstract skill in clinics, it includes a lot of acupuncture—moxibustion manipulations of experienced outstanding doctors which have not been classified into the abstract skill. But the methods are the most brimming with vigour and individual character in clinical skills, and even many of them have become clinically unique and specifc treatment means. As they are not popular in clinics and need to be further researched to make them finalized in the pattern and to fully express them, they are not included in the abstract skill category in this book. We try to collect and introduce more outstanding doctors' specific manipulation methods as many as possible in this book so as to enrich the abstract skills and clinical skills. In fact, in the current peried, with the deficiency of research of standardization of acupuncture—moxibustion techniques, the abstract skill still bears a comparatively strong personal imprint, and the abstract skills introduced in this book, therefore, need to be further discussed and supplemented. We hope specialists and doctors of acupuncture and moxibustion, both at home and abroad, give us constructive guidance so as to estalish jointly a more perfect and rigorous acupuncture—moxibustion technique system.

Additionally, as considering that Chinese acupuncture and moxibustion are spreading to all over the world, we compile this book in bilingual form, i.e. in Chinese and English languages, and use the original complex forms of the Chinese characters in this book instead of their simplified forms in order to meet the needs of people in and out of China of learning and grasping Chinese acupuncture—moxibustion techniques. It is deeply hoped that this idea can be helpful to international academic exchange of acupuncture and moxibustion.

It should be pointed out that Mr. Wang Yifang, the responsible editor of this book plays an important role in compiling this book. We are deeply indebted to him for his help in making the writing plan, determining the writing outline, readjusting the writing construction, polishing the Chinese language, and revising the illustrations.

The publication of this book is also a result of support and help of many respected scholars from acupuncture—moxibustion field and publshing field. The foreward of introducing this book is written by Prof. Wang Xuetai, Chairman of the World Federation of Acupuncture and Moxibustion Societies, with pleasure. Prof. Quan Ruchen, copy editor of Chinese Great Encyclopaedia Press, read through the English manuscript carefully and gave helpful suggestions. Mr. Zhao Shixiong of Science Press gave enthusiastic guidance in technical design to edit this book. All their help are greatly beneficial to this book. Taking this opportunity we express our heartfelt thanks to them.

Yan Jie, Yin Ganglin
At Changsha, Hunan, China
November 10, 1991

目 录

上篇　预备知识

第一章　经络腧穴概要 …………… (1)
  第一节　经络概述 ………………… (1)
    一、经络系统的组成 ……………… (1)
    二、经络的作用 …………………… (5)
  第二节　腧穴概述 ………………… (6)
    一、腧穴分类 ……………………… (6)
    二、常用特定穴含义与功用 ……… (7)
    三、腧穴定位法 …………………… (14)
  第三节　十四经循行及常用腧穴 … (24)
    一、手太阴肺经 …………………… (24)
      中府　尺泽　孔最　列缺　经渠　太渊
      鱼际　少商
    二、手阳明大肠经 ………………… (30)
      商阳　二间　三间　合谷　阳溪　偏历
      温溜　手三里　曲池　臂臑　肩髃　扶突
      迎香
    三、足阳明胃经 …………………… (38)
      承泣　四白　地仓　颊车　下关　头维
      人迎　乳根　天枢　水道　归来　髀关
      伏兔　梁丘　犊鼻　足三里　上巨虚　条
      口　下巨虚　丰隆　解溪　冲阳　陷谷
      内庭　厉兑
    四、足太阴脾经 …………………… (52)
      隐白　大都　太白　公孙　商丘　三阴交
      地机　阴陵泉　血海　大横　大包
    五、手少阴心经 …………………… (60)
      极泉　少海　灵道　通里　阴郄　神门
      少府　少冲

    六、手太阳小肠经 ………………… (65)
      少泽　前谷　后溪　腕骨　阳谷　养老
      支正　小海　肩贞　天宗　肩外俞　颧
      髎　听宫
    七、足太阳膀胱经 ………………… (73)
      睛明　攒竹　天柱　大杼　风门　肺俞
      厥阴俞　心俞　膈俞　肝俞　胆俞　脾俞
      胃俞　三焦俞　肾俞　大肠俞　小肠俞
      膀胱俞　次髎　承扶　殷门　委阳　委
      中　膏肓俞　志室　秩边　承山　飞扬
      跗阳　昆仑　申脉　金门　京骨　束骨
      足通谷　至阴
    八、足少阴肾经 …………………… (90)
      涌泉　然谷　太溪　大钟　水泉　照海
      复溜　交信　筑宾　阴谷　俞府
    九、手厥阴心包经 ………………… (97)
      天池　曲泽　郄门　间使　内关　大陵
      劳宫　中冲
    十、手少阳三焦经 ………………… (103)
      关冲　液门　中渚　阳池　外关　支沟
      会宗　天井　肩髎　翳风　角孙　耳门
      丝竹空
    十一、足少阳胆经 ………………… (111)
      瞳子髎　听会　率谷　阳白　风池　肩井
      日月　京门　带脉　环跳　风市　膝阳
      关　阳陵泉　阳交　外丘　光明　阳辅
      悬钟　丘墟　足临泣　侠溪　足窍阴
    十二、足厥阴肝经 ………………… (124)
      大敦　行间　太冲　中封　蠡沟　中都

· 1 ·

　　　　曲泉　章门　期门
　十三、任脉 …………………………(131)
　　　　会阴　中极　关元　石门　气海　神阙
　　　　下脘　中脘　巨阙　鸠尾　膻中　天突
　　　　廉泉　承浆
　十四、督脉 …………………………(139)
　　　　长强　腰阳关　命门　至阳　陶道　大椎
　　　　哑门　风府　百会　上星　素髎　水沟
　　　　龈交
　第四节　常用经外奇穴 ………………(147)
　　一、头颈部 …………………………(147)
　　　　四神聪　印堂　太阳　鱼腰　球后　牵正
　　　　翳明　安眠
　　二、躯干部 …………………………(150)
　　　　定喘、夹脊
　　三、四肢部 …………………………(151)
　　　　十宣　八邪　四缝　八风　阑尾穴　胆囊
　　　　穴　膝眼　鹤顶

第二章　耳针、头针、腕踝针分区
　　　　与穴位定位 …………………(157)
　第一节　耳廓表面解剖及耳穴定位 …(157)
　　一、耳廓表面的解剖 ………………(157)
　　二、耳穴分布规律、定位及适应症 …(159)
　第二节　常用头针刺激区定位与主治病症……
　　………………………………………(169)
　　一、运动区 …………………………(169)
　　二、感觉区 …………………………(171)
　　三、舞蹈震颤控制区 ………………(172)
　　四、晕听区 …………………………(172)
　　五、言语二区 ………………………(172)

　　六、言语三区 ………………………(172)
　　七、运用区 …………………………(173)
　　八、足运感区 ………………………(173)
　　九、视区 ……………………………(173)
　　十、平衡区 …………………………(174)
　　十一、胃区 …………………………(174)
　　十二、胸腔区 ………………………(174)
　　十三、生殖区 ………………………(175)
　【附】"中国头皮针施术部位标准化方案"
　　………………………………………(175)
　第三节　腕踝针刺激点定位与主治病症………
　　………………………………………(180)

第三章　常用针具、器械及消毒法
　　………………………………………(184)
　第一节　常用针具 ……………………(184)
　　一、毫针 ……………………………(184)
　　二、三棱针 …………………………(186)
　　三、皮内针 …………………………(187)
　　四、皮肤针 …………………………(188)
　　五、火针 ……………………………(188)
　　六、鍉针 ……………………………(189)
　第二节　常用器械及材料 ……………(189)
　　一、电针器 …………………………(189)
　　二、耳穴探测器 ……………………(190)
　　三、其他器材 ………………………(191)
　第三节　常用消毒方法 ………………(196)
　　一、针具消毒 ………………………(196)
　　二、施术部位消毒 …………………(197)
　　三、医生手指消毒 …………………(197)

下篇　针灸技法

第四章　针灸技法述要 …………(201)
　第一节　毫针 …………………………(201)
　　一、针刺练习 ………………………(201)
　　二、选择体位 ………………………(206)

　　三、进针法 …………………………(209)
　　　1.单手进针 ………………………(209)
　　　2.双手进针 ………………………(209)
　　　　指切进针法　舒张进针法　提捏进针法

　　　　挟持进针法　套管进针法
　四、针刺角度与深度 …………………(212)
　五、治神、守神与得气 ………………(214)
　六、行针法 ……………………………(215)
　　（一）基本手法 ……………………(215)
　　　　提插法　捻转法
　　（二）辅助手法 ……………………(216)
　　　　循行　摄法　弹法　刮法　飞法　摇法
　　　　盘法　按法　抽法　敲法　推法
　　（三）补泻手法 ……………………(220)
　　　　捻转补泻　提插补泻　疾徐补泻　迎随
　　　　补泻　呼吸补泻　开合补泻　平补平泻
　　　　烧山火与透天凉　进火与进水　阴中
　　　　隐阳与阳中隐阴
　　（四）其他手法 ……………………(226)
　　　　青龙摆尾　白虎摇头　苍龟探穴　赤凤
　　　　迎源　子午捣臼　龙虎交战　龙虎升降
　　　　进气法　留气法　抽添法
　七、留针与出针 ………………………(239)
　八、异常情况处理与注意事项 ………(240)
　　（一）异常情况处理 ………………(240)
　　（二）注意事项 ……………………(241)
　　（三）针刺事故的预防 ……………(241)
第二节　三棱针 ……………………………(248)
　一、适应范围 …………………………(248)
　二、实用技法 …………………………(249)
　三、注意事项 …………………………(251)
第三节　皮内针 ……………………………(251)
　一、适应范围 …………………………(251)
　二、实用技法 …………………………(252)
　三、注意事项 …………………………(253)
第四节　皮肤针 ……………………………(254)
　一、适应范围 …………………………(254)
　二、实用技法 …………………………(254)
　三、刺激部位 …………………………(255)
　四、注意事项 …………………………(257)
第五节　鍉针 ………………………………(258)
　一、适应范围 …………………………(258)

　二、实用技法 …………………………(258)
第六节　火针 ………………………………(260)
　一、适应范围 …………………………(260)
　二、实用技法 …………………………(261)
　三、注意事项 …………………………(262)
第七节　电针 ………………………………(263)
　一、实用技法 …………………………(263)
　二、波型选择与适应范围 ……………(265)
　三、注意事项 …………………………(266)
第八节　水针 ………………………………(267)
　一、适应范围 …………………………(267)
　二、实用技法 …………………………(267)
　三、注意事项 …………………………(270)
第九节　耳针 ………………………………(271)
　一、实用技法 …………………………(271)
　二、注意事项 …………………………(277)
第十节　头针 ………………………………(278)
　一、特点与适应范围 …………………(278)
　二、实用技法 …………………………(279)
　三、注意事项 …………………………(282)
第十一节　腕踝针 …………………………(283)
第十二节　灸法 ……………………………(284)
　一、常用灸法 …………………………(284)
　二、艾灸补泻 …………………………(295)
　三、施灸禁忌及注意事项 ……………(295)
【附】拔罐法 ………………………………(297)

第五章　针灸技法的临床运用

…………………………………………………(304)
第一节　内科病症 …………………………(307)
　一、流行性腮腺炎 ……………………(307)
　二、急性传染性肝炎 …………………(310)
　三、细菌性痢疾 ………………………(312)
　四、疟疾 ………………………………(314)
　五、感冒 ………………………………(317)
　六、急、慢性支气管炎 ………………(321)
　七、支气管哮喘 ………………………(324)

八、急、慢性胃炎 …………………… (327)
九、胃、十二指肠溃疡 ………………… (330)
十、胃下垂 ……………………………… (333)
十一、膈肌痉挛 ………………………… (335)
十二、肠炎 ……………………………… (337)
十三、阑尾炎 …………………………… (340)
十四、急性胆道疾患 …………………… (343)
十五、脱肛 ……………………………… (346)
十六、痔疮 ……………………………… (348)
十七、高血压病 ………………………… (351)
十八、心绞痛 …………………………… (353)
十九、高脂血症 ………………………… (355)
二十、心律失常 ………………………… (356)
二十一、脑血管意外 …………………… (358)
二十二、癫痫 …………………………… (363)
二十三、神经衰弱 ……………………… (365)
二十四、癔病 …………………………… (367)
二十五、精神分裂症 …………………… (369)
二十六、三叉神经痛 …………………… (371)
二十七、周围性面神经麻痹 …………… (374)
二十八、坐骨神经痛 …………………… (377)
二十九、肋间神经痛 …………………… (380)
三十、前列腺炎 ………………………… (382)
三十一、遗尿 …………………………… (384)
三十二、尿潴留 ………………………… (386)
三十三、男性不育症及性功能障碍 …… (389)
三十四、关节炎 ………………………… (392)
【附】肩关节周围炎 …………………… (392)
三十五、落枕 …………………………… (396)
三十六、肥胖 …………………………… (398)

第二节 妇产科病症 …………………… (400)
　一、痛经 ……………………………… (400)
　二、更年期综合征 …………………… (402)
　三、带下 ……………………………… (404)
　四、胎位不正 ………………………… (407)
第三节 皮肤与外伤科病症 …………… (407)
　一、急性乳腺炎 ……………………… (407)
　二、多发性疖肿 ……………………… (411)
　三、神经性皮炎 ……………………… (413)
　四、湿疹 ……………………………… (416)
　五、荨麻疹 …………………………… (417)
　六、带状疱疹 ………………………… (420)
　七、痤疮 ……………………………… (423)
　八、脱发 ……………………………… (425)
　九、软组织损伤 ……………………… (426)
　十、腱鞘囊肿 ………………………… (430)
第四节 眼、耳、鼻、咽喉病症 ……… (431)
　一、鼻炎 ……………………………… (431)
　二、急性扁桃体炎 …………………… (434)
　三、急性眼结膜炎 …………………… (436)
　四、近视 ……………………………… (439)
　五、牙痛 ……………………………… (440)
　六、耳鸣、耳聋 ……………………… (443)
　七、耳源性眩晕 ……………………… (445)
第五节 急症 …………………………… (448)
　一、休克 ……………………………… (448)
　二、中暑 ……………………………… (450)
附录1. 主要参考书籍 ………………… (452)
附录2. 图录 …………………………… (456)

CONTENTS

PART ONE

PREPARATORY KNOWLEDGES FOR APPLICATION OF SKILL OF ACUPUNCTURE AND MOXIBUSTION

CHAPTER ONE THE SUMMARY OF MERIDIANS, COLLATERALS AND ACUPOINTS ················ (1)

SECTION 1 MERIDIANS AND THEIR COLLATERALS ················ (2)

I. THE COMPOSITION OF THE MERIDIAN AND COLLATERAL SYSTEM ············ (3)

II. FUNCTIONS OF THE MERIDIAN AND COLLATERALS ··················· (5)

SECTION 2 ACUPOINTS ··········· (6)

I. CLASSIFICATION OF ACUPOINTS ························· (6)

  1. Acupoints of the Fourteen Meridians
  2. Extraordinary points
  3. Ashi points

II. MEANINGS AND FUNCTIONS OF THE COMMONLY USED SPECIFIC POINTS ········· (8)

  1. Five Shu Points
  2. Yuan—Source and Luo—Connecting Points
  3. Back—Shu and Front—Mu Points
  4. Xi—Cleft Points
  5. Eight—Influential Points
  6. Lower Confluent Points
  7. Eight Confluence Points

III. METHODS OF LOCATING ACUPOINTS ·································· (15)

  1. Surface Anatomical Landmarks
  2. Bone Proportional Measurement
  3. Finger Measurement

SECTION 3 THE COURSES AND COMMONLY USED ACUPOINTS OF THE FOURTEEN MERIDIANS ········ (27)

I. THE LUNG MERIDIAN OF HAND—TAIYIN ·································· (27)

  1. The Course
  2. The Commonly Used Acupoints
    Zhongfu (LU 1), Chize (LU 5), kongzui (LU 6), Lieque (LU 7), Jingqu (LU 8), Taiyuan (LU 9), Yuji (LU 10), Shaoshang (LU 11)
  3. An Outline of Indications of the Commonly Used Acupoints

II. THE LARGE INTESTINE MERIDIAN OF HAND—YANGMING ··············· (34)

  1. The Course
  2. The Commonly Used Acupoints
    Shangyang (LI 1), Erjian (LI 2), Sanjian (LI

· 5 ·

3), Hegu (LI 4), Yangxi (LI 5), Pianli (LI 6), Wenliu (LI 7), Shaousanli (LI 10), Quchi (LI 11), Binao (LI 14), Jianyu (LI 15), Futu (LI 18), Yingxiang (LI 20)
3. An Outline of Indications of the Commonly Used Acupoints of the Meridian

Ⅲ. THE STOMACH MERIDIAN OF FOOT—YANGMING ·················· (45)
1. The Course
2. The Commonly Used Acupoints
Chengqi (ST 1), Sibai (ST 2), Dicang (ST 4), Jiache (ST 6), Xiaguan (ST 7), Touwei (ST 8), Renying (ST 9), Rugen (ST 18), Tianshu (ST 25), Shuidao (ST 28), Guilai (ST29), Biguan (ST 31), Futu (ST 32), Liangqiu (ST 34), Dubi (ST 35), Zusanli (ST 36), Shangjuxu (ST 37), Tiaokou (ST 38), Xiajuxu (ST 39), Fenglong (ST 40), Jiexi (ST 41), Chongyang (ST 42), Xiangu (ST 43), Neiting (ST 44), Lidui (ST 45)
3. An Outline of Indications of the Commonly Used Acupoints of the Meridian

Ⅳ. THE SPLEEN MERIDIAN OF FOOT—TAIYIN ·················· (56)
1. The Course
2. The Commonly Used Acupoints
Yinbai (SP 1), Dadun (SP 2), Taibai (SP 3), Gongsun (SP 4), Shangqiu (SP 5), Sanyinjiao (SP 6), Diji (SP 8), Yinlingquan (SP 9), Xuehai (SP 10), Daheng (SP 15), Dabao (SP 21)
3. An Outiline of Indications of the Commonly Used Acupoints of the Meridian

Ⅴ. THE HEART MERIDIAN OF HAND—SHAOYIN ·················· (62)
1. The Course
2. The Commonly Used Acupoints
Jiquan (HT 1), Shaohai (HT 3), Lingdao (HT 4), Tongli (HT 5), Yinxi (HT 6), Shenmen (HT 7), Shaofu (HT 8), Shaochong (HT 9)
3. An Outline of Indications of the Commonly Used Acupoints of the Meridian

Ⅵ. THE SMALL INTESTINE MERIDIAN OF HAND—TAIYANG ·················· (69)
1. The Course
2. The Commonly Used Acupoints
Shaoze (SI 1), Qiangu (SI 2), Houxi (SI 3), Wangu (SI 4), Yanggu (SI 5), Yanglao (SI 6), Zhizheng (SI 7), Xiaohai (SI 8), Jianzhen (SI 9), Tianzong (SI 11), Jianwaishu (SI 14), Quanliao (SI 18), Tinggong (SI 19)
3. An Outline of Indications of the Commonly Used Acupoints of the Meridian

Ⅶ. THE BLADDER MERIDIAN OF FOOT—TAIYANG ·················· (81)
1. The Course
2. The Commonly Used Acupoints
Jingming (BL 1), Cuanzhu (BL 2), Tianzhu (BL 10), Dashu (BL 11), Fengmen (BL 12), Feishu (BL 13), Jueyinshu (BL 14), Xinshu (BL 15), Geshu (BL 17), Ganshu (BL 18), Danshu (BL 19), Pishu (BL 20), Weishu (BL 21), Sanjiaoshu (BL 22), Shenshu (BL 23), Dachangshu (BL 25), Xiaochangshu (BL 27), Pangguangshu (BL 28), Ciliao (BL 32), Chengfu (BL 36), Yinmen (BL 37), Weiyang (BL 39), Weizhong (BL 40), Gaohuang (BL 43), Zhishi (BL 52), Zhibian (BL 54), Chengshan (BL 57), Feiyang (BL 58), Fuyang (BL 59), Kunlun (BL 60), Shenmai (BL 62), Jinmen (BL 63), Jinggu (BL 64), Shugu (BL 65), Zutonggu (BL 66), Zhiyin (BL 67)
3. An Outline of Indications of the Commonly Used Acupoints of the Meridian

Ⅷ. THE KIDNEY MERIDIAN OF FOOT—SHAOYIN ·················· (94)
1. The Coures
2. The Commmonly Used Acupoints
Yongquan (KI 1), Rangu (KI 2), Taixi (KI 3), Dazhong (KI 4), Shuiquan (KI 5), Zhaohai (KI 6), Fuliu (KI 7), Jiaoxin (KI 8), Zhubin (KI 9), Yingu (KI 10), Shufu (KI 27)
3. An Outline of Indications of the Commonly Used

Acupoints of the Meridian

IX. THE PERICARDIUM MERIDIAN OF HAND—JUEYIN ·················· (100)
1. The Course
2. The Commonly Used Acupoints
   Tianchi (PC 1), Quze (PC 3), Ximen (PC 4), Jianshi (PC 5), Neiguan (PC 6), Daling (PC 7), Laogong (PC 8), Zhongchong (PC 9)
3. An Ontline of Indications of the Commonly Used Acupoints of the Meridian

X. THE SANJIAO (TRIPLE ENERGIZER) MERIDIAN OF HAND—SHAOYANG ·········· (107)
1. The Course
2. The Commonly Used Acupoints
   Guanchong (SJ 1), Yemen (SJ 2), Zhongzhu (SJ 3), Yangchi (SJ 4), Waiguan (SJ 5), Zhigou (SJ 6), Huizong (SJ 7), Tianjing (SJ 10), Jianliao (SJ 14), Yifeng (SJ 17), Jiaosun (SJ 20), Ermen (SJ 21), Sizhukong (SJ 23)
3. An Outline of Indications of the Commonly Used Acupoints of the Meridian

XI. THE GALLBLADDER MERIDIAN OF FOOT—SHAOYANG ··············· (119)
1. The Course
2. The Commonly Used Acupoints
   Tongziliao (GB 1), Tinghui (GB 2), Shuaigu (GB 8), Yangbai (GB 14), Fengchi (GB 20), Jianjing (GB 21), Riyue (GB24), Jingmen (GB25), Daimai (GB26), Huantiao (GB 30), Fengshi (GB 31), Xiyangguan (GB 33), Yanglingquan (GB 34), Yangjiao (GB 35), Waiqiu (GB 36), Guangming (GB 37), Yangfu (GB 38), Xuanzhong (GB 39), Qiuxu (GB 40), Zulinqi (GB 41), Xiaxi (GB 43), Zuqiaoyin (GB 44)
3. An Outline of Indications of the Commonly Used Acupoints of the Meridian

XII. THE LIVER MERIDIAN OF FOOT—JUEYIN ·························· (128)
1. The Course
2. The Commonly Used Acupoints
   Dadun (LR 1), Xingjian (LR 2), Taichong (LR 3), Zhongfeng (LR 4), Ligou (LR 5), Zhongdu (LR 6), Ququan (LR 8), Zhangmen (LR 13), Qimen (LR 14)
3. An Outline of Indications of the Commonly Used Acupoints of the Meridian

XIII. THE REN MERIDIAN (CONCEPTION VESSEL) ·················· (136)
1. The Course
2. THe Commonly Used Acupoints
   Huiyin (RN 1), Zhongji (RN 3), Guanyuan (RN 4), Shimen (RN 5), Qihai (RN 6), Shenque (RN 8), Xiawan (RN 10), Zhongwan (RN 12), Juque (RN 14), Jiuwei (RN 15), Danzhong (RN 17), Tiantu (RN 22), Lianquan (RN 23), Chengjiang (RN 24)
3. An Outline of Indication of the Commonly Used Acupoints of the Meridian

XIV. THE DU MERIDIAN (GOVERNOR VESSEL) ·················· (144)
1. The Course
2. The Commonly Uesd Acupoints
   Changqiang (DU 1), Yaoyangguan (DU 3), Mingmen (DU 4), Zhiyang (DU 9), Taodao (DU 13), Dazhui (DU 14), Yamen (DU 15), Fengfu (DU 16), Baihui (DU 20), Shangxing (DU 23), Shenting (DU 24), Suliao (DU 25), Shuigou (DU 26), Yinjiao (DU 28)
3. An Outline of Indications of the Commonly Used Acupoints

SECTION 4   THE COMMONLY USED EXTRA POLNTS ············· (153)
1. The Points on the Head and Neck Region
   Sishencong (EX—HN 1), Yintang (EX—HN 3), Taiyang (EX—HN 5), Yuyao (EX—HN 4), Qiuhou (EX-HN 7), Qianzheng (EX-HN 16), Yiming (EX—HN 14), Anmian (EX—HN 17)
2. The Points on the Trunk
   Dingchuan (EX—B 1), Jiaji (EX—B 2)
3. The Points on the Four Extremities
   Shixuan (EX—UE 11), Baxie (EX—UE 9),

Sifeng (EX—UE 10), Bafeng (EX—LE 10), Lanwei (EX—LE 7), Dannan (EX—LE 6), Xiyan (EX—LE 4 and 5), Heding (EX—LE 2)

CHAPTER TWO LOCATION AND INDICATIONS OF OTOPOINTS, SCALP ACUPUNCTURE LINES AND WRIST—ANKLE ACUPUNCTURE POINTS .... (157)

SECTION 1 ANATOMICAL TERMINOLOGY OF THE AURICULAR SURFACE AND LOCATION AND INDICATIONS OF OTOPOINTS .... (158)

I. ANATOMICAL TERMINOLOGY OF THE AURICULAR SURFACE .... (158)

II. DISTRIBUTION, LOCATION AND INDICATIONS OF THE OTOPOLNTS .... (159)

SECTION 2 LOCATION AND INDICATIONS OF COMMONLY USED SCALP ACUPUNCTURE LINES ...... (171)

I. MOTER AREA .... (171)
II. SENSORY AREA .... (172)
III. CHOREIFORM TREMOR CONTROL AREA .... (172)
IV. VERTIGO AND AURAL AREA .... (172)
V. SPEECH AREA 2 .... (172)
VI. SPEECH AREA 3 .... (172)
VII. PRAXIA AREA .... (173)
VIII. FOOT—KINESTHETIC SENSORY AREA .... (173)
IX. VISUAL AREA .... (173)
X. EQUILIBRIUM AREA .... (174)
XI. STOMACH AREA .... (174)
XII. THORACIC AREA .... (175)
XIII. GENETIC AREA .... (175)

APPENDIX: STANDARD NOMENCLATURE OF CHINESE SCALP ACUPUNCTURE LINES .... (175)

I. FOREHEAD REGION .... (176)
 1. Middle Line of Forehead
 2. Line 1 Lateral to Forehead
 3. Line 2 Lateral to Forehead
 4. Line 3 Lateral to Forehead

II. VERTEX REGION .... (177)
 5. Middle Line of Vertex
 6. Anterior Oblique Line of Vertex—Temporal
 7. Posterior Obique Line of Vertex—Temporal
 8. Line 1 Lateral to Vertex
 9. Line 2 Lateral to Vertex

III. TEMPORAL REGION .... (178)
 10. Anterior Temporal Line
 11. Posterior Temporal Line

IV. OCCIPITAL REGION .... (180)
 12. Upper—Middle Line of Occiput
 13. Upper—Lateral Line of Occiput
 14. Lower—Lareral Line of Occiput

SECTION 3 LOCATION AND INDICATIONS OF WRIST—ANKLE ACUPUNCTRE POINTS .... (180)

CHAPTER THREE COMMONLY USED INSTRUMENTS IN ACUPUNCTURE AND MOXIBUSTION AND STERILIZATION .... (184)

SECTION 1 COMMONLY USED NEEDLE APPARATUSES .... (185)

I. EILIFORM NEEDLE .... (185)
 1. The Structure
 2. The Gange

II. THREE—EDGED NEEDLE .... (186)

III. INTRADERMAL NEEDLE .... (187)
 1. The Wheat—Granule—Shaped or Circle—Shaped Needle
 2. The Thumb—Pin—Shaped Needle

IV. SKIN NEEDLE .... (188)
V. HOT NEEDLE .... (188)
VI. DULL NEDDLE .... (189)

SECTION 2   COMMONLY USED OTHER INSTRU-
              MENTS AND MATERIALS ……
              ……………………………… (190)
Ⅰ. ELECTROACUPUNCTURE APPARATUS ……
   ……………………………………… (190)
Ⅱ. ELECTRIC UNIT FOR PROBING THE OTO-
    POINTS ……………………… (191)
Ⅲ. OTHER INSTRUMENTS AND MATERIALS ……
   ……………………………………… (195)
  1. Syringe
  2. Syringe Needle
  3. Commonly Used Injections
  4. Equipments and Drugs for Sterilization
  5. Materials for Moxibustion
  6. Jars
  7. Materials for Sticking and Pressing Method on Oto-
     points
SECTION 3   COMMON METHODS OF STERILIZA-
              TION …………………… (197)
Ⅰ. STERILIZATION OF THE NEEDLE APPARATUS-
    ES ……………………………… (197)
  1. By Autoclave
  2. By Soaking in the Drug Fluid
Ⅱ. STERILIZATION OF THE SKIN AREAS TO BE
    PUNCTURED ………………………… (197)
Ⅲ. STERILIZATION OF THE OPERATOR'S FIN-
    GERS ………………………………… (198)

PART TWO

SKILL OF ACUPUNCTURE & MOXIBUSTION

CHAPTER FOUR   A GENERAL DISCUS-
SION ON THE SKILL OF ACUPUNC-
TURE AND MOXIBUSTION ………
……………………………………… (201)

SECTION 1   ACUPUNCTURE WITH THE FILI-
             FORM NEEDLE ……… (204)
Ⅰ. NEEDLING PRACTLCE …………… (204)
  1. Commonly Used Methods of Holding the Needle
   (1) Holding the Needle with Two Fingers
   (2) Holding the Needle with Three Fingers
   (3) Holding the Needle with Four Fingers
  2. Practice of the Finger Force and Manipulations
   (1) Practicing the Finger Force
   (2) Practicing the Manipulations
   a. Twirling and rotating the needle
   b. Lifting and thrusting the needle
Ⅱ. POSTURE OF THE PATIENT ………… (208)
  1. The Supine Posture
  2. The Prone Posture
  3. The Lateral Recumbent Posture
  4. The Supine Sitting Posture
  5. The Prone Sitting Posture
  6. The Lateral Sitting Posture
Ⅲ. METHODS OF INSERTION OF THE NEEDLE
   ……………………………………… (210)
  1. Insertion with One Hand
  2. Insertion with Both Hands
   (1) Inserting the Needle Aided by the Pressure from
       the Finger of the Pressing Hand
   (2) Inserting the Needle with Fingers Stretching the
       Skin
   (3) Inserting the Needle By Pinching up the Skin
   (4) Inserting the Needle by Gripping it
   (5) Inserting the Needle with the Help of the Tube
Ⅳ. ANGLE AND DEPTH OF INSERTION ………
   ……………………………………… (213)
  1. Angle of Needle Insertion

(1) Perpendicular Puncture
(2) Oblique Puncture
(3) Horizontal Puncture
2. Depth of Needle Insertion
Ⅴ. REGULATION AND CONCENTRATION OF THE VITALITY AND ARRIVAL OF QI ...... (214)
Ⅵ. NEEDLE MANIPULATIONS .... (228)
1. Basic Manipulations
(1) Lifting and Thrusting
(2) Twirling and Rotating
2. Auxillary Manipulations
(1) Massaging along the Meridian
(2) Pinching along the Meridian
(3) Flicking Method
(4) Scraping Method
(5) Flying Method
(6) Shaking Method
(7) Circling Method
(8) Fressing Method
(9) Withdrawing Method
(10) Tapping Method
(11) Pushing Method
3. Reinforcing and Reducing Manipulations
(1) The Basic Reinforcing and Reducing Methods
a. Reinforcing and reducing by twirliing and rotating the needle
b. Reinforcing and reducing by lifting and thrusting the needle
c. Reinforcing and reducing achieved by rapid and slow insertion and withdrawal of the needle
d. Reinforcing and reducing achieved by puncturing along and against the direction of the meridian
e. Reinforcing and reducing achieved by manipulating the needle in cooperation with the patient's respiration
f. Reinforcing and reducing achieved by keeping the needle hole open or close
g. Uniform reinforcing and reducing
(2) The Commonly Used Comprehensive Reinforcing and Reducing Methods
a. Heat — producing needling and cool — producing needling
b. Fire (yang) — producing needling and water (yin) - producing needling
c. Yin occluding in yang and yang occluding in yin
4. Other Manipulations
(1) Green Dragon Shaking Tail
(2) White Tiger Shaking Head
(3) Green Tortoise Seeking for Cave
(4) Red Phenix Meeting Resource
(5) Zi Wu Dao Jiu Needling
(6) Dragon—Tiger Fighting
(7) Dragon—Tiger Ascending—Descending Method
(8) Qi—Enterring Method
(9) Qi—Retaining Method
(10) Chou Tian Method
Ⅶ. RETAINING AND WITHDRAWING THE NEEDLE .... (239)
1. Retaining the Needle
2. Withdrawing the Needle
Ⅷ. PRECAUTIONS AND MANAGEMENT OF POSSIBLE ACCIDENTS IN ACUPUNCTURE AND MOXIBUSTION TREATMENT .... (243)
1. Management of Possible Accidents
(1) Stuck Needle
(2) Bent Needle
(3) Broken Needle
(4) Needlng Fainting
(5) Hematoma
(6) Sequela
2. Precautions
3. Preventions of Acupuncture Accidents
(1) Traumatic Pneumothorax
(2) Injury of the Heart, Liver, Spleen, Kidney and Some Other Internal Organs
(3) Injury of the Brain and Spinal Cord

SECTION 2 ACUPUNCTURE WITH THE THREE—EDGED NEEDLE .... (249)
Ⅰ. INDICATIONS .... (249)
Ⅱ. MANIPULATIONS .... (250)
1. Spot Pricking
2. Scattering Pricking

   3. Fibrous—Tissue—Broken Pricking
Ⅱ. PRECAUTIONS ·················· (251)
SECTION 3   ACUPUNCTURE WITH THE INTRA-DERMAL NEEDLE ········· (251)
Ⅰ. INDICATIONS ·················· (252)
Ⅱ. MANIPULATIONS ·················· (253)
Ⅲ. PRECAUTIONS ·················· (253)
SECTION 4 ACUPUNCTURE WITH THE SKIN NEEDLE ·················· (254)
Ⅰ. INDICATIONS ·················· (254)
Ⅱ. MANIPULATIONS ·················· (255)
Ⅲ. STIMULATING AREAS ·············· (256)
  1. The Routine Area
  2. The Corresponding Meridian Area
  3. The Corresponding Points
  4. The Affected Area
Ⅳ. PRECAUTIONS ·················· (257)
SECTION 5   ACUPUNCTURE WITH THE DULL NEEDLE ·············· (258)
Ⅰ. INDICATIONS ·················· (258)
Ⅱ. MANIPULATIONS ·················· (259)
SECTION 6   ACUPUNCTURE WITH THE HOT NEEDLE ·············· (260)
Ⅰ. INDICATIONS ·················· (261)
Ⅱ. MANIPULATIONS ·················· (261)
  1. Deep Puncture
  2. Shallow Puncture
Ⅲ. PRECAUTIONS ·················· (262)
SECTION 7   ELECTROACUPUNCTURE ········ ·················· (264)
Ⅰ. MANIPULATIONS ·················· (264)
Ⅱ. SELECTION AND INDICATIONS OF THE WAVE FORMS ·················· (265)
High frequency (dense wave); Low frequency (sparse wave); Irregular wave (alternately dense and sparse wave); Intermittent wave; Sawtooth wave
Ⅲ. PRECAUTIONS ·················· (266)
SECTION 8   HYDRO — ACUPUNCTURE (POINT INJECTION) ·············· (267)
Ⅰ. INDICATIONS ·················· (267)

Ⅱ. MANIPULATIONS ·················· (269)
Ⅲ. PRECAUTIONS ·················· (270)
SECTION 9   OTOPUNCTURE ············ (274)
Ⅰ. MANIPULATIONS ·················· (274)
  1. Detecting the Otopoint
  (1) Observe with the Naked Eye
  (2) Detecting the Tender Spot
  (3) Detecting Electrical Changes
  2. Sterilization
  3. Methods of Stimulation
  (1) Punctuer with the Filiform Needle
  (2) Mounting
  (3) Puncture with the Plum—blossom Needle
  (4) Pricking to Cause Bleeding
Ⅱ. PRECAUTIONS ·················· (277)
SECTION 10   SCALP ACUPUNCTURE ·················· (278)
Ⅰ. THE CHARACTERISTICS AND INDICATIONS ·················· (278)
Ⅱ. MANIPULATIONS ·················· (281)
  1. Insertion of the Needle
  2. Manipulation of the Needle
  3. Withdrawal of the Needle
Ⅲ. PRECAUTIONS ·················· (282)
SECTION 11   WRIST—ANKLE ACUPUNCTURE ·················· (283)
SECTION 12   MOXIBUSTION ······· (289)
Ⅰ. COMMONLY USED MOXIBUSTION TECHNIQUES ·················· (290)
  1. Moxibustion with Moxa Cone
  (1) Direct Moxibustion
  a. Non—scarring moxibustion
  b. Scarring moxibstion
  (2) Indirect Moxibustion
  a. Ginger moxibustion
  b. Garlic moxibustion
  c. Salt moxibustion
  d. Monkshood moxibustion
  2. Moxibustion with Moxa Stick
  (1) Mild—Warming Moxibustion

  (2) Rounding Moxibustion
  (3) Sparrow—Pecking Moxibustion
 3. Moxibustion with Warming Needle
 4. Rush—Burning Moxibustion
 5. Crude Herb Moxibustion
  (1) Mashed Garlic Moxibustion
  (2) Castor Seed Moxibustion
  (3) Fructus Euodiae Moxibustion
Ⅱ. REINFORCING AND REDUCING IN MOXIBUS-
  TION THERAPY ················· (295)
Ⅲ. CONTRAINDICATIONS AND PRECAUTIONS
  ···························· (296)
APPENDIX: CUPPING METHOD ········ (297)
Ⅰ. INDICATIONS ·················· (297)
Ⅱ. MANIPULATIONS ··············· (300)
 1. Cup—Placing Method
  (1) Fire—Throwing Method
  (2) Fire Twinkling Method
  (3) Cotton—Attaching Method
  (4) Material—Placing Method
 2. Cup—Manipulating Method
  (1) Retaining Cupping
  (2) Successive Flash Cupping (Quick Cupping)
  (3) Moving Cupping
  (4) Cupping with the Needle Inside the Jar
  (5) Blood—Letting Puncture and Cupping
Ⅲ. PRECAUTIONS ················ (303)

CHAPTER FIVE   CLINICAL APPLICA-TION OF SKILL OF ACUPUNCTURE & MOXIBUSTION ············· (304)

SECTION 1   DISEASES OR SYNDROMES IN IN-
    TERNAL MEDICINE ······ (308)
 1. Mumps
 2. Acute Infectious Hepatitis
 3. Bacillary Dysentery
 4. Malaria
 5. Common Cold
 6. Bronchitis
 7. Bronchial Asthma

 8. Gastritis
 9. Gastric And Duodenal Ulcer
 10. Gastroptosis
 11. Phrenospasm
 12. Enteritis
 13. Appendicitis
 14. Acute Biliary Disorders
 15. Prolapse of Rectum
 16. Hemorrhoid
 17. Hypertension
 18. Angina Pectoris
 19. Hyperlipemia
 20. Arrhythmia
 21. Cerebrovascular Accident
 22. Epilepsy
 23. Neurasthenia
 24. Hysteria
 25. Schizophrenia
 26. Trigeminal Neuralgia
 27. Peripheral Facial Paralysis
 28. Sciatica
 29. Intercostal Neuralgia
 30. Prostatitis
 31. Enuresis
 32. Retention of Urine
 33. Male Infertility (Appendix: Sexual Disoders)
 34. Arthrits (Appendix: Periarthritis of Shoulder Joint)
 35. Stiff Neck
 36. Obesity
SECTION 2   CYNECOLOGICAL DISEASES ·······
  ···························· (400)
 1. Dysmenorrhea
 2. Menopausal Syndrome
 3. Morbid Leukorrhea
 4. Malposition of Fetus
SECTION 3   DISEASES OR SYNDROMES IN DER-
    MATOLOGY, SURGERY, AND
    TRAUMATOLOGY ········ (409)
 1. Acute Mastitis
 2. Multiple Boils

3. Neurodermatitis
4. Eczema
5. Urticaria
6. Herpes Zoster
7. Acne
8. Baldness
9. Soft Tissue Injury
10. Ganglion

SECTION 4   DISEASES OF EYE, EARS, NOSE AND THROAT ············ (432)

1. Rhinitis
2. Acute Tonsillitis
3. Acute Conjunctivitis
4. Myopia
5. Toothache
6. Tinnitus and Deafness
7. Aural Vertigo

SECTION 5   EMERGENCY DISEASES ·················· (449)

1. Shock
2. Sunstroke

APPENDIX 1: BIBLIOGRAPHY ············ (454)

APPENDIX 2: CROSS INDEX OF THE FIGURES ································ (459)

上篇
预备知识

PART ONE
PREPARATION
KNOWLEDGE

for Application of Techniques of Acupuncture And Moxibustion

第一章
经络腧穴概要

CHAPTER ONE
THE SUMMARY OF MERIDIAN COLLATERALS AND ACUPOINTS

第一节 经络概述

在中医学基本理论体系中,经络是人体运行气血的通路,是经脉和络脉的总称。直行的主干为经,细小的分支为络。它们纵横交错分布于全身,把人体脏腑和各种组织器官紧密地联系起来,构成一个有机的整体。并与脏腑、气血、营卫等共同组成中医学的基本理论。经络理论对于指导中医各科临床实践,尤其是针灸学科更为重要。故早在《灵枢·经脉》篇中,就有"经脉者,所以能决死生。处百病,调虚实,不可不通"的记载。

一、经络系统的组成

经络系统包括十二经脉、奇经八脉、十二经别、十五络脉、孙络、浮络以及十二经筋、十二皮部等。

十二经脉是经络系统中的主体,故又称十二正经。内属于相应的脏腑,外络于躯干、头面、四肢。根据经脉起止在手或在足,循行于四肢外侧(阳面)或内侧(阴面),与所属十二脏腑的名称,以及阴阳消长、衍化的理论等,分为手足太阴、少阴、厥阴;太阳、少阳、阳明,共十二条。例如止于手,循行于上肢内侧,隶属于肺脏的经脉,称为手太阴肺经。止于足,循行于下肢外侧,隶属于胃腑的经脉,称为足阳明胃经。

十二经对称地分布于人体两侧,阳经主表,属腑络脏,分布于四肢外侧及头面、躯干;阴经主里,属脏络腑,分布于四肢内侧及腹胸,其中手的三条阴经从胸至手;手的三条阳经从手上头;足的三条阳经从头走足;足的三条阴经从足至腹胸。为此,阴经与阳经在四肢末端衔接,阳经与阳经在头面部衔接,阴经与阴经在胸部衔接。使十二经脉的气血流注周而复始,如环无端。此外,十二经脉还有一脏配一腑的阴阳表里属络关系,如手太阴肺经与手阳明大肠经;手厥阴心包经与手少阳三焦经;手少阴心经与手太阳小

· 1 ·

肠经；足阳明胃经与足太阴脾经；足厥阴肝经与足少阳胆经；足少阴肾经与足太阳膀胱经等互为表里。十二经脉每条经都有穴位分布在体表相应的循行线路上，既是疾病的反应点，也是针灸的施术点。

奇经八脉是十二经脉之外的特殊通路，共有八条。即督脉、任脉、冲脉、带脉、阴维脉、阳维脉、阴跷脉、阳跷脉。由于督脉与任脉也有专穴分布在体表循行线上，故常与十二经脉合称为十四经，是针灸学中的重点，为临床实践必不可少.

经络系统中的十二经别，是十二正经别行深入体腔的分支；十五络脉乃十二经脉在四肢部各分出的一条络脉，加上任脉、督脉在躯干部各分出的一条络脉，及脾经分出的一条大络，共十五条，称为十五络；十二经筋是十二经脉之气，结、聚、散、络于筋肉关节的体系；十二皮部乃十二经脉功能活动反应于体表的部分。

SECTION 1 MERIDIANS AND THEIR COLLATERALS

The meridians and their collaterals are the passages through which qi, a traditional Chinese medicine (TCM) term referring to both the refined materials which are highly nutritious and circulate in the body and the functional activities of the viscera and tissues, and blood circulate, the meridians being the trunk running straight in the body and the collaterals being the branch. The meridians and collaterals distribute through the whole body, and connect interiorly with the zang—fu organs (viscera)[1] and exteriorly with the tissues and organs at the body surface so as to make the human body organic integral. The theories referring to the meridians and their collaterals, as well as the zang—fu organs, qi[2] and blood, and ying and wei (the nutrient principles and the defense princples) consist of the basic part of TCM theories. The theory of meridian and collateral is important in guiding the clinical practice of TCM, especially the clinical practice of acupuncture and moxibustion.

---

[1] Zang and fu organs, viscera, including the five solid organs—the heart, the liver, the spleen, the lung, and the kidney, six hollow organs—the gallbladder, the stomach, the small intestine, the large intestine, the bladder and the tri—jiao, and extraordinary fu—organs— the brain, marrow, bone, vessels, gallbladder and uterus. Although the most zang and fu organs in traditional Chinese Medicine (TCM) share the same names with the corresponding internal organs in modern medicine, and are roughly in accordance with those in modern medicine in the morphosis and anatomy, they are largely different from those in modern medicine. The kidney in TCM, for example, has the function of being in charge of the genital, urinary and endocrinal activitises, etc, and is closely related to the respiratory system, the digestive system, the body fluid metabolism, the hemopoietic system, growth and development, and the physiologic activities of hearing. So a zang or fu organ in TCM mainly refers to a functional unit which controls some functional activities of some systems of human body.

[2] Qi refers to the following three meanings:
a. vital energy, the refined nutritive substance flowing within the body, such as qi (essence) of water and food, and the inspired air; b. functional activity, generally denoting the function of the internal organs and tissues, eg, qi of the five zang (solid) —organs, qi of the six fu (hollow) —organs; c. one of the affected phases or stages in acute febrile disease.

As early as in the book Ling Shu (Acupuncture Classic, one of the two parts of "The Yellow Emperor's Internal Classic", an important medical literature for the study of acupuncture and medical theories of the Warring States Period in China), in its chapter "Meridians and Vessels", it is recorded that "Meridians and veccels play the role to determine one's life and death, act against diseases, and adjust deficiency or excess in the body. So they should be kept to be passed freely."

I. THE COMPOSITION OF THE MERIDIAN AND COLLATERAL SYSTEM

The meridian and collateral system, i. e. the channel system, comprises the twelve regular meridians or twelve mridians, eight extra meridians, branches of the twelve meridians, fifteen collaterals, mini—collaterals, and floating collaterals, as well as the twelve musculofascia of the meridians and twelve skin areas of the meridians.

The twelve meridians, usually termed the twelve regular meridians, are the main part of the channel system, which respectively pertain to an internal organ interiorly and connect with the trunk, head and limbs exteriorly. They are named after the limbs where they run from or to and the zang or fu organs they pertain to, and according to the anterior aspect (i. e. yang surface) or medial aspect (i. e. yin surface) they run along and the theory of the growth and decline of yin and yang,① Taiyin, Shaoyin, Jueyin, Taiyang, Shaoyang, and Yangming② are termed to them. For example, the meridian pertaining to the lung and running along the medial aspect of the upper limb and ending at the hand is termed the Lung Meridian of Hand—Taiyin; that running to the foot and along the lateral aspect of the lower limb and ending at the foot, and pertaining to the stomach, the Stomach Meridian of Foot—Yangming.

The twelve meridians are distributed symmetrically at two sides of the body. The yang meridians master the exterior, pertain to the fu organs (hollow viscera) and connect with the zang organs (parenchymatous or solid viscera), distributing at the anterior aspect of the limbs, head and face, and trunk. The ying meridians dominate the interior, pertain to

---

① yin and yang are general terms for two opposite aspects of matters and phenomena in the nature, which are interrelated and opposed to each other. They present not only two diferent matters in opposition but two oppsite aspects in the same entity. In traditional Chinese Medicine, they are used to summerize and explain the problems in the fields of anatomy, physiolgy, pathology, diagnosis, treatment, etc. Generally speaking, matters and phenomena, whick are dynamic, external, upward, ascending, brilliant, progressive, hyperactive, or pertaining to funntional activities belong to the category of Yang. Those which are static, internal, downward, descending, dull, retrogressive, hypoactive, or pertaining to materials, belong to that of Yin.

② Taiyin means that the yin—qi is flourishing; Shaoyin refers to thot the yin—qi is diminishing; Jueyin means that the yin—qi at the final stage of development. Taiyang refers to that the yang—qi is flourishing; Shaoyang means to that the yang—qi is diminishing; and Yangming rfers to that the yang—qi is at the final stage of development.

the zang organs and connect with the fu organs, distributing at the medial aspect of the limbs and abdomen and chest. The three yin meridians of hand run from the chest to the hand, while the three yang meridians of the hand from the hand upwards to the head; the three yang meridians of foot run from the head to the foot, while the three yin meridians of foot from the foot to the abdomen and chest. So the yin meridians connect with the yang meridians at the distal end of the limbs, the yang meridian with the yang meridian at the head and face; the yin meridian with the yin meridian at the chest. Through the connection of the meridians the qi and blood of the channels circulate without any terminal point.

As each of the twelve meridians pertains to one zang organ and connects with one fu organ, the zang and the fu organs being a couple, or pertains to one fu organ and connects with one zang organ, the two organs being a couple too, there is a yin—yang, exterior—interior, pertaining — conncting relationship in each pair of the meridians. Namely, the Lung Meridian of Hand—Taiyin is the reciprocal internal counterpart of the Large Intestine Meridian of Hand—Yangming, and vice versa; the Pericardium Meridian of Hand—Jueyin, the reciprocal internal counterpart of the Sanjiao (Triple Energizer) Meridian of Hand — Shaoyang and vice versa; the Heart Meridian of Hand — Shaoyin, the reciprocal internal counterpart of the Small intestine Meridian of Hand—Taiyang and vice versa; the Stomach Meridian of Foot—yangming, the reciprocal extenal counterpart of the Spleen Meridian of Foot—Taiyin and vice versa; the Liver Meridian of Foot—Jueyin, the reciprocal internal counterpart of the Gallbladder Meridian of Foot—Shaoyang and vice versa; and the Kidney Meridian of Foot — Shaoyin, the reciprocal internal counterpart of the Bladder Meridian of Foot—Taiyang and vice versa.

Each of the twelve meridians has its own acupoints distributed along its running course on the corresponding body surface. The acupoint is not only the spot where the disease is reflected, but also the point where the acpuncture and moxibustion are performed on, namely the treatment spot.

The eight extra meridians are the special passages besides the twelve meridians, which are the Ren Meridian (Conception Vessel, Renmai, Ren Channel), Du Meridian (Governor Versssel, Dumai, Du Channel), Chong Channel (Chongmai, Strategic Channel), Dai Channel (Daimai, Girdle Channel), Yinwei Channel (the regulating meridian of yin), Yangwei Channel (the regulating meridian of yang), Yinqiao Channel (the motility meridian of yin) and Yangqiao Channel (the motility meridian of yang). Most of the eight extra meridians don't have their own acupoints but points in the twelve meridians. But, the Governor Vessel and the Conception Vessel have their own specific acupoints. Moreoover, the Governor Vessel running along the median line of the back is considered as "the sea of the yang channels", and the Conception Vessel running along the midline of the chest and abdomen taken as "the sea of the yin channels". Therefore, these two channels are put together with the twelve meridians under the term "the fourteen channels" which are a key point in the science of the acupuncture & moxibustion, and play an importat role in the clinical practice.

The twelve branches of the meridians in the channel system, each of which gives off from each of the twelve meridians at the area proximal to the elbow or knee of the limbs, run deep into the body cavity and emerge to the body surface at the head and neck. After emerging the branch of a yang meridian joins the yang meridian which it belongs to, and the branch of a yin meridian joins the yang meridian which is exteriorly—interiorly related to the yin meridian which it belongs to, resulting in that "all branches of the twelve meridians merge into the six yang meridians." The fifteen collaterals refer to the branches giving off respectively from the Luo—Connecting points of each of the twelve meridians and from the Governor and Conception Vessels, plus a large one (the major collateral of the spleen) from the spleen. The twelve musculofascia channels refer to a system of the collaterals distributed to the muscles and joints, at which the qi of the twelve meridians is to join, collect and spread. The skin areas of the twelve meridians refer to a system of the collaterals distributed to the body surface areas in which the condition of the function of the twelve meridians may be reflected.

二、经络的作用

经络学说是中医理论的重要组成部分，它具有联络脏腑和肢体，运行气血营养周身，传导感应，调整虚实，保卫机体抗御外邪的作用。当人体功能低下时，经络能将外邪由体表传注于脏腑，反之，亦能将内脏的病理变化反应于体表，医生通过压按或探测穴位的反应，以及根据病变所在的部位，症候表现，可推测疾病所累及的经络与脏腑。如牙痛、口臭、胃脘胀满，中脘穴处有压痛，根据这些症状表现与发病部位，及压按诊察反应的穴位，可以判定病在足阳明胃经。结合局部与远端循经、对症选穴，调整经络气血及内脏功能，从而达到防病保健、治疗疾病的目的。

II. FUNCTIONS OF THE MERIDIANS AND COLLATERALS

The theory of the channel is an important part of the theories of TCM. The meridians and their collaterals have functions to link the internal organs with the limbs, to carry qi and blood to nourish the body, to conduct the sensation to adjust excess or deficiency in the body, and to prevent the body from the attacks by exogenous evils.[①] When the function of the body resistance is lower, through the meridians and their collaterals the exogenous evil may be transported from the body surface into the internal zang and fu

---

① Exogenous evils, also termed exopathogen or exogenous pathogenic factor, refer to the environmental pathogenic factor (wind, cold, summer—heat, dampness, dryness, fire) and other epidemic factors.

organs, and the pathologic changes of the internal organs may be reflected to the body surface since the meridians and their collaterals interiorly link with the zang and fu organs and exteriorly with the limbs and joints. As this reason, whether the meridian or the zang or fu organ is involved by disease may be known by pressing or probing the acupoints, in combination with consideration of the diseased area and manifestations. For example, a patient with toothache, foul breath, fullness of gastric region, tenderness at Zhongwan (RN12, a point at the lower abdomen) may be diagnosed as disorder of the Stomach Meridian of Foot — Yangming. Finally, the purpose to pervent and treat diseases and to keep healthy may be reached by application of acupuncture & moxibustion to abjust the function of the meridians and collaterals, blood and qi, and internal organs.

第二节 腧穴概述

一、腧穴分类

腧穴是人体脏腑经络之气输注于体表的部位，也是针灸施术的部位。一般分为以下三类：

1. 十四经经穴：简称经穴。分布在十二经与任、督脉的循行线路上，均有一定的名称及定位，具有主治本经病症的共同作用。

2. 经外奇穴：简称奇穴。是在十四经经穴确定后又陆续发现的一些穴位，它们尚未列入十四经系统，但有奇效故称经外奇穴，亦有一定名称及定位。

3. 阿是穴：其称呼首见于《千金方》，它没有固定的位置及具体的名称，而是以压痛点或其他反应点作为针灸的施术部位。

SECTION 2 ACUPOINTS

I. CLASSIFICATION OF THE ACUPOINTS

The acupoint is the site through which the qi of the zang and fu organs and of the meridians is transported to the body surface, and at which acupuncture and moxibustion are performed. Generally, the acupoints may be classified into three groups.

1. *The Acupoints of the Fourteen Meridians*

The acupoint of the fourteen meridians is termed "acupoint of the meridian" for short, which is situated along the twelve meridians, Conception Vessel, and Governor Vessel, and has the specific name and location. The acupoints belonging to the same meridian have the common fnction in treament of the disorders of the meridian along which the acupoints are situated.

2. *The Extra Acupoints*

The extra points, also termed extraordinary points and abridged as Ex., are discovered in succession after the acupoints of the fourteen meridians are defined.

They can exert the extraordinary curative effect and have defined locations and names, but not listed in the system of the foureen meridians.

3. *The Ashi Points*

The term "Ashi point" is seen in "Thousand Golden Prescriptions" at first. The Ashi points have neither definite location nor names. They are nothing but the tender or sensitive spots which are selected as the puncture points for treatment purpose.

二、常用特定穴的含义与功用

特定穴是指十四经中具有特殊治疗作用的经穴，它们各有其特定的名称。

1. 五腧穴：十二经在四肢肘膝关节以下各有五个重要经穴，分别称为井、荥、输、经、合。古人把经气运行过程，用自然界的流水由小到大，由浅入深的变化来形容，将五腧穴按井、荥、输、经、合的顺序，从四肢末端向肘膝方向依次排列。由于五腧穴又与五行相配属，故亦称五行腧（穴位见表1—1.2）。

表1—1 六阴经的五腧穴

穴名 经名	井(木)	荥(火)	输(土)	经(金)	合(水)
肺(金)	少商	鱼际	太渊 T	经渠	尺泽 ⊥
肾(水)	涌泉 ⊥	然谷	太溪	复溜 T	阴谷
肝(木)	大敦	行间 ⊥	太冲	中封	曲泉 T
心(火)	少冲 T	少府	神门 ⊥	灵道	少海
脾(土)	隐白	大都 T	太白	商丘 ⊥	阴陵泉
心包(相火)	中冲 T	劳宫	大陵 ⊥	间使	曲泽

注：表内"T"符号代表母子补泻法中的母穴；"⊥"符号代表母子补泻法中的子穴。下表同。

表1—2 六阳经的五腧穴

穴名 经名	井(金)	荥(水)	输(木)	经(火)	合(土)
大肠(金)	商阳	二间 ⊥	三间	阳溪	曲池 T
膀胱(水)	至阴 T	通谷	束骨 ⊥	昆仑	委中
胆(木)	窍阴	侠溪 T	足临泣	阳辅 ⊥	阳陵泉
小肠(火)	少泽	前谷	后溪 T	阳谷	小海 ⊥
胃(土)	厉兑 ⊥	内庭	陷谷	解溪 T	足三里
三焦(相火)	关冲	液门	中渚 T	支沟	天井 ⊥

临床上常用五腧穴对症治疗，即井穴能开窍，多用来急救；荥穴能泻热，可治疗一切热证；输穴治疗经脉的痛证；经穴既用来治经脉病如寒热，亦治疗脏腑病如喘咳等；合穴多用来治疗六腑的病症。

除外，还用作母子补泻，即根据木、火、土、金、水五行相生中"生我者母""我生者子"，以及"虚则补其母"、"实则泻其子"的原则进行选穴。如肺属金，肺气虚的病症可以取其生金的母穴输土太渊；反之，肺气实的病症可以取其金所生的子穴合水尺泽，如此类推，各经母子穴见表1—1.2。

2. 原络穴：原穴是脏腑原气输注经过留止的部位；络穴有联络的意思，是表里两经联络的处所，十二经各有一个原穴与络穴，其中任、督二脉又各有一络穴，加上脾的大络总计十五络（穴位见表1—3）。

临床上原穴多用来治疗或诊察内脏病；络穴用来治疗表里两经的疾患。原穴与络穴还可配合运用，称原络配穴法。如肺病可取本经原穴太渊，配合相表里的大肠经络穴偏历。

3. 俞、募穴：俞穴是脏腑之气输注于背部的穴位，又称背俞穴；募穴是脏腑之气输注于胸腹部的穴位。十二经中各有一个背俞穴及募穴（穴位见表1—3）。

临床上,脏病与相关的官窍病多取背俞穴治疗,如咳嗽、胸闷或鼻塞可取肺俞穴治疗,腑病多取募穴治疗,如肠鸣腹泻取天枢穴治疗。俞穴与募穴还可配合运用,称俞募配穴,可帮助诊察疾病及治疗相关的脏腑病。如腹泻可取大肠背俞穴大肠俞及募穴天枢。

4. 郄穴: 郄穴是经脉之气深聚的部位,每一经均有一个郄穴(穴位见表1—3)。

临床上多用来治疗急性痛证与炎症,如急性胃痛或乳腺炎可取胃经郄穴梁丘。

表1—3 原、络、俞、募、郄穴

穴名 经名	原穴	络穴	俞穴	募穴	郄穴
肺经	太渊	列缺	肺俞	中府	孔最
大肠经	合谷	偏历	大肠俞	天枢	温溜
胃经	冲阳	丰隆	胃俞	中脘	梁丘
脾经	太白	公孙	脾俞	章门	地机
心经	神门	通里	心俞	巨阙	阴郄
小肠经	腕骨	支正	小肠俞	关元	养老
膀胱经	京骨	飞扬	膀胱俞	中极	金门
肾经	太溪	大钟	肾俞	京门	水泉
心包经	大陵	内关	厥阴俞	膻中	郄门
三焦经	阳池	外关	三焦俞	石门	会宗
胆经	丘墟	光明	胆俞	日月	外丘
肝经	太冲	蠡沟	肝俞	期门	中都

附:任脉络穴鸠尾,督脉络穴长强,脾之大络大包穴。

5. 八会穴:是人体脏腑、气、血、筋、脉、骨、髓等精气的聚会处即:

脏会—章门　　腑会—中脘
气会—膻中　　血会—膈俞
骨会—大杼　　髓会—绝骨(悬钟)
筋会—阳陵泉　脉会—太渊

临床上常用来治疗脏、腑、气、血、骨、髓、筋、脉等相关方面的疾患,如血会膈俞,故凡属一切血病均可取膈俞穴进行治疗。

6. 下合穴:是指手三阳经的脉气与下肢相通的合穴,即手阳明大肠经的下合穴上巨虚;手太阳小肠经的下合穴下巨虚;手少阳三焦经的下合穴委阳。均可用来治疗相关的腑病,如腹泻可取大肠经下合穴上巨虚治疗。

7. 八脉交会穴:是四肢部正经通向奇经八脉的八个穴位,可治奇经病及相应部位的病症。如后溪通督脉,故督脉的脊柱强痛、角弓反张可取后溪穴治疗,如此类推,其八脉交会穴的配合运用见下表。

公孙通冲脉 ⎫
内关通阴维脉 ⎭ 主治心、胸、胃病症

后溪通督脉 ⎫
申脉通阳跷脉 ⎭ 主治目内眦、颈项、耳、肩部病症

足临泣通带脉 ⎫
外关通阳维脉 ⎭ 主治目外眦、耳后、颊、颈、肩部病症

列缺通任脉 ⎫
照海通阴跷脉 ⎭ 主治肺、咽喉、胸膈病症

II. MEANINGS AND FUNCTIONS OF THE COMMONLY USED SPECIFIC POINTS

Among the acupoints of the fourteen meridians there are some ones with the specific roles in treatment, which respectively have their specific names and clinical indications.

1. *The Five Shu Points*

The five shu points refer to the five important acupoints of each of the twelve meridians situated distal to the elbow and knee of the limds, named Jing — Well, Ying — Spring, Shu — Steream, Jing — River and He — Sea points. The ancient writers compared the flow of qi in the channel to that of water in the nature and used the terms for description of the natural course of the water flowing in a river from the small to the large, and from the shallow to the deep to designate the particular acupoints of the different sites along the course of the meridian. They are arranged from the distal end of the limbs to the elbow or knee, in the order of Jing, Ying, Shu, Jing and He. As they are coordinated with the five elements, they are also named the acupoints of the five elements. The five elements refer to metal, wood, water, fire, and earth. The Chinese ancients thought that these five kinds of materials were the indispensable and most fundamental elements in constituting the Universe. There existed enhancing, inhibiting and restraining relationships among them. They were also in constant motion and change. In TCM, they are used to explain and expand a series of medical problems by comparing with and deducing from such properties and mutual relationships. The theory of the five elements[①] can be used to explain and expand the properties of the five shu points, so the term point of tive element is given to the five shu points. The five shu points are seen in the Table 1—1 and 1—2.

Note: In the follwing tables, the mark "T" represents the "mother point" and the mark "⊥" represents the "son point" in the application of the theory of reinforcing and reducing according to the "mother—son relation".

The five shu points are usually selected for the expectant treatment in clinic. To the treatment of the emergency condition, the Jing—Well point is frequently employed because it can serve to induce resuscitation; to the febrile diseases, the Ying—Spring point usually selected as it

Tab. 1—1 Five Shu Points of the Six Yin Meridians

point meridian	Jing (Wood)	Ying (Fire)	Shu (Earth)	Jing (Metal)	He (Water)
Lung (Metal)	Shaoshang (LU 11)	Yuji (LU 10)	Taiyuan T (LU 9)	Jingqu (LU 8)	Chize (LU 5) ⊥
Kidney (Water)	Yongquan ⊥ (KI 1)	Rangu (KI 2)	Taixi (KI 3)	Fuliu T (KI 7)	Yingu (KI 10)
Liver (Wood)	Dadun (LR 1)	Xingjian (LR 2) ⊥	Taichong (LR 3)	Zhongfeng (LR 4)	Ququan T (LR 8)
Heart (Fire)	Shaochong T (HT 9)	Shaofu (HT 8)	Shenmen (HT 7) ⊥	Lindao (HT 4)	Shaohai (HT 3)
Spleen (Earth)	Yinbai (SP 1)	Dadu T (SP 2)	Taibai (SP 3)	Shangqiu (SP 5) ⊥	Yinlingquan (SP 9)
Pericardium (prime—minister fire)	Zhongchong T (PC 9)	Laogong (PC 8)	Daling (PC 7) ⊥	Jianshi (PC 5)	Quze (PC 3)

---

① The theory of five elements is one of the philosophic theories integrated with medical practice in ancient China, expounding the unity of the human body and matters, and the physiopathological relationship between the five zang—organs.

Tab. 1—2 **Five Shu points of the Six Yang Meridians**

meridian \ point	Jimg—Well (metal)	Ying—Spring (water)	Shu—Stream (wood)	Jing—River (fire)	He—Sea (earth)
Large Intsetine (Metal)	Shangyang LI 1	Erjian (LI 2) ⊥	Sanjian (LI 3)	Yangxi (LI 5)	Quchi T (LI 11)
Bladder (Water)	Zhiyin T (BL 67)	Zutonggu (BL 66)	Shugu (BL 65) ⊥	Kunlun (BL 60)	Weizhong (BL 40)
Gallbladder (Wood)	Zuqiaoyin (GB 44)	Xiaxi T (GB 43)	Zulinqi (GB 41)	Yangfu (GB 38) ⊥	Yanglingquan (GB 34)
Small Intestine (Fire)	Shaoze (SI 1)	Qiangu (SI 2)	Houxi T (SI 3)	Yanggu (SI 5)	Xiaohai (SI 8) ⊥
Stomach (Earth)	Lidui ⊥ (ST 45)	Neiting (ST 44)	Xiangu (ST 43)	Jiexi T (ST 41)	Zusanli (ST 36)
Sanjiao (Triple Energizer, prime—Minister Fire)	Guanchong (SJ 1)	Yemen (SJ 2)	Zhongzhu T (SJ 3)	Zhigou (SJ 6)	Tianjiang (SJ 10) ⊥

can serve to purge the heat; to the painful syndromes, the Shu—Stream point usually selected; to the disorders of the meridian such as cold and fever, and to the problems of the viscera such as asthma and cough, the Jin—River point usually selected; and to the disorders of the six fu organs, the He—sea point usually selected.

Additionally, the five shu points are also selected for reinforcing and reducing[①] according to the theory of mother—son relation in the theory of the five elements.[②] As the five shu points are correlated respectively to the five elements as shown on the Tab 1 and 2, the selection of the points can be based on the mother-child relationship of the five elements. Namely, the five shu points are employed according to the principle in the theoy of the five elements that "in two elements between which these is the mother-child relation, the element promoting the other is known as mother and the element being promoted as son", and "deficiency of the son element is treated by reinforcing its mother element and excess of the mother element by reducing its son element". For example, the lung

---

① Reinforcing refers to a treatment method of reinforcing and nourishing the deficiency of Qi, blood, Yin and Yang; reducing refers to a treatment method of purging and dispelling pathogenic factors.

② The Chinese ancients thought that the five kinds of materials—metal, wood, water, fire, and earth—were the indispensable and most fundamental elements in constituting the Universe. There existed enhancing, inhibiting and restraining relationships among them. They were also in constant motion and change. In traditional Chinese medicine, they are usesd to explain and expand a series of medical problems by comparing with and deducing from such properties and mutual relationships.

pertains to the metal, so deficiency of the lung③ may be treated by selection of Taiyuan (LU 9) because Taiyuan (LU 9) is the Shu—Stream (earth) point of the five shu points of the Lung Meridian and the earth cun serve to promote the metal. Oppositely, excess of the lung④ may be treated by selection of Chize (LU 5), the He—Sea (water) point of the five shu points of the Lung Meridian because the water is promoted by the metal and the metal is the mother element of the water, on the analogy of this. (The mother and son acupoints of the five shu points of each of the twelve meridian are seen on the table 1—1 and 1—2)

2. Yuan—Source and Luo—Connecting Points

Yuan means orginal, the Yuan—Source point is the site where the original qi of zang and fu organs infuses, collects and retains. Luo means connecting, the Luo—Connecting point is the site where the two meridians which are exteriorly—interiorly related link with each other. Each of the twelve meridians has a Yuan—Source point, and each of them and of the Conception and Governor Vessels and of the major collateral of the spleen has a Luo—Connecting point, making 15 in total. (The Luo—Connecting and Yuan—Source points are seen on the Table 1—3)

The Yuan—Source points are frequently employed in treatment and diagnosis of the diseases of the internal organs in clinic, while the Luo—Connecting points usually selected for disorders involving the two exteriorly—interiorly related meridians. The Yuan—Source points can be used in combination with the Luo—Connecting points, this method being called combined selection of the Yuan—Source and Luo—Connecting points. For example, the lung disorders can be treated with Taiyuan (LU 9) which is the Ynan—Source point of the Lung Meridian, and Pianli (LI 6) which is the Luo—Connecting point of the Large Intestine Meridian because the Lung and Large Intestine Meridians are externally—internally related.

3. The Back—Shu and Front—Mu Points

The Back—Shu points are the sites where the qi of the zang and fu organs is infused at the back. The Front—Mu pionts are the sites where qi of the zang and fu organs is infused at the chest and abdomen. Each of the twelve meridians has a Back—Shu and a Front—Mu point. (the Back—Shu and Front—Mu points are seen on Tab. 1—3)

In clinic, Back—Shu points are usual-

---

③ Deficiency of the lung includes deficiency of yin and insufficiency of Qi of the lung. The former is manifested by dry cough, afternoon fever, night sweats, flushed cheeks, heet inpalms and soles, dry throat with hoarseness, red and dry tongue, faint and rapid pulse. The latter is manifested by shortness of breath, low and weak voice, aversion to wind, perspiration, pale complexion, weak pulse.

④ Excess of the lung refers to a morbid condition due to invasion of the lung by whelming pathogenic factors, manifested by cough with copious whitish or yellow sputum, feeling of stuffiness in the chest, greasy or slimy coating of the tongue, often seen in bronchitis and bronchiectasis, and pneumonia.

ly used to treat disorders of the zang organs and their related orifices. For example, cough, oppressed feeling in the chest or stuffy nose, which belong to disorders of the lung, can be treated by selection of Feishu (BL 13), the Back—Shu point of the Lung Meridian. The Front—Mu points are usually selected for treating fu organ disorders. For example, borborymus and diarrhea are treated by selection of Tianshu (ST 25), the Front-Mu point of the Large Intestine Meridian. The Back-Shu and Front-Mu points can be used in combination, this method being called association of the Back—Shu with the Front—Mu points, which can aid in diagnosis and treatment of the disorders of the related zang and fu organs. For example, diarrhea is treated by selection of Dachangshu (BL 25) and Tianshu (ST 25), the Back—Shu and Ftont—Mu points of the Larrge Intestine Meridian.

Tab. 1—3 Yuan—Source, Luo—Connecting, Back—Shu, Front-Mu and Xi—Cleft points

point \ meridian	Yuan—Source	Luo—Connecting	Back—Shu	Front—Mu	Xi—Cleft
Lung	Taiyuan (LU9)	Lieque (LU7)	Feishu (BL13)	Zhongfu (LU1)	Kongzui (LU6)
Large Intestine	Hegu (LI4)	Pianli (LI6)	Dachangshu (BL25)	Tianshu (ST25)	Wenliu (LI7)
Stomach	Chongyang (ST42)	Fenglong (ST40)	Weishu (BL21)	ZHongwan (RN12)	Liangqiu (ST34)
Spleen	Taibai (SP3)	Gongsun (SP4)	Pishu (BL20)	Zhangmen (LR13)	Diji (SP8)
Heart	Shenmen (HT7)	Tongli (HT5)	Xinshu (BL15)	Juque (RN14)	Yinxi (HT6)
Small Intestine	Wangu (SI4)	Zhizheng (SI7)	Xiaochangshu (BL27)	Guanyuan (RN4)	Yanglao (SI6)
Bladder	Jinggu (BL64)	Feiyang (BL58)	Pangguanshu (BL28)	Zhongji (RN3)	Jinmen (BL63)
Kidney	Taixi (KI3)	Dazhong (KI4)	Shenshu (BL23)	Jingmen (GB25)	Shuiquan (KI5)
pericardium	Daling (PC7)	Neiguan (PC6)	Jueyinshu (BL14)	Danzhong (RN17)	Ximen (PC4)
Trple Energizer (Sanjiao)	Yangchi (SJ4)	Waiguan (SJ5)	Sanjiaoshu (BL22)	Shimen (RN5)	Huizong (SJ7)
Galldladder	Qiuxu (GB40)	Guangming (GB37)	Danshu (BL19)	Riyue (GB24)	Waiqiu (GB36)
Liver	Taichong (LR3)	Ligou (LR5)	Ganshu (BL18)	Qimen (LR14)	Zhongdu (LR6)

4. The Xi—Cleft Points

The Xi—Cleft point is the site where the qi of the meridian is deep converged. There is a Xi—Cleft point in each of the twelve meridians. (The points seen on Tab. 1—3)

In clinic, the Xi—Cleft points are usually used in treating acute inflammation and pain. For example, acute stomachache or acute mastitis, Liangqiu (ST34), the Xi—Cleft point of the Stomach Meridian, is selected.

Note: In Tab3, the Luo—Connecting point of the Conception Vessel is Jiuwei (RN 15); the Governor Vessel, Changqiang (DU 1); and the major collateral or the spleen, Dabao (SP 21).

5. Eignt Influential Points

The eight influential points are the sites where the energy of zang, fu qi, blood, bone, marrow, tendon and blood vessels joint and collect. They include the follows:

The influential point of the primordial enegy of the zang organ———— . Zhangmen (LR 13)

The influential point of the primordial energy of the fu organ———— Zhongwan (RN 12)

The inflnential point of qi————Dangzhong (RN 17)

The influental point of blood————Gashu (BL 17)

The influential point of bone————Dashu (BL 11)

The influential point of marrow————Xuanzhong (GB 39)

The influential point of tendon————Yanglingquan (GB 34)

The influential point of blood vessel————Taiyan (LU 9)

In clinic, the eight influential points are usually used in treating diseases which they are related to, namely, Zhangmen (LR 13), related to the zang organ, is frequently selected for treatment of diseases in the zang organs, Geshu (BL 17), related to the blood, may be selected for hemorrhagic disorders, and so on.

6. The Lower Confluent Points

The lower conflent points are the spots where the qi of the three yang meridians of the hand is confluent at the lower extremities. The lower confluent point of the Large Intestine Meridian of Hand—Yangming is Shangjuxu (ST 37), while Xiajuxu (ST 39) is of the Small Intestine Meridian of Hand—Taiyang and Weiyang (BL 53) is of the Triple Energizer Meridian of Hand—Shaoyang. They are employed to treat disorders of the fu organs which are related to. For example, Shangjuxu (ST 37), the lower confluent point of the Large Intestine Meridian, can be used in treating diarrhea, a problem of the stomach and large intestine.

7. Eighy Confluence Points

The eight confluence points refer to the acupoints located at the extremities and connecting the eight extra meridians with the twelve meridians. They are indicated in diseases of the extra meridians and corresponding areas. For example, Houxi (SI 3), one of the confluence points, connecting the Governor Vessel, is usually selected in treatment of disorders of the Governor Vessel, Such as spinal stiffness and

· 13 ·

pain, opisthotonos. The coordinated application of the eight confluence points are as follwoing:

Gongsun (SP 4) connecting Chong Channel
Neiguan (PC 6) Connecting Yinwei Channel
— Indicated in disorders of heart, chest and stomach

Houxi (SI 3) connecting Du Meridian (Governor Vessel)
Shenmai (BL 62) connecting Yangqiao Channel
— Indicated in disorders of inner canthus, nape, ear, shoulder and back

Zulinqi (GB 41) connectng Dai Channel
Waiguan (SJ 5) connecting Yangwei Channel
— Indicated in disorders of outer canthus, posterior ear, cheek, neck and shoulder

Lieque (LU 7) connecting Ren Meridian (Conception Vessel)
Zhaohai (KI 6) connecting Yinqiao Channel
— Indicated in disorders of lung, throat. chest and diaphragm

三、腧穴的定位法

1. 体表解剖标志定位法：是以体表解剖学的各种体表标志为依据来确定经穴位置的方法。体表解剖标志，可分为固定的标志和活动的标志两种。

固定的标志，指各部由骨节和肌肉所形成的突起或凹陷，五官轮廓，发际，指（趾）甲、乳头、脐窝等。例如，腓骨头前下方定阳陵泉；三角肌尖端部定臂臑；眉头定攒竹；两眉之中间定印堂；两乳头之中间定膻中等。

活动的标志，指各部关节、肌肉、肌腱、皮肤随着活动而出现的空隙、凹陷、皱纹、尖端等。例如，听宫，在耳屏与下颌关节之间，微张口呈凹陷处；曲池，在屈肘时，肘横纹外侧端凹陷处。

全身各部的主要体表解剖标志如下：

头部
①前发际正中（头部有发部位的前缘正中）；
②后发际正中（头部有发部位的后缘正中）；
③额角（发角）（前发际额部曲角处）；
④完骨（颞骨乳突）。

面部：
①眉间（印堂）（两眉头之间的中点处）；
②瞳孔（正坐平视，瞳孔中央）或目中（目内眦至外眦连线的中点处）。

颈、项部：
①喉结（喉头凸起处）；
②第七颈椎棘突。

胸部：
①胸骨上窝（胸骨切迹上方凹陷处）；
②胸剑联合中点（胸骨体和剑突结合部）；
③乳头（乳头的中央）。

腹部：
①脐中（神阙）（脐窝的中央）；
②耻骨联合上缘（耻骨联合上缘与前正中线的交点处）；
③髂前上棘（髂骨嵴前部的上方突起

处)。

侧胸、侧腹部：
①腋窝顶点（腋窝正中央最高点）；
②第十一肋端（第十一肋骨游离端）。

背、腰、骶部：
①第七颈椎棘突；
②胸椎棘突1～12、腰椎棘突1～5、骶正中嵴、尾骨；
③肩胛岗根部点（肩胛骨内侧缘近脊柱侧点）；
④肩峰角（肩峰外侧缘与肩胛冈连续处）；
⑤髂后上棘（髂骨嵴后部的上方突起处）。

上肢：
①腋前纹头（腋窝皱襞前端）
②腋后纹头（腋窝皱襞后端）
③肘横纹；
④肘尖（尺骨鹰嘴）；
⑤腕掌、背侧横纹（尺、桡二骨茎突远端连线上的横纹）。

下肢：
①髀枢（股骨大转子）；
②股骨内侧髁（内辅骨上）；
③胫骨内侧髁（外辅骨上）；
④臀下横纹（臀与大腿的移行部）；
⑤犊鼻（外膝眼）（髌韧带外侧凹陷处的中央）；
⑥腘横纹（腘窝处横纹）；
⑦内踝尖（内踝向内侧的凸起处）、
⑧外踝尖（外踝向外侧的凸起处）。

2. "骨度"折量定位法：是以体表骨节为主要标志折量全身各部的长度和宽度，定出分寸，用于经穴定位的方法。即以《灵枢·骨度》规定的人体各部分寸为基础，并结合历代学者创用的折量分寸（将设定的两骨节点之间的长度折量为一定的等分，每一等分为1寸，十等分为1尺），作为定穴的依据。全身主要"骨度"折量寸见表1—4、图1—1。

3. 指寸定位法：是依据患者本人手指所规定的分寸以量取腧穴的方法。

中指同身寸　以患者的中指中节桡侧两端纹头（拇、中指屈曲成环形）之间的距离为1寸（图1—2）。

拇指同身寸　以患者拇指的指间关节的宽度作为1寸（图1—3）。

横指同身寸（一夫法）　患者尺侧手四指并拢，以其中指中关节横纹为准，其四指的宽度作为三寸（图1—4）。

具体取穴时，应当在骨度折量定位法的基础上，参照被取穴对象自身的手指进行比量，并结合一些简便的活动标志取穴方法，如垂手中指端所到处取风市（图1—5①）；两手虎口自然平直交叉，食指尖所到处取列缺（图1—5②）等，以确定经穴的标准部位。故下述腧穴中所涉及的寸、均非现代市寸。

Ⅲ. METHODS OF LOCATING ACUPOINTS

There are three methods for locating points, surface anatomical landmarks, bone proportional measurement and finger measurement. They should be used in combination, but the first one is the fundamental and the other two the supplemental ones.

1. *Surface Anatomical Landmarks*

Theis is a method to determine the location of points on the basis of anatomical landmarks on the body surface, which are divided into the fixed and movable landmarks.

表1—4 常用"骨度"折量寸

部位	起止点	折量寸	度量法	说明
头面部	前发际正中→后发际正中	12	直寸	用于确定头部经穴的纵向距离
	眉间(印堂)→前发际正中	3	直寸	用于确定前或后发际及其头部经穴的纵向距离
	第七颈椎棘突下(大椎)→后发际正中	3	直寸	
	眉间(印堂)→后发际正中→第七颈椎棘突下(大椎)	18	直寸	
	前两额发角(头维)之间	9	横寸	用于确定头前部经穴的横向距离
	耳后两乳突(完骨)之间	9	横寸	用于确定头后部经穴的横向距离
胸腹胁部	胸骨上窝(天突)→胸剑联合中点(岐骨)	9	直寸	用于确定胸部任脉穴的纵向距离
	胸剑联合中点(岐骨)→脐中	8	直寸	用于确定上腹部经穴的纵向距离
	脐中→耻骨联合上缘(曲骨)	5	直寸	用于确定下腹部经穴的纵向距离
	两乳之间	8	横寸	用于确定胸腹部经穴的横向距离
	腋窝顶点→第11肋游离端(章门)	12	直寸	用于确定胁部经穴的横向距离
背腰部	肩胛骨内缘→后正中线	3	横寸	用于确定背腰部经穴的横向距离
	肩峰缘→后正中线	8	横寸	用于确定肩背部经穴的横向距离
上肢部	腋前、后纹头→肘横纹(平肘尖)	9	直寸	用于确定臂部经穴的纵向距离
	肘横纹(平肘尖)→腕掌(背)侧横纹	12	直寸	用于确定前臂部经穴的纵向距离
下肢部	耻骨联合上缘→股骨内上髁上缘	18	直寸	用于确定下肢内侧足三阴经穴的纵向距离
	胫骨内侧髁下方→内踝尖	13	直寸	
	股骨大转子→腘横纹	19	直寸	用于确定下肢外后侧足三阳经穴的纵向距离.(臀沟→腘横纹,相当14寸)
	腘横纹→外踝尖	16	直寸	用于确定下肢外后侧足三阳经穴的纵向距离

The fixed landmarks include the prominences and depressions formed by the joints and muscles, the configuration of the five sense organs, hairline, fingernails and toenails, nipples and umbilicus. For instance, Yang—lingquan (GB 34) is in the depression anterior and inferior to the head of the fibula; Binao (LI 14) is at the end of the insertion of the deltoid muscle; Cuanzhu (BL 2) is at the medial end of the eyebrow; Yintang (Extra point) is midway detween the eyebrows; and Danzhong (RN 17) is at the midpoint between the nipples.

经络腧穴概要

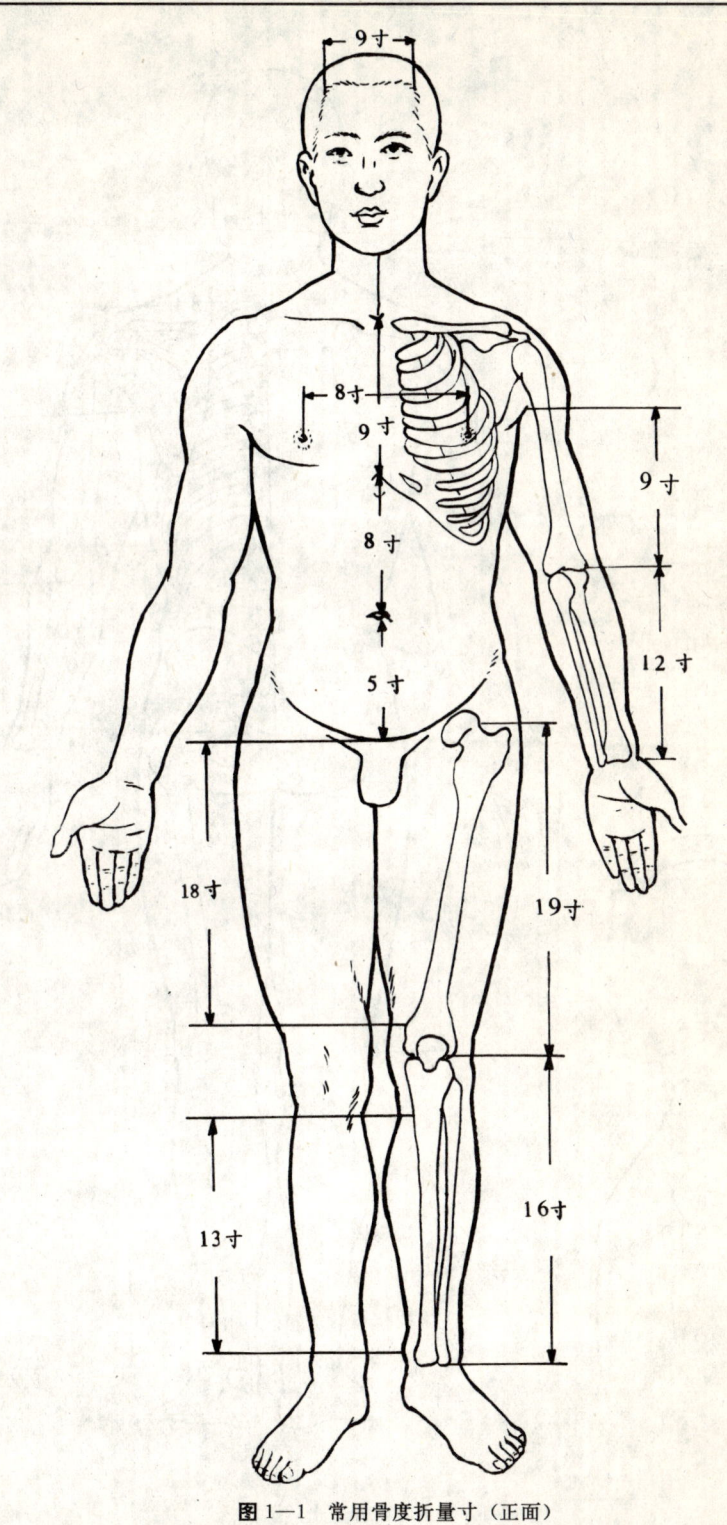

图 1—1　常用骨度折量寸（正面）
Fig. 1—1 Commonly Used Bone—Measurements (Front)

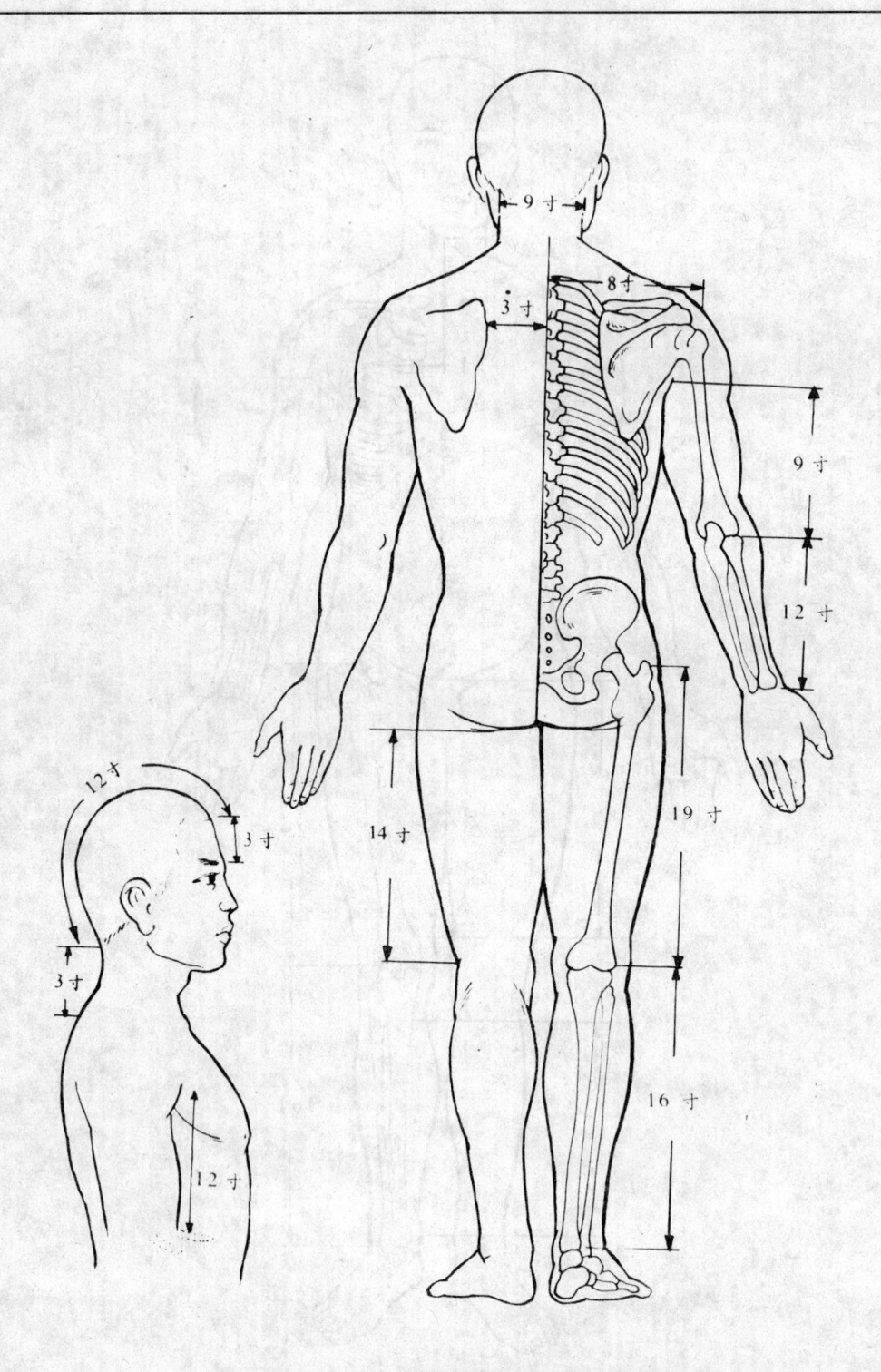

图 1—1　常用骨度折量寸（背面）
Fig. 1—1 Commonly Used Bone—Measurements (Back)

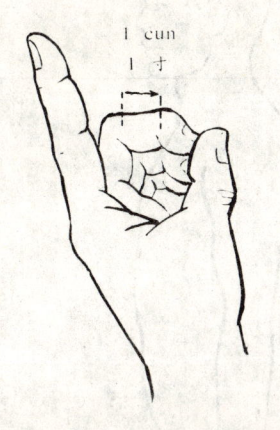

图 1—2 中指同身寸 图 1—3 拇指同身寸 图 1—4 横指同身寸（一夫法）
Fig. 1—2 Middle Finger Measurement   Fig. 1—3 Thumb Measurement   Fig. 1—4 Four—Finger Measurement

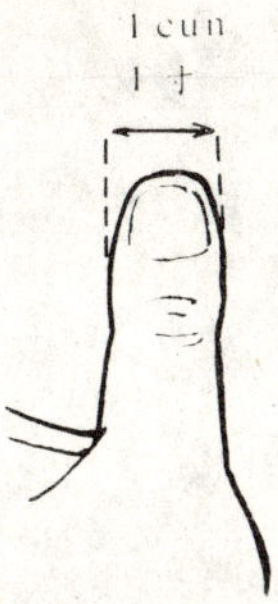

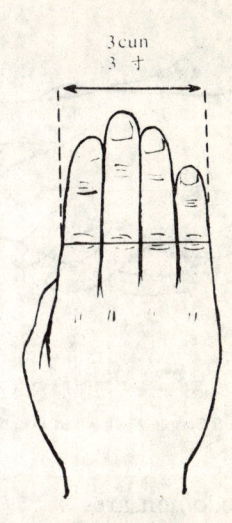

The movable landmarks refer to the clefts, depressions, wrinkles or prominences appearing on the joints, muscles, tendons and skin during motion. For example, Tinggong (SI 19) is between the tragus and mandibular join, where a depression is formed when the mouth is slightly open; Quchi (LI 11) is in the depression at the lateral end of the cubital crease when the elbow is flexed.

The major anatomical landmark on the human body surface are listed as follows:

On the head are:

1) the midpoint of the anterior hairine;

2) the midpoint of the posterior hairline;

3) the corner of the forehead (at the corner of anterior hairline); and

4) the mastoid process.

On the face are:

1) Yintang (Extra point) (at the midpoint between the eyebrows); and

2) the pupil (in the erect sitting position and looking straight forward), or the center of the eye (at the midpoint of the line between the inner and outer canthi).

On the neck is:

1) the laryngeal protuberance.

On the chest are:

1) the suprasternal fossa (in the deeeepression above the suprasternal notch);

2) the midpoint of sternoxyphoid symphysis (at the conjunction of the sternum and xyphoid process); and

3) the nipple (the center of the nipple)

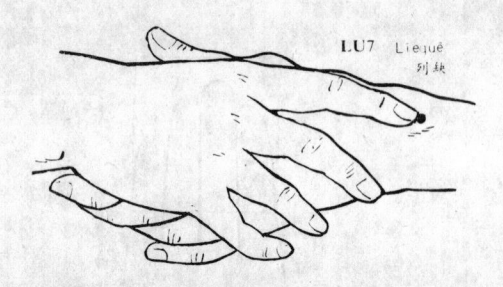

Fig. 1—5 Simple Methods in Locating Points (Lieque)

On the abdomen are:

1) the umbilicus (Shenque, RN 8) (the center of the umbilicus);

2) the upper border of the pubic symphysis at the crossing point of the upper border of the pubic symphysis and the anterior midline); and

3) the anterior superior iliac spine.

On the lateral side of the chest and abdomen are:

1) the apex of the axilla (the highest point of the axillary fossa); and

2) the free end of the 11th rib.

On the back, low back and sacrum are:

1) the spinous process of the 7th cervical vertebra;

2) the spinous processes from the 1st to the 12th thoracic vertebrae and from the 1st to the 5th lumbar vertebrae, the median sacral crest and the coccyx;

3) the medial and the scapular spine (on the medial border of the scapula);

4) the acromial angle; and

5) the posterior superior iliac spine.

On the upper limbs are:

1) anterior axillary fold (the anterior end of the axillary crease);

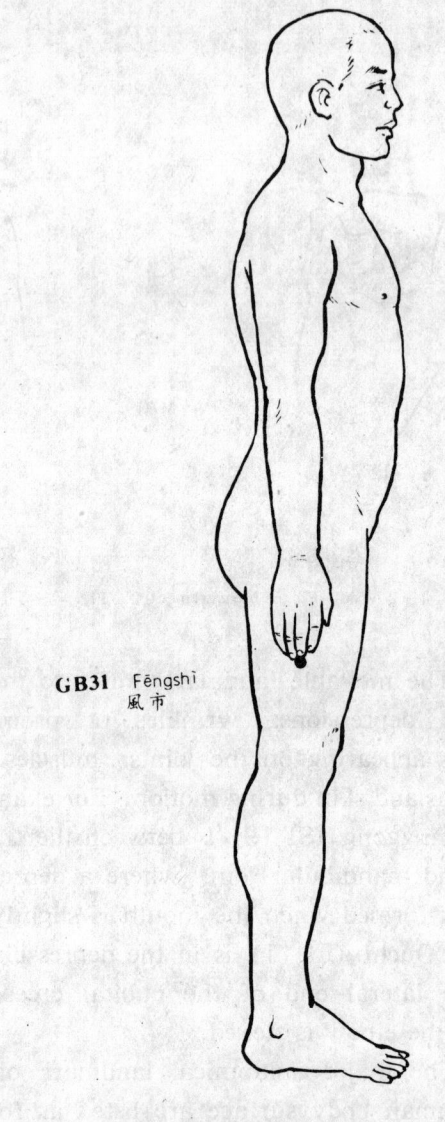

Fig. 1—5 Simple Methods in Locating Points (Fengshi)

2) the posterior axillary fold (the posterior end of the axillary crease);

3) the cubital crease;

4) the tip of the elbow (olecranon);

5) the dorsal and palmar creases of the wrist (the styloid crease between the

distal ends of the styloid processes of the ulna and radius).

On the lower limbs are:

1) the greater trochanter of the femur;

2) the medial epicondyle of the femur;

3) the medial epicondye of the tibia;

4) the inferior gluteal crease (the border detween the buttocks and thigh);

5) Dubi (ST 35) (in the center of the depression lateral to the patella ligamnt);

6) the popliteal crease;

7) the tip of the medial malleolus;

8) the tip of the lateral malleous.

2. *Bone Proportional Measurment*

In this method the joints are taken as the main landmarks to measure the length and width of various portions of the human body. The proportional measurement of various portions of the human body defined in the Miraculous Pivot (Ling Shu) is taken as the basis for the locaion of points in combination with the modified methods introdced by the acupuncturists through the ages. The length between two joints is divided into several epual portions, each portion as one cun and 10 portions as one chi. "Cun" (寸) is used as a length unit in China, 1 cun = 3.3 cm.

Obviously, in location of acupoints in clinical practice of acupuncture and moxibustion, "cun" is taken as the unit of the proportional measurement and finger measurement. As this reason, the length of cun on different patients' bodys can be actually differnt in length.

The descriptions of the portions of the human body in traditional Chinese medicine are not always the same as those in modern anatomy. The palmar (flexor) side of the upper limbs is named the "medial side", where the three yin meridians of the hand are distributed, while the dorsal (extensor) side is known as the "lateral side", where the three yang meridians of the hand are distributed. The side of the lower limbs facing the sagittal plane of the body is called the "media side", where the three yin meridians of the foot are distributed, while the sides where the three yang meridians of the foot are distrbuted are the "lateral side" and the "posterior side".

The main bone proportional measurements are listed in the follwing table.

3. *Finger Measurement*

This is a method to locate the points by measuring the distance with either the length or width of the patient's finger(s).

Table 1—4: Bone Proportional Measurement

Position	Origin and end points	Poririon (cun)	Method of measurement	Remarks
Head and face	From the midpoint of the anterior hairline to the midpoint of the posterior hairline	12	Longitudinal measurement	Used for measuring the longitudinal distance of the points of the head
	From Yintang (EX — HN3) to the midpoint of the anterior hairline	3	Longitudinal measuruement	Used for measuring the longitudinal distance of the points on the anterior and posterior hairline and the head
	From the point below the spinous process of the 7th cervical vertebra (Dazhui, DU 14) to the midpoint of the posterior hairline	3	Longitudinal measuruement	
	From Yintang (EX — HN3) to the midpoint of the posterior hairline and then to the point below the spinous process of the 7th cevical vertebra (Dazhui, DU 14)	18	Longitudinal measurement	
	Between the corners of the forehead (Touwei, ST 8)	9	Transverse measurement	Used for measuring the transverse distance of the points on the anterior part of the head
	Between the bilateral mastoid processes	9	Transverse measurement	Uded for measuring the transverse distance of the points on the posterior part of the head
Chest, abdomen and hypochondrium	From the suprasternal fossa (Tiantu, RN22) to the midpoint of the sternoxyphoid symphysis	9	Longitudinal measurement	Used for measueing the longitudinal distance of the points of Ren Meridian (Conception Vessel) on the chest
	From the midpoint of the sternoxyphoid symphysis to the centre of the umbilicus	8	Longitudinal measurement	Used for measuruing the longitudinal distance of the points on the upper abdomen
	From the centre of the umbilicus to the upper border of the pubic symphysis (Qugu, RN 2)	5	Longitudinal measurement	Used for measuruing the longitudinal distance of the points on the lower abdomen
	Between the two nipples	8	Transverse measurement	Used for measuring the transverse distance of the points on the chest and abdomen
	From the apex of the axilla to the free end of the 11th rib (Zhangmen, LR 13)	12	Longitudinal measurement	Used for measuring the longitudinal distance of the points on the hypochondrium
Back and low back	From the medial border of the scapula to the posterior midline	3	Transverse measurement	Used for measuring the transverse distance of the points on the back
	From the acromial angle to the posterior midline	8	Transverse measurement	Used for measuring the transverse distance of the points on the shoulder and back

Position	Origin and end points	Poririon (cun)	Method of measurement	Remarks
Upper limbs	From the anterior and posterior axillar folds to the cubital crease	9	Longitudinal measrement	Used for measuring the longitudinal distance of the points on the arm
	From the cubital crease to the dorsal crease of the wrist	12	Longitudinal measurement	Used for measuring the longitudinal distance of the points in the forearm
lower limbs	From the upper border of the pubic symphysis to the upper border of the medial epicondyle of the femur	18	Longitudinal measurement	Used for measuring the longitudinal distance of the points on the three yin meridians of the foot on the medial side of the lower limbs
	From the lower border of the medial epicondyle of the tibia to the tip of the medial malleolus	13	Longitudinal measurement	
	From the greater trochanter to the popliteal crease	19	Longitudinal measurement	Used for measuring the longitudinal distance of the points on the three yang meridians of the foot on the lateroposterior side of the lower limbs (the distance from the gluteal groove to the popliteal crease is equivalent to 14 cun)
	From the politeal crease to the tip of the lateral malleolus	16	Longitudinal mesurement	Used for measuring the longitudinal distance of the points on the three yang meridians of the foot on the latero—posterior side of the lower limds

1) Middle finger measurement: When the middle finger is flexed, the distance between the radial ends of the two interphalangeal crease of the patient's middle finger is taken as 1 cun (See Fig. 1—2).

2) Thumb measurement: The width of the interphalangeal joint of the patient's thumb is taken as 1 cun (See Fig. 1—3).

3) Four—Finger measurement: When the four fingers (index, middle, ring and little fingers) keep close, their width on the level of the proximal interphalangeal crease of the middle finger is taken as 3 cun (See Fig. 1—4).

This method is mainly used for locating the points of the lower limbs. When locating the points, this method should be used in combination with some simple movable landmarks on the basis of the bone proportional measurement.

Additionally, there are simle methods for the location of some points, which are a way to locate the points by the patient's simple action accordinated with. Fengshi (GB 31), for example, is where the tip of the middle finger touches when the patient stands erect with the hands at laxation (See Fig. 1—5); and when the index fingers and thumbs of the both hands are crossed naturally and horizontally, Lieque (LU1) is where the tip of the index finger touches (See Fig1—5).

第三节 十四经循行及常用腧穴

一、手太阴肺经（共11穴）

（一）经脉循行

1. 起于中焦，向下联络大肠；2. 回过来沿着胃的上口；3. 通过横膈；4. 属肺；5. 从肺与喉相连系的部位横行出来；6. 沿上臂内的桡侧；7. 下行到肘中；8. 再沿前臂内的桡侧下行；9. 进入桡动脉搏动处；10. 经鱼际；11. 沿鱼际边缘；12. 至拇指桡侧端。

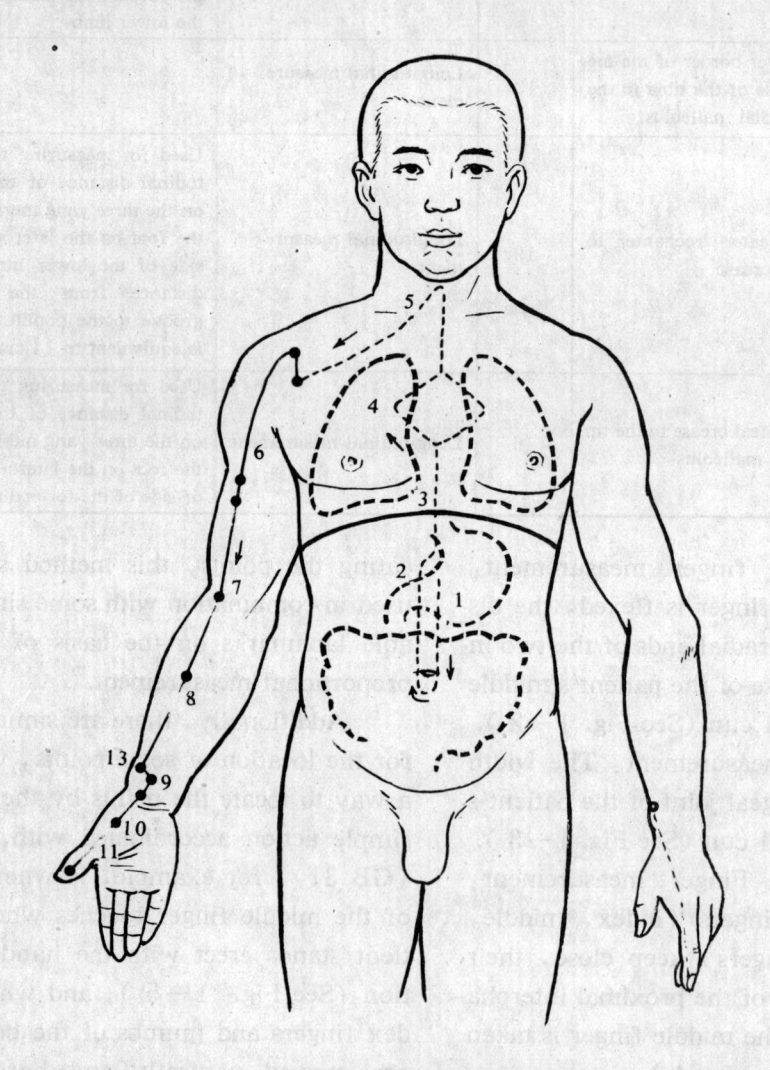

图1—6 手太阴肺经循行示意图

Fig. 1—6 The Running Course of the Lung Meridian of Hand Taiyin

支脉：13. 从腕后列缺穴分出来走向食指桡侧端，与手阳明大肠经相交接。

体表穴位分布线：起于胸部外上方中府穴，沿上肢内侧的桡侧缘下行至腕后桡动脉处，经鱼际边缘终于拇指桡侧端少商穴。

体内相关的组织脏器：肺、大肠、喉咙。

（二）本经常用腧穴

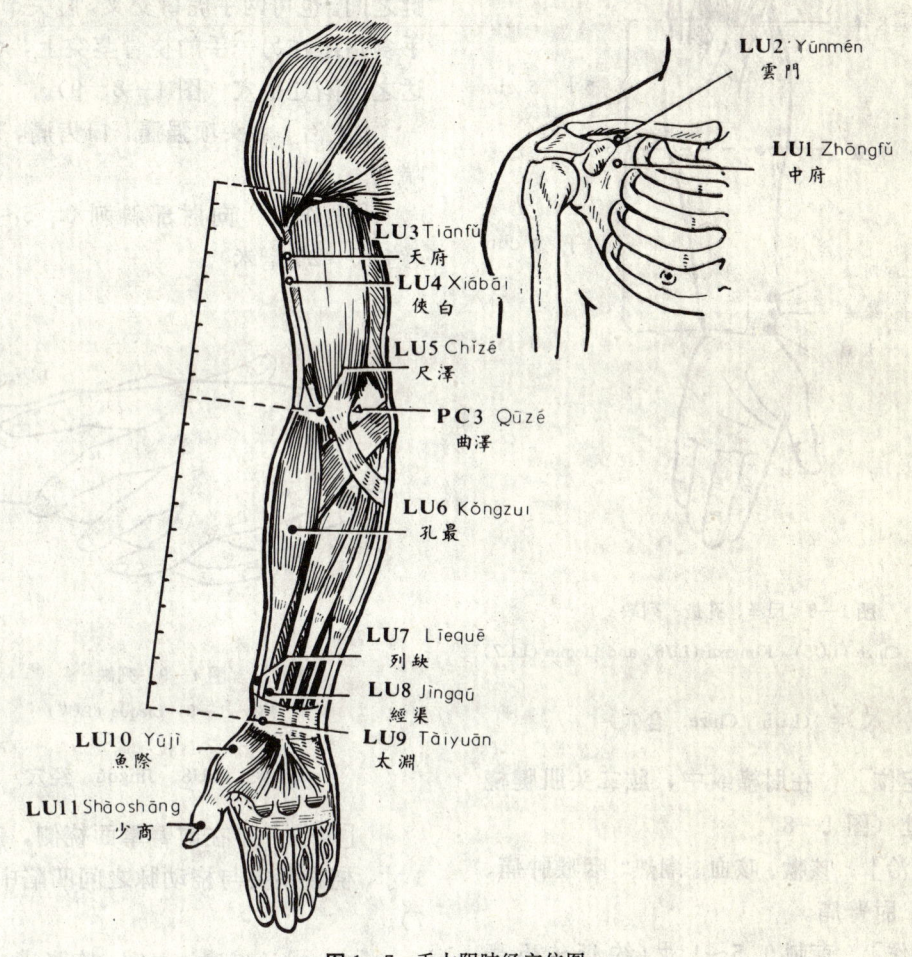

图 1-7 手太阴肺经穴位图
Fig. 1-7 Acupoints of the Lung Meridian

注：图中黑点表示常用穴，黑圈表示非常用穴，以下各图均同。
Note：In this figure and the following figures, ". " represents the commonly used acupoint, while "。" represents the non-commonly used acupoint.

中府 （LU1 Zhōngfǔ 募穴）

[定位] 胸前壁外上方，距前正中线旁开6寸，平第一肋间隙（图1-7）。

[主治] 咳嗽、喘息、胸痛、肺胀满。

[操作] 向外斜刺或平刺0.5～0.8寸（约15～20毫米），不可向内斜刺，以防伤及肺脏。（小儿、老人针刺深度酌减，以下各穴

均同）

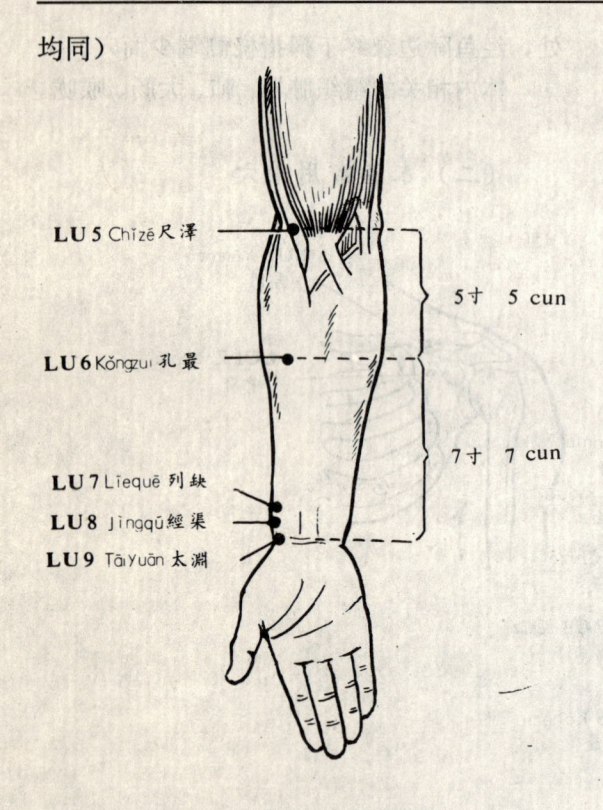

图 1—8 尺泽、孔最、列缺
Fig. 1—8 Chize (LU5), Kongzui (LU6) and Lieque (LU7)

尺泽（LU5 Chǐzé 合穴）

［定位］　在肘横纹中，肱二头肌腱桡侧凹陷处（图 1—8）。

［主治］　咳嗽、咳血、潮热、咽喉肿痛、胸胀痛、肘臂痛。

［操作］　直刺 0.5～1 寸（约 15～25 毫米）

孔最（LU6 Kǒngzuì 郄穴）

［定位］　在前臂掌面桡侧，尺泽穴与太渊穴连线上，腕横纹上 7 寸（图 1—8）。

［主治］　咳嗽、气喘、咯血、咽喉肿痛、失音、痔疮。

［操作］　直刺 0.5～1 寸（约 15～25 毫米）。

列缺（LU7 Lièquē 络穴，八脉交会穴）

［定位］　在前臂桡侧缘，桡骨茎突上方，腕横纹上 1.5 寸。当肱桡肌与拇长展肌腱之间。也可两手虎口交叉，腕关节伸直，一手食指压在另一手的桡骨茎突上，食指尖所达之凹陷处是穴（图 1—8、9）。

［主治］　头项强痛，口齿痛，咳嗽，气喘。

［操作］　向肘部斜刺 0.5～0.8 寸（约 15～20 毫米）。

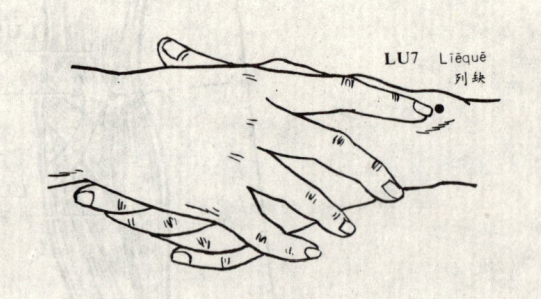

图 1—9　列缺
Fig. 1—9 Lieque (LU7)

经渠（LU8 Jīngqú 经穴）

［定位］　在前臂掌面桡侧，腕横纹上 1 寸，桡骨茎突与桡动脉之间凹陷中（图 1—7）。

［主治］　咳嗽、气喘、胸胀满、手腕痛。

［操作］　避开血管，直刺 0.3～0.5 寸（约 9～15 毫米）。

太渊（LU9 Tàiyuān 原穴、输穴、八会穴）

［定位］　在腕掌侧横纹桡侧，桡动脉搏动处（图 1—7）。

［主治］　咳嗽、气喘、咯血、胸痛、腕痛、无脉症。

［操作］　避开血管，直刺 0.3～0.5 寸

（约9～15毫米）。

鱼际（LU10 Yújì 荥穴）

［定位］ 在手拇指本节（第1掌指关节）后陷处。约当第1掌骨中点桡侧，赤白肉际处（图1—7）。

［主治］ 咳嗽、咳血、失音、咽喉肿痛、身热。

［操作］ 直刺0.5～0.8寸（约15～20毫米）。

少商（LU11 Shàoshāng 井穴）

［定位］ 手拇指末节桡侧指甲角旁约0.1寸（图1—7）。

［主治］ 咽喉肿痛，鼻衄、发热、昏迷、癫狂。

［操作］ 浅刺0.1寸（约3毫米），或三棱针点刺出血。

（三）常用经穴主治提要

本经腧穴能主治与肺、喉有关的病症，如咳嗽、气喘、胸胀满疼痛、咽喉疼痛。其中中府、太渊、经渠主要治肺气虚引起的喘咳、多痰；尺泽、鱼际治肺实热引起的咳嗽、咽痛；孔最治咳嗽、咯血及痔疮下血；列缺治外感咳嗽及头项强痛；少商治咽喉肿痛等。

SECTION 3 THE COURSES AND COMMONLY USED ACUPOINTS OF THE FOURTEEN MERIDIANS

I. THE LUNG MERIDIAN OF HAND —TAIYIN (11 points in total)

1. *The Course*

It originates in the Middle Warmer (i. e. Middle—jiao, referring to the abdominal cavity above the level of the umbilicus with its contents, including the spleen and stomach), and runs downwards to connect with the large intestine (1). Turning back to run along the cardiac orifice (2), it passes through the diaphragm (3), and enters its pertaining organ————the lung (4). From the portion connecting the trachea with the larynx it comes out transversely (5), passes downwards along the radial side of the medial aspect of the upper arm (6) and runs through the cubital fossa (7). Then, it goes continuously downwards along the radial side of the medial aspect of the forearm (8), and enters the site where radial pulse is felt (9). Passing through Yuji (LU 11) (10), it goes along the border of the thenar (11), and ends at the radial side of the tip of the thumb (12).

Its branch proximal tio the wrist gives off from Lieque (LU 7), and runs to the radial side of the tip of the index finger to connect with the Large Intestine Meridian of Hand —Yangming (13).

The line made up by the acupoints distributed on the body surface: It originates from Zhongfu (LU 1) at the latero—superior aspect of the chest, runs along the radial border of the medial aspect of the upper limb and goes downwards to the site where the radial artery beats. Then, it passes along the margin of the thenar and ends at the tip of the radial side of the thumb at Shaoshang (LU 11).

The inner organs concerned: The

lung, intestine and throat.

2. *The Commonly Used Acupoints*

Zhongfu (LU 1, Front—Mu point)

Location: At the latero—superior aspect of the anterior wall of the chest, 6 cun lateral to the anterior midline, 1 cun below Yunmen (LU 2), at the level of the 1st intercostal space (See Fig. 1—7).

Indications: Cough, dyspnea, pain in the chest, distension and fullness in the chest.

Method: Puncture obliquely or horizontally 0.5—0.8 cun ① (15—20mm) towards the lateral side of the chest. It is forbidden to puncture obliquely towards the interior aspect of the chest, otherwise the lung may be injured. Moxibustion is applicable.

Chize (LU 5, He—Sea point)

Location: In the cubital crease, in the depression of the radial side of the tendon of the biceps muscle of the arm (See Fig. 1—8).

Indications: Cough, hemoptysis, hectic fever, swelling and sore throat, fullness and distenion in the chest, pain in the elbow and arm.

Method: Puncture perpendicularly 0.5-1.0 cun (15—25mm).

Kongzui (LU 6, Xi—Cleft point)

Location: On the radial side of trhe palmar suface of the forearm, and on the line connecting Chize (LU 5) and Taiyuan (LU 9), 7 cun above the wrist furrow (See Fig. 1—8).

Indications: Cough, asthma, hemoptysis, swelling and sore throat, aphonia, hemorrhoids.

Method: Puncture perpendicularly 0 5—1.0 cun (15—25mm). Moxibustion is applicable.

Lieque (LU 7, Luo—Connecting point, Confluence point)

Location: On the radial side of the forearm, proximal to the styloid process of the radius, 1.5 cun proximal to the wrist furrow, betwen the brachioradeial muscle and the tendon of the long abductor muscle of the thunb. Or, when the index fingers and thumds of both hands are crossed with the wrist joint extended and index finger of one hand placed on the styloid process of the radius of the other, the acupoint is in the depression on the dorsum on the wrist right under the tip of the index finger (See Fig. 1—8, 1—9).

---

① In addition to as the unit of bone proportional measurement and finger measurement in location of acupoints, "cun" is also taken as the unit of length of the acupuncture needle and depth of puncture. When measuring the length of a needle or depth of puncture, generally, 15 mm is taken as 0.5 cun, but 25mm as 1 cun. See Chapter Three in detail.

Indications: Headahce, stiffness of the neck, pain in the tooth and mouth, cough, asthma.
Method: Puncture obliquely toward elbow 0.5—0.8 cun (15—20mm). Moxibustion is applicable.

Jingqu (LU 8, Jing—River point)

Location: On the radial side of the palmar surface of the forearm, 1 cun proximal to the transverse crease of the wrist, in the depression between the radial artery and the medial aspect of the styloid process of the radius (See Fig. 1—7).
Indications: Cough, asthma, distenion and fullness in the chest, apin in the wrist and hand.
Method: Puncture perpendicularly 0.3—0.5 cun (9—15mm), avoiding the radial artery.

Taiyuan (LU 9, Yuan—Source and Shu—Stream point, Influential point dominating vesssels)

Location: At the radial end of the crease of the wrist, where the pulsation of the radial artery is palpable (See Fig. 1—7).
Indications: Cough, astnma, hemoptysis, pain in the chest, pain in the wrist, pulselessness.
Method: Puncture perpendicularly 0.3—0.5 cun (9—15mm), avoiding the radial artery. Moxibustion is applicable.

Yuji (LU 10, Ying—Spring point)

Location: In the depression proximal to the 1st metacarpophalangeal joint, on the radial side of the midpoint of the 1st metacarpal bone, and at the dorso—ventral boundary of the hand (See Fig. 1—7).
Indications: Cough, hemoptysis, aphonia, swelling and sore throat, fever.
Method: Puncture perpendicularly 0.5—0.8 cun (15—20mm). Moxibustion is applicable.

Shaoshang (LU 11, Jing—Well point)

Location: On the radial side of the distal segment of the thumb, about 0.1 cun from the corner of the fingernail (See Fig. 1—7).
Indications: Swelling and sore throat, epistaxis, fever, coma, mania and epilepsy.
Method: Puncture shallowly 0.1 cun (about 3mm) or prick with the three—edged needle to cause bleeding.

3. An Ontline of Indications of the Commonly Used Acupoints of the Meridian

The acupoints of this meridian can be employed in treating disorders of the lung and throat, such as cough, asthma, fullness and pain in the chest, sore throat. In the concrete, Zhongfu (LU 1), Taiyuan (LU 9), and Lieque (LU 8) are mainly indicated in asthma and cough with much sputum due to deficiency of Lung — qi; Chize (LU 5) and Yuji (LU 10), in cough and sore throat due to excess and heat condifion of the lung; Kongzui (LU6), in cough, hemoptysis, and hemorrhoids with bleeding; Lieque (LU 7), in cough and neck stiffness and headache due to attack by exogenous pathogenic factor; and Shaoshang (LU 1), in swelling and sore throat.

二、手阳明大肠经（共20穴）

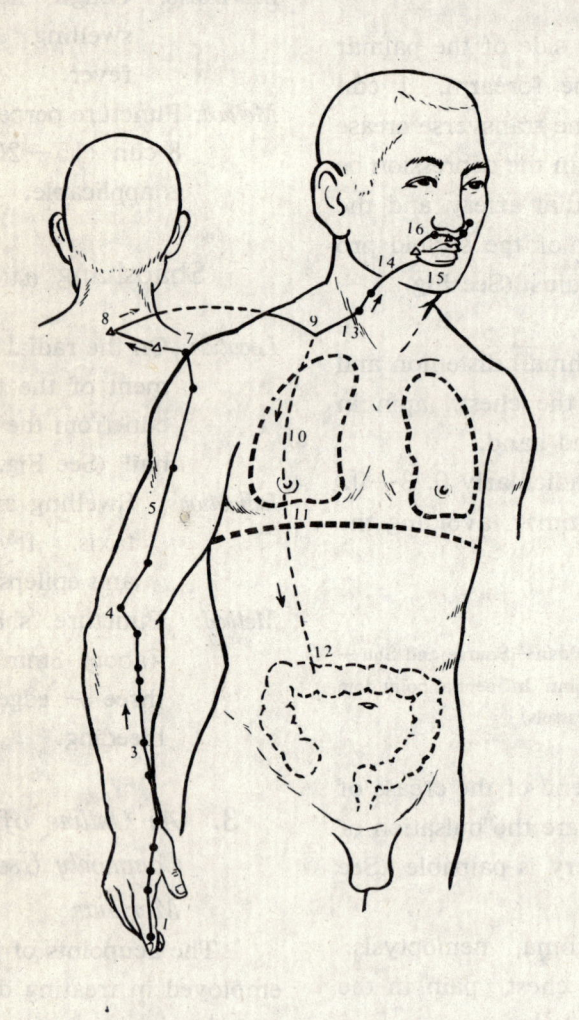

图1—10 手阳明大肠经循行示意图
Fig. 1—10 The Running Course of the Large Intestine Meridian of Hand—Yangming

（一）经脉循行

1. 起于食指末端商阳穴；2. 沿着食指内（桡）侧向上，通过第一、二掌骨之间，向上进入拇长伸肌腱与拇短伸肌腱间的凹陷处；3. 再沿前臂外侧桡侧缘；4. 行至肘部外侧；5. 沿着上臂外侧前缘；6. 向上进入肩端；7. 沿肩峰前缘；8. 向上出于颈椎"手足三阳经聚会处"（大椎）；9. 再向下行至锁骨上窝部；10. 联络肺脏；11. 向下通过横膈；12. 属于大肠。

支脉：13. 从锁骨上窝部上走颈部；14. 通过面颊；15. 进入下齿龈；16. 回绕至上嘴唇，交叉于人中处，左脉向右，右脉向左，分布在鼻孔两侧迎香穴，与足阳明胃经相接。

体表穴位分布线：起于食指桡侧端商阳穴，沿着上肢外侧桡侧缘，上行至肩、颈、通过面颊、回绕至上嘴唇，止于对侧鼻旁迎香穴。

体内相关的组织脏器：大肠、肺、下齿龈。

（二）本经常用腧穴

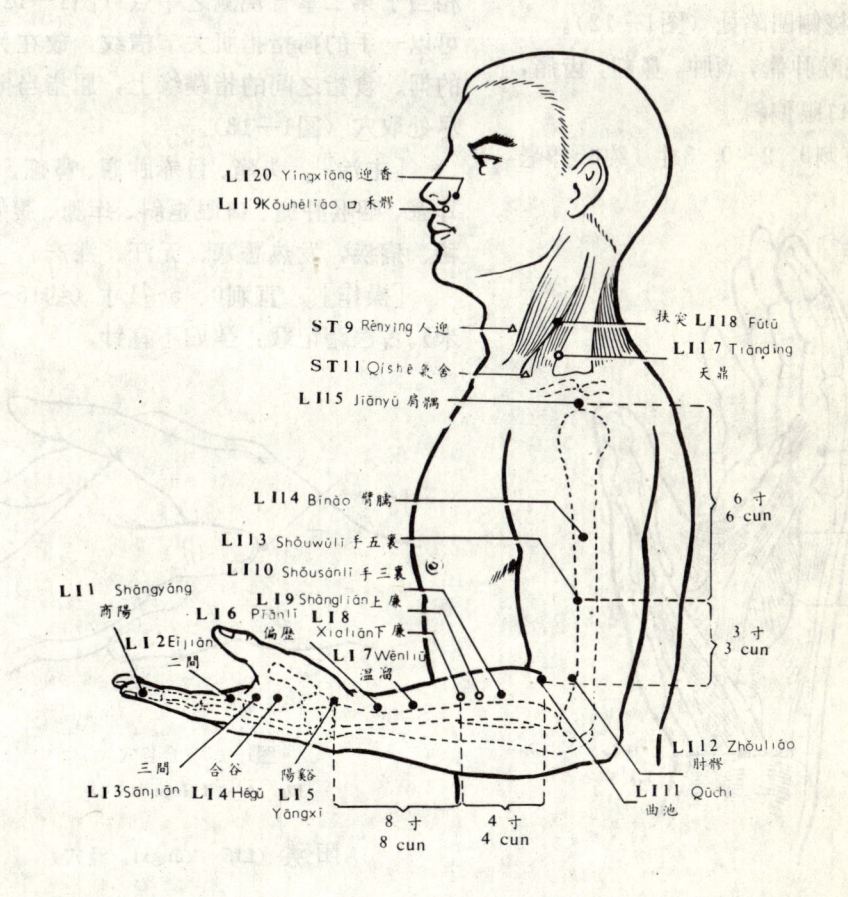

图1—11 手阳明大肠经穴位图

Fig. 1—11 Acupoints of the Large Intestine Meridian of Hand—Yangming

商阳 (LI1 Shāngyáng 井穴)

[定位] 食指末节桡侧指甲角旁0.1寸许（图1—11）。

[主治] 咽喉肿痛，颌肿，耳聋，齿痛，手指麻木，热病，昏厥。

[操作] 浅刺0.1寸（约3毫米）或点刺出血。

二间 (LI2 Erjiān 荥穴)

[定位] 微握拳，在食指本节（第二掌指关节）前，桡侧凹陷处（图1—12）。

[主治] 咽喉肿痛，颌肿，鼻衄，齿痛，身热，肩背痛，口眼偏斜。

[操作] 直刺0.2～0.3寸（约6～9毫米）。

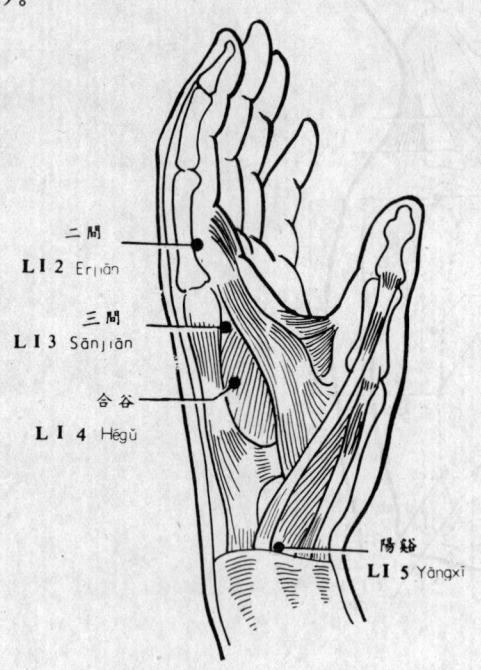

图1—12 二间、三间、合谷、阳溪
Fig. 1—12 Erjian (LI 2), Sanjian (LI3), Hegu (LI 4) and Yangxi (LI5)

三间 (LI3 Sānjiān 输穴)

[定位] 微握拳，在食指本节，（第二掌指关节）后桡侧凹陷处（图1—12）。

[主治] 目痛、齿痛、咽喉肿痛、腹满、肠鸣、腹泄。

[操作] 直刺0.5～0.8寸（约15～20毫米）。

合谷 (LI4 Hégǔ 原穴)

[定位] 手背，第一、二掌骨之间，约相当于第二掌骨桡侧之中点（图1—12），亦可以一手的拇指指肌关节横纹，放在另一手的拇、食指之间的指蹼缘上，屈指当拇指尖尽处取穴（图1—13）。

[主治] 头痛、目赤肿痛、鼻衄、齿痛、耳聋、咽喉肿痛、口眼歪斜、痄腮、腹痛、便秘、痢疾，发热恶寒、无汗、滞产。

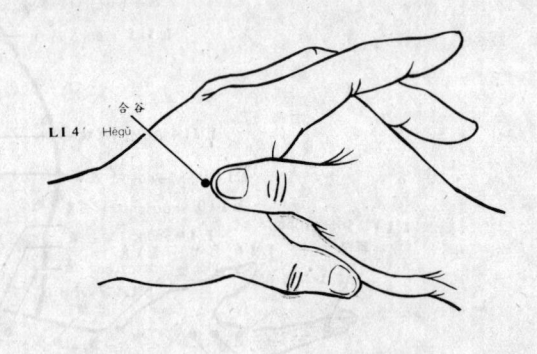

[操作] 直刺0.5～1寸（约15～25毫米）。古医藉记载：孕妇不宜针。

图1—13 合谷穴
Fig. 1—13 Hegu (LI 4)

阳溪 (LI5 Yángxī 经穴)

[定位] 在腕背横纹桡侧，当拇指翘起时，拇短伸肌腱与拇长伸肌腱之间的凹陷中（图1—12）。

[主治] 头痛、咽喉肿痛、目赤、耳聋、

经络腧穴概要

耳鸣、齿痛、臂腕痛。

［操作］ 直刺0.3～0.5寸（约9～15毫米）。

偏历 (LI6 Piānlì 络穴)

［定位］ 屈肘，在前臂背面桡侧，当阳溪穴与曲池穴连线上，腕横纹上3寸处（图1—11）。

［主治］ 目赤、耳聋、耳鸣、鼻衄、喉痛、口眼㖞斜、手臂酸痛。

［操作］ 直刺或斜刺0.3～0.5寸（约9～15毫米）。

温溜 (LI7 Wēnliū 郄穴)

［定位］ 侧腕屈肘，在前臂背面桡侧，当阳溪穴与曲池的连线上，腕横纹上5寸处（图1—11）。

［主治］ 头痛、面肿、鼻衄、咽喉肿痛、肩背酸痛、肠鸣腹痛。

［操作］ 直刺0.5～0.8寸（约15～20毫米）。

手三里 (LI10 Shǒusānlǐ)

［定位］ 侧腕屈肘，在前臂背面桡侧，当阳溪穴与曲池穴连线上，肘横纹下2寸处（图1—11）。

［主治］ 齿痛、颊肿、偏瘫、腹痛、腹泻。

［操作］ 直刺0.5～0.8寸（约15～20毫米）。

曲池 (LI11 Qūchí 合穴)

［定位］ 侧腕屈肘，在肘横纹外侧端，当尺泽与肱骨外上髁连线的中点取穴（图1—11）。

［主治］ 热病、咽喉肿痛、齿痛、目赤肿痛、荨麻疹、手臂肿痛、上肢不遂、腹痛吐泻。

［操作］ 直刺1～1.5寸（约25～40毫米）。

臂臑 (LI14 Bìnào)

［定位］ 在臂外侧，三角肌止点处，当曲池与肩髃连线上，曲池上7寸（图1—14）。

［主治］ 肩臂痛、颈项拘急、目疾、颈颔淋巴结核。

［操作］ 直刺或向上斜刺1～1.5寸（约25～40毫米）。

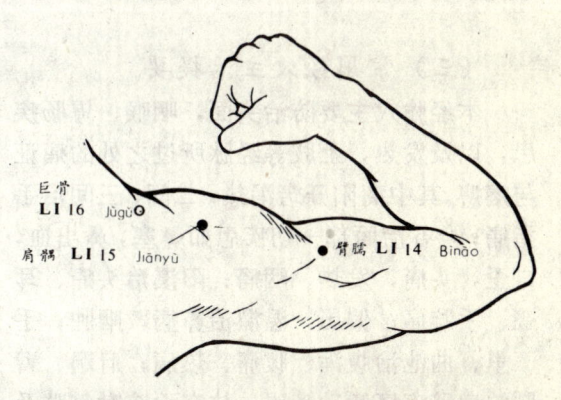

图1—14 臂臑、肩髃
Fig. 1—14 Jianyu (LI 15) and Binao (LI 14)

肩髃 (LI15 Jiānyú)

［定位］ 在肩部，三角肌上，臂外展，或向前平伸时，当肩峰前下方凹陷处（图1—14）。

［主治］ 肩臂疼痛，手臂挛急，半身不遂，颈颔淋巴结核。

［操作］ 直刺或向下斜刺0.8～1.5寸（约20～40毫米）。

扶突 (LI18 Fútū)

［定位］ 在颈外侧部，结喉旁，当胸锁乳突肌的前、后缘之间（图1—11）。

［主治］ 咳嗽气喘、咽喉肿痛。

［操作］ 直刺0.5～0.8寸（约15～20毫米）。

迎香 (LI20 Yíxiāng)

［定位］ 在鼻翼外缘中点旁开，当鼻唇沟中取穴（图1—11）。

［主治］ 鼻塞、不闻香臭、鼻出血、口眼歪斜。

［操作］ 直刺0.1～0.2寸（约3～6毫米），或斜刺0.3～0.5寸（约9～15毫米），不宜灸。

（三）常用经穴主治提要

本经腧穴主要防治头面，咽喉、胃肠疾患，以及发热，上肢等经脉所过之处的痛证与痿痹。其中商阳开窍泻热；二间、三间治手指痛；合谷治面部一切疾患如鼻塞，鼻出血，口歪，头痛，发热，咽痛；阳溪治头痛、耳聋、手腕痛；偏历，温溜治鼻病，咽肿；手三里、曲池治腹泻、腹痛、热病；肩髃、臂臑治肩臂疼痛活动障碍；扶突治咳嗽气喘及头部病；迎香通鼻窍。

II. THE LARGE INTESTINE MERIDIAN OF HAND — YANGMING (20 acupoints in total)

1. The Course

It starts from the tip of the index finger at Shangyang (LI 1) (1). Running upwards along the radial side of the index finger, and passing through the 1st inter—metacarpal space, it dips into the depression between the tendon of m. extensor pollicis longus and brevis (2), and goes along the radial border of the lateral aspect of the forearm (3) to reach the lateral side of the elbow (4). It goes upwards along the latero—anterior border (5) to the highest point of the shoulder (6). Then, it goes along the anterior border of the acromion (7), and ascends to come out at the confluence point where the three yang meridians of hand and foot meet, i. e. at Dazhui (DU 14) (8). Then, it descends into the supraclavicular fossa (9) to connect with the lung (10), and goes downwards through th the diaphragm (11) to enter the large intestine, its pretaining organ (12).

Its branch giving off from the supraclavcular fossa ascends along the neck (13) and passes through the cheek (14) to enter the lower gums (15). Then, it curvse around the upper lip and crosses at the philtrum with the opposite one. From there, it ends at the opposite side of the naris at Yingxiang (LI 20), where it connects with the Stomacn Meridian of Foot—Yangming (16).

The line made up by the acup oints distributed on the body surface: It originates from the radial end of the index finger at Shangyang (LI 1), runs upward along the radial border of the lateral side of the upper limb to the shoulder and neck, and goes through the cheek. It curves around the upper lip and ends at Yingxiang (LI 20) at the opposite side of the naris.

The inner organs concerned: The large intestine, lung, and lower gums.

2. The Commonly Used Acupoints of this Meridian

Shangyang (LI 1, Jing—Well point)

Location: At the radial side of the distal segment of the index finger, about 0.1 cun from the corner of the nail (See Fig. 1—11).

Indications: Swelling and sore throat, swelling in the submaxillary region, deafness, toothache, numbness of fingers, febrile diseases, loss of consciousness.

Method: Puncture shallowly 0.1 cun (about 3mm) or prick with the three—edged neeble to cause bleeding.

Erjian (LI 2, Ying—Spring point)

Location: with the fist made, at the dorso—ventral boundary, in the depression of the radial side of the index finger, distal to the 2nd metacarpal—phalangal joint (See Fig. 1—12).

Indications: Swelling and sore throat, swelling in the submaxillary region, epistaxis, toothache, pain in the shoulder and back, deviation of the mouth and eye.

Method: Puncture perpendicularly 0.2—0.3 cun (6—9mm). Moxibustion is applicable.

Sanjian (LI 3, Shu—Stream poimt)

Location: In the depression of the radial side, proximal to the 2nd metacarpophangeal joint when a loose fist is made (See Fig. 1—12).

Indications: Pain in the eye, toothache, swelling and sore throat, fullness in the abdomen, borborygmus, diarrhea.

Method: Punctre perpendicularly 0.5—0.8 cun (15—20mm) Moxibustion is applicable.

Hegu (LI 4, Yuan—Source point)

Location: Between the 1st and 2nd metacarpal bones, on the radial side of the midpoint of the 2nd metacarpal bone, and on the dorsum of the hand (See Fig. 1—12). or, make the patient place the interphalangel crease of the palmar surface of the thumb of one hand on the margin of the web between the thumb and index finger of the other hand. The point is located just beneath the tip of the thumb when the thumb is at flexion (See Fih. 1—13).

Indications: Headache, redness, swelling and pain of the eye, epistaxis, toothache, deafness, swelling and sore throat, facial paralysis, mumps, abdominal pain, constipation, dysentery, fever, chills, no sweating, dystocia.

Method: Puncture perpendicularly 0.5—1.0 cun (15—25mm). Moxibustion is applicable.

Note: According to the ancient medical books, this point should not be punctured to the pregnant women.

Yangxi (LI 5, Jing—River point)

Location: At the radial end of the carpal transverse crease, in the depression between the tendons of m. extensor pollicis brevis and longus when the thumb is titled upward (See Fig. 1—12).
Indications: Headache, swelling and sore throat, redness of eye, deafness, tinnitus, toothache, pain in the arm and wrist.
Method: Puncture perpendicularly 0.3—0.5 cun (9—15mm) Moxibustion is applicable.

Pianli (LI 6, Luo—Connecting point)

Location: On the radial side of the dorsal surface of the forearm and on the line connecting Yangxi (LI 5) and Quchi (LI 11), 3 cun proximal to Yangxi (LI 5) when the elbow is flexed (See Fig. 1—11).
Indications: Epistaxis, swelling and sore throat, redness of the eye, deafness, tinnitus, facial paralysis, aching in the upper arm.
Method: Puncture perpendiculaly or obliquely 0.3—0.5 cun (9—15mm). Moxibustion is applicable.

Wenliu (LI 7, Xi—Cleft point)

Location: On the radial side of the dorsal surface of the forearm and on the line connecting Yangxi (LI 5) and Quchi (LI 11), 5 cun proximal to Yangxi (LI 5) when the elbow is flexed (See Fig. 1—11).
Indications: Headache, facial swelling, epistaxis, swelling and sore throat, aching in the back and shoulder, borborygmus and abdominal pain.
Method: Puncture perpendicularly 0.5—0.8 cun (15—20mm) Moxibustion is applicable.

Shousanli (LI 10)

Location: With the elbow flexed, on the radial side of the dorsal sarface of the forearm and on the line connecting Yangxi (LI 5) and Quchi (LI 11), 2 cun distal to Quchi (LI 11) (See Fig. 1—11).
Indications: Toothache, swelling cheek, hemiplegia, abdominal pain, diarrhea.
Method: Puncture perpendicularly 0.5—0.8 cun (15—20mm). Moxibustion is applicable.

Quchi (LI 11, He—Sea point)

Location: Make the patient flex the elbow at the right angle, at the lateral end of the cubital crease and at the midpoint of the line connecting the radial end of the transverse cubital crease and the external humeral epicondyle (See Fig. 1—11).
Indications: Febrile diseases, swelling and sore throat, toothache, redness and swelling and pain in the eye, eczema, swelling and pain

of the arm, paralysis of the upper limbs, abdominal pain, vomiting and diarrhea.

Method: Puncture perpendicularly 1.0—1.5 cun (25—40mm). Moxibustion is applicable.

Binao (LI 14)

Location: On the lateral side of the arm, at the insertion of the deltoid muscle and on the line connecting Quchi (LI 11) and Jianyu (LI 15), 7 cun above Quchi (LI 11) (See Fig. 1—14).

Indications: Pain in the shoulder and arm, stiffness of the neck, eye disorders, tuberculous cervical lymphadenitis.

Method: Puncture perpendicularly or odliquely upwards 1.0—1.5 cun (25—40mm). Moxibustion is applicable.

Jiangyu (LI 15)

Location: On the shoulder, superior to the deltoid muscle, in the depression anterior and inferior to the acromion when the arm is abducted or raised on the level of the shoulder (See Fig. 1-14).

Indications: Pain of the shoulder and arm, contructure of the arm, hemiplegia, tuberculous cervical lymphadenitis.

Method: Puncture perpendicularly or obliquely downwards 0.8-1.5 cun (20-40mm). Moxibustion is applicable.

Futu (LI 18)

Location: Asking the patient to sit upright and raise the head slightly, 3 cun lateral to the Adam's apple, at the midpoint between the sternal head and the clavicular head of m. sternocleidomastoideus (See Fig. 1-11).

Indications: Cough with asthma, swelling and sore throat.

Method: Puncture perpendicularly 0.5-0.8 cun (15-20mm). Moxibustion is appliccable.

Yingxiang (LI 20)

Location: Lateral to the midpoint of the lateral border of the ala nasi in the nasolabial groove (See Fig. 1—11).

Indications: Nasal stuffiness without smelling, epistaxis, deviation of the mouth and eye.

Method: Puncture perpendicularly 0.1—0.2 cun (3—6mm), or obliquely 0.2—0.5 cun (9—15mm), The moxidustion is forbidden.

3. *An Outline of Indications of the Commonly Used Acupoints*

The points of this meridian are mainly employed in preventing and treating disorders of the head and face, throat, stomach and intestines, and fever. they are also indicated in painful disorders and flaccidity in the upper limbs, which are on the pathway of the meridian. In the concrete, Shangyang (LI 1) is used to induce resuscitation and expel pathogenic heat; Erjian (LI 2) and Sanjian (LI 3) indicated in pain in the finger, while Hegu (LI 3), in facial disorders such as nasal stuffiness, epistaxis, deviation of the mouth, headache, fever, and sore throat; Yangxi (LI 5); in headache, deafness and pain in the wrist; Pianli (LI 6) and Wenliu (LI 7), in nasal disorders, swelling throat; Shousanli (LI 7), and Quchi (LI 11), in diarrhea, abdominal pain, and febrile diseases; Jianyu (LI 15) and Binao (LI 14), in pain and motor disorders of the shoulder; Futu (LI 18), in cough, asthma, and neck problem; and Yingxiang (LI 20), in stuffiness of the nose.

三、足阳明胃经（共45穴）

（一）经脉循行

1. 起于鼻旁，上行鼻根部；2. 与旁边足太阳经交会；3. 向下沿鼻外侧；4. 入上齿龈；5. 回出来环绕口唇；6. 下交颏唇沟；7. 向后沿下颌；8. 至下颌角；9. 上耳前；10. 沿发际；11. 到前额。

面部支脉：12. 从下颌大迎穴前下行颈动脉人迎穴处，沿喉咙；13. 进入缺盆；14. 向下通过横膈；15. 属于胃，联络脾。

缺盆支脉：16. 经乳头；17. 向下挟肚脐旁，进入少腹气冲。

胃下口支脉：18. 沿腹里下到气冲与前支会合；19. 下行髋关节前；20. 抵股四头肌伏兔处；21. 下膝髌、22. 沿胫骨外侧前缘下行；23. 经足背；24. 止于二趾外端。

胫部支脉：25. 从膝下3寸分出；26、下行进入中趾外端。

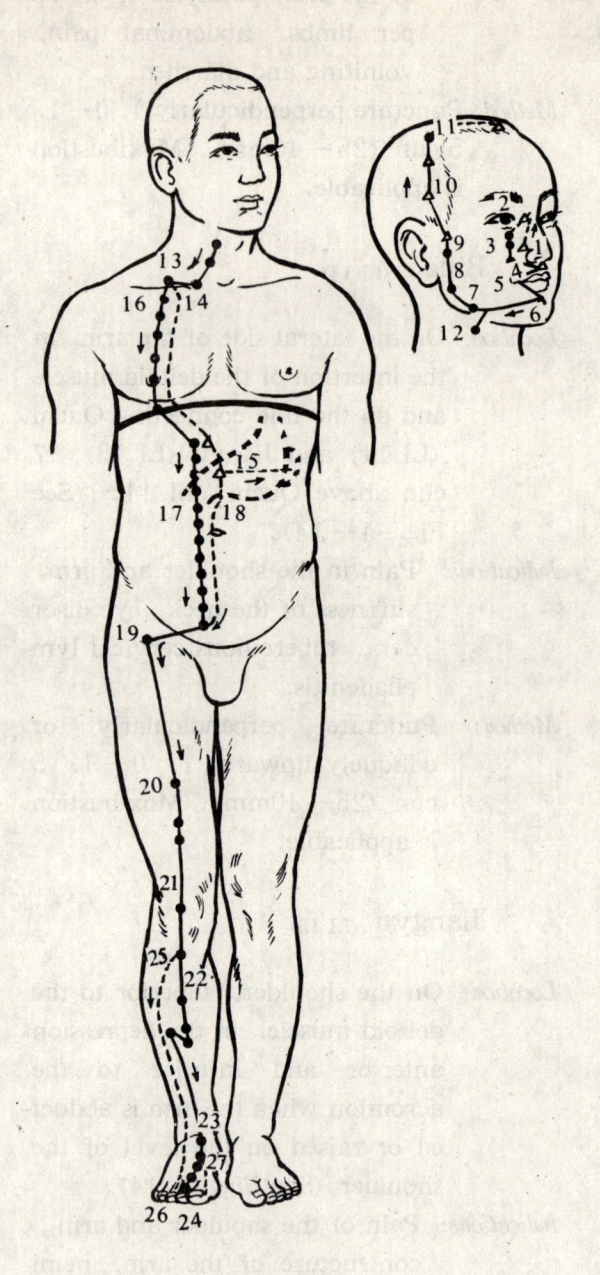

图1—15 足阳明胃经循行示意图

Fig. 1—15 The Running Course of the Stomach Meridian of Foot—Yangming

足背支脉：27. 从足背冲阳分出，进入大趾内侧端，与足太阴脾交接。

体表穴位分布线：起于眼下承泣穴，绕面颊经耳前上头角头维穴；另一支从下颌角下颈，沿胸正中线旁开4寸，腹正中线旁开2寸下行，经下肢外侧前缘通过足背、止于二趾趾甲角外端厉兑穴。

体内相关的组织脏器：脾、胃、喉咙。

（二）本经常用腧穴

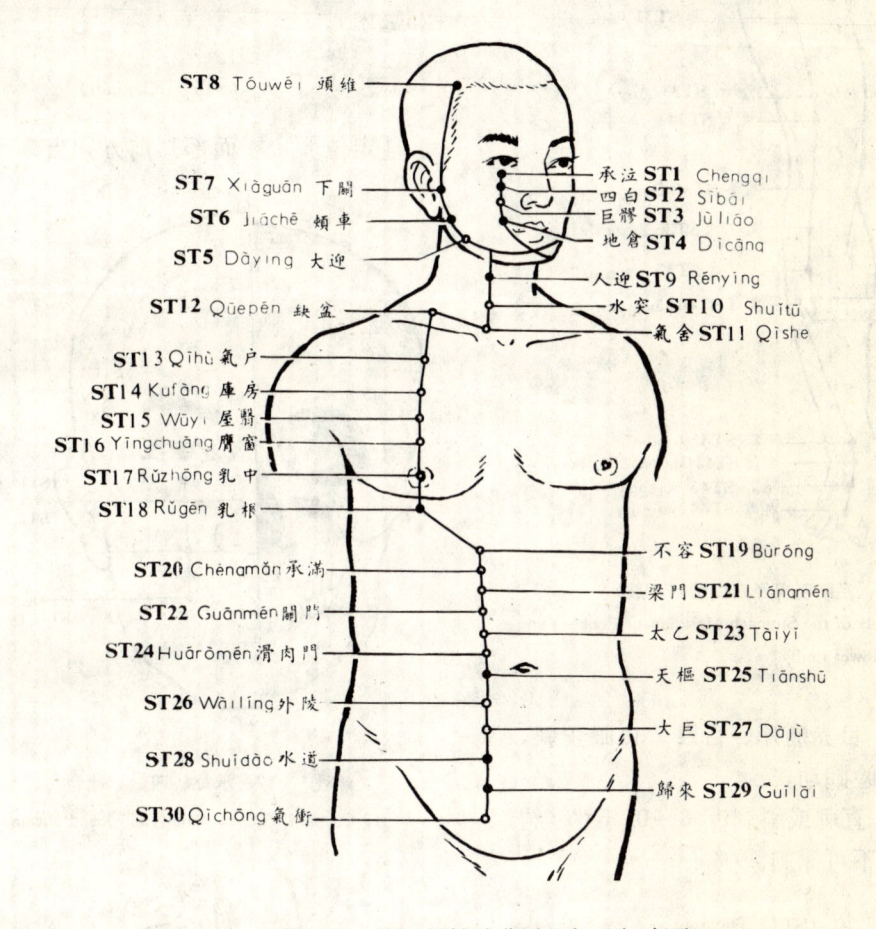

图1—16 足阳明胃经穴位图（头、面、躯干）

Fig. 1—16 Acupoints of the Stomach Meridian of Foot—Yangming (head、face、truck)

承泣 (ST1 Chéngqì)

[定位] 在面部，瞳孔直下，当眼眶下缘与眼球之间取穴（图1—17）。

[主治] 眼睑瞤动，口眼歪斜，目赤肿痛，迎风流泪，夜盲等目疾。

[操作] 医生左手拇指向上轻推眼球，紧靠眶缘缓慢直刺0.5～1寸（约15～20毫米）（图1—18）。不宜提插，以防刺破血管引起血肿；禁灸。

四白 (ST2 Sìbái)

[定位] 在面部，瞳孔直下，眶下孔凹陷中（图1—17）。

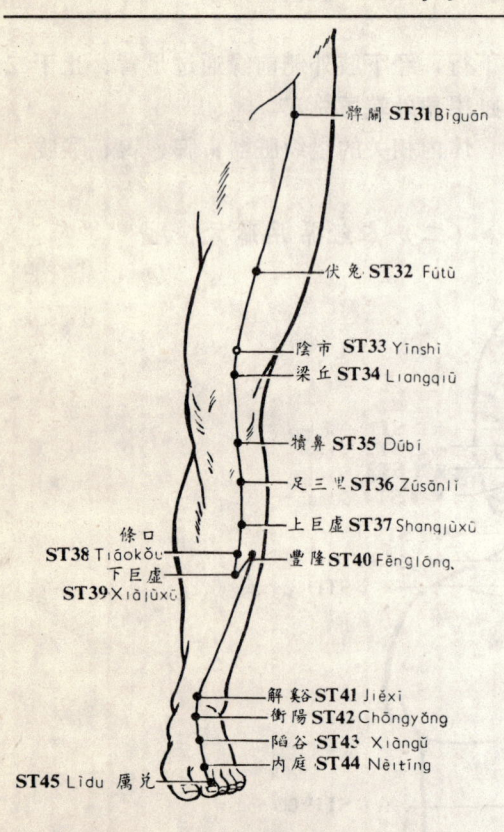

图1—16 足阳明胃经穴位图（下肢）
Fig. 1—16 Acupoints of the Stomach Meridian of Foot—Yangming (lower limb)

［主治］ 目赤痛痒、目翳、口眼歪斜，头面疼痛，眼睑瞤动。

［操作］ 直刺或斜刺0.3～0.5寸（约9～15毫米），不可深刺。

地仓（ST4 Dìcāng）

［定位］ 在面部，口角外侧，上直瞳孔（图1—17）。

［主治］ 口歪，流涎，口腔溃疡。

［操作］ 直刺0.2寸（约6毫米），或向颊车方向平刺0.5～0.8寸（约15～20毫米）。

颊车（ST6 Jiáchē）

［定位］ 在面颊部，下颌角前上方一横指（中指）凹陷中，咀嚼时咬肌隆起按之凹陷处（图1—19）。

［主治］ 口噤不开，口歪，齿痛，颊肿。

［操作］ 直刺0.3～0.5寸（约9～15毫米），或向地仓方向斜刺0.5～1寸（约15～25毫米）。

下关（ST7 Xiàguān）

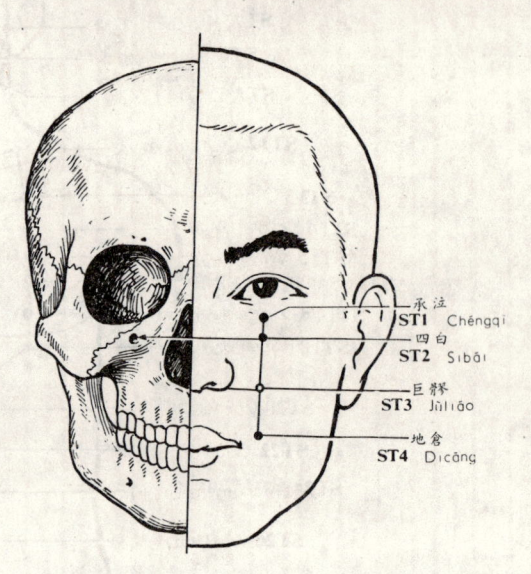

［定位］ 在面部耳前方，当颧弓与下

图1—17 承泣、四白、地仓
Fig. 1—17 Chengqi (ST1), Sidai (ST2) and Dicang (ST4)

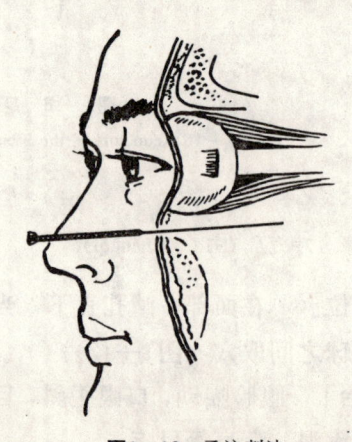

图1—18 承泣刺法
Fig. 1—18 Needling at Chengqi (ST 1)

颌切迹所形成的凹陷中，合口有空，张口即闭（图1—19）。

［主治］ 牙痛、面疼、牙关紧闭、耳疾、下颌关节炎。

［操作］ 直刺0.3～0.5寸（约9～15毫米）。

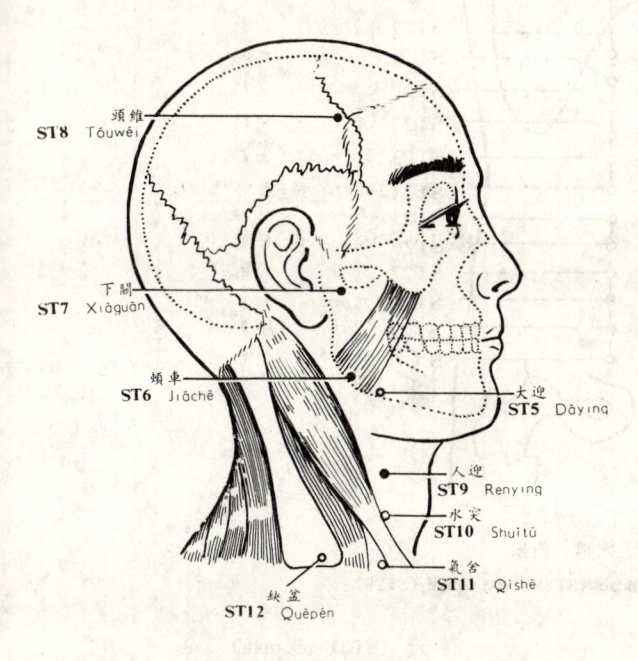

图1—19 颊车、下关、头维、人迎

Fig. 1—19 Jiache (ST6), Xiaguan (ST 1), Touwei (ST8) and Renying (ST9)

头维 (ST8 Tóuwéi)

［定位］ 在头侧部，额角发际上0.5寸，头正中线旁4.5寸（图1—19）。

［主治］ 头痛、目眩、眼疾。

［操作］ 向下或向后平刺0.5～1寸（约15～25毫米）。

人迎 (ST9 Rényíng)

［定位］ 在颈部，喉结旁，当胸锁乳突肌前缘，颈总动脉搏动处（图1—19）。

［主治］ 咽喉肿痛、气喘、高血压、半身不遂。

［操作］ 避开动脉直刺0.5～1寸（约15～25毫米）。

乳根 (ST18 Rǔgēn)

［定位］ 在胸部，乳头直下，乳房根部，第五肋间隙，距前正中线4寸（图1—20）。

［主治］ 喘咳、胸闷、胸痛、乳腺炎、乳汁少。

［操作］ 治乳房病向上斜刺或平刺0.5～0.8寸（约15～20毫米）；治胸闷，咳喘向胸骨处平刺0.5～0.8寸（约15～20毫米），不可垂直深刺，以防伤及肺脏。

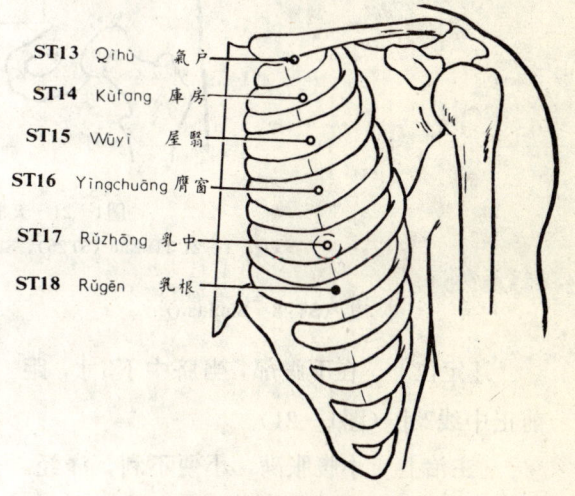

图1—20 乳根穴

Fig. 1—20 Rugen (ST 18)

天枢 (ST25 Tiānshū 募穴)

［定位］ 仰卧，在腹中部，距脐中2寸，（图1—21）。

［主治］ 绕脐痛，腹胀，肠鸣泄泻，便闭，痢疾。

［操作］ 直刺1～1.5寸（约25～40毫米）。

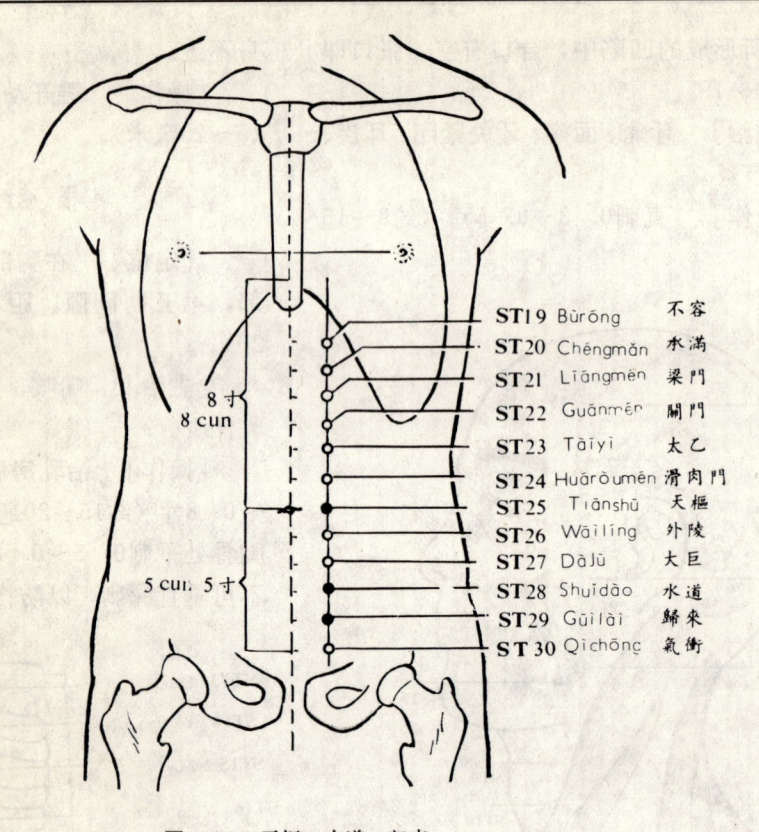

图1—21 天枢、水道、归来
Fig. 1—21 Tianshu (ST25), Shuidao (ST28) and Guilai (ST29)

水道 (ST28 Shuǐdào)

［定位］ 在下腹部，当脐中下3寸，距前正中线2寸（图1—21）。

［主治］ 小腹胀满，小便不利，痛经。

［操作］ 直刺1～1.5寸（约25～40毫米）。

归来 (ST29 Guīlái)

［定位］ 在下腹部，当脐中下4寸，距前正中线2寸（图1—21）。

［主治］ 腹痛、疝气、月经不调，子宫脱垂等妇科疾患。

［操作］ 直刺1～1.5寸（约25～40毫米）。

髀关 (ST31 Bìguān)

［定位］ 在大腿前面，当髂前上棘与髌底外侧端的连线上，屈股时，平会阴，居缝匠肌外侧凹陷处（图1—22）。

［主治］ 腰腿疼痛，下肢麻痹，挛急。

［操作］ 直刺1～1.5寸（约25～40毫米）。

伏兔 (ST32 Fútù)

［定位］ 在大腿前面，当髂前上棘与髌底外侧端的连线上，髌底上6寸（图1—22）。另有简便取穴，即医师将掌根对准髌骨上缘，手指伸直朝下按去，中指所到之处是穴（图1—23）。

［主治］ 腿膝冷痛，痿痹，腹胀。

[操作] 直刺1~2寸（约25~50毫米）。

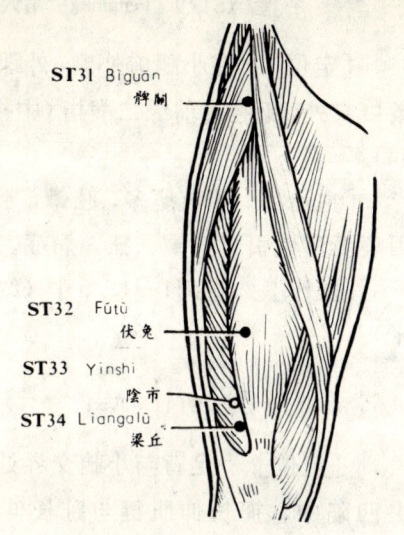

图1—22 髀关、伏兔、梁丘
Fig. 1—22 Biguan (ST31), Futu (ST32) and Liangqiu (ST34)

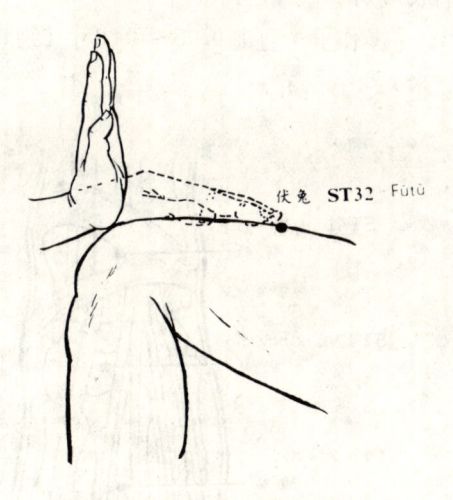

图1—23 伏兔穴简便取穴法
Fig. 1—23 Simple Way for Locating Futu (ST32)

梁丘 (ST34 Liángqiū 郄穴)

[定位] 屈膝，在大腿前面，当髂前上棘与髌底外侧端的连线上，髌底上2寸（图1—22）。

[主治] 膝肿痛、胃痛、乳腺炎。

[操作] 直刺1~1.2寸（约25~30毫米）。

犊鼻 (ST35 Dúbí)

[定位] 屈膝，在膝部，髌骨与髌韧带外侧凹陷中（图1—24）。

[主治] 膝痛、下肢痿痹，屈伸不利。

[操作] 稍向髌韧带内方斜刺0.5~1.2寸（约15~30毫米）。

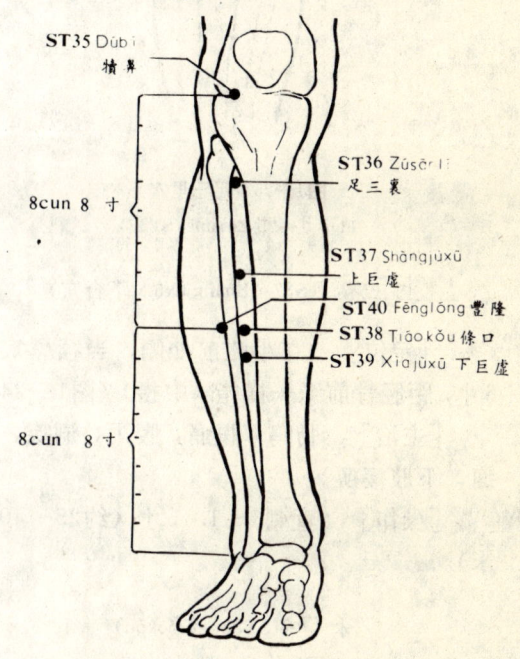

图1—24 足阳明胃经下肢常用穴
Fig. 1—24 Acupoints of the Stomach Meridian of Foot—Yangming at the Lower Limb

足三里 (ST36 Zúsānlǐ 合穴)

[定位] 在小腿前外侧，犊鼻穴下3寸，距胫骨前缘一横指（中指）处，（图1—24、25）。简便取穴：屈膝，令患者掌心对准髌骨正中，手指自然下垂，中指所到处外开一横指是穴。

[主治] 胃痛、肠鸣、腹胀、泄泻，便闭，痢疾等消化功能失调病症，以及乳腺炎，癫狂。亦为强身保健穴。

［操作］　直刺1～2寸（约25～50毫米）。

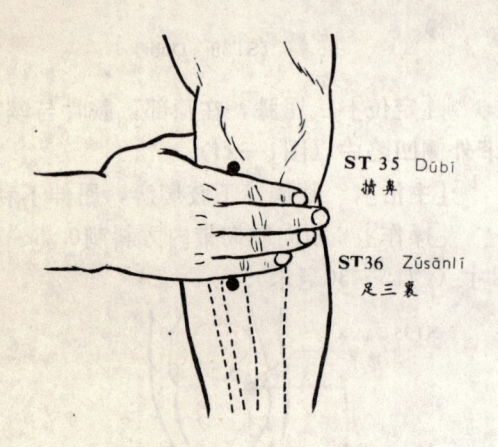

图1-25　足三里穴
Fig. 1－25 Zusanli (ST36)

上巨墟（S37 Shàngjùxū　下合穴）

［定位］　在小腿前外侧，当犊鼻穴下6寸，距胫骨前缘一横指（中指）（图1—24）。

［主治］　肠鸣，腹痛，腹泻，痢疾，肠痈，下肢痿痹。

［操作］　直刺1～1.5寸（约25～40毫米）。

条口（ST38 Tiáokǒu）

［定位］　在小腿前外侧，犊鼻穴下8寸，距胫骨前缘一横指（中指）（图1—24）。

［主治］　下肢痿痹，转筋，肩臂痛。

［操作］　直刺1～1.5寸（约25～40毫米）。

下巨墟（ST39 Xiàjùxū　下合穴）

［定位］　在小腿前外侧，当犊鼻穴下9寸，距胫骨前缘一横指（中指）（图1—24）。

［主治］　小腹痛，泄泻，痢疾，下肢痿痹，腰脊痛引睾丸。

［操作］　直刺1～1.5寸（约25～40毫米）。

丰隆（ST40 Fēnglóng　络穴）

［定位］　在小腿前外侧，外踝尖上8寸，条口穴外，距胫骨前缘二横指（中指）（图1—24）。

［主治］　喘咳痰多，眩晕，呕吐，以及因痰涎壅盛引起的癫、狂、痫症。

［操作］　直刺1～1.5寸（约25～40毫米）。

解溪（ST41 Jiěxī　经穴）

［定位］　足背与小腿交界处的横纹中央凹陷中，拇长伸肌腱与趾长伸肌腱之间（图1—26）。

［主治］　头痛，癫狂，目赤面赤，腹胀，下肢痿痹。

［操作］　直刺0.5～0.8寸（约15～20毫米）。

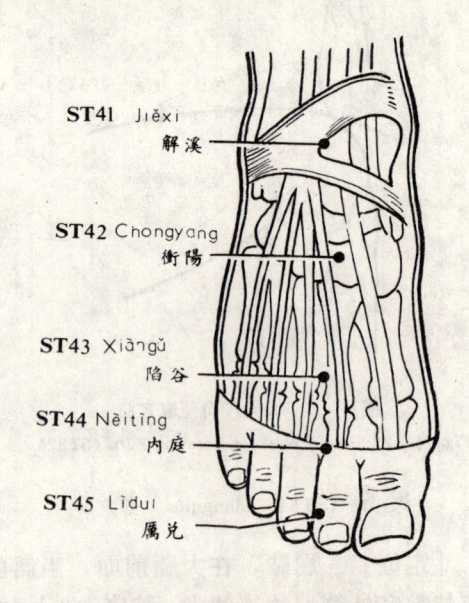

图1—26　足阳明胃经足部常用穴
Fig. 1－26 Commonly Used Acupoints of the Stomanh Meridian of Foot—Yangming at the Foot

冲阳 (ST42 Chōngyáng 原穴)

［定位］ 在足背最高处，足背动脉搏动处，当拇长伸肌腱与趾长伸肌腱之间（图1—26）。

［主治］ 口歪，面肿，齿痛，癫，狂，痛，足痿无力。

［操作］ 避开动脉，直刺0.3～0.5寸（约9～15毫米）。

陷谷 (ST43 Xiàngǔ 输穴)

［定位］ 在足背，第二、三跖骨结合部之前的凹陷中（图1—26）。

［主治］ 面浮身肿，肠鸣腹痛，足背肿痛。

［操作］ 直刺或斜向上刺0.5～1寸（约15～25毫米）。

内庭 (ST44 Nèitíng 荥穴)

［定位］ 足背，当2、3趾间趾蹼缘后方赤白肉际处（图1—26）。

［主治］ 口歪、齿痛、咽喉肿痛、鼻衄、腹胀、腹泻、热病。

［操作］ 直刺或向上斜刺0.5～0.8寸（约15～20毫米）。

厉兑 (ST45 Lìduì 井穴)

［定位］ 在足第二趾末节外侧，距趾甲角0.1寸（图1—26）。

［主治］ 面肿、热病、癫、狂、鼻衄、咽痛。

［操作］ 浅刺0.1寸（约3毫米）。

（三）常用经穴主治提要

本经腧穴均能主治与胃有关的消化方面疾病。如胃痛、腹痛、肠鸣、腹胀、腹泻、痢疾、便闭等。其中解溪、内庭穴还能泄胃热，治癫、狂、鼻衄；丰隆除痰解郁；梁丘善治乳腺肿痛。

头面部腧穴及远端的内庭、上巨墟等穴，治口眼歪斜，面肿痛。

除外，本经腧穴尚能治胃经循行经过之处的痛症及痿痹。

III. THE STOMACH MERIDIAN OF FOOT — YANGMING (45 points in total)

1. *The Course*

It originates from the either side of the ala nasi and ascends to the root of the nose (1), where it meets the Bladder Meridian of Foot—Taiyang (2). Running downwards along the lateral side of the nose, it enters the upper gum (4). Emerging, it winds around the lips (5) and descends to meet the mentolabial groove (6). Then, running backwards along the lower jaw (7), it reaches the angle of the mandible (8). Then, it ascends in front of the auricle (9), goes along the anterior hairline (10) and reaches the forehead (11).

The facial branch starting in front of Dayin (ST5) runs downwards to Renyin (ST9). From there, it goes along the throat (12) and enters the supraclavicular fossa (13). Descending, it passes through the diaphargm (14), enters the stomach, its pertaining organ, and connects with the spleen (15).

The branch arising in the supraclavicular fossa runs downwards through the nipple (16), and descends by the umbilicus to enter Qichong (ST30) on the lower abdomen (17).

The branch arising around the lower orifice of the stomach descends inside the abdomen and joins the previous branch of the meridian at Qichong (ST30) (18). Running downwards, it goes in front of the hip joint (19), reaaches Futu (ST32) at the femur (20), and passes through the knee (21). From there, it continues downwards along the anterior border of the lateral aspect of the tibia (22), passes through the dorsum of the foot (23), and ends at the lateral aspect of the tip of the 2nd toe (24).

The tibial branch comes out 3 cun below the knee (25), and enters the lateral side of the tip of the middle toe (26).

The branch arising in the dorsum of the foot starts at Chongyang (ST42) (27) and terminates at the medial side of the tip of the big toe, where it connects with the Spleen Meridian of Foot—Taiyin.

The line made up by the acupoints distributed on the body surface: It starts from Chengqi (ST1) below the eye, and runs around the cheek and in front of the anricle. Then, it ascends to Touwei (ST8) at the corner of the forehead. The branch comes out from the angle of the mandible, runs downwards to the neck, and descends along the line 4 cun lateral to the midline of the chest and 2 cun lateral to the mid line of the abdomen. Then it goes downwards along the lateral anterior border of the lower limb, passes through the dorsum of the foot and ends at Lidui (ST45) at the lateral side of the tip of the corner of the nail of the 2nd toe.

The inner organs concerned: The spleen, stomach, throat.

2. *The Commonly Used Acupoints*

Chengqi (ST1)

Location: On the face, when the patient's eyes looking straight forward, directly below the pupil and between the eyeball and infraorbital ridge (See Fig. 1—17).

Inodications: Flickering of the eyeball, deviation of the mouth and eye, epiphora induced by wind, night blindness, and some other eye problems.

Method: Push the eyeball gently upwards with the thumb of the left hand, insert the needle close to the infraorbital margin perpendicu—larly slowly 0.5—1.0 cun (15—25mm) (See Fig. 1—18). It is not allowed to lift or thrust the needle so as to avoid injuring the blood vessels and causing hemotoma. Moxibustion is prohihibited.

Sibai (ST2)

Location: On the face, when the patient's eyes looking straight forward, at the depression of the infraorbital foramen, and 1 cun below the pupil (See Fig. 1—17).

Indications: Pain and itching in the eye, nebule or macule of the cornea, deviation of the mouth and eye, pain in the head and face, flickering of the eye lids.

Method: Puncture perpendicularly or obliquely 0.3—0.5 cun (9—15mm). Deep puncture is not advisable.

Dicang (ST4)

Location: On the face, when the patient's eyes looking straight forward, about 0.4 cun lateral to the corner of the mouth, directly below the pupil (See Fig. 1—17).

Indications: Deviation of the mouth, sialosis, canker sore.

Method: Puncture perpendicularly 0.2 cun (about 6mm), or horizontally 0.5—0.8 cun (15—20mm) towards Jiache (ST6). Moxidustion is applicable.

Jiache (ST6)

Location: On the cheek, one finger breadth (middle finger) anterior and superior to the mandibular angle, in the depression where the masseter muscle is prominent (See Fig. 1—19).

Indications: Lockjaw, deviation of the mouth, toothache, swelling in the cheek.

Method: Puncture perpendicularly 0.3—0.5 cun, or obliquely 0.5—1.0 cun (15—25mm) toward Dicang (ST4). Moxibustion is applicadle.

Xiaguan (ST7)

Location: On the face, anterior to the ear, in the depression between the zygomatic arch and mandibular notch. It is where there is a hole with the mouth closed and nothing with the mouth opened (See Fig. 1—19)

Indications: toothache, facial pain, lockjaw, ear disorders, mandibular arthritis.

Method: Puncture perpendicularly 0.3—0.5 cun (9—15mm). Moxibustion is applicable.

Towwei (ST8)

Location: On the lateral side of the head, 0.5 cun directly above the anterior hairline at the corner of the forehead, and 4.5 cun lateral to the midline of the head (See Fig. 1—19).

Indications: Headache, dizziness, eye disorders.

Method: Puncture horizontally 0.5—1.0 cun (15—20mm) downwards or backwards.

Renying (ST9)

Location: On the neck, 1.5 cun lateral to the Adam's apple, at the anterior border of m. sternocleidomastoideus where the pulsation of the common carotid artery is palpable (See Fig. 1—19).

Indications: Swelling and sore throat, asthma, hypertension, hemiplegia.

Method: Puncture perpendicularly 0.5—1.

0 cun (15—25mm), avoiding the common carotid artery.

Rugen (ST18)

Location: On the chest, directly below the nipple, on the lower border of the breast, in the 5th intercostal space, 4 cun lateral to the anterior midline (See Fig. 1—20).

Indications: Cough, asthma, oppression feeling in the chest, pain in the chest, mastitis, insuffieincy of lactation.

Method: Puncture obliquely or horizontally 0. 5—0. 8 cun (15—20mm) upwards in treating disorders of the breast, horizontally 0. 5-0. 8 cun (15-20mm) towards the sternum in treating cough and asthma and oppression feeling in the chest. It is prohibiited to puncture perpendicularly deep so as to avoid injuring the lung. Moxidustion is applicable.

Tianshu (ST25, Front—Mu point)

Location: On the middle abdomen, 2 cun lateral to the center of the umbilicus, at the m. pararectus with the supine position selected (See Fig. 1—21).

Indications: Pain around the umbilicus, abdminal distension, borborygmus and diarrhea, constipation, dysentery.

Method: Puncture perpendicularly 1. 0—0. 5 cun (25—40mm). Moxibustion is applicable.

Shuidao (ST28)

Location: On the lower abdomen, 3 cun directly below Tianshu (ST25), 2 cun lateral to the midline of the abdomen (See Fig. 1—21).

Indications: Distension and fullness in the lower abdomen, dysuria, dysmenorrhea.

Method: Puncture perpendicularly 1. 0—1. 5 cun (25—40mm). Moxibustion is applicable.

Guilai (ST29)

Location: On the lower abdomen, 4 cun directly below Tianshu (ST25), 2 cun lateral to the midline of the abdomen (See Fig. 1—21).

Indications: Abdominal pain, hernia, disorders of the gyneocology such as ahnornal menstruation, prolapse of the uterus.

Method: Puncture perpendicularly 1. 0—1. 5 cun (25—40mm). Moxibustion is applicable.

Biguan (ST31)

Location: On the anterior side of the thigh and at the line connecting the anterior superior iliac spine and the superiolateral corner of the patella, at the level of the perineum when the thigh is flexed, in the depression lateral to the sartorius muscle (See Fig. 1—22).

Indications: Pain in the leg and waist, numduess or contructure of the lower limds.

Method: Puncture perpendicularly 1.0—1.5 cun (25—40mm). Moxibustion is applicable.

Futu (ST32)

Location: On the anterior side of the thigh and on the line conneting the anterior superior iliac spine and the superiolateral corner of the pattela, 6 cun above this corner (See Fig. 1—22). The simple way for the location: The point is where the doctor's middle finger of one hand reaches when the doctor presses the upper border of the patella with the root of the palm of that hand and stresses downwards with all fingers of that hand (See Fig. 1—23).

Indications: Cold and pain in the leg and knee, flaccidity and arthralgia, distension in the abdomen.

Method: Punctere perpendicularly 1.0—2.0 cun (25—50mm). Moxibustion is applicable.

Liangqiu (ST34, Xi—Cleft point)

Location: With the knee flexed, on the line connecting the anterior superior iliac spine and the superiolateral corner of the patella, 2 cun proximal to this corner (See Fig. 1—22).

Indications: Swelling and pain in the knee, stomachache, mastitis.

Method: Puncture perpendicularly 1.0—1.2 cun (25—30mm). Moxibustion is applicable.

Dubi (ST35)

Location: With the knee flexed, on the knee, at the lower border of the patella, in the depression lateral to the patella and its ligament (See Fig. 1—24).

Indications: Pain in the knee, flaccidity and arthralgia and disorders in movenent of the lower limbs.

Method: Puncture obliquely 0.5—1.2 cun (25—30mm) slightly towards the medial side of the patellar ligament. Moxibustion is applicable.

Zusanli (ST36, He—Sea point)

Location: On the anteriolateral side of the leg, 3 cun below Dubi (ST35), one finger — breadth lateral to the anterior crest of the tibia (See Fig. 1—24, 1—25). Simple way: Ask the patient to flex the knee, and to press the center of his patella with the center of his palm with the fingers hung down naturally, the point is where the tip of the middle finger of the hand reaches.

Indications: Disorders of digestive function, such as stomachache, borborygmus, abdominal distension, diarrhea, constipation, dysentery, as well as mastitis, insanity.

Note: This is an important point for tonification, used to keep the body healthy and stronger.

Method: Puncture perpendicularly 1.0—2.

0 cun (25—50mm). Moxibustion is applicable.

Shangjuxu (ST37, Lower Confluent point of the Large Intestine Meridian)

Location: On the anteriolateral side of the leg, 6 cun below Dubi (ST 35), one finger breadth (middle finger) from the anterior crest of the tibia (See Fig. 1—24).
Indications: Borborygmus, abdominal pain, diarrhea, dysentery, apendicitis, flaccidity and arthralgia of the lower limbs.
Method: Puncture perpendicularly 1.0—1.5 cun (25—40mm). Moxibustion is applicable.

Tiaokou (ST38)

Location: On the anteriolateral side of the leg, 8 cun distal to Dubi (ST35), about at the midpoint of the line connecting Dudi (ST35) and the tip of the external malleolus, one finger — breadth lateral to the anterior crest of the tidia (See Fig. 1—24).
Indications: Flaccidity and arthralgia of the lower limbs, muscular cramp in the calf, pain in the sh—oulder and arm.
Method: Puncture perpendicularly 1.0—1.5 cun (25—40mm). Moxibustion is applicable.

Xiajuxu (ST39, Lower Confluent point of the Small Inteine Meridian)

Location: On the anteriolateral side of the leg, 9 cun below Dubi (ST 35), one finger breadth (middle finger) from the antnerior crest of the tibia (See Fig. 1—24).
Indications: Pain in the lower abdomen, dysentery, flaccidity and arthralgia of the lower limds, pain in the lower back spreading to the testicle.
Method: Puncture perpendicularly 1.0—1.5 cun (25—40mm). Moxibustion is applicable.

Fenglong (ST40, Luo—Connecting point)

Location: On the anteriolateral side of the leg, 8 cun proximal to the tip of the lateral malleolus, 1 cun lateral to Tiaokou (S 38), and two finger bredths (middle finger) from the anterior crest of the tibia (See Fig. 1—24).
Indications: Asthma and cough with much sputum, dizziness, vomiting, disorders caused by accumulation of sputum such as insanity, mania and epilepsy.
Method: Puncture perpendicularly 1.0—1.5 cun (25—40mm). Moxibustion is applicable.

Jiexi (ST41, Jing—River point)

Location: At the central depression of the crease between the instep of the foot and leg, between the tendons of m. extensor digitorum longus and hallucis longus (See —Fig. 1—26).

Indications: Headache, epilepsy and mania, redness in the eye and face, abdominal distension, flaccidity and arthralgia of the lower limbs.

Method: Puncture perpendicularly 0.5—0.8 cun (15—20mm). Moxibustion is applicable.

Chongyang (ST42, Yuan—Source point)

Location: On the dome of the instep of the foot, between the tendons of the long extensor muscle of the great toe and the long extensor muscle of the toes, where the pulsation of the dorsal artery of the foot is palpable (See Fig. 1—26).

Indications: Deviation of the mouth, swelling of the face, toothache, insanity, mania and epilepsy, atrophic disability of the lower limds

Method: Puncture perpendicularly 0.3—0.5 cun (9—15mm), avoiding the artery. Moxibustion is applicable.

Xiangu (ST43, Shu—Stream point)

Location: On the instep of the foot, at the depression distal to the commissure of the 2nd and 3rd metatarsal bones (See Fig. 1—26).

Indications: Facial or general edma, borborygmus and abdominal pain, swelling and pain of the dorsum of the foot.

Method: Puncture perpendicularly or obliquely 0.5—1.0 cun (15—25mm) upwards. Moxidution is applicable.

Neiting (ST44, Ying—Spring point)

Location: At the dorsum of the foot, at the junction of the red and white skin proximal to the margin of the web between the 2nd and 3rd toes (See Fig. 1—26)

Indications: Deviation of the mouth, toothache, swelling and sore throat, epistaxis, abdominal distension, diarrhea, febrile diseaes.

Method: Puncture perpendicularly or obliquely upwards 0.5—0.8 cun (15—20mm). Moxibustion is applicable.

Lidui (ST45, Jing—Well point)

Location: At the lateral side of the distal segment of the 2nd toe, 0.1 cun from the corner of the nail (See Fig. 1—26).

Indications: Facial edema, febrile diseases, insanity, epistaxis, mania, sore theoat.

Method: punctture shallowly 0.1 cun (about 3mm). Moxibustion is applicable.

3. *An Outline of Indications of the Commonly Used Acupoints*

The acupoints of this meridian can be employed in treating disorders of the digestive system, which are related to the stomach, such as stomachache, abdominal pain, borborgmus, abdominal distension, diarrhea, dysentery, constipation, etc. In concrete, Jiexi (ST41) and Neiting (ST44) are indicated in insanity, epistaxis and mania by reducing stomach — heat; Fenglong (ST40) is used to eliminate sputum and relieve stagnant qi; Liangqiu (ST34) is indicated in swelling and pain of the breast; the acupoints distributed on the head and face, as well as on the distal area of the lower limb such as Neiting (ST44) and Shangjuxu (ST39) are indicated in deviation of the mouth and eye, swelling and pain of the face. Additionally, the acupoints of this meridian can be used to treat painful syndromes and flaccidity and arthralgia of the portions of the body where the pathway of this meridian is at.

四、足太阴脾经（共21穴）

（一）经脉循行

1. 起于足大趾末端隐白穴；2. 沿着大趾内侧赤白肉际，经过第一跖趾关节后面；3. 上行至内踝前面；4. 再上小腿内侧中；5. 沿着胫骨后面；6. 在内踝上8寸处交出于足厥阴经的前面；7. 向上经膝股部内侧前缘；8. 进入腹部；9. 属于脾脏，联络胃；10. 向上通过横膈；11. 挟咽喉部；12. 连系舌根并分散于舌下。

支脉：13. 从胃向上通过横膈；14. 流注于心中，与手少阴心经相接。

体表穴位分布线：起于足大趾内端隐白穴，沿第一趾、跖骨内缘，经内踝前面，在内踝上8寸处交于足厥阴经之前，沿下肢内侧前缘，上循腹正中线旁开4寸，胸正中线旁开

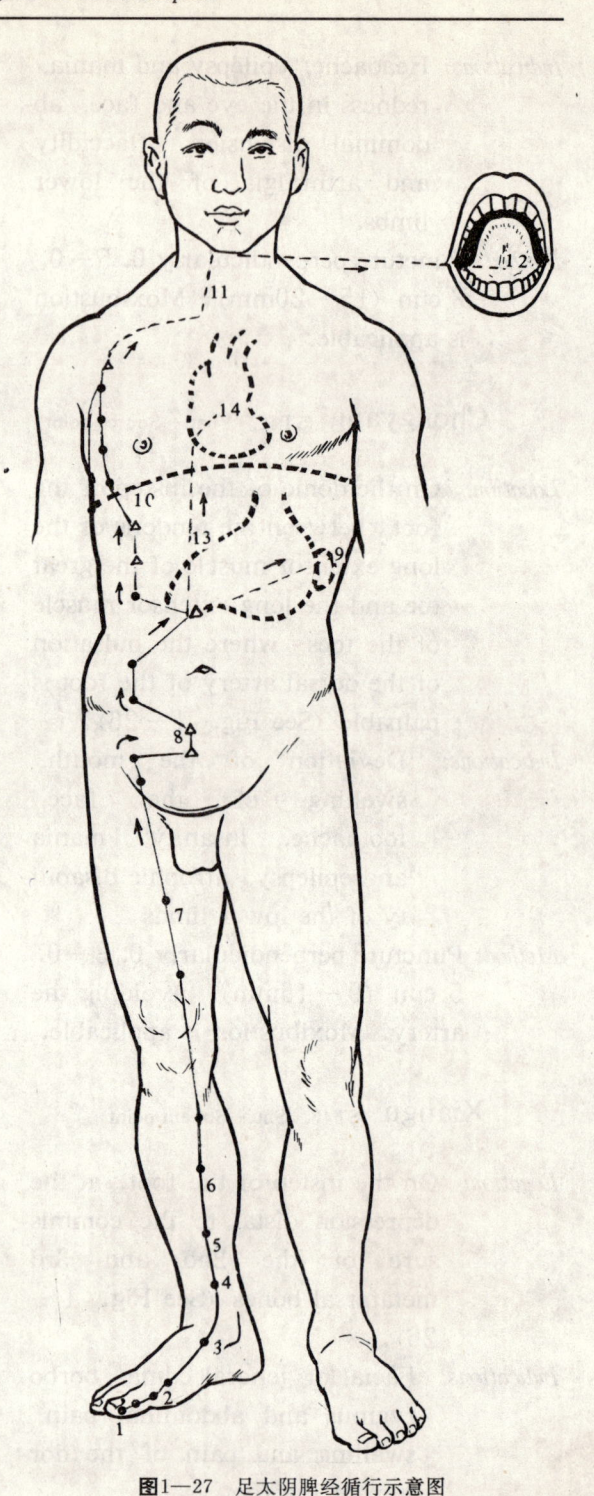

图1—27 足太阴脾经循行示意图

Fig. 1—27 The Running Course of the Spleen Meridian of Foot—Taiyin

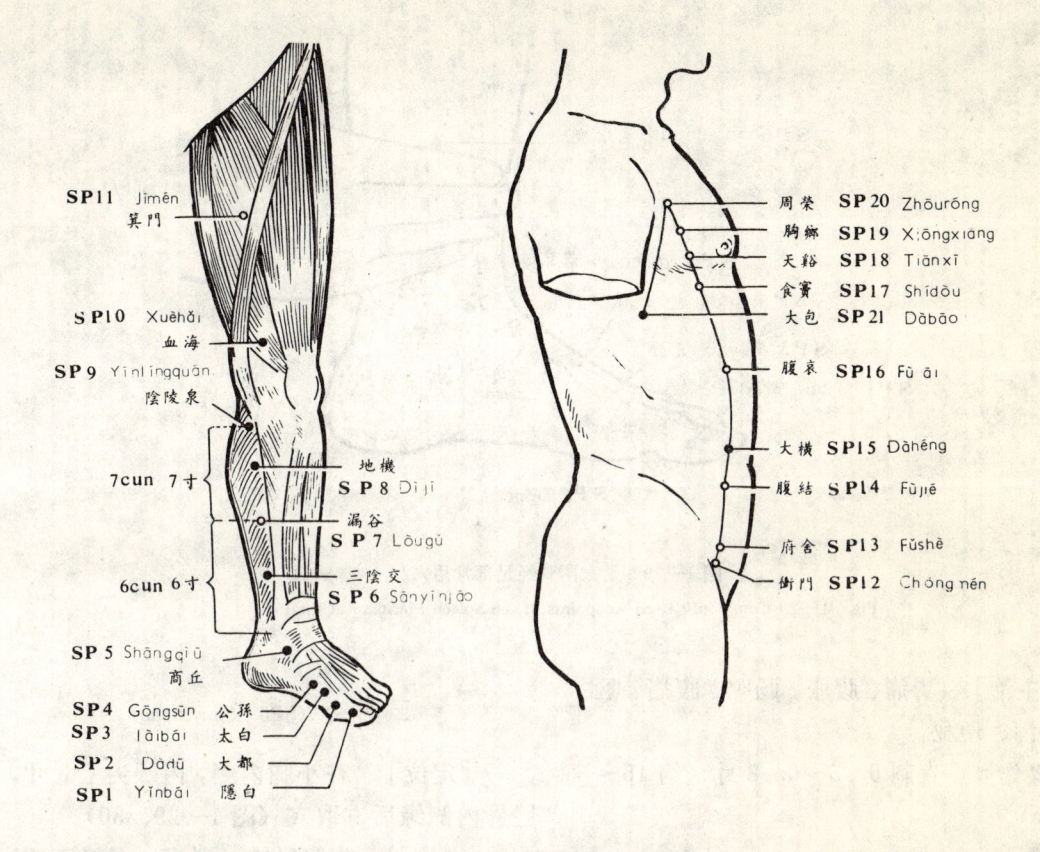

图1—28 足太阴脾经穴位图
Fig. 1—28 Acupints of the Spleen Meridian of Foot—Taiyin

6寸，止于腋下大包穴。

体内相关的组织脏器：脾、胃、心、咽、舌。

（二）本经常用腧穴

隐白穴（SP1 Yǐnbái 井穴）

[定位] 在足大趾末节内侧，距趾甲角0.1寸（图1—29）。

[主治] 腹胀、崩漏、便血、吐血、衄血、尿血、慢惊风、昏厥。

[操作] 浅刺0.1寸（约3毫米）或用三棱针点刺出血；或灸。

大都（SP2 Dàdū 荥穴）

[定位] 在足内侧缘，当足大趾本节（第一跖趾关节）前下方赤白肉际凹陷处（图1—29）。

[主治] 胃痛、腹胀、呕逆、泄泻、便秘、热病汗不出。

[操作] 直刺0.3～0.5寸（约9～15毫米）。

太白（SP3 Tàibái 输穴，原穴）

[定位] 在足内侧缘，当足大趾本节（第1跖趾关节）后下方赤白肉际凹陷处（图1—29）。

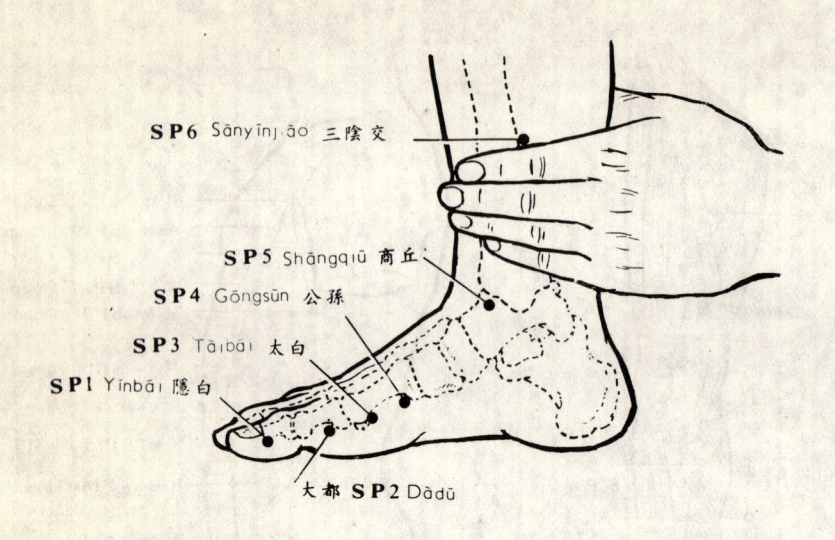

图 1—29　足太阴脾经足部常用穴

Fig. 1—29 Commonly Used Acupoints of the Spleen Meridian at the Foot

　［主治］　胃痛、腹胀、肠鸣、腹痛、呕吐、泄泻、便秘。
　［操作］　直刺 0.5～0.8 寸（约 15～20 毫米）。

　公孙（SP4　Gōngsūn　络穴、八脉交会穴）

　［定位］　在足内侧缘，第一跖骨基底部的前下方（图 1—29）。
　［主治］　胃痛、呕吐、腹胀、腹痛、泄泻、水肿。
　［操作］　直刺 0.5～1.2 寸（约 15～30 毫米）。

　　商丘（SP5　Shāngqiū　经穴）

　［定位］　在内踝前下方凹陷中。当舟骨结节与内踝尖连线之中点取穴（图 1—29）。
　［主治］　腹胀、肠鸣、泄泻、黄疸、便秘、足踝痛。
　［操作］　直刺 0.3～0.5 寸（约 9～15 毫米）。

　　三阴交（SP6　Sānyīnjiāo）

　［定位］　在小腿内侧，内踝尖上 3 寸，胫骨内侧缘后方取穴（图 1—29、30）。
　［主治］　腹胀肠鸣、泄泻、月经不调，崩漏，阴挺，不孕，滞产，遗精，阳萎，失眠，下肢痿痹。
　［操作］　直刺 1～1.5 寸（约 25～40 毫米）。

　　地机（SP8　Dìjī　郄穴）

　［定位］　在小腿内侧，阴陵泉穴下 3 寸，在阴陵泉与内踝尖的连线上取穴（图 1—30）。
　［主治］　腹胀，腹痛，泄泻，月经不调，痛经，小便不利，水肿。
　［操作］　直刺 1～1.5 寸（约 25～40 毫米）。

　　阴陵泉（SP9　Yīnlíngquán　合穴）

　［定位］　在上腿内侧，当胫骨内侧踝

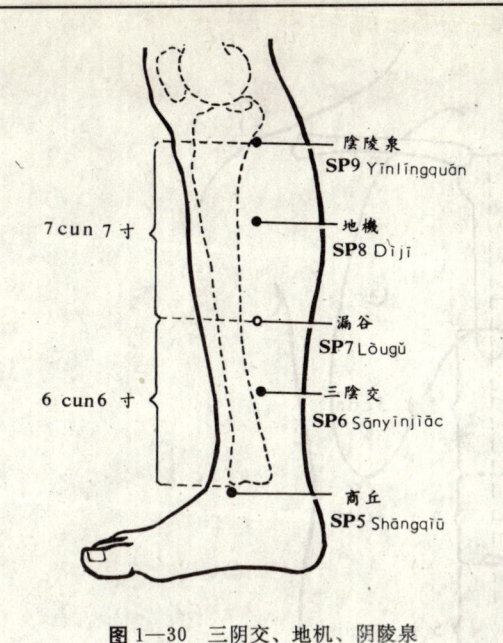

经络腧穴概要

图1—30 三阴交、地机、阴陵泉
Fig. 1—30 Sanyinjiao (SP 6), Diji (SP 8) and Yinlingquan (SP9)

后下方凹陷处（图1—30）。

[主治] 腹胀、泄泻、水肿、黄疸、小便不利或失禁，膝痛。

[操作] 直刺1～2寸（约25～50毫米）。

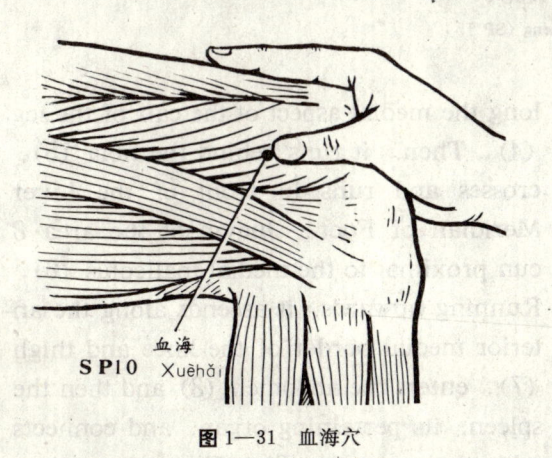

图1—31 血海穴
Fig. 1—31 Xuehai (SP 10)

血海 (SP10 Xuěhǎi)

[定位] 屈膝，在大腿内侧，髌底内侧端上2寸，股四头肌内侧头的隆起处（图1—28）；或以左手掌心按于患者右膝髌骨上缘，二至五指向上伸直，拇指约呈45°斜置，拇指尖下即是该穴（图1—31）。

[主治] 月经不调，痛经，经闭，崩漏，湿疹，丹毒，股内侧痛。

[操作] 直刺1～1.5寸（约25～40毫米）。

大横 (SP15 Dàhéng)

[定位] 仰卧，在腹中部，距脐中4寸（1—32）。

[主治] 腹痛、泄泻、便结。

[操作] 直刺0.8～1.2寸（约20～30毫米）。

大包 (SP21 Dàbāo 络穴)

[定位] 在侧胸部，腋中线上，第六肋间隙中取穴（图1—28）。

[主治] 气喘，胸胁痛。

[操作] 斜刺0.5～0.8寸（约15～20毫米）。不可直刺，深刺，以防刺伤肺脏。

（三）常用经穴主治提要

本经经穴主要用于防治脾胃功能失调的消化系统病，如呕吐，胃痛、泄泻、痢疾，以及肝胆疾患与各种血症和经脉所过处病变。如公孙，大都，太白治胃痛、腹痛、吐泄；隐白治崩漏；三阴交调理脾、肝、肾经气，除治消化不良外，尚治一切妇科及男性生殖病，并且可治肾，肝阴虚之失眠多梦；阴陵泉治"脾"转输功能失调病，如水肿腹胀，黄疸以及膝痛；血海调治一切血证、兼治湿疹、隐疹；大横治腹泻、便秘；大包治气喘，胸胁痛。

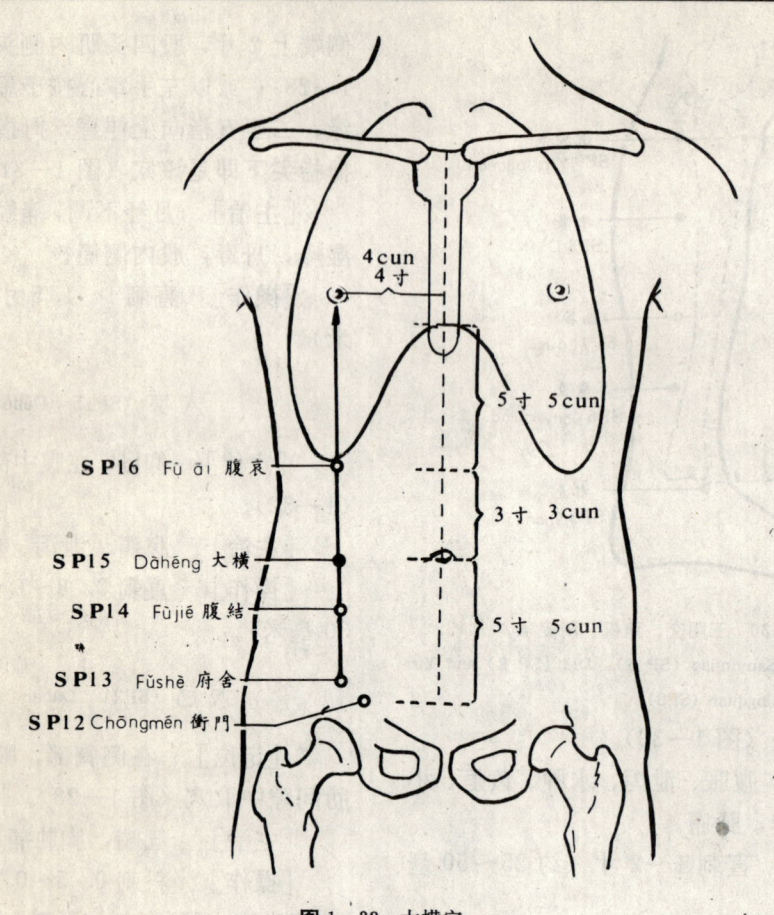

Fig. 1—32 Daheng (SP 15)

IV. THE SPLEEN MERIDIAN OF FOOT —TAIYIN (21 acupoints in total)

1. *The Course*

It originates from Yinbai (SP 1) at the tip of the great toe (1). Then, it runs along the dorso—ventral boundary at the medial aspect of the great toe and passes behind the first metatarsal phalangeal joint (2). Ftom there, it ascends in front of the medial malleolus (3), and runs upwards along the medial aspect ot the calf of the leg (4). Then, it runs behind the tibia (5), crosses and runs in front of the Liver Meridian of Foot — Jueyin at the area 8 cun proximal to the medial malleolus (6). Running upwards, it ascends along the anterior medial border of the knee and thigh (7), enters the abdomen (8) and then the spleen, its pertaining organ, and connects with the stomach (9). From there it ascends, passing through the diaphragm (10), and running alongside the esophagus (11). When it reaches the root of the tongue, it spreads over the sublingual region (12).

The branch starting from the stomach ascends through the diaphragm (13), and disappears into the heart to connect with the Heart Meridian of Hand — Shaoyin (14).

The line made up dy distrtibution of the acupoints of this meridian: It starts from Yinbai (SP1) at the tip of the medial border of the great toe, runs along the medial border of the fisrt phalanx and the first metatarsal bone, and passes in front of the medial malleolus. Ascending, it crosses and runs in front of the Liver Meridian of Foot — Jueyin at the area 8 cun above the medial malleolus. Ascending again, it runs along the anterior medial border of the lower limb and along the line 4 cun lateral to the abdominal midline and 6 cun lateral to the midline of the chest, and ends at Dabao (SP 21) below the axillus.

The inner organs concerned: The spleen, stomach, heart, throat, and tongue.

2. *The Commonly Used Acupoints*

Yinbai (SP 1, Jing—Well point)

Location: On the medial side of the distal segment of the big toe, adout 0.1 cun posterior to the corner of the nail of the big toe (See Fig. 1—29).

Indications: Abdominal distension, bloody stool, hemoturia, hematemesis, apistaxis, chronic convulsion, coma, metrorrhagia and metrostaxis.

Method: Puncture shallowly 0.1 cun (about 3mm), or prick with the three — edged needle to cause bleeding, or apply moxibustion.

Dadu (SP 2, Ying—Spring point)

Location: At the medial side of the big toe, at the dorso—ventral boundary, antero — inferior to the first metatarsal phalangeal joint (See Fig. 1—29).

Indications: Stomachache, abdominal distension, vomiting, diarrhea, constipation, febrile diseases without sweating.

Method: Punctre perpendicularly 0.3—0.5 cun (9—15mm). Moxibustion is applicable.

Taibai (SP 3, Shu—Stream point and Yuan —Source point)

Location: On the medial border of the foot, posterior and inferior to the 1st metatarsal phalangeal joint, in the dorso — ventral boundary of the foot (See fin. 1—29).

Indications: Stomachache, abdominal distension, borborygmus, abdominal pain, vomiting, diarrhea, constipation.

Method: Puncture perpendicularly 0.5—0.8 cun (15—20mm). Moxibustion is applicable.

Gongsun (SP 4, Luo — Connecting point, Confluence point)

Location: On the medial border of the foot, antero—inferior to the proximal end of the 1st metatarsal bone, at the dorso—ventral boundary of the foot (See Fig. 1—29).
Indications: Stomachache, vomiting, abdominal distension and pain, diarrhea, edema.
Method: Punture perpendicularly 0.6—1.2 cun (15-30mm). Moxibustion is applicable.

Shangqiu (SP 5, Jing—River point)

Location: At the depression antero—inferior to the medial malleolus, at the midpoint of the line connecting the tip of the medial malleolus with the tubercle of the scaphoid bone (See Fig. 1—29).
Indications: Abdominal distension, borborygmus, diarrhea, jaundice, constipation, pain in the ankel joint.
Method: Puncture perpendicularly 0.3—0.5 cun (9—15mm). Moxibustion is applicable.

Sanyinjiao (SP 6)

Location: On the medial side of the leg, 3 cun proximal to the tip of the medial malleolus, posterior to the medial border of the tidia (See Fig. 1—29, 1—30).
Indications: Abdominal distension, borborygmus, diarrhea, abnormal menstruation, metrorrhagia and metrostaxis, prolapse of the uterus, sterility, difficult labour, emission, impotence, insomnia, flaccidity and arthralgia of the lower limbs.
Method: Puncture perpendicularly 1.0—1.5 cun (25—40mm). Moxibustion is applicable.

Diji (SP 8, Xi—Cleft point)

Location: On the medial side of the leg, 3 cun distal to Yinlingquan (SP 9), at the line connecting Yinlingquan (SP 9) and San—yinjiao (SP 6) (See Fig. 1—30).
Indications: Abdominal distension and pain, diarrhea, abnormal menstruation, dysmenorrhea, dysuria, edema.
Method: Puncture perpendicularly 1.0—1.5 cun (25-40mm). Moxibustion is applicable.

Yinlingquan (SP 9, He—Sea point)

Location: On the medial side of the leg, in the depression posterior and inferior to the medial condyle of the tibia (See Fig. 1—30).
Indications: Abdominal distesion, diarrhea, edema, jaundice, dysuria or incontinence of urine, pain in the knee.
Method: Puncture perpendicularly 1.0—2.0 cun (25—50mm). Moxibustion is applicable.

Xuehai (SP 10)

Location: When the knee is flexed, on the medial side of the thigh, 2 cun proximal to the supero—internal border of the patella, on the bulge of the medial portion of m. quadriceps femoris of the thigh (See Fig. 1—28). Or, the operator puts his left hand over the patient's right patella with the center of the palm just on the upper border of the patella, and 2nd — 5th fingers directed upwards and the thumd at the angle of 45°with the index finger, the spot beneath the tip of the thumb is the location (See Fig. 1—31).

Indications: Abnormal menstruation, dysmenorrhea, amenorrhea, metrorrhagia and metrostaxis, eczema, erysipelas, pain in the medial aspect of the thigh.

Method: Puncture perendicularly 1.0—1.5 cun (25—40mm). Moxibustion is applicable.

Daheng (SP 15)

Location: On the middle abdomen, 4 cun lateral to the center of the umbilicus (See Fig. 1—32).

Indications: Abdominal pain, diarrhea, constipation.

Method: Puncture perpendicularly 0.8—1.2 cun (20—30mm). Moxibustion is applicable.

Dabao (SP 21, Luo—Connecting point)

Location: On the lateral side of the chest and on the mid-axillary line, in the 6th intercostal space (See Fig. 1—28).

Indications: Asthma, pain in the chest and hypochondrium.

Method: Puncture obliquely 0.5—0.8 cun (15—20mm). Perpendicular and deep puncture is prohibited, so as to prevent injuring the lung. Moxibustion is applicable.

3. *An Outline of Indications of the Commonly Used Acupoints*

The acupoints of this meridian are mainly used in preventing and treating the disorders of digestive system due to dysfunction of the spleen and stomach, such as vomiting, stomachache, diarrhea, dysentery, and in disorders of the liver and gallbladder and blood troubles, as well as disorders appearing on the pathway of the meridian. In concrete, Gongsun (SP 4), Dadu (SP 2), and Taibai (SP 3) are indicated in stomachache, abdominal pain, and vomiting; Yinbai (SP 1), in metrorrhagia and metrostaxis. As Sanyinjiao (SP 6) can serve to adjust the qi of the Spleen, Liver and Kidney Meridians, it is indicated in, besides dyspepsia, diseases of the gynecology and genital disorders of man, as well as imsomnia with dreaminess due to deficiency of yin of the kidney and liver; Yinlingquan (SP 9), in disorders of function of transportation and transformation of the spleen, such as edema, abdominal distension, jaundice, pain in the knees; Xuehai (SP 10), in diarrhea, constipation; and Dabao (SP 21), in asthma, pain in the chest and hypochondrium.

五、手少阴心经（共9穴）

（一）经脉循行

1. 起于心中，出属心系（心与其他脏器相联系的部位）；2. 通过横膈向下联络小肠；3. 心系向上的脉；4. 挟着咽喉上行；5. 联系于目系（眼球联系于脑的部位）；6. 心系直行的脉：上行于肺部，向下出于腋窝部极泉穴；7. 再向下沿着上臂掌侧面尺侧缘；8. 到达肘窝，沿着前臂尺侧缘；9. 抵达掌后腕豆骨部；10. 再进入掌内四、五掌骨间；11. 止于小指桡侧少冲穴，与手太阳小肠经相接。

体表穴位分布线：起于腋下极泉穴，沿臂掌侧面尺侧缘，入掌内四、五掌骨间，止于小指桡侧少冲穴。

体内相关的组织脏器：心、小肠、肺、咽喉、眼。

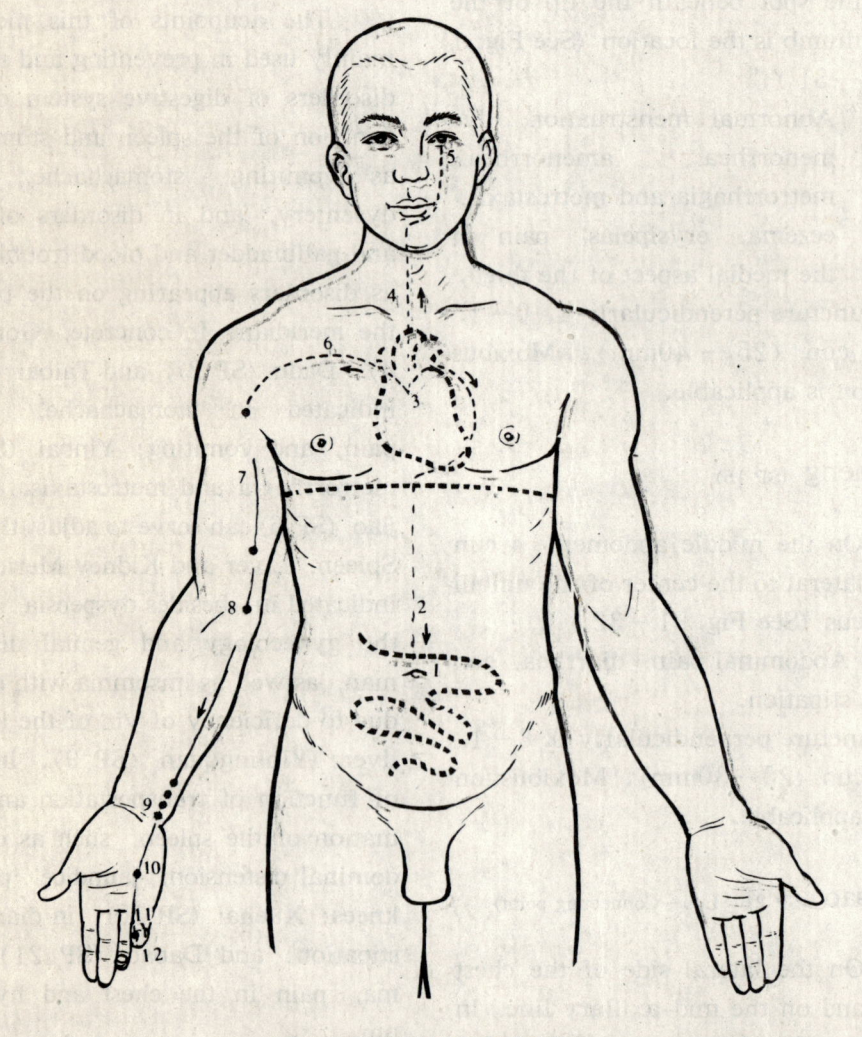

图 1—33 手少阴心经循行示意图
Fig. 1—33 The Running Course of the Heart Meridian of Hand—Shaoyin

（二）本经常用腧穴

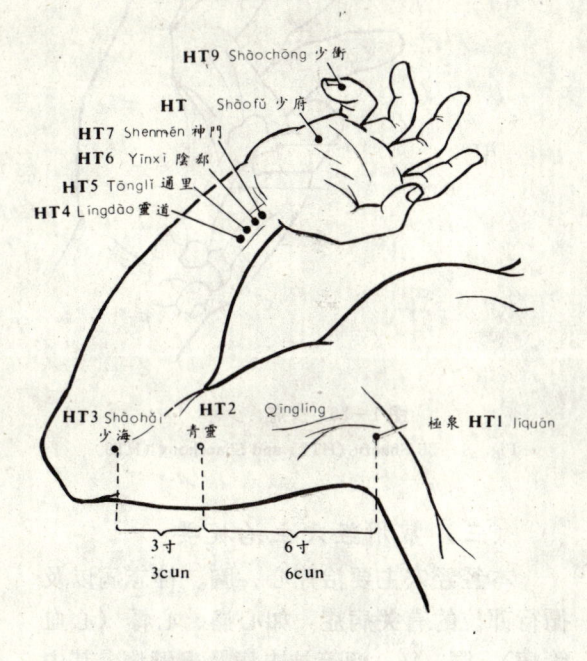

图 1—34 手少阴心经穴位图
Fig. 1—34 Acupoints of the Heart Meridian of Hand—Shaoyin

极泉 （HT1 Jíquán）

［定位］ 上臂外展，在腋窝顶点，腋动脉跳动处（图1—34）。

［主治］ 心痛、胸闷、心悸、咽干烦渴、胁肋疼痛、淋巴结肿大、肩臂疼痛。

［操作］ 避开腋动脉，直刺0.2～0.3寸（约6～9毫米）。

少海 （HT3 Shàohǎi）

［定位］ 屈肘，当肘横纹内侧端与肱骨内上髁连线之中点取穴（图1—34）。

［主治］ 心痛、淋巴结肿大、腋胁痛、癫、狂、痫症。

［操作］ 直刺0.5～1寸（约15～25毫米）。

灵道 （HT4 Língdào 经穴）

［定位］ 在前臂掌侧，在腕横纹上1.5寸，尺侧腕屈肌腱的桡侧缘取穴（图1—35）。

［主治］ 心痛、心悸、舌强不语，突然不能发声，肘臂疼痛。

［操作］ 直刺0.3～0.5寸（9～15毫米）。

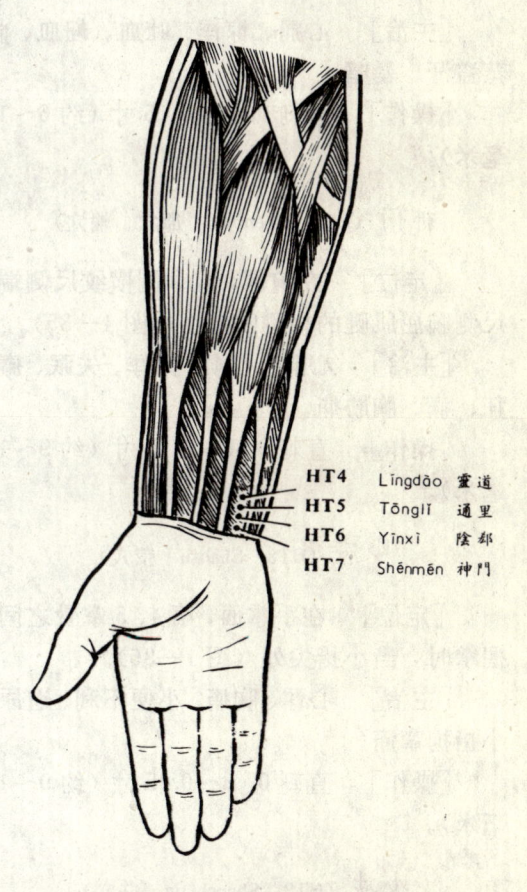

图1—35 灵道、通里、阴郄、神门
Fig. 1-35 Lingdao (HT4), Tongli (HT5), Yinxi (HT6) and Shenmen (HT7)

通里 （HT5 Tōnglǐ 络穴）

［定位］ 在前臂掌侧，在腕横纹上1寸，

尺侧腕屈肌腱的桡侧缘取穴（图1—35）。

[主治] 心悸、舌强不语、暴喑，腕臂痛。

[操作] 直刺0.2～0.5寸（约6～15毫米）。

阴郄（HT6 Yīnxì 郄穴）

[定位] 在前臂掌侧，在腕横纹上0.5寸，尺侧腕屈肌腱的桡侧缘取穴（图1—35）。

[主治] 心痛、惊悸、吐血、衄血、骨蒸盗汗、暴喑。

[操作] 直刺0.2～0.5寸（约6～15毫米）。

神门（HT7 Shénmén 原穴、输穴）

[定位] 在腕部，腕掌侧横纹尺侧端，尺侧腕屈肌腱的桡侧凹陷处（图1—35）。

[主治] 心痛、心烦、惊悸、失眠、癫、狂、痫、胸胁痛。

[操作] 直刺0.3～0.5寸（约9～15毫米）。

少府（HT8 Shàofǔ 荥穴）

[定位] 在手掌面，第4、5掌骨之间，握拳时，当小指尖处（图1—36）。

[主治] 心悸、胸痛、小便不利、遗尿、小指拘挛痛。

[操作] 直刺0.3～0.5寸（约9～15毫米）。

少冲（HT9 Shàochōng 井穴）

[定位] 手小指末节桡侧，距指甲角0.1寸（图1—36）。

[主治] 心悸，心痛，胸胁痛，癫，狂，中风昏迷，热病。

[操作] 浅刺0.1寸（约3毫米），或点刺出血。

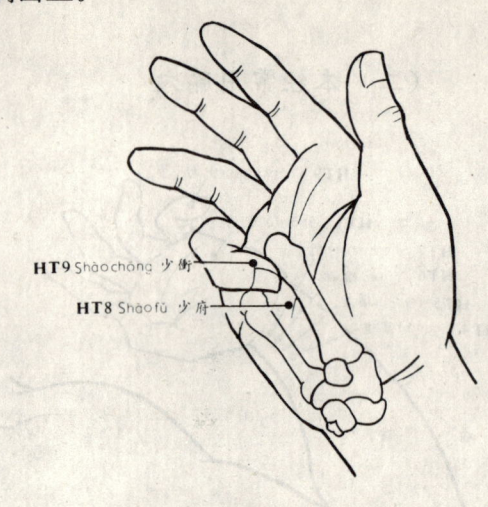

图1—36 少府、少冲
Fig. 1—36 Shaofu (HT8) and Shaochong (HT9)

（三）常用经穴主治提要

本经经穴主要治疗心、胸、神志病以及循行部位的有关病症，如心痛、心悸（心血管病），癫、狂、痫等神志病及肩臂痛。其中少冲、少海、神门穴治癫、狂、痫证；少海、灵道、通里、阴郄除治心痛、心悸外，尚能治暴喑；阴郄治盗汗，吐血。

V. THE HEART MERIDIAN OF HAND — SHAOYIN (9 acupoints in total)

1. The Course

It starts from the heart. Emerging, it runs to the "heart system", the connction between the heart and other viscera (1). It passes through the diaphragm and goes downwards to connect with the small intestine (2).

The ascending branch starting from

the "heart system" (3) runs upwards alongside the esophagus (4), and connects with the "eye system", the connection between the eyeball and brain (5).

The vertical branch starting from the "heart system" runs upwards to the lung. Then, it turns downwards and emerges at Jiquan (HT1) at the axilla (6). From there it runs downwards along the ulnar border of the palm surface of the upper arm (7) to the cubital fossa. Then, it descends along the ulnar border of the forearm (8) to the carpus proximal to the palm (9), and enters the area between the 4th and 5th metacarpal bones of the palm (10). It ends at Shaochong (HT9) at the radial side of the little finger, where it connects with the Small Intestine Meridian of Hand—Taiyang (11).

The line made up by the acupoints distributed on the body surface: It originates from the axilla at Jiquan (HT1), passes along the ulnar border of the palmar surface of the arm, and enters the area between the 4th and 5th metacarpal bones of the palm. Then, it ends at Shaochong (HT9) at the radial side of the little finger.

The inner organs concerned: The heart, small intestine, lung, throat, and eye.

2. *The Commonly Used Acupoints*

Jiquan (HT1)

Location: At the apex of the axillary fossa, where the pulsation of the axillary artery is palpable (See Fig. 1—34).

Indications: Cardiac pain, oppressed feeling in the chest, palpitation, dry throat with excessive thirst, pain in the chest and hypochondrium, scrofula, pain in the shoulder and arm.

Method: Puncture perpendicularly 0.2-0.3 cun (6—9mm), avoiding the axillary artery. Moxibustion is applicable.

Shaohai (HT3, He—Sea point)

Location: When the elbow is flexed, at the midpoint of the line connecting the ulnar end of the transverse cubital crease and the medial epicondyle of the humerus (See Fig. 1—34).

Indications: Cardiac pain, scrofula, pain in the axilla and hypochondrium, epilepsy, mania.

Method: Puncture perpendicularly 0.5—1.0 cun (15—25mm). Moxibustion is applicable.

Lindao (HT4, Jing-River point)

Location: On the palmar side of the forearm, 1.5 cun proximal to the transverse crease of the wrist, at the radial border of the tendon of m. flexor carpi ulnaris (See Fig. 1-35).

Indications: Cardiac pain, palpitation, stiff tongue with aphonia, sudden aphonia, pain in the elbow and arm.

Method: Puncture perpendicularly 0.3-0.

5 cun (9-15mm). Moxibustion is applicable.

Tongli (HT5, Luo—Connecting point)

Location: On the palmar side of the forearm, 1 cun proximal to the transverse crease of the wrist, at the radial border of the tendon of m. flexor carpi ulnaris (See Fig. 1—35).
Indications: Palpitaion, stiff tongue with aphonia, sudden aphonia, pain in the wrist and arm.
Method: Puncture perpendicularly 0.2—0.5 cun (6—15mm). Moxibustion is applicable.

Yinxi (HT6 Xi—Cleft point)

Location: On the palmar side of the forearm, 0.5 cun proximal to the transverse crease of the wrist, at the radial border of the tendon of m. flexor carpi ulnaris (See Fig. 1—35).
Indications: Cardiac pain, palpitation with fright, hematemesis, epistaxis, sudden aphonia, hectic night sweating.
Method: Puncture perpendicularly 0.2—0.5 cun (6—15mm). Moxibustion is applicable.

Shenmen (HT7, Yuan—Source and Shu—Stream point)

Location: On the wrist, at the ulnar end of the crease of the wrist, in the depression of the radial side of the tendon of the ulnar flexor muscle of the wrist (See Fig. 1—35).
Indications: Cardiac pain, restlessness, palpitation, insomnia, epilepsy, mania, pain in the chest and hypochondrium.
Method: Puncture perpendicularly 0.3—0.5 cun (9—15mm). Moxibustion is applicable.

Shaofu (HT8, Ying—Spring point)

Location: In the palm, between the 4th and 5th metacarpal bones, at the part of the palm touching the tip of the little finger when a fist is made (See Fig. 1—36).
Indications: Palpitaion, pain in the chest, enuresis, dysuria, spasmodic pain in the little finger.
Method: Punctre perpendicularly 0.3—0.5 cun (9—15mm). Moxibustion is applicable.

Shaochong (HT9, Jing—River point)

Location: At the radial side of the distal segment of the little finger, about 0.1 cun posterior to the corner of the nail (See Fig. 1—36).
Indications: Palpitation, cardiac pain, pain in the chest and hypochondriac region, epilepsy, mania, appoplectic coma, febrile diseases.
Method: Puncture shallowly 0.1 cun (about 3mm) or prick with the three—edged needle to cause bleeding. Moxibustion is applicable.

3. *An Outline of Indications of the Commonly Used Acupoints*

The acupoints of this meridian are mainly used in treatment of disorders of the heart and chest, and mental disorders, as well as symptoms appearing on the pathway of the meridian, such as cardiac pain and palpitation which belong to cardiovascular problem, mania and epilepsy, and pain in the shoulder and arm. In the concrete, Shaochong (HT1), Shaohai (HT3), and Shenmen (HT7) are indicated in mania and epilepsy; Shaohai (HT3), Lidao (HT4), Tongli (HT5) and Yinxi (HT6), in cardiac pain and palpitation, as well as sudden aphonia; and Yinxi (HT6), in night sweating and hematemesis.

六、手太阳小肠经（共 19 穴）

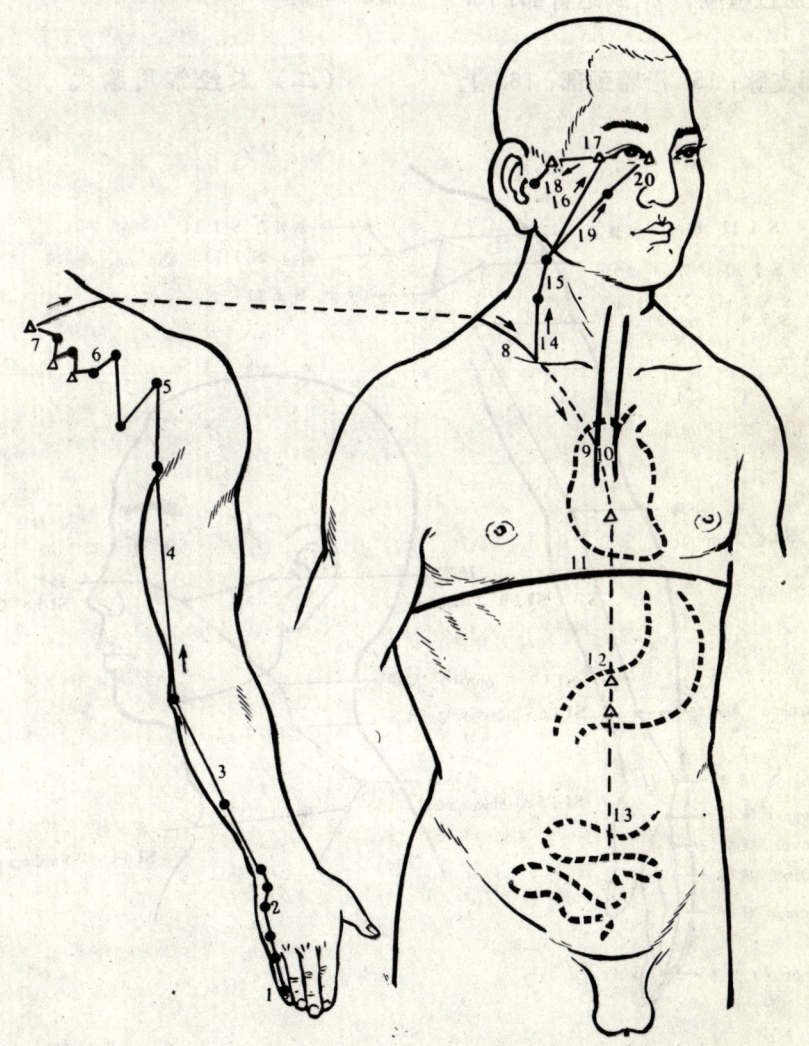

图 1—37　手太阳小肠经循行示意图
Fig. 1—37 The Running Course of the Small Intestine Meridian of Hand—Taiyang

Summary of Meridians, Collaterals and Acupoints

（一）经脉循行

1. 起于手小指外侧端少泽穴；2. 沿着手背外侧至腕部，出于尺骨茎突；3. 再直上沿着前臂外侧尺侧缘，经过尺骨鹰嘴与肱骨内上髁之间；4. 沿着上臂外侧后缘；5. 出于肩关节后；6. 绕行肩胛部；7. 交会于大椎穴；8. 向下进入缺盆部；9. 联络心脏；10. 沿着食管；11. 通过横膈；12. 到达胃部；13. 属于小肠。

14. 缺盆部支脉；15. 沿着颈部；16. 上行至面颊部；17. 到达目外眦；18. 回转入耳前听宫穴。

19. 颊部支脉：上行目眶下，抵于鼻旁；20. 行至目内眦睛明穴，与足太阳膀胱经相接。

体表穴位分布线：起于小指尺侧少泽穴，沿上肢外侧尺侧缘上行、出肩关节后，绕肩胛，经过颈部到达面颊部，止于耳前听宫穴。

体内相关的组织脏器：心、胃、小肠、咽、目、耳。

（二）本经常用腧穴

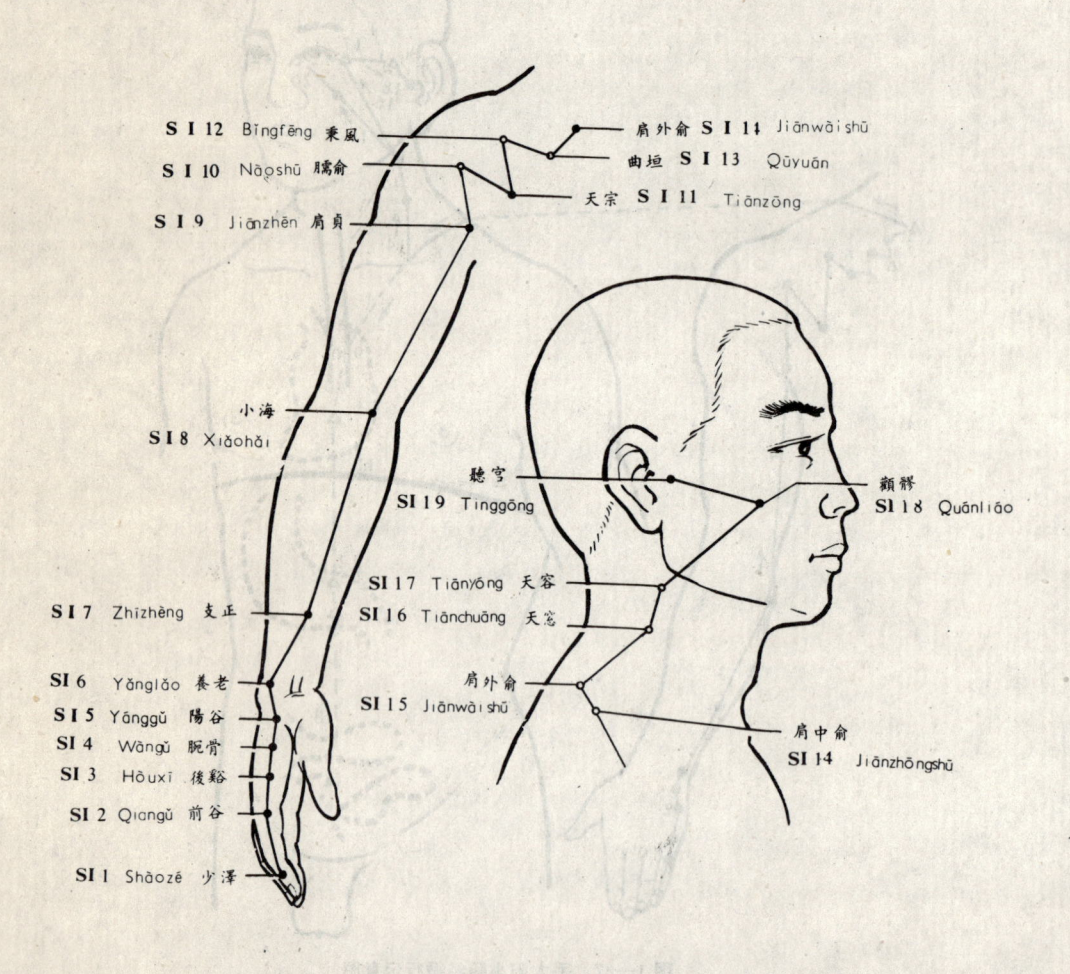

图 1—38 手太阳小肠经穴位图

Fig. 1—38 The Acupoints of the Small Intestine Meridian of Hand—Taiyang

少泽 (SI1 Shàozé 井穴)

［定位］ 在手小指末节尺侧，距指甲角0.1寸（图1—39）。

［主治］ 热病，中风昏迷，咽喉肿痛，目翳，目痛，耳聋，乳痈，乳汁少。

［操作］ 浅刺0.1寸（约3毫米），或点刺出血。

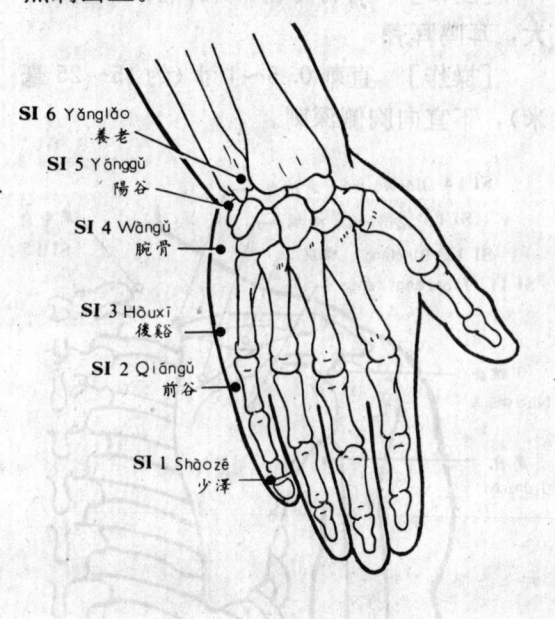

图1—39 手太阳小肠经手部常用穴
Fig. 1—39 Commonly Used Acupoints of the Small Intestine Meridian at the Hand

前谷 (SI2 Qiángǔ 荥穴)

［定位］ 在手尺侧，微握拳，当小指本节（第五掌指关节）前的掌指横纹头赤白肉际（图1—39）。

［主治］ 目痛、目翳、耳鸣、咽喉肿痛、热病、产后无乳。

［操作］ 直刺0.3～0.5寸（约9～15毫米），不宜用直接灸。

后溪 (SI3 Hòuxī 输穴、八脉交会穴)

［定位］ 在手掌尺侧，微握拳，当小指本节（第五掌指关节）后的远侧掌横纹头赤白肉际（图1—39）。

［主治］ 头项强痛、目翳、耳聋、腰背痛、癫、狂、痫、疟疾。

［操作］ 直刺0.5～1寸（约15～25毫米）。

腕骨 (SI4 Wàngǔ 原穴)

［定位］ 在手掌尺侧，当第5掌骨基底与钩骨之间的凹陷处，赤白肉际（图1—39）。

［主治］ 头痛项强、目翳耳鸣、热病、疟疾、手指挛缩、臂痛。

［操作］ 直刺0.3～0.5寸（约9～15毫米）。

阳谷 (SI5 Yánggǔ 经穴)

［定位］ 腕背横纹尺侧端，尺骨茎突与三角骨之间的凹陷中（图1—39）。

［主治］ 头痛、目赤肿痛、耳鸣耳聋、癫、狂、痫、热病、腕痛。

［操作］ 直刺0.3～0.5寸（约9～15毫米），不宜用直接灸。

养老 (SI6 Yánglǎo 郄穴)

［定位］ 在前臂背面尺侧，当尺骨小

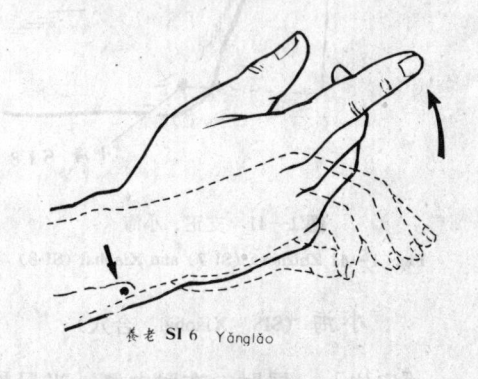

图1—40 养老穴取穴图
Fig. 1—40 The Way of Locating Yanglao (ST 6)

头近端桡侧凹陷中（图1—40）。

[主治] 目视不明，急性腰痛，肩背肘臂酸痛。

[操作] 直刺或斜刺0.5～0.8寸（约15～20毫米）。

支正 (SI7 Zhīzhèng 络穴)

[定位] 在前臂背面尺侧，腕背横纹上五寸，当阳谷穴与小海穴的连线上取穴（图1—41）。

[主治] 头痛、项强、癫、狂、热病、肘臂小指痛。

[操作] 直刺0.3～0.5寸（约9～15毫米）。

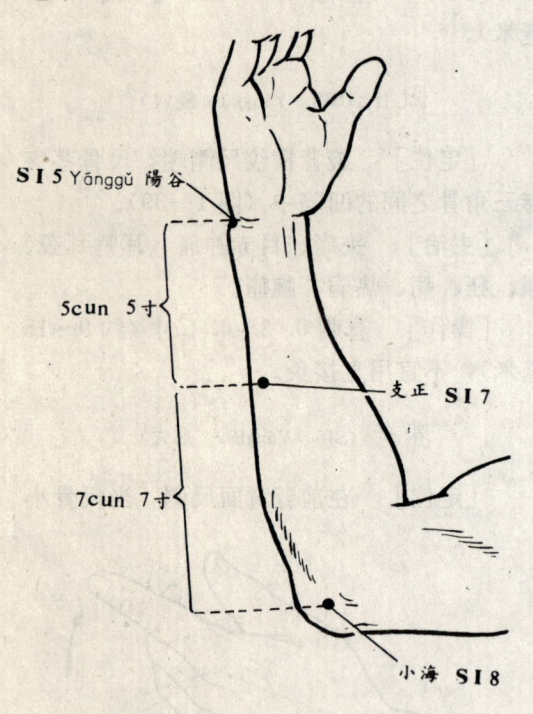

图1—41 支正、小海
Fig. 1—41 Zhizheng (SI 7) and Xiaohai (SI 8)

小海 (SI8 Xiǎohǎi 合穴)

[定位] 屈肘，在肘内侧，当尺骨鹰嘴与肱骨内上髁之间凹陷处取穴（图1—41）

[主治] 颈项肩背疼痛、癫、狂、痫。

[操作] 直刺0.3～0.5寸（约9～15毫米）。

肩贞 (SI9 Jiānzhēn)

[定位] 肩关节后下方，臂内收时，腋后纹头上1寸（图1—42）。

[主治] 肩臂疼痛，肩胛痛，淋巴结肿大，耳鸣耳聋。

[操作] 直刺0.5～1寸（约15～25毫米），不宜向胸侧深刺。

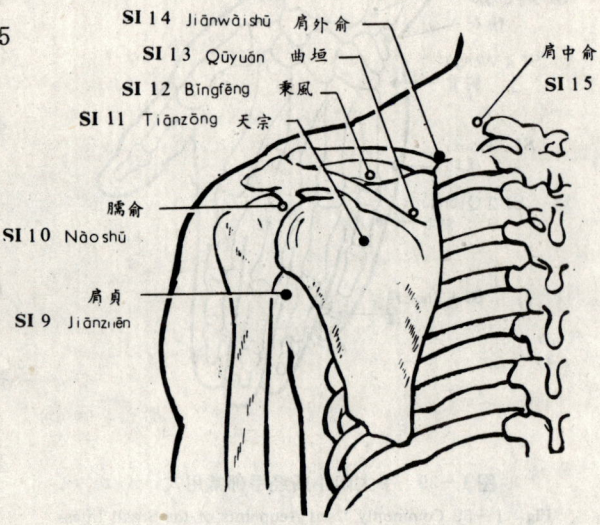

图1—42 肩贞、天宗、肩外俞
Fig. 1—42 Jianzhen (SI 9), Tianzong (SI 11) and Jianwaishu (SI 14)

天宗 (SI11 Tiānzōng)

[定位] 在肩胛部，当岗下窝的中央凹陷处，与第四胸椎相平，（图1—42）。

[主治] 肩胛肘臂疼痛。

[操作] 直刺或斜刺0.5～1寸（约15～25毫米）。

肩外俞 (SI14 Jiānwàishū)

[定位] 在背部，当第一胸椎棘突下

旁开3寸(图1—42)。

[主治] 肩背疼痛,颈项强痛。

[操作] 斜刺0.3~0.5寸(约9~15毫米),不宜深刺,以免损伤肺脏,引起气胸。

颧髎 (SI18 Quánliáo)

[定位] 在面部,目外眦直下,颧骨下缘凹陷中(图1—43)。

[主治] 口眼歪斜,眼睑跳动,颊肿,齿痛,三叉神经痛。

[操作] 直刺0.3~0.5寸(约9~15毫米),斜刺或平刺0.5~1寸(约15~25毫米),不宜用直接灸。

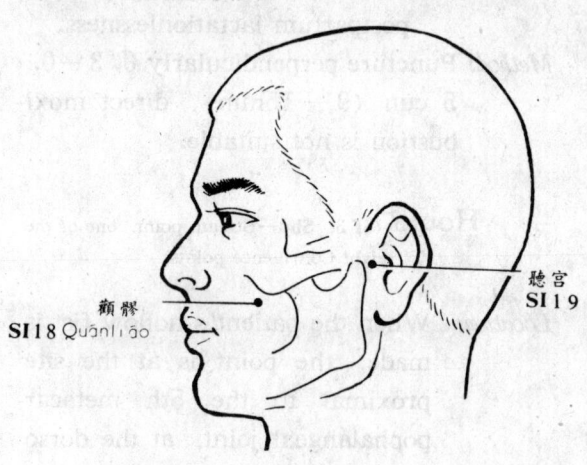

图1—43 颧髎,听宫

Fig. 1—43 Quanliao (SI 18) and Tinggong (SI 19)

听宫 (SI19 Tīnggōng)

[定位] 在面部,耳屏前,下颌骨髁状突的后方,张口时呈凹陷处(图1—43)。

[主治] 耳鸣、耳聋、聤耳、齿痛、癫狂。

[操作] 张口,直刺1~1.2寸(约25~30毫米),不宜直接灸。

(三)常用经穴主治提要

本经经穴主要用于防治神志病,头面、耳、目病及肩臂外侧后缘痛。其中后溪、前谷、腕骨、阳谷、支正、小海治头痛,目赤肿痛与癫狂痫症;少泽开窍泄热,并治乳少;养老治目视不明;听宫治耳鸣耳聋;颧髎治齿痛;天宗治肩背痛。

VI. THE SMALL INTESTINE MERIDIAN OF HAND — TAIYANG (19 acupoints in total)

1. *The Course*

It starts from Shaoze (SI 1) at the ulnar side of the tip of the little finger (1), runs along the ulnar side of the dorsum of the hand to the wrist, and passes through the styloid process of the ulna (2). From there, it ascends along the ulnar border of the lateral side of the forearm, passes between the olecranon of the ulna and the medial epicondyle of the humerus (3), and runs upwards along the posterior border of the lateral aspect of the upper arm (4) to the posterior area of the shoulder joint (5). Circling around the scapular region (6), it meets Dazhui (DU 14) (7). Then, it runs downwards into the supraclavicular fossa (8) to connect with the heart (9). From there, it goes downwards along the esophagus (10), passes through the diaphragm (11), reaches the stomach (12), and finally enters the small intestine, its pertaining organ (13).

The branch arising in the supraclavicular fossa (14) runs along the neck (15), and ascends to the cheek (16). Then, it reaches the outer canthus (17). From there it turns to end at Tinggong (SI 19) in front of the ear (18).

The branch arising in the cheek (19) ascends to the infraorbital region, and to the side of the nose. Then, it runs to the inner canthus at Jingming (BL1) and connects with Bladder Meridian of Foot — Taiyang (20).

The line made up by distribution of the acupoints of this meridian on the body surface: It originates from Shaoze (SI 1) at the ulnar side of the little finger, and passses upwards along the ulnar border of the lateral side of the upper limb. Then, it passes behind the shoulder joint, circles around the scapular region, passes through the neck to the cheek, and ends at Tinggong (SI 19) in the front of the auricle.

The inner organs concerned: The heart, stomach, small intestine, throat, eye, and ear.

2. The Commonly Used Acupoints

Shaoze (SI 1, Jing—Well point)

Location: At the ulnar side of the distal segment of the little finger, about 0.1 cun proximal to the corner of the nail (See Fig. 1—39).

Indications: Febrile diseases, apoplectic coma, swelling and sore throat, nebula of the cornea, pain in the eye, deafness, acute mastitis, lack of lactation.

Method: Puncture shallowly 0.1 cun (about 3mm) or prick with the three — edged needle to cause bleeding. Moxibustion is applicable.

Qiangu (SI 2, Ying—Spring point)

Location: When the patient making a loose fist, the point is at the dorso—ventral boundary of the uluar border of the hand, at the ulnar end of the crease of the 5th metacarpal phalangeal joint (See Fig. 1—39).

Indications: Pain in the eye, nebula of the cornea, tinnitus, swelling and sore throat, febrile diseases, postpartum lactationlessness.

Method: Puncture perpendicularly 0.3—0.5 cun (9—15mm), direct moxibustion is not suitable.

Houxi (SI 3, Shu—Stream point, one of the eight Confluence points)

Location: When the patient's hollow fist is made, the point is at the site proximal to the 5th metacarpophalangeal joint, at the dorso—ventral boundary of the hand at the ulnar side and at the ulnar end of the distal palmar crease (See Fig. 1-39).

Indications: Stiffness and pain in the neck and head, nebula of the cornea, deafness, pain in the back and waist, epilepsy, mania, malaria.

Method: Puncture perpendicularly 0.5—1.0 cun (15—25mm). Moxibustion is applicable.

Wangu (SI 4, Yuan—Source point)

Location: On the ulanr border of the hand, in the depression between the proximal end of the 5th metacarpal bone and hamate bone, and at the dorso—ventral boundary of the hand (See Fig. 1—39).
Indications: Stiffness and pain in the neck and head, nebula of the cornea, tinnitus, febrile diseases, malaria, contracture of the finger, pain in the arm.
Method: Puncture perpendicularly 0.3—0.5 cun (9—15mm). Moxibustion is applicable.

Yanggu (SI 5, Jing—Kiver point)

Location: On the ulnar end of the transverse crease of the dorsum of the wrist, in the depression detween the styloid process of the ulna and the triangular bone (See Fig. 1—39).
Indications: Headache, redness and swelling and pain in the eye, tinnitus and deafness, epilepsy, mania, febrile diseases, pain in the wrist.
Method: Puncture perpendicularly 0.3—0.5 cun (9—15mm). Moxibustion is applicadle, but direct moxibustion is inadvisable.

Yanglao (SI 6, Xi—Cleft point)

Location: On the ulnar side of the posterior surface of the forearm, in the depression proximal to and on the radial side of the head of the ulua (See Fig. 1—40).
Indications: Blurring of vision, acute lumbago, aching of the shoulder, back, elbow and arm.
Method: Puncture perpendicularly or obliquely 0.5—0.8 cun (15—20mm). Moxibustion is applicable.

Zhizheng (SI 7, Luo—Connecting point)

Location: 5 cun proximal to the dorsal transverse crease of the wrist, on the ulnar side of the posterior surface of the forearm, at the line connecting Yanggu (SI 5) and Xiaohai (SI 8) (See Fig. 1—41).
Indications: Headache, neck rigidity, epilepsy, mania, febrile diseases, pain in the elbow, arm, and little finger.
Method: Puncture perpendicularly 0.3—0.5 cun (9—15mm). Moxibustion is applicable.

Xiaohai (SI 8, He—Sea point)

Location: On the medial side of the elbow, in the depression between the olecranon of the ulna and the medial epicondyle of the humerus (See Fig. 1—41).
Indications: Pain in the neck, shoulder and back, epilepsy, mania.
Method: Puncture perpendicularly 0.3—0.5 cun (9—15mm). Moxibustion is applicale.

Jianzhen (SI 9)

Location: Posterior—interior to the shoulder

joint, 1 cun superior to the posterior end of the axillary fold when the upper limb is adducted (See Fig. 1—42).

Indications: Pain in the shoulder and arm, pain in the scapular region, scrofula, tinnitus and deafness.

Method: Puncture perpendicularly 0.5—1.0 cun (15—25mm). Avoid puncturing towards the chest deep. Moxibustion is applicable.

Tianzong (SI 11)

Location: On the scapula, in the depression of the center of the subscapular fossa, and on the level of the 4th thoracic vertebra. Or at the junction point of the upper 1/3 and middle 1/3 of the line connecting the lower border of the scapular spine and the inferior angle of the scapula (See Fig. 1—42).

Indications: Pain in the scapula and elbow and arm.

Method: Puncture perpendicularly or obliquely 0.5—1.0 cun (15—25mm). Moxibustion is applicale.

Jianwaishu (SI 14)

Location: On the back, 3 cun lateral to the midsternal line, paralle to the interspace between the spinous process of the 1st and 2nd thoracic vertedrae (See Fig. 1—42).

Indications: Pain in the shoulder and back, stiffness and pain in the neck.

Method: Puncture obliquely 0.5—0.8 cun (15—20mm). Avoid puncturing deep, otherwise the lung may be injured and the pneumothorax caused. Moxibustion is applicable.

Quanliao (SI 18)

Location: Ask the patient to sit upright with the eyes looking horizontally, on the face, directly below the outer canthus, in the depression on the lower border of the zygoma (See Fig. 1—43).

Indications: Deviation of the mouth and eye, flickering of the eyelids, edema of the cheek, toothache, trigeminal neuralgia.

Method: Punture perpendicularly 0.3—0.5 cun (9—15mm) or obliquely or horizontally 0.5—1.0 cun (15—25mm). Direct moxibustion is inadvisable.

Tinggong (SI 19)

Location: On the face, anterior to the tragus and posterior to the mandibular condyloid process, in the depression found when the mouth is open (See Fig. 1—43).

Indications: Tinnitus, deafness, otorrhea, toothache, epilepsy and mania.

Method: Ask the patient to open his mouth, puncture perpendicularly 1.0—1.5 cun (25—40mm). Direct moxibustion is inadvisable.

3. *An Outline of Indications of the Commonly Used Points*

The points of this meridian are mainly employed in preventing and treating mental disorders and disorders of head and face, ear, and eye, as well as pain at the posterior border of the lateral aspect of the shoulder and arm. In the concrete, Houxi (SI 3), Qiangu (SI 2), Wangu (SI 4), Yanggu (SI 5), Zhizheng (SI 7) and Xiaohai (SI 8) are indicated in headache, redness, swelling and pain of the eye, epilepsy and mania; Shoaze (SI 1) is used to induce resuscitation and to purge pathogenic heat and to treat lack of lactation; Yanglao (SI 5) is indicated in blurring of sight; Tinggong (SI 19), in tinnitus and deafness; Quanliao (SI 18), in toothache, and Tianzong (SI 11), in pain in the shoulder and back.

七、足太阳膀胱经（共67穴）

（一）经脉循行

1. 起于目内眦睛明穴；2. 上行到额部；3. 交会于巅顶百会穴；4. 巅顶部支脉：从头顶到耳上角；5. 巅顶部直行的脉：从头顶入里通于脑；6. 回出来分开下行到项部后面；7. 沿着肩胛部内侧，挟脊柱；8. 直下抵达腰部；9. 沿着脊旁肌肉进入体腔；10. 联络肾脏；11. 属于膀胱；12. 腰部的支脉：从腰部向下行，经过臀部；13. 进入腘窝中；14. 后项的支脉：通过肩胛骨内缘直下；15. 经过臀部下行；16. 沿着大腿后外侧；17. 直向下行，与腰部下来的支脉会合于腘窝中；18. 再向下行，通过腓肠肌；19. 出于外踝的后面；20. 沿着第五跖骨粗隆；21. 到足小趾外侧末端至阴穴，与足少阴经相接。

体表穴位分布线：从目内眦睛明穴，经眉头直上，至头正中线旁开处，下后项挟脊旁开1.5寸，3寸两线下行至臀，沿大腿后面会合于腘窝，再沿小腿后面，下行至外踝后，经足背外侧，止于足小趾外侧端至阴穴。

体内相关的组织脏器：膀胱、肾、脑。

（二）本经常用腧穴

睛明（BL1 Jīngmíng）

[定位] 在面部，目内眦角稍上方凹陷处（图1—46）。

[主治] 目赤肿痛，视物不明，近视，夜盲等一切目疾。

[操作] 嘱患者闭目，医者左手将眼球轻轻推向外侧固定，右手将针沿眼眶边缘缓慢直刺入0.5～1寸（约15～25毫米），不捻转，不提插（或只轻微地捻转和提插）。出针后按压针孔片刻，以防出血。一般不留针，禁灸。

攒竹（BL2 Cuánzhú＆zǎnzhú）

[定位] 在面部，眉头陷中，眶上切迹处（图1—46）。

[主治] 眉棱骨痛，目视不明，目赤肿痛，近视，流泪，眼睑下垂。

[操作] 向眉中平刺0.3～0.5寸（约9～15毫米），禁灸。

天柱（BL10 Tiānzhù）

[定位] 在项部，大筋（斜方肌）外缘之后发际凹陷中，约当后发际正中旁开1.3寸（图1—47）。

[主治] 头痛项强，鼻塞肩背痛。

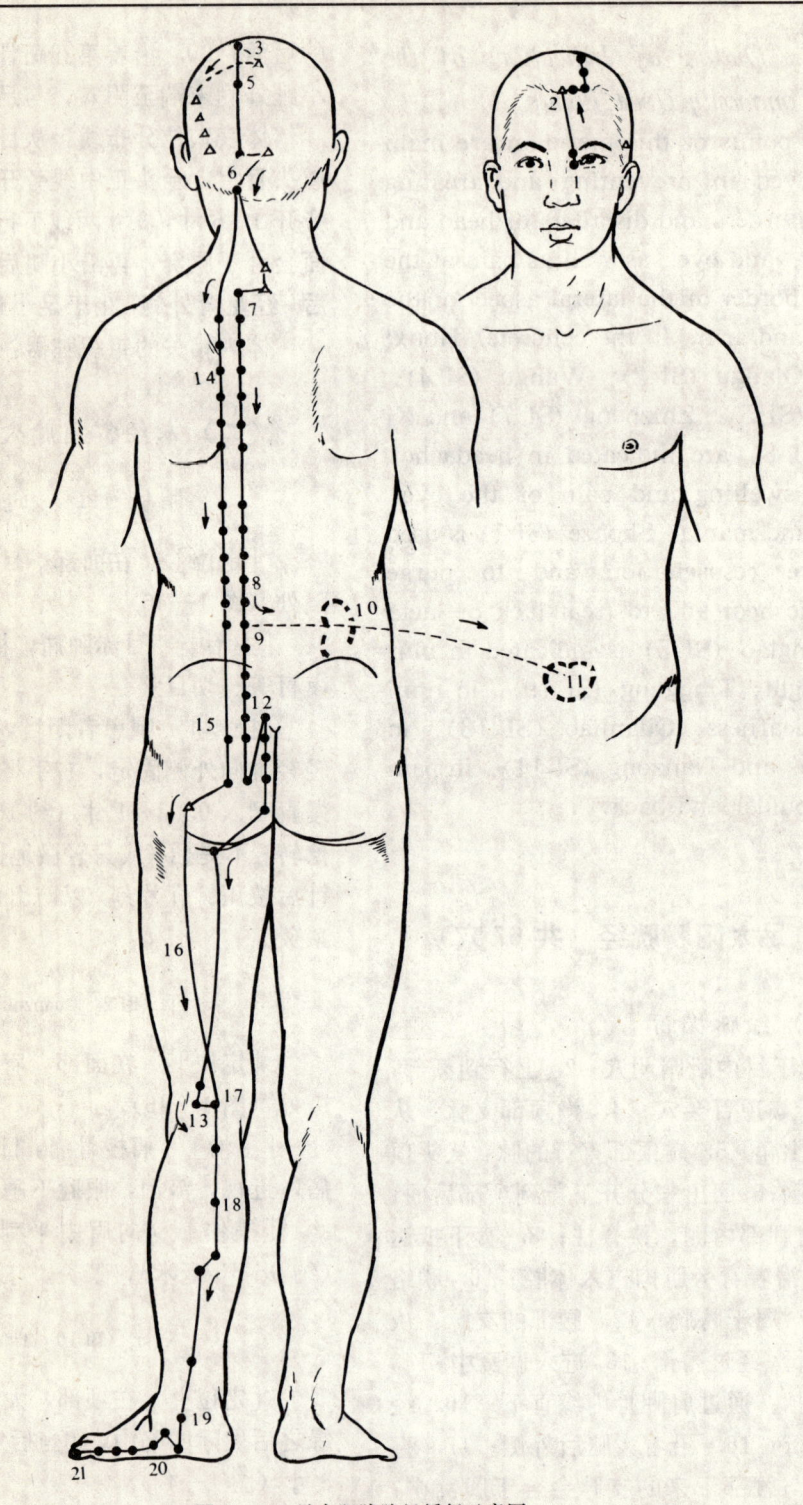

图 1—44 足太阳膀胱经循行示意图

Fig. 1—44 The Running Course of the Bladder Meridian of Foot—Taiyang

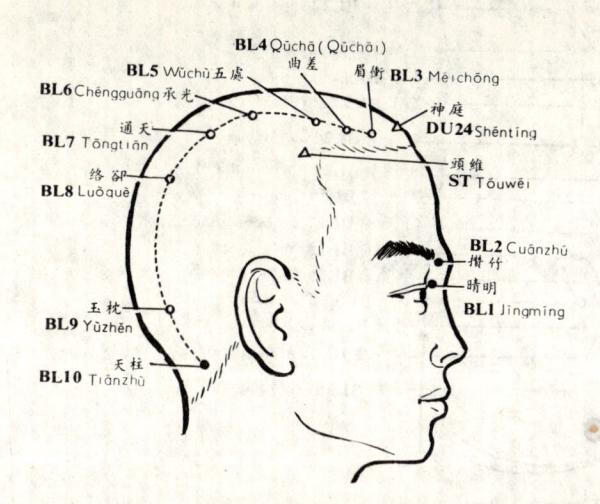

[操作] 直刺或斜刺 0.5～0.8 寸（约 15～20 毫米），不可向内上方深刺，以免伤及延髓。

大杼（BL11 Dàzhú 骨会穴）

[定位] 在背部，第一胸椎棘突下，旁开 1.5 寸处（图 1—48）。

[主治] 咳嗽、发热、颈项强急、肩胛酸痛。

[操作] 向棘间斜刺 0.5～0.8 寸（约 15～20 毫米），背部腧穴深刺恐伤内脏。

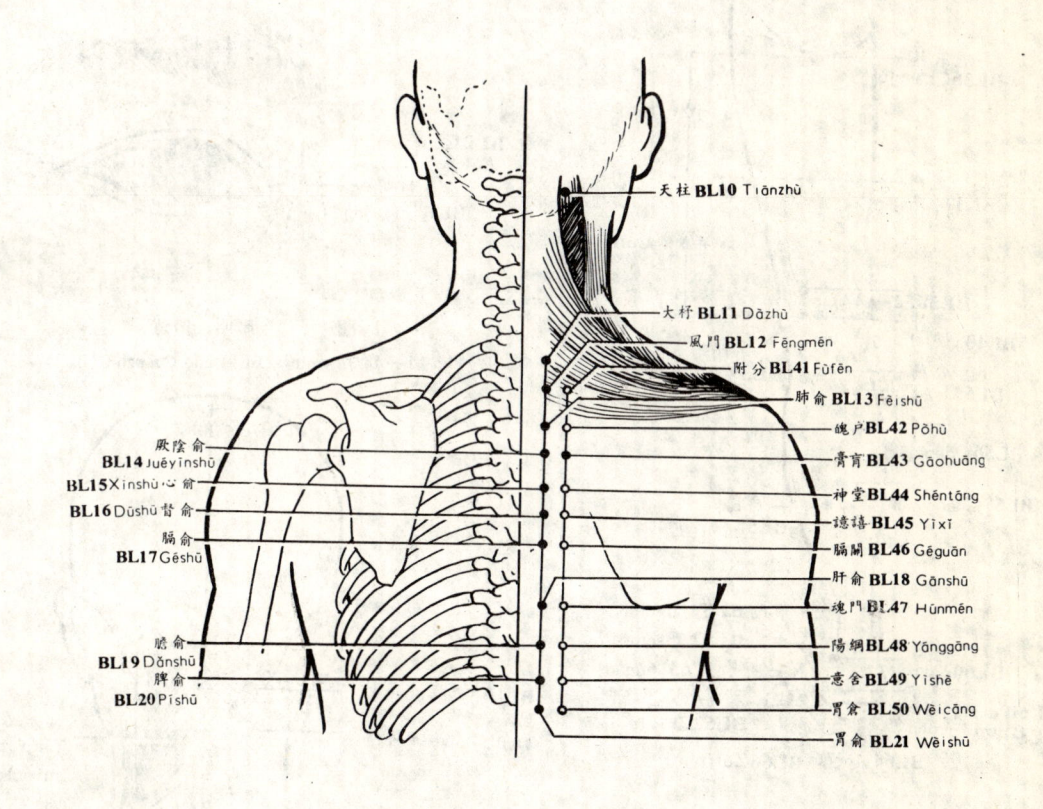

图 1—45① 足太阳膀胱经穴位图

Fig1—45① Acupoints of the Bladder Meridian of Foot—Taiyang

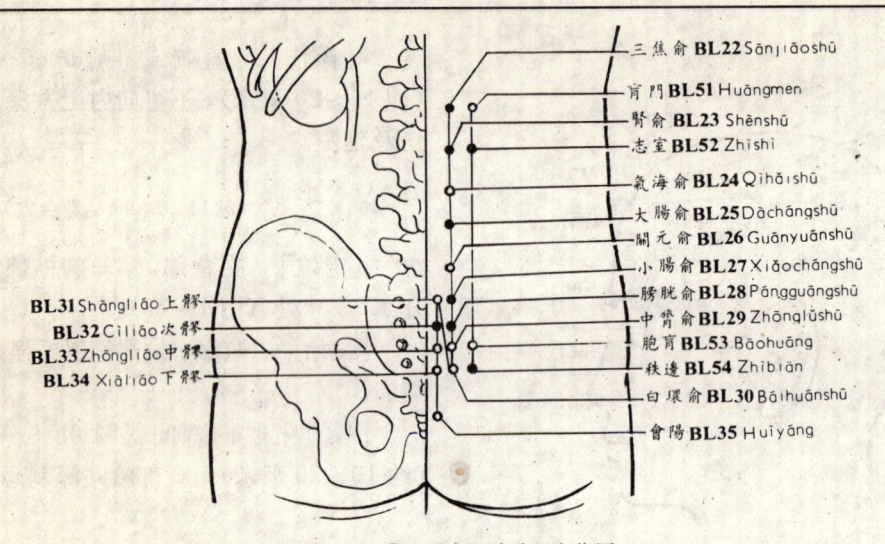

图 1—45② 足太阳膀胱经穴位图
Fig1—45② Acupoints of the Bladder Meridian of Foot—Taiyang

图 1—46 晴明、攒竹
Fig. 1—46 Jingming (BL1) and Cuanzhu (BL2)

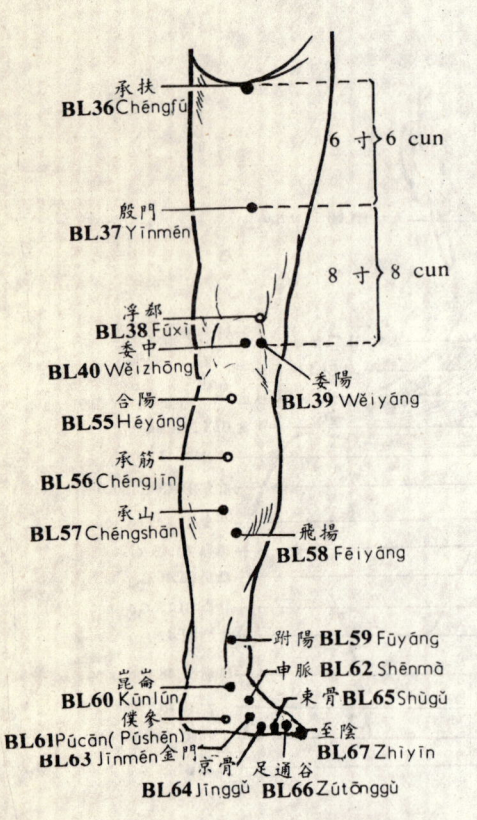

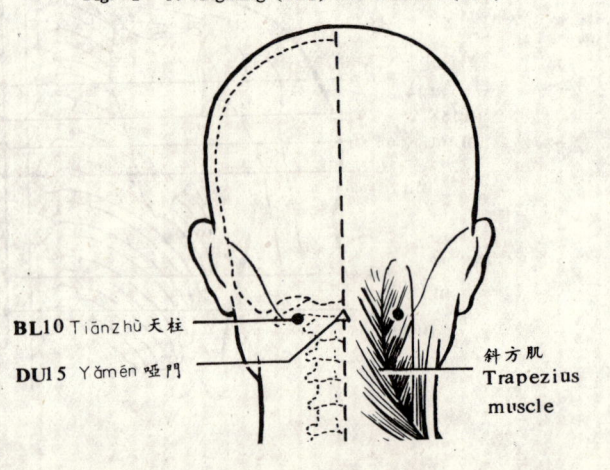

图 1—45③ 足太阳膀胱经穴位图
Fig1—45③ Acupoints of the Bladder Meridian of Foot—Taiyang

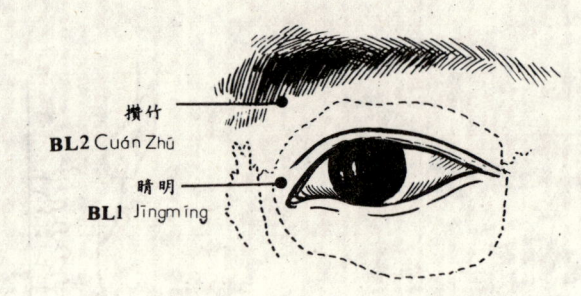

图 1—47 天柱穴
Fig. 1—47 Tianzhu (BL 10)

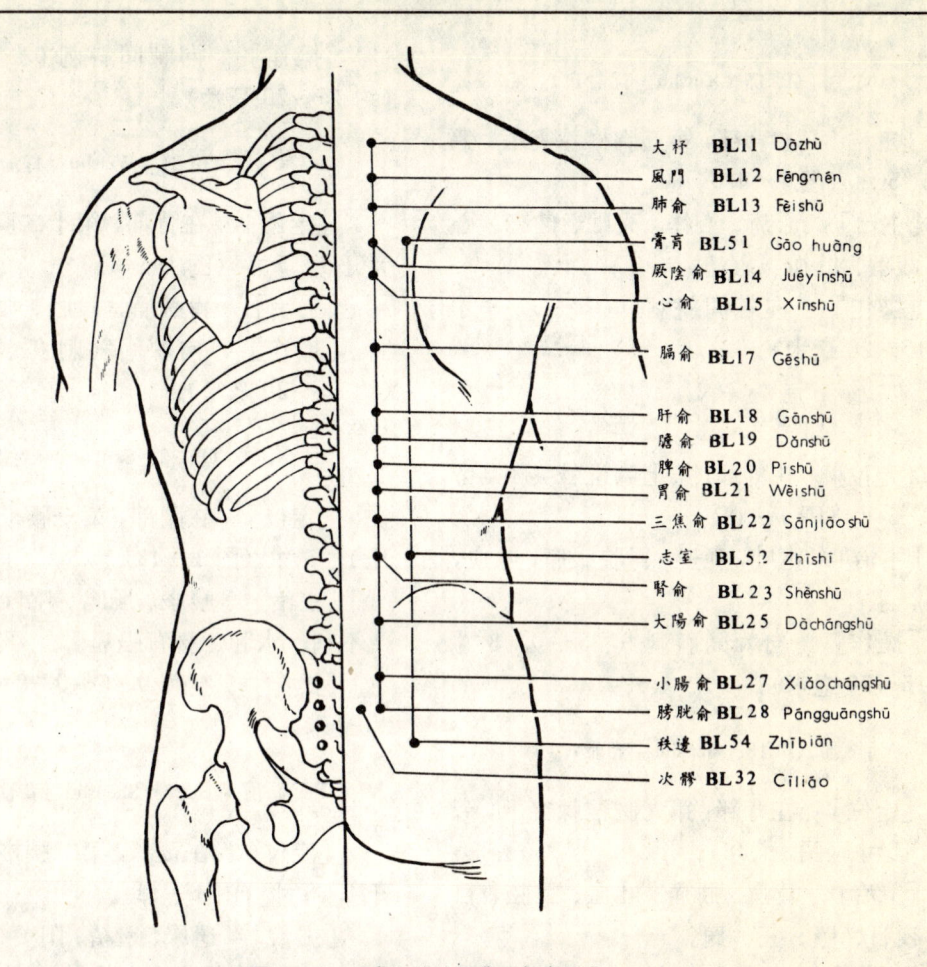

图 1—48　足太阳膀胱经背腰部常用穴
Fig. 1—48 Commonly Used Acupoints of the Bladder Meridian at the Back

风门 (BL12 Fēngmén)

［定位］　在背部，第二胸椎棘突下，旁开 1.5 寸（图 1—48）。

［主治］　伤风咳嗽，发热头痛，鼻塞，项强，胸背痛。

［操作］　向棘间斜刺 0.5～0.8 寸（约 15～20 毫米）。

肺俞 (BL13 Fèishū 背俞穴)

［定位］　在背部，第三胸椎棘突下，旁开 1.5 寸（图 1—48）。

［主治］　咳嗽、气喘、胸满、吐血、潮热盗汗。

［操作］　向棘间斜刺 0.5～0.8 寸（约 15～20 毫米）。

厥阴俞 (BL14 Juéyīnshū 背俞穴)

［定位］　在背部，第四胸椎棘突下，旁开 1.5 寸（图 1—48）。

［主治］　咳嗽、心悸、心痛、胸闷、呕吐。

［操作］　向棘间斜刺 0.5～0.8 寸（约 15～20 毫米）。

· 77 ·

心俞 (BL15 Xīnshù 背俞穴)

［定位］ 在背部，第五胸椎棘突下，旁开1.5寸（图1—48）。

［主治］ 心痛、心悸、失眠、健忘、心烦、咳嗽、吐血、癫痫。

［操作］ 向棘间斜刺0.5～0.8寸（约15～20毫米）。

膈俞 (BL17 Géshù 血会穴)

［定位］ 在背部，第七胸椎棘突下，旁开1.5寸（图1—48）。

［主治］ 呕吐，呃逆，胃脘胀痛，吐血，潮热，盗汗。

［操作］ 向棘间斜刺0.5～0.8寸（约15～20毫米）。

肝俞 (BL18 Gānshù 背俞穴)

［定位］ 在背部，第九胸椎棘突下，旁开1.5寸（图1—48）。

［主治］ 黄疸、胁痛、吐血、目眩、目赤、夜盲、癫、狂、痫。

［操作］ 向棘间斜刺0.5～0.8寸（约15～20毫米）。

胆俞 (BL19 Dǎnshù 背俞穴)

［定位］ 在背部，第十胸椎棘突下，旁开1.5寸（图1—48）。

［主治］ 黄疸、口苦、胁痛、呕吐。

［操作］ 向棘间斜刺0.5～0.8寸（约15～20毫米）。

脾俞 (BL20 Píshù 背俞穴)

［定位］ 在背部，第十一胸椎棘突下，旁开1.5寸（图1—48）。

［主治］ 腹胀、呕吐、泄泻、水肿、便血。

［操作］ 向棘间斜刺0.5～0.8寸（约15～20毫米）。

胃俞 (BL21 Wèishù 背俞穴)

［定位］ 在背部，第十二胸椎棘突下，旁开1.5寸（图1—48）。

［主治］ 胃脘痛、腹胀、呕吐、肠鸣。

［操作］ 向棘间斜刺0.5～0.8寸（约15～20毫米）。

三焦俞 (BL22 Sānjiāoshù 背俞穴)

［定位］ 在腰部，第一腰椎棘突下，旁开1.5寸（图1—48）

［主治］ 腹胀、肠鸣、呕吐、腹泻、小便不利、水肿、腰背强痛。

［操作］ 直刺0.5～0.8寸（约15～20毫米）。

肾俞 (BL23 Shènshù 背俞穴)

［定位］ 在腰部，第二腰椎棘突下，旁开1.5寸（图1—48）。

［主治］ 遗尿、遗精、阳萎、小便频数、月经不调、小便不利、水肿、耳鸣、腰痛。

［操作］ 直刺1～1.2寸（约25～30毫米）。

大肠俞 (BL25 Dàchángshù 背俞穴)

［定位］ 在腰部，第四腰椎棘突下，旁开1.5寸（图1—48）。

［主治］ 腹痛、腹胀、泄泻、便秘、腰背疼痛。

［操作］ 直刺1～1.2寸（约25～30毫米）。

小肠俞 (BL27 Xiǎochángshù 背俞穴)

［定位］ 在骶部，当骶正中嵴旁1.5寸，平第一骶后孔（图1—48）。

［主治］ 小腹胀痛，泄泻，遗尿，尿血，遗精，白带，疝气。

［操作］ 直刺1～1.2寸（约25～30毫米）。

膀胱俞（BL28 Pángguāngshū 背俞穴）

［定位］ 在骶部，当骶正中嵴旁1.5寸，平第二骶后孔（图1—48）。

［主治］ 小便不利，遗尿，腹痛泄泻，便秘，腰脊强痛。

［操作］ 直刺1～1.5寸（约25～40毫米）

次髎（BL32 Cìliáo）

［定位］ 在骶部，当髂后上棘内下方，适对第二骶后孔处（图1—48）。

［主治］ 腰痛、月经不调、痛经、赤白带下、疝气、小便不利、下肢痿痹。

［操作］ 直刺1～1.5寸（约25～40毫米）

承扶（BL36 Chéngfú）

［定位］ 大腿后面，臀下横纹中点（图1—49）。

［主治］ 痔疾，腰骶臀股部疼痛。

［操作］ 直刺1～2寸（约25～50毫米）。

殷门（BL37 Yīnmén）

［定位］ 在大腿后面，承扶穴与委中穴连线上，承扶穴下6寸（图1—49）。

［主治］ 腰脊强痛、下肢痿痹。

［操作］ 直刺1～2寸（约25～40毫米）。

委阳（BL39 Wěiyáng 三焦下合穴）

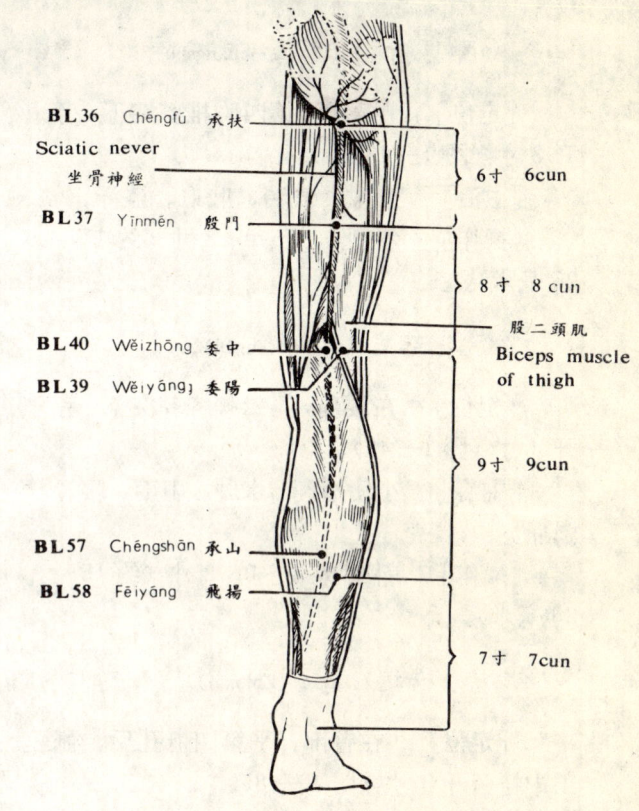

［定位］ 腘横纹外侧端、股二头肌腱内侧（图1—49）。

图1—49 足太阳膀胱经下肢常用穴

Fig. 1 — 49 Commonly Used Acupoints of the Bladder Meridian at the Lower Limb

［主治］ 小腹胀满、小便不利、腰脊强痛、腿足拘挛疼痛。

［操作］ 直刺0.5～1寸（约15～25毫米）。

委中（BL40 Wěizhōng 合穴）

［定位］ 在腘横纹中点，当股二头肌腱与半腱肌肌腱的中间（图1—49）。

［主治］ 腰痛、腹痛、下肢痿痹、吐泻、小便不利、丹毒。

［操作］ 直刺0.5～1寸（约15～25毫米），或三棱针点刺出血。

膏肓俞（BL43 Gāohuāngshù）

［定位］ 在背部，第四胸椎棘突下，旁开3寸（图1—48）。

［主治］ 咳嗽、气喘、吐血、盗汗。

［操作］ 斜刺0.5～0.8寸（约15～25毫米）。

志室（BL52 Zhìshì）

［定位］ 在腰部，第二腰椎棘突下，旁开3寸（图1—48）。

［主治］ 小便不利、水肿、阳萎、腰脊强痛。

［操作］ 斜刺0.5～0.8寸（约15～20毫米）。

秩边（BL54 Zhìbiān）

［定位］ 在臀部，平第四骶孔后，骶正中嵴旁开3寸（图1—48）。

［主治］ 小便不利、便秘、腰骶痛、下肢痿痹。

［操作］ 直刺1.5～2寸（约40～50毫米）。

承山（BL57 Chéngshā）

［定位］ 在小腿后面正中，委中与昆仑之间，当伸直小腿或足跟上提时腓肠肌肌腹下出现尖角凹陷处（图1—49）。

［主治］ 腿痛转筋，腰痛、背痛、痔疾、便秘、脚气。

［操作］ 直刺1～1.2寸（约25～30毫米0。

飞扬（BL58 Fēiyáng 络穴）

［定位］ 在小腿后面，当外踝后，昆仑穴直上7寸，承山外下方1寸处（图1—49）。

［主治］ 腰腿疼痛、头痛。

［操作］ 直刺1～1.2寸（约25～40毫米）。

跗阳（BL59 Fūyáng 郄穴）

［定位］ 在小腿后面，外踝后，昆仑穴直上3寸（图1—50）。

［主治］ 头痛、腰骶疼痛、下肢痿痹。

［操作］ 直刺0.5～1寸（约15～25毫米）。

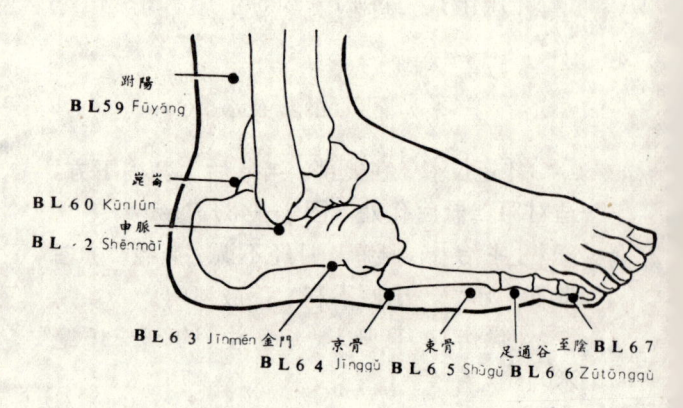

图1—50 足太阳膀胱经足部常用穴

Fig. 1—50 Commonly Used Acupoints of the Bladder Meridian at the Foot

昆仑（BL60 Kūnlún 经穴）

［定位］ 在足部外踝后方，当跟腱与外踝尖之间凹陷处（图1—50）。

［主治］ 头痛、项强、目眩、腰痛、难产、癫痫。

［操作］ 直刺0.5～0.8寸（约15～20毫米）。

申脉（BL62 Shēnmài 八脉交会穴）

［定位］ 在足外侧部，外踝直下方凹陷中（图1—50）。

［主治］ 头痛、目赤、失眠、眩晕、腰

腿酸痛、癫、狂、痫。

[操作] 直刺0.3~0.5寸（约9~15毫米）。

金门 (BL63 Jīnmén 郄穴)

[定位] 在足外侧，当外踝前缘直下，骰骨下缘处（图1—50）。

[主治] 头痛、癫痫。

[操作] 直刺0.3~0.5寸（约9~15毫米）。

京骨 (BL64 Jīnggǔ 原穴)

[定位] 足外侧，第五跖骨粗隆下，赤白肉际处取穴（图1—50）。

[主治] 头痛、项强、腰腿痛、癫痫。

[操作] 直刺0.3~0.5寸（约9~15毫米）。

束骨 (BL65 Shùgǔ 输穴)

[定位] 足外侧，足小趾本节（第5趾关节）的后方，赤白肉际处（图1—50）。

[主治] 头痛、项强、目眩、腰腿痛、癫狂。

[操作] 直刺0.3~0.5寸（约9~15毫米）。

足通谷 (BL66 Zútōnggǔ 荥穴)

[定位] 在足外侧，足小趾本节（第5跖趾关节）的前方，赤白肉际处（图1—50）。

[主治] 头痛、项强、目眩、鼻衄、癫狂。

[操作] 直刺0.2~0.3寸（约6~9毫米）。

至阴 (BL67 Zhìyīn 井穴)

[定位] 足小趾末节外侧，距趾甲角0.1寸（图1—50）。

[主治] 头痛、目痛、鼻塞、鼻衄、难产、胎位不正。

[操作] 浅刺0.1寸（约3毫米）。胎位不正可用灸法。

（三）常用经穴主治提要

本经腧穴主治头、项、目、背、腰、下肢病证及神志方面的病，背部的腧穴还主治与其相关的脏腑病证和有关的组织器官病证。如头痛、项强、目赤肿痛、胸背痛、腰痛、下肢痿痹、咳嗽、吐血、心痛、胁痛、胃脘痛、腹胀、呕吐、泄泻、小便不利、月经不调、癫、狂、痫等。其中睛明、攒竹、天柱治头痛、目疾；大杼、风门治伤风咳嗽；肺俞、厥阴俞、心俞、膈俞、膏肓俞治咳嗽、吐血，心悸等呼吸及心血管神志方面病；肝俞、胆俞治胁痛；脾俞、胃俞治胃脘痛，腹胀，呕吐，泄泻；三焦俞、大肠俞、小肠俞治腹胀，泄泻；肾俞、志室、次髎治月经不调、小便失常，遗精；膀胱俞治腰脊强痛、遗尿；承扶、殷门治腰痛；委阳、委中、秩边治小便不利、腰腿痛；飞扬、跗阳、昆仑治头痛，腰痛；申脉、金门、京骨、束骨、通谷、至阴治头痛、目疾、项强、癫、狂、痫；承山治便秘、腿痛转筋、痔疾等。

VII. THE BLADDER MERIDIAN OF FOOT—TAIYANG (67 points in total).

1. *The Course*

It starts from Jingming (BL 1) at the inner canthus (1). Ascending to the forehead (2), it meets Baihui (DU 20) at the vertex (3).

The branch arising at the vertex runs to the temple (4).

Another branch arising at the vertex which is straight enters and communicates with the brain (5). Then, it emerges and bifurcates to desced to the posterior aspect of the neck (6). Running downwards along the medial side of the scapula and parallel to the vertebral coloum (7), it reaches the lumbar region (8), and enters the body cavity via the paravertebral muscle (9) to connect with the kidney (10). Then, it enters the urinary bladder, its pertaining organ (11).

The branch arising in the lumbar region runs downwards through the gluteal region (12), and ends at the center of the popliteal fossa (13).

The branch arising at the nape passes downwards along the medial border of the scapula (14). Passing through the gluteal region (15) downwards along the posterolateral aspect of the thigh (16), it meets the branch from the lumbar region at the center of the popliteal fossa (17). From there, it runs downwards through the gastrocnemius (18) to the posterior aspect of the external malleolus (19). Then, it runs along the tuberosity of the 5th metatarsal bone (20) to reach zhiyin (BL 67) at the lateral border of the tip of the small toe, where it connects with the Kidney Meridian of Foot—Shaoyin (21).

The line made up by the acupoints distributed over the body surface: It starts at Jingming (BL1) at the inner canthus, ascends through the medial end of the eyebrow to the side of the midline of the head, then descends through the back of the neck. From there, it divides into two to go respectively downwards along the two lines which are 1.5 cun and 3.0 cun lateral to the vertebral column to the gluteal region, and along the posterior aspect of the thigh, and to join each other in the popliteal fossa. From there, it goes downwards along the posterior aspect of the lower leg to the posterior aspect of the external malleolus, and passes through the lateral side of the dorsum of the foot. Then, it ends at Zhiyin (BL67) at the lateral border of the tip of the little toe.

The inner organs concerned: The urinary bladder, kidney, brain.

2. *The Commonly Used Acupoints*

Jingming (BL1)

Location: On the face, in the depression 0.1 cun superior to the inner canthus (See Fig. 1—46).

Indications: Redness and swelling and pain in the eye, blurring vision, myopia, night blindness, some other eye problems.

Method: Ask the patient to close his eyes, fix the patient's eyeball by gently pushing it laterally with the left hand, insert the needle slowly with the right hand and perpendicularly insert it close to the orbital wall, inserting 0.5—1.0 cun (15 — 25mm) deep without twirling, lifting, or thrusting the needle. But gentle twirling, lifting, or thrusting manipulation may be allowed. Press the needle hole for a moment after withdrawal of the needle, otherwise bleeding may be caused. Generally, it is not advisable to retain the needle, and moxibustion is prohibited.

Cuanzhu (Zanzhu BL2)

Location: On the face, in the depression at the medial end of the eyebrow, at the supraorbital notch (See Fig. 1—46).

Indications: Pain in the supercillary ridge, blurring vision, redness and swelling and pain in the eye, myopia, lacrimation, ptosis of the eyelids.

Method: Puncture horizontally 0.3—0.5 cun (9—15mm) towards the middle of the eyebrow. Moxibustion is contraindicated.

Tianzhu (BL10)

Location: On the nape, 0.5 cun above the posterior hairline, 1.3 cun lateral to the posterior midline, at the depression at the lateral border of m. trapezius (See Fig. 1—47).

Indications: headache and stiff neck, nasal stuffiness, pain in the shoulder and back.

Method: Puncture perpendicularly or obliquely 0.5—0.8 cun (15—20mm), avoiding puncturing deep toward the medial and superior area, otherwise the bulb may be injured.

Dazhu (BL11, Influent point of bone)

Location: On the back, 1.5 cun lateral to the posterior midline, below the spinous process of the 1st thoracic vertebra (See Fig. 1—48).

Indications: Cough, fever, stiffness and rigidity of the neck, aching of the scapular region.

Method: Puncture obliquely 0.5—0.8 cun (15—20mm) toward the interspace of the spines, never puncture deep otherwise the lung may be injured. Moxibustion is applicable.

Fengmen (BL12)

Location: On the back, 1.5 cun lateral to the posterior midline, below the spinous process of the 2nd thoracic vertebra (See Fig. 1—48).

Indications: Common cold with cough, fever and headache, nasal stuffiness, stiff neck, pain in the chest and back.

Method: Puncture obliquely 0.5—0.8 cun (15—20mm) toward the interspace of the spines. Moxibustion is applicable.

Feishu (BL13, Back—Shu point of the lung)

Location: On the back, 1.5 cun lateral to the posterior midline, below the spinous process of the 3rd thoracic vertebra (See Fig. 1—48).

Indications: Cough, asthma, fullness of the chest, hematemesis, hemoplysis, hectic fever.
Method: Puncture obliquely 0.5—0.8 cun (15 — 20mm) toward the interspace of the spines. Moxibustion is applicable.

Jueyinshu (BL14, Back—Shu point of the pericardium)

Location: On the back, 1.5 cun lateral to the posterior midline, below the spinous process of the 4th thoracic vertebra (See Fig. 1—48).
Indications: Cough, palpitation, cardiac pain, oppressed feeling in the chest, vomiting.
Method: Punctre obliquely 0.5—0.8 cun (15 — 20mm) toward the interspace of the spines. Moxibustion is applicable.

Xinshu (BL15, Back — Shu point of the heart)

Location: On the back, 1.5 cun lateral to the posterior midline, below the spinous process of the 5th thoracic vertebra (See Fig. 1—48).
Indications: Cardiac pain, palpitation, insomnia, amnesia, restlessness, cough, hematemsis, hemoptysis, epilepsy.
Method: Puncture obliquely 0.5—0.8 cun (15 — 20mm) toward the interspace of the spines. Moxibustion is applicable.

Geshu (BL17, Influential point relating to the blood)

Location: On the back, 1.5 cun lateral to the posterior midline, below the spinous process of the 7th thoracic vertebra (See Fig. 1—48).
Indications: Vomiting, hiccup, distension and fullness in the stomach, hematemesis, hemoptysis, hectic fever, night sweating.
Method: Puncture obliquely 0.5—0.8 cun (15 — 20mm) toward the interspace of the spines. Moxibustion is applicable.

Ganshu (BL18, Back—Shu point of the liver)

Location: On the back, 1.5 cun lateral to the posterior midline, below the spinous process of the 9th thoracic vertebra (See Fig. 1—48).
Indications: Jaundice, hypochondriac pain, hematemesis, hemoptysis, dizziness, nyctalopia, mania, epilepsy, redness of the eye.
Method: Puncture obliquely 0.5—0.8 cun (15 — 20mm) toward the interspace fo the spines. Moxibustion is applicable.

Danshu (BL19, Back—Shu point of the gall—bladder)

Location: On the back, 1.5 cun lateral to the posterior midline, below the spinous process of the 10th thoracic vertebra (See Fig. 1—48).

Indications: Jaundice, bitter taste in the mouth, hypochondriac pain, vomiting.

Method: Puncture obliquely 0.5—0.8 cun (15—20mm) toward the interspace of the spines. Moxibustion is applicable.

Pishu (BL20, Back—Shu point of the spleen)

Location: On the back, 1.5 cun lateral to the posterior midline, below the spinous process of the 11th thoracic vertebra (See Fig. 1—48).

Indications: Abdominal distension, vomiting, diarrhea, edema, bloody stool.

Method: Puncture obliquely 0.5—0.8 cun (15—20mm) toward the interspace of the spines. Moxibustion is applicable.

Weishu (BL21, Back—Shu point of the stomach)

Location: On the back, 1.5 cun lateral to the posterior midline, below the spinous process of the 12th thoracic vertebra (See Fig. 1—48).

Indications: Stomachache, abdominal distension, vomiting, borborygmus.

Method: Puncture obliquely 0.5—0.8 cun (15—20mm) toward the interspace between the spines. Moxibustion is applicable.

Sanjiaoshu (BL22, Back—Shu point of the triple energizer)

Location: On the low back, 1.5 cun lateral to the posterior midline, below the spinous process of the 1st lumbar vertebra (See Fig. 1—48).

Indications: Abdominal distension, borborygmus, vomiting, diarrhea, dysuria, edema, pain in the lumbar region and back.

Method: Puncture perpendicularly 0.5—0.8 cun (15—20mm). Moxibustion is applicable.

Shenshu (BL23, Back—Shu point of the kidney)

Location: On the low back, 1.5 cun lateral to the posterior midline, below the spinous process of the 2nd lumbar vertebra (See Fig. 1—48).

Indications: Enuresis, emission, impotence, frequent urination, irregular menstruation, dysuria, edema, tinnitus, lumbago.

Method: Puncture perpendicularly 1.0—1.2 cun (25—30mm). Moxibustion is applicable.

Dachangshu (BL25, Back—Shu point of the large intestine)

Location: On the low back, 1.5 cun lateral to the posterior midline, below the spinous process of the 4th lumbar vertebra (See Fig. 1—48).

Indications: Abdominal pain and distension, diarrhea, constipation, pain in

the back and lumbar region.
Method: Puncture perpendicularly 1.0—1.2 cun (25—30mm). Moxibustion is applicable.

Xiaochangshu (BL27, Back—Shu point of the small intestine)

Location: On the sacrum and on the level of the 1st posterior sacral foramen, 1.5 cun lateral to the median sacral crest (See Fig. 1—48).

Indications: Lower abdominal distension and pain, diarrhea, enuresis, hematuria, emission, leukorrhea, hernia.

Method: Puncture perpendicularly 1.0—1.2 cun (25—30mm). Moxibustion is applicable.

Pangguangshu (BL28, Back—Shu point of bladder)

Location: On the sacrum and on the level of the 2nd posterior sacral foramen, 1.5 cun lateral to the median sacral crest (See Fig. 1—48).

Indications: Dysuria, enuresis, abdominal pain and diarrhea, constipation, stiffness and pain of the lower back.

Method: Puncture perpendicularly 1.0—1.2 cun (25—30mm). Moxibustion is applicable.

Ciliao (BL32)

Location: On the sacrum, at the 2nd posterior sacral foramen, medial and inferior to the posterior superior iliac spine and the Governor Vessel (See Fig. 1—48).

Indications: Lumbago, abnormal menstruation, dysmenorrhea, leukorrhea with reddish discharge, hernia, dysuria, flaccidity and arthralgia of the lower limbs.

Method: Puncture perpendicularly 1.0—1.5 cun (25—40mm). Moxibustion is applicable.

Chengfu (BL36)

Location: On the posterior side of the thigh and on the midpoint of the inferior transverse gluteal fold (See Fig. 1—49).

Indications: Hemorrhoids, pain in the lumbar, sacral, gluteal and femoral regions.

Method: Puncture perpendicularly 1.0—2.0 cun (25—50mm). Moxibustion is applicable.

Yinmen (BL37)

Location: On the posterior side of the thigh and on the line connecting Chengfu (BL36) and Weizhong (BL40), 6 cun distal to Chengfu (BL36) (See Fig. 1—49).

Indications: Stiffness and pain of the lumbar region, flaccidity and arthralgia of the lower limbs.

Method: Puncture perpendicularly 1.0—2.0 cun (25—50mm). Moxibustion is applicable.

Weiyang (BL39, Lower Confluent point of

the Triple Energizer Meridian)

Location: At the lateral end of the transverse popliteal fold, on the medial border of the tendon of m. biceps femoris with knee the flexed (See Fig. 1—49).

Indications: Lower abdominal distension and fullness, dysuria, stiffness and pain of the lower back, muscular spasm and pain in the calf and foot.

Method: Puncture perpendicularly 0.5—1.0 cun (15—25mm). Moxibustion is applicable.

Weizhong (BL40, He-Sea point)

Location: At the midpoint of the transverse popliteal fold, between the tendons of the biceps muscle of the thigh and the semitendinous muscle (See Fig. 1—49).

Indications: Lumbago, abdominal pain, flaccidity and arthralgia of the lower limbs, vomiting and diarrhea, dysuria, erysipelas.

Method: Puncture perpendicularly 0.5—1.0 cun (15—25mm). Or prick with the three—edged needle to cause bleeding.

Gaohuang (BL43)

Location: On the back, 3 cun lateral to the posterior midline, level with the interspace between the 4th and 5th thoracic vertebrae, at the medial border of the scapula (See Fig. 1—48).

Indications: Cough, asthma, hematemesis, hemoptysis, night sweating.

Method: Puncture obliquely 0.5—0.8 cun (15—20mm). Moxibustion is applicable.

Zhishi (BL52)

Location: On the lower back, 3 cun lateral to the posterior midine, level with the interspace between the 2nd and 3rd lumbar vertebrae (See Fig. 1—48).

Indications: Dysuria, edema, impotence, stiffness and pain of the lower back.

Method: Puncture obliquely 0.5—0.8 cun (15—20mm). Moxibustion is applicable.

Zhibian (BL54)

Location: On the buttock and on the level of the 4th posterior sacvel foramen, 3 cun lateral to the median sacral crest (See Fig. 1—48).

Indications: Dysuria, constipation, pain in the lumbar and sacral regions, flaccidity and arthralgia of the lower limbs.

Method: Puncture perpendicularly 1.5—2.0 cun (25—50mm). Moxibustion is applicable.

Chengshan (BL 57)

Location: On the posterior midline of the leg, between Weizhong (BL 40) and Kunlun (BL 60), in pointed depression formed below the gastrocnemius muscle belly when the leg is stretched or the heel is lifted (See Fig. 1—49).

Indications: Pain and muscular cramp in the calf, lumbago, pain in the back, hemorrhoids, constipation, beriberi.

Method: Puncture perpendicularly about 1.0 cun (25mm). Moxibustion is applicable.

Feiyang (BL 58, Luo—Connecting point)

Location: On the posterior side of the leg, 7 cun proximal to Kunlun (B 60), 1 cun inferior lateral to Chengshan (BL 51) (See Fig. 1—49).

Indications: Pain in the lower back and leg, headache.

Method: Puncture perpendicularly 1.0—1.5 cun (25—40mm). Moxibustion is applicable.

Fuyang (BL 59, Xi—Cleft point of the Yangqiao Channel)

Location: On the posterior side of the leg, posterior to the lateral malleolus, 3 cun directly above Kunlun (BL 60) (See Fig. 1—50).

Indications: Headache, pain in the lumbar and sacral regions, flaccidity and arthralgia of the lower limbs.

Method: Puncture perpendicularly 0.5—1.0 cun (15—25mm). Moxibustion is applicable.

Kunlun (BL 60, Jing—River point)

Location: Posterior to the lateral malleolus, at the depression between the tendon of m. calcaneus and the tip of the external malleolus (See Fig. 1—50).

Indications: Headache, stiffness of the neck, dizziness, lumbago, difficult labour, epilepsy.

Method: Puncture perpendicularly 0.5—0.8 cun (15—20mm). Moxibustion is applicable.

Shenmai (BL 62, one of the Eight Confluence points)

Location: On the lateral side of the foot, in the depression directly below the external malleolus (See Fig. 1—50).

Indications: Headache, redness in the eye, insomnia, dizziness, aching of the lower back and leg, epilepsy, mania.

Method: Puncture perpendicularly 0.3—0.5 cun (9—15mm). Moxibustion is applicable.

Jinmen (BL63, Xi—Cleft point)

Location: On the lateral side of the foot, directly below the anterior border of the external malleolus, on the lower border of the cuboid bone (See Fig. 1—50).

Indications: Headche, epilepsy.

Method: Puncture perpendicularly 0.3—0.5 cun (9—15mm). Moxibustion is applicable.

Jinggu (BL 64, Yuan—Source point)

Location: At the lateral aspect of the tarsus of the foot, below the tuberosity of the 5th metatarsal bone, at the dorso—ventral boundary of the foot (See Fig. 1—50).
Indications: Headache, stiffness of the neck, pain in the lower back and leg, epilepsy.
Method: Puncture perpendicularly 0.3—0.5 cun (9—15mm). Moxibustion is applicable.

Shugu (BL 65, Shu—Stream point)

Location: At the lateral aspect of the tarsus of the foot, posterior to the 5th metatarsophalangeal joint at the dorso—ventral boundary of the foot (See Fig. 1—50).
Indications: Headache, stiffness of neck, dizziness, pain in the lower back and leg, epilepsy and mania.
Method: Puncture perpendicularly 0.3—0.5 cun (9—15mm). Moxibustion is applicable.

Zutonggu (BL 66, Ying—Spring point)

Location: On the lateral side of the foot, anterior to the 5th metatarsal phalangeal joint, at the dorso—ventral boundary of the foot (See Fig. 1—50).
Indications: Headache, stiff neck, dizziness, epilepsy, mania, epistaxis.
Method: Puncture perpendicularly 0.2—0.3 cun (6—9mm). Moxibustion is applicable.

Zhiyin (BL 67, Jing—Well point)

Location: At the lateral side of the distal segment of the small toe, about 0.1 cun posterior to the corner of the nail (See Fig. 1—50).
Indications: Headache, pain in the eye, nasal stuffiness, epilepsy, epitaxis, difficult labour, malposition of the fetus.
Method: Puncture shallowly 0.1 cun (about 3mm). For malposition of the fetus moxibustion should be applied.

3. *An Outline of Indications of the Commonly Used Acupoints*

The acupoints of this meridian are mainly used in treatment of disorders of head, neck, eye, back, waist, and lower limb, as well as mental disorders. Of them, those on the back are indicated in disorders of the concerned zang and fu organs, as well as diseases of some body portions, such as headache, stiff neck, redness and swelling and pain of eye, pain in chest and back, lumbago, flaccidity and arthralgia of the lower limb, cough, hematemesis and hemoptysis, cardiac pain, hypochondriac pain, stomachache, abdominal distension, vomiting, diarrhea, dysuria, irregular menstruation, epilepsy and mania. In the concrete, usually, Jingming (BL1), Cuanzhu (BL2) and Tianzhu (BL10) are indicated in headache, eye disorders; Dashu (BL11) and Fengmen (BL12), in common cold with cough; Feishu (BL13), Jueyinshu (BL14), Xinshu (BL15), Geshu

(BL17), and Gaohuang (BL43), in cough, hematemsis and hemoptysis, palpitation, and some other symptomes which are related to the respiratary system, cardiovascular system and the brain; Ganshu (BL20) and Danshu (BL19), in hypochondriac pain; Pishu (BL20) and Weishu (BL21), in stomachache, abdominal distension, vomiting, diarrhea; Sanjiaoshu (BL22), Dachangshu (BL25), and Xiaochangshu (BL27), in abdominal distension, diarrhea; Shenshu (BL23), Zhishi (BL52), and Ciliao (BL32), in irreglar menstruation, dysuia, emission; Pangguangshu (BL28), in stiffness and psin of the lumbosacral region, enuresis; Chengfu (BL36) and Jinmen (BL37), in lumbago; Weizhong (BL40), Weiyang (BL39), and Zhibian (BL54), in dysuria and pain in the waist and leg; Feiyang (BL58), Fuyang (BL59), and Kunlun (BL60), in headache and lumbago; Shenmai (BL62), Jinmen (BL63), Jingu (BL64), Shugu (BL65), Zutonggu (BL66), and Zhiyin (BL67), in headache, eye disorders, stiff neck, epilepsy and mania; and Chengshan (BL57), in constipation, pain and muscular scramp of the leg, and hemorrhoids.

八、足少阴肾经（共27穴）

（一）经脉循行

1. 起于足小趾之下，斜向足心涌泉穴；2. 出于舟骨粗隆下；3. 沿着内踝后面；4. 进入足跟；5. 再向上行于小腿肚内侧；6. 出腘窝的内侧；7. 上行于股内后缘；8. 贯通脊柱，属于肾脏；9. 联络膀胱；10. 肾脏部直行的脉；11. 从肾向上通过肝和横膈；12. 进入肺中；13. 沿着喉咙；14. 挟于舌根部；15. 肺部支脉：从肺部出来，联络心脏，流注于胸中，与手厥阴心包经相接。

体表穴位分布线：起于足心涌泉穴，绕内踝后，沿下肢内侧后缘，入小腹，挟腹正中线旁开5分，胸正中线旁开2寸，止于锁骨下俞府穴。

体内相关的组织脏器：肾、膀胱、肝、肺、心、脊柱、喉咙、舌根。

（二）本经常用腧穴

涌泉（KI1 Yǒngquán 井穴）

［定位］ 在足底部，卷足时足前部凹陷处，约当足底2、3趾趾缝纹头端与足跟连线的前三分之一与后三分之二交点上（图1—52）。

［主治］ 咽喉肿痛、小便不利、便秘、昏厥、头痛、目眩、小儿惊风、癫、狂。

［操作］ 直刺0.5～1寸（约15～25毫米）。

然谷（KI2 Ránggǔ 荥穴）

［定位］ 在足内侧缘，足舟骨粗隆下方，赤白肉际（图1—53）。

［主治］ 月经不调、遗精、咳血、消渴。

［操作］ 直刺0.5～1寸（约15～25毫米）。

太溪（KI3 Tàixī 输穴，原穴）

［定位］ 在足内侧，内踝后方，足内踝尖与跟腱之间的凹陷中（图1—53）。

［主治］ 咽喉肿痛、咳血、月经不调、齿痛、失眠、耳鸣。

［操作］ 直刺0.5～1寸（约20毫米）。

经络腧穴概要

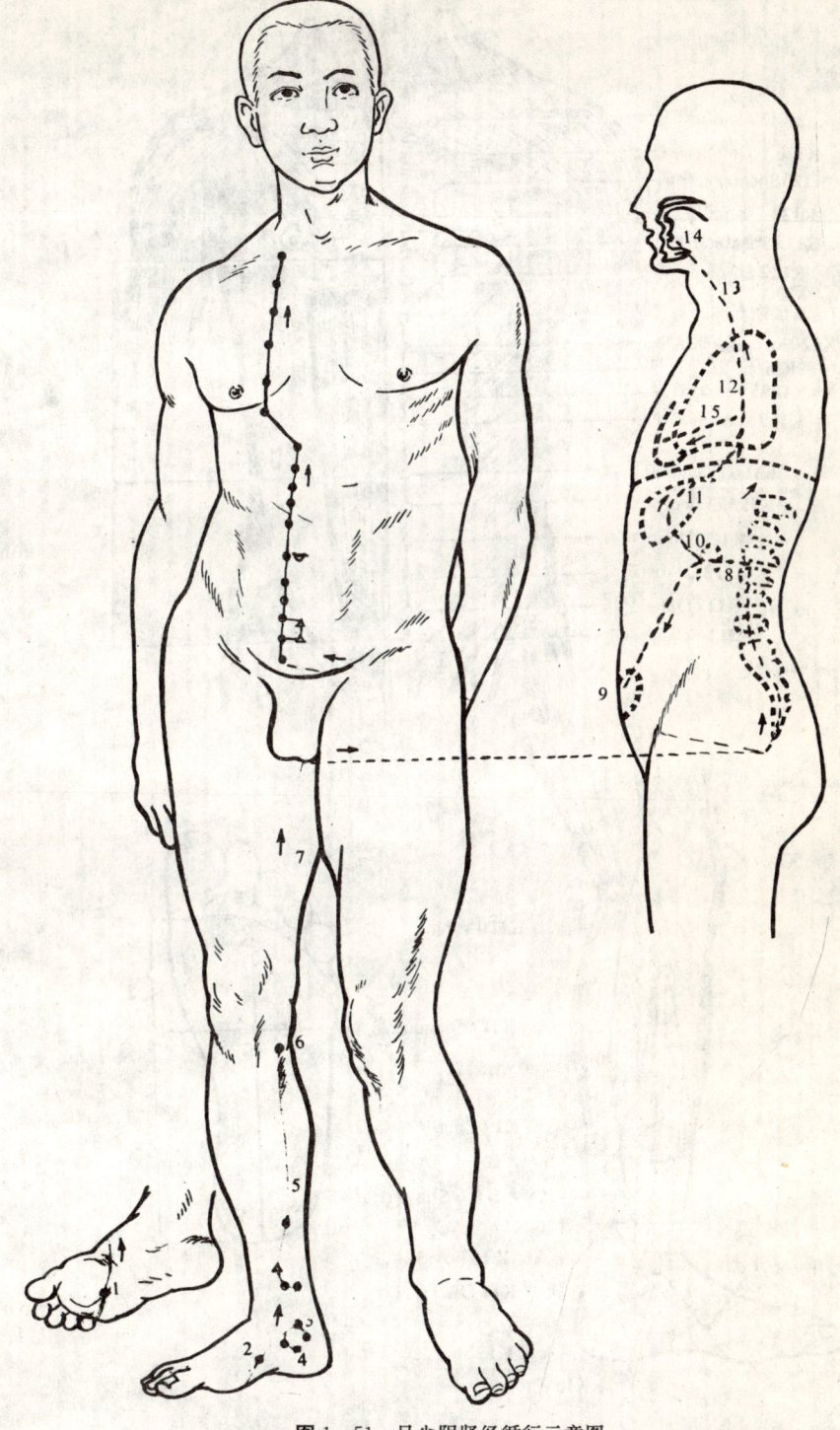

图 1—51 足少阴肾经循行示意图
Fig. 1—51 The Running Course of the Kidney Meridian of Foot—Shaoyin

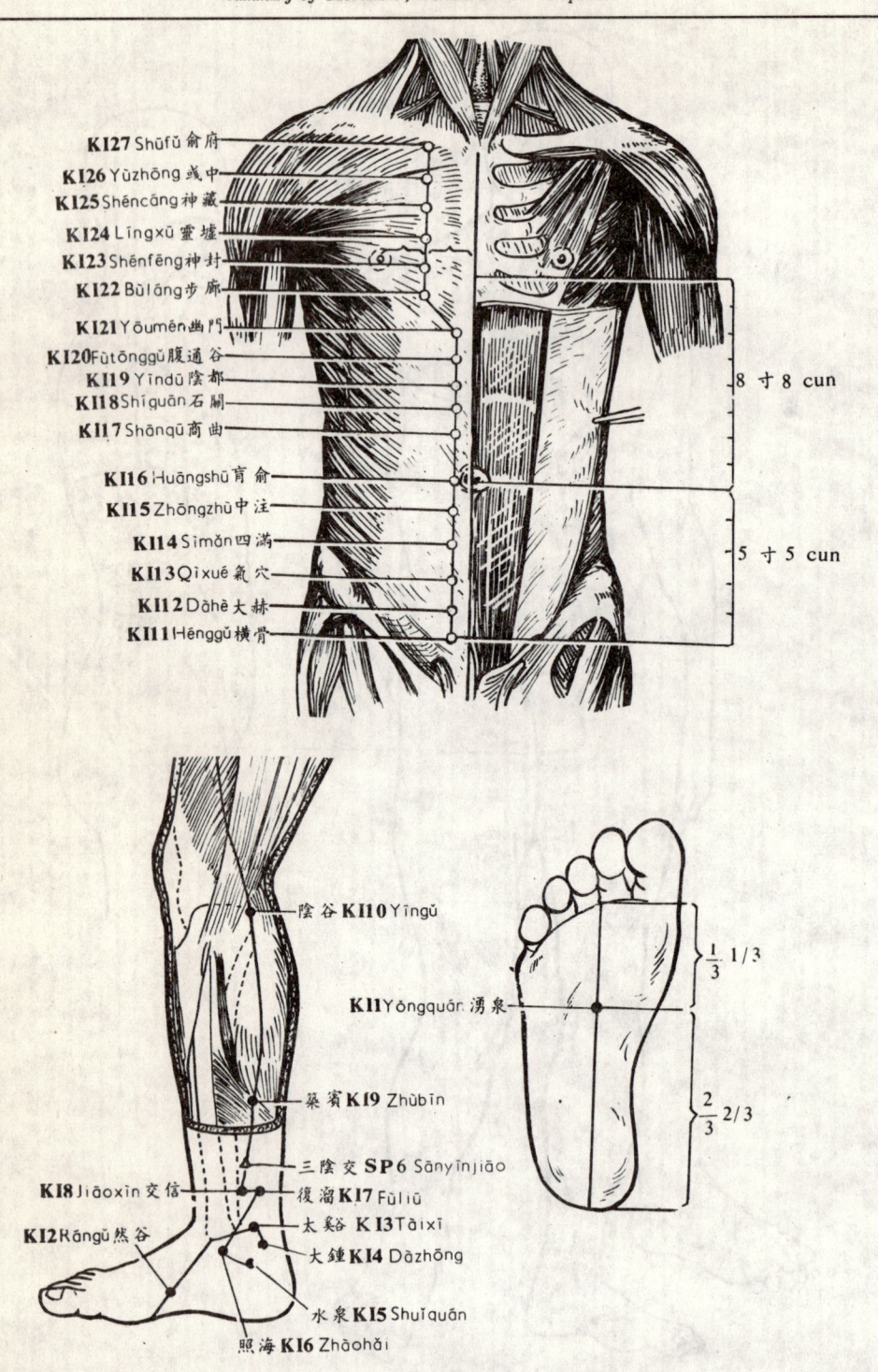

图 1—52 足少阴肾经穴位图
Fig. 1—52 The Acupoints of the Kidney Meridian of Foot-Shaoyin

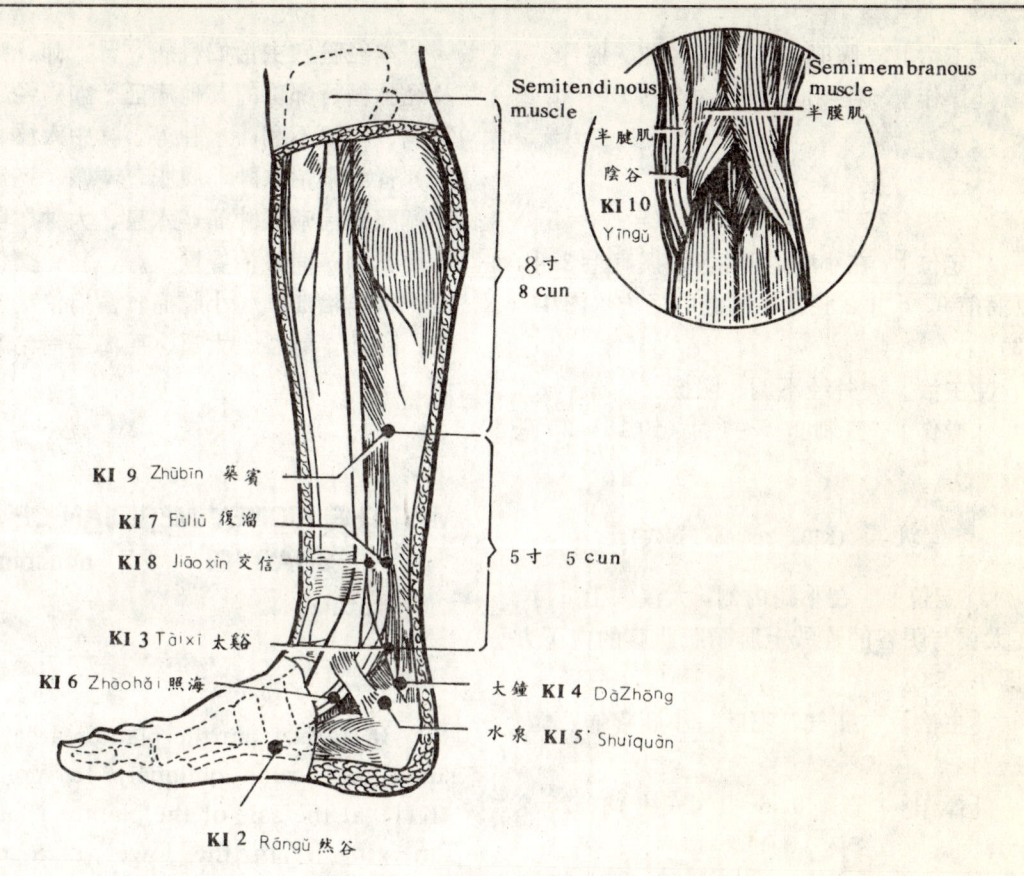

图 1—53 足少阴肾经下肢常用穴
Fig. 1—53 Commonly Used Acupoints of the Kidney Meridian at the Lower Limb

大钟（KI4 Dàzhōng 络穴）

［定位］ 在足内侧，内踝后下方，当跟腱附着部的内侧前方凹陷处（图1—53）。

［主治］ 癃闭、遗尿、便秘、足跟痛、痴呆。

［操作］ 直刺0.3～0.5寸（约9～15毫米）。

水泉（KI5 Shuǐquán 郄穴）

［定位］ 在足内侧，内踝后下方，当太溪直下1寸，跟骨结节的内侧凹陷处（图1—53）。

［主治］ 月经不调、痛经、小便不利。

［操作］ 直刺0.3～0.5寸（约9～15毫米）。

照海（KI6 Zhàohǎi）

［定位］ 在足内侧，内踝尖下方之凹陷中（图1—53）。

［主治］ 咽喉干痛、月经不调、便秘、癫、狂、失眠。

［操作］ 直刺0.3～0.5寸（约9～15毫米）。

复溜（KI7 Fùliū 经穴）

［定位］ 在小腿内侧，太溪直上2寸，当跟腱之前方取穴（图1—53）。

［主治］ 腹胀、泄泻、水肿、盗汗。
［操作］ 直刺0.6～1寸（约18～25毫米）。

交信 (KI8 Jiāoxìn)

［定位］ 在小腿内侧，当太溪直上2寸，复溜前0.5寸，胫骨内侧缘的后方（图1—53）。
［主治］ 月经不调、阴挺。
［操作］ 直刺0.6～1寸（约18～25毫米）。

筑宾 (KI9 Zhúbīn 郄穴)

［定位］ 在小腿内侧，太溪穴上5寸。在太溪与阴谷的连线上腓肠肌肌腹的内下方（图1—53）。
［主治］ 疝气、呕吐、小腿疼痛、癫、狂。
［操作］ 直刺0.6～1寸（约18～25毫米）。

阴谷 (KI10 Yīngǔ 合穴)

［定位］ 在腘窝内侧，屈膝时，在半腱肌肌腱和半膜肌肌腱之间取穴（图1—53）。
［主治］ 阳萎、崩漏、小便不利。
［操作］ 直刺0.6～1寸（约18～25毫米）。

俞府 (KI27 Shūfǔ)

［定位］ 在胸部，锁骨下缘，前正中线旁开2寸（图1—52）。
［主治］ 咳嗽、气喘、胸痛。
［操作］ 斜刺或平刺0.5～0.8寸（约15～20毫米），不可深刺，以防伤及内脏。

（三）常用经穴主治提要

本经腧穴主治妇科病，肾、肺、咽喉病及经脉循行部位的其他病证。如痛经、月经不调、小便不利、水肿等。其中太溪、复溜穴补肾壮阳治水肿，腹胀、喘咳、盗汗、自汗；照海治咽喉肿痛；水泉、大钟、阴谷治小便不利；涌泉治昏厥、癫、狂；交信治阴挺；筑宾治疝气、小腿痛；俞府治喘咳、胸痛；除外，然谷、太溪、照海等尚治月经不调。

VIII. THE KIDNEY MERIDIAN OF FOOT — SHAOYIN (27 acupoints in total)

1. The Course

It starts from the plantar area of the small toe, runs obliquely to Yongquan (KI1) at the sole of the plantar foot (1). Emerging from the lower area of the tuberosity of the navicular bone (2) and running behind the medial malleolus (3), it enters the heel (4). Then, it ascends along the medial side of the calf of the leg (5) to the medial side of the popliteal fossa (6), and goes further upwards along the posterior medial border of the thigh (7) towards the vertebral column. It connects with the kidney, its pertaining organ (8), and communicates with the urinary bladder (9).

The trunk starting from the kidney (10) ascends and passes through the liver and the diaphragm (11), and enters the lung (12). Then, it further ascends along the throat (13), and terminates at the root of the tongue (14).

The branch starting from the lung

comes out from the lung to connect with the heart. Then, it distributes in the chest to connect with the Pericardium Meridian of Hand—Jueyin. (15).

The line made up by the acupoints distributed on the body surface: It starts from the sole at Yongquan (Ki1), runs behind the medial malleolus, and ascends along the posterior border of the medial side of the lower limb to reach the lower abdomen. Then, it further ascends along the line 0.5 cun lateral to the midline of the abdomen and 2.0 cun lateral to the midline of the chest, and ends at the point Shufu (KI27) below the clavicle.

The inner organs concerned: The kidney, urinary bladder, liver, lung, heart, vertebral column, throat, and the root of the tongue.

2. *The Commonly Used Acupoints*

Yongquan (KI1, Jing-Well point)

Location: On the sole, in the depression appearing on the anterior part of the sole when the foot is in the plantar flexion, approxiately at the junction of the anterior third and posterior two—thirds of the line connecting the base of the 2nd and 3rd toes and the heel (See Fig. 1—52).
Indications: Swelling and sore throat, dysuria, constipation, loss of consciousness, headache, dizziness, infantile convulsion, epilepsy and mania.
Method: Puncture perpendicularly 0.5—1.0 cun (15—25mm). Moxibustion is applicable.

Rangu (KI2, Ying—Spring point)

Location: On the medial border of the foot, below the tuberosity of the navicular bone, and at the junction of the red and white skin (See Fig. 1—53).
Indication: Abnormal menstuation, emission, hemoptysis, diabetes.
Method: Puncture perpendicularly 0.5—0.9 cun (15—25mm). Moxibustion is applicable.

Taixi (KI3, Shu—Stream and Yuan—Source point)

Location: On the medial side of the foot, posterior to the medial malleolus, at the depression betwen the tip of the medial malleolus and the tendon of m. calcaneus (See Fig. 1—53).
Indications: Swelling and sore throat, hemoptysis, abnormal menstruation, toothache, insomnia, tinnitus.
Method: Puncture perpendicularly 0.5—1.0 cun (15—25mm). Moxibustion is applicable.

Dazhong (KI4, Luo—Connecting point)

Location: On the medial side of the foot, posterior and inferior to the medial malleolus, in the depression of the medial side of and anterior to the attachment of the

Achilles tendon (See Fig. 1—53).

Indications: Uroschesis, enuresis, constipation, pain in the heel, dementia.

Method: Puncture perpendicularly 0.3—0.5 cun (9—15mm). Moxibustion is applicable.

Shuiquan (KI5 Xi—Cleft point)

Location: On the medial side of the foot, posterior and inferior to the medial malleolus, 1 cun directly below Taixi (KI3), in the depression of the medial side of the tuberosity of the calcaneum (See Fig. 1—53).

Indications: Abnormal menstuation, dysmenorrhea, dysuria.

Method: Puncture perpendicularly 0.3—0.5 cun (9—15mm). Moxibustion is applicable.

Zhaohai (KI6, one of the Eight Confluence points)

Location: On the medial side of the foot, in the depression of the lower border of the medial malleolus (See Fig. 1—53).

Indications: Dry and sore throat, abnormal menstruation, constipation, epilepsy and mania, insomnia.

Method: Puncture perpendicularly 0.3-0.5 cun (9-15mm). Moxibustion is applicable.

Fuliu (KI7, Jing-River point)

Location: On the medial side of the leg, 2 cun above Taixi (KI3), anterior to the tendon calcaneus (See Fig. 1—53).

Indications: Abdominal distension, diarrhea, edema, night sweating.

Method: Puncture perpendicularly 0.5—1.0 cun (15—25mm). Moxibustion is applicable.

Jiaoxin (KI8, Xi—Cleft point of the Yinqiao Channel)

Location: On the medial side of the leg, 2 cun above Taixi (KI 3) and 0.5 cun anterior to Fuliu (KI 7), posterior to the medial border of the tibia (See Fig. 1—53).

Indications: Abnormal menstruation, prolapse of the uterus.

Method: Puncture perpendicularly 0.6—1.0 cun (15—25mm). Moxibustion is applicable.

Zhubin (KI9, Xi—Cleft point of the Yinwei Channel)

Location: On the medial side of the leg, 5 cun proximal to Taixi (KI3), at the line connecting Taixi (KI3) and Yingu (KI10), medial and inferior to the gastrocnemius muscle belly (See Fig. 1—53).

Indications: Hernia, vomiting, pain in the leg, epilepsy, mania.

Method: Puncture perpendicularly 0.6—1.0 cun (15—25mm). Moxibustion is applicable.

Yingu (KI10, He—Sea point)

Location: When the knee is flexed, the point is at the medial side of the transverse popliteal fossa, at the same level as Weizhong (B40), between the tendons of m. semitendinosus and semimembranosus (See Fig. 1—53).

Indications: Impotence, metrorrhagia, metrostaxis, dysuria.

Method: Puncture perpendicularly 0.6—1.0 cun (15—25mm). Moxibustion is applicable.

Shufu (KI27)

Location: On the chest, below the lower border of the clavicle, 2 cun lateral to the midsternal line (See Fig. 1—52).

Indications: Cough, asthma, pain in the chest

Method: Puncture obliquely or horizontally 0.5—0.8 cun (15—20mm), avoiding deep puncture so as to prevent the internal organs from being injured. Moxibustion is applicable.

3. *An Outline of Indications of the Commonly Used Acupoints*

The acupoints of this meridian are mainly used in treatment of disorders of the gynecology, and diseases of the lung, kidney and throat, as well as some other symptoms appearing on the pathway of this meridian, such as dysmenorrhea, abnormal menstruation, dysuria, edema. In the concrete, Taixi (KI3) and Fuliu (KI7) are used to reinforce the kidney and strengthen kidney—yang for treatment of edema, abdominal distension, asthma, nigtht sweating, and spontaneous perspiration; Zhaohai (KI6) is indicated in sore throat; Shuiquan (KI5), Dazhong (KI4), and Yingu (KI10), in dysuria; Yongquan (KI1), in syncope and insanity; Jiaoxin (KI6), in prolapse of uterus; Zhubin (KI9), in pain of the lower leg; Shufu (KI27), in asthma and cough, pain in the chest; and Rangu (KI2) and Taixi (KI3) and Zhaohai (KI6), in abnormal menstruation.

九、手厥阴心包经（共9穴）

（一）经脉循行：

1. 起于胸中，出属心包络；2. 向下通过横膈；3. 从胸至腹，依次联络上、中、下三焦。

4. 胸部支脉：沿着胸中；5. 出走于胁部，向下至腋下三寸处（天池穴）；6. 再向上抵达腋窝中；7. 沿着上臂内侧，行于手太阴和手少阴之间；8. 再进入肘窝中；9. 向下行于前臂掌长肌腱与桡侧腕屈肌腱之间；10. 进入掌中；11. 沿着中指到指端（中冲穴）。

12. 掌中支脉：从劳宫分出，沿着无名指到指端（关冲穴），与手少阳三焦经相接。

体表穴位分布线：起于乳头外侧天池穴，上行腋窝、沿着上肢内侧之中，下两筋间，进入掌中，止于中指之端中冲穴。

体内相关的组织脏器：心包、三焦。

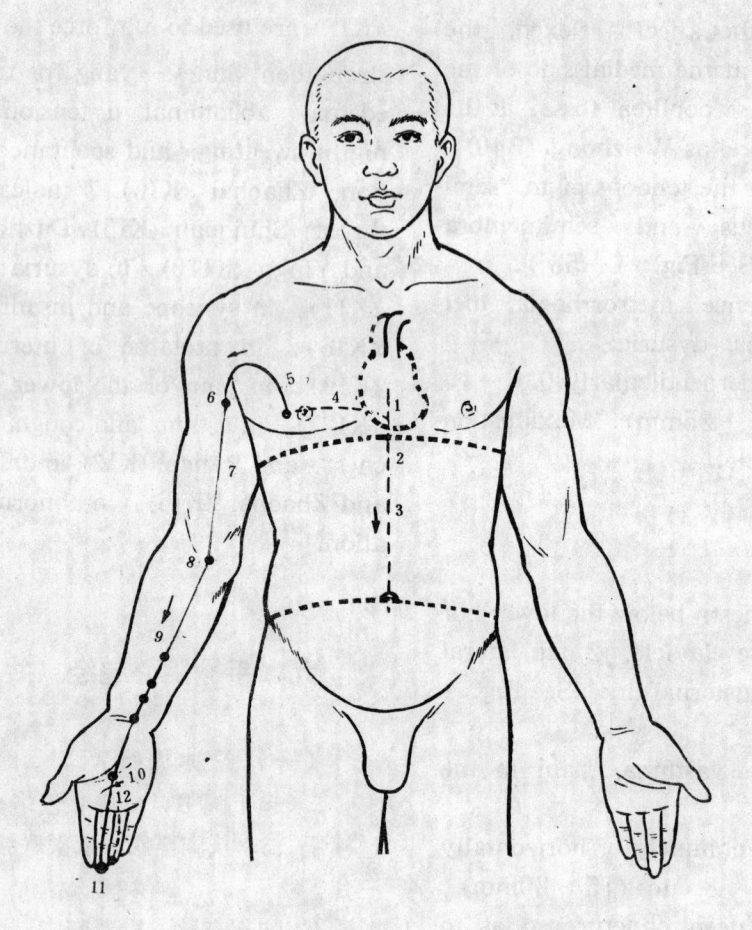

图 1—54 手厥阴心包经循行示意图
Fig. 1—54. The Running Course of the Pericardium Meridian of Hand—Jueyin

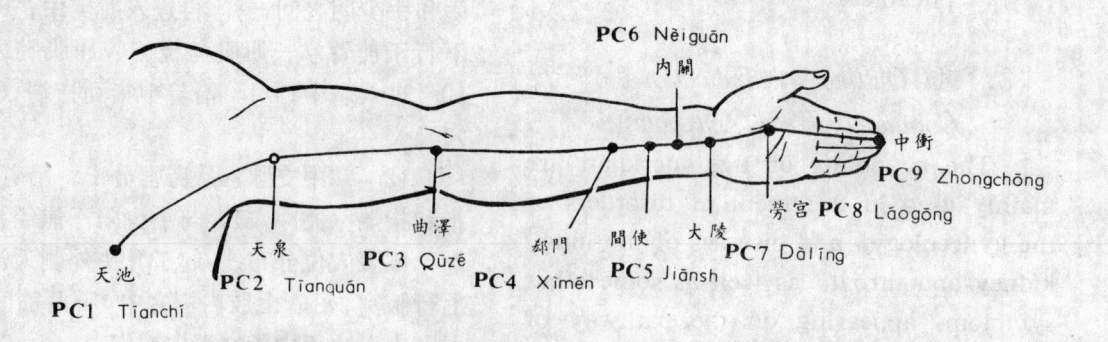

图 1—55 手厥阴心包经穴位图
Fig. 1—55 The Acupoints of the Pericardium Meridian of Hand—Jueyin

（二）本经常用腧穴

天池 (PC1　Tiānchí)

[定位]　在胸部，第四肋间隙中，乳头外侧1寸，前正中线旁开5寸（图1—55）。

[主治]　胸闷、瘰疬。

[操作]　斜刺或平刺0.3～0.5寸（约9～15毫米），不可深刺，以防刺伤肺脏。

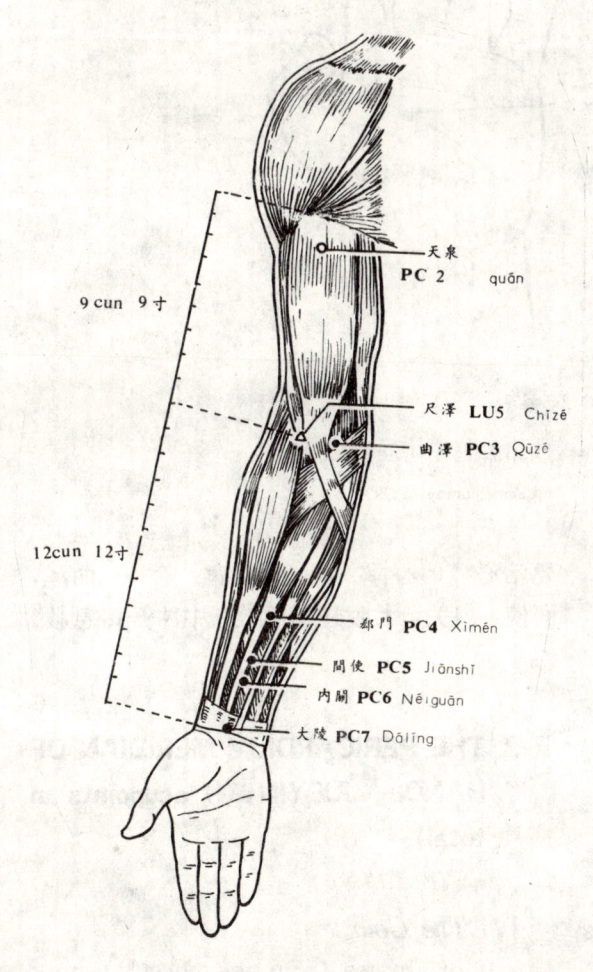

图1—56　手厥阴心包经上肢常用穴
Fig. 1—56 Commonly Used Acupoints of the Pericardium Meridian at the Upper Limb

曲泽 (PC3　Qūzé)

[定位]　在肘横纹中，肱二头肌腱的尺侧缘（图1—56）。

[主治]　心痛、胃痛、呕吐、热病。

[操作]　直刺0.8～1寸（约20～25毫米），或用三棱针刺血。

郄门 (PC4　Xìmén　郄穴)

[定位]　在前臂掌侧，腕横纹上5寸，当曲泽穴与大陵穴的连线上，（图1—56）。

[主治]　心痛、心悸、呕血。

[操作]　直刺0.5～1寸（约15～25毫米）。

间使 (PC5　Jiānshǐ　经穴)

[定位]　在前臂掌侧，腕横纹上3寸，当曲泽与大陵的连线上，掌长肌腱与桡侧腕屈肌腱之间取穴（图1—56）。

[主治]　心痛、呕吐、癫、狂、痫、疟疾。

[操作]　直刺0.5～1寸（约15～25毫米）。

内关 (PC6　Nèiguān　络穴、八脉交会穴)

[定位]　在前臂掌侧，当曲泽与大陵的连线上，腕横纹上2寸，掌长肌腱与桡侧腕屈肌腱之间（图1—56）。

[主治]　心痛、心悸、胸闷、呕吐、癫痫、热病。

[操作]　直刺0.5～1寸（约15～25毫米）。

大陵 (PC7　Dàlíng　输穴、原穴)

[定位]　腕掌横纹正中，当掌长肌腱与桡侧腕屈肌腱之间取穴（图1—56）。

[主治]　心痛、呕吐、癫狂、疮疡。

［操作］ 直刺0.3～0.5寸（约9～15毫米）。

劳宫（PC8 Láogōng 荥穴）

［定位］ 在手掌心，当2、3掌骨之间偏于第3掌骨，握拳屈指时中指尖处（图1—57）。

［主治］ 心痛、癫、狂、痫、口疮。
［操作］ 直刺0.3～0.5寸（约9～15毫米）。

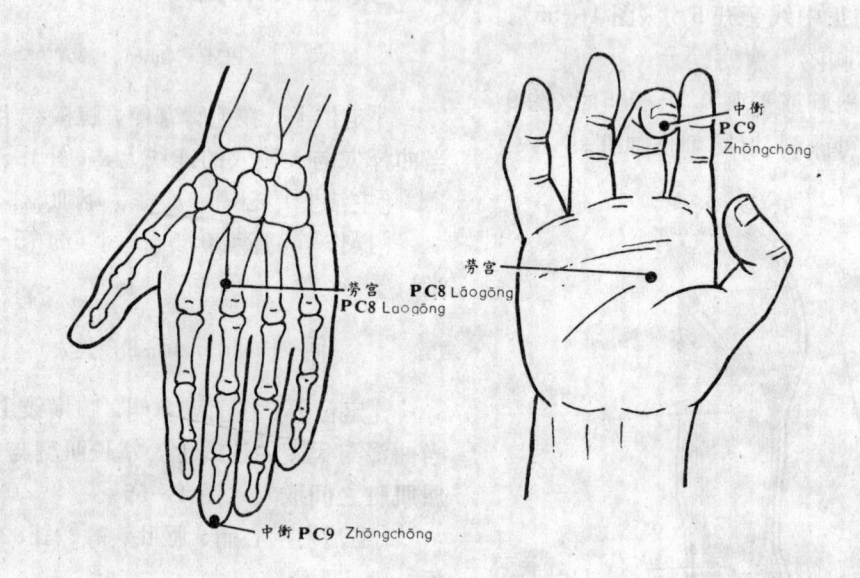

图1—57 劳宫、中冲
Fig. 1—57 Laogong (PC8) and Zhongchong (PC9)

中冲（PC9 Zhōngchōng 井穴）

［定位］ 手中指末节尖端之中央取穴（图1—57）。

［主治］ 心痛、昏迷、热病。
［操作］ 浅刺0.1寸（约3毫米）或点刺出血。

（三）常用经穴主治提要

本经腧穴主治心、胸、胃、神志病及经脉循行部位的病证，如心烦、心悸、心痛、胸闷、癫狂、以及肘臂挛急、掌心热等。其中曲泽、郄门、间使、内关、大陵、劳宫，主要治心痛、心悸、癫、狂、痫；除外，曲泽，间使，内关，大陵还治呕吐；中冲开窍急救。

Ⅸ. THE PERICARDIUM MERIDIAN OF HAND — JUEYIN (9 acupoints in total)

1. *The Course*

It originates from the chest. Emerging, it enters its pertaining organ, the pericardium (1). Then, it descends through the diaphragm (2) to the abdomen, and connects successively with the upper, middle, and lower warmers (i. e. sanjiao, triple energizer) in the order from the chest to the abdomen (3).

The branch starting from the chest runs inside the chest (4), emerges at the lateral aspect of the chest, and descends to the point 3 cun below the armpit at Tianchi (PC1) (5). Then, it ascends to the armpit (6). From there, it runs downwards along the medial aspect of the upper arm and between the meridians of Hand—Taiyin and Hand—Shaoyin (7) to the cubital fossa (8). Then it further descends between the tendons of m. palmaris longus and m. flexor carpi radialis of the forearm (9) to the palm (10). From there, it runs along the middle finger to its tip at Zhongchong (PC9) (11).

The beanch starting from the palm originates from Laogong (PC8), and runs along the ring finger to its tip at Guangchong (SJ1) where it connects with the Triple Energizer Meridian of Hand — Shaoyang (12).

The line made up by the distribution of the acupoints of this meridian on the body surface: It starts from Tianchi (PC1) at the point lateral to the nipple, and ascends to the axilla, Then, it runs downwards between the tendons of the m. palmaris longus and m. flexor carpi radialis at the meidal aspect of the arm to the palm. Finally, it ends at Zhongchong (PC8) at the tip of the middle finger.

The inner organs concerned: The pericardium, Sanjiao.

2. *The Commonly Used Acupoints*

Tianchi (PC1)

Location: On the chest, in the 4th intercostal space, 1 cun lateral to the nipple and 5 cun lateral to the anterior midline (See Fig. 1—55).

Indications: Oppressed feeling in the chest, tuberculous cervical lymphadenitis.

Method: Puncture obliquely or horzontally 0.3—0.5 cun (9—15mm). Deep puncture is prohibited, otherwise the lung may be injured. Moxibustion is applicable.

Quze (PC3, He—Sea point)

Location: At the midpoint of the cubital crease, on the ulnar side of the tendon of the biceps muscle of the arm (See Fig. 1—56).

Indications: Cardiac pain, stomachache, vomiting, febrile diseases.

Method: Puncture perpendicularly 0.8—1.0 cun (20—25mm), or prick with the three—edged needie to cause bleeding. Moxibustion is applicable.

Ximen (PC4, Xi—Cleft point)

Location: On the palmar side of the forearm, 5 cun proximal to the transverse crease of the wrist, at the line connecting Quze (PC3) with Daling (PC7), between the tendons of m. palmaris longus and m. flexor carpi radialis (See Fig. 1—56).

Indications: Cardiac pain, palpitation, hematemesis.

Method: Puncture perpendicularly 0.5—1.0 cun (15—25mm). Moxibustion is applicable.

Jianshi (PC5, Jing—River point)

Location: On the palmar side of the forearm and on the line connecting Quze (PC3) and Daling (PC7), 3 cun proximal to the transverse crease of the wrist, between the tendons of m. palmaris longus and m. flexor carpi radialis (See Fig. 1—56).

Indications: Cardiac pain, vomiting, epilepsy, mania, malaria.

Method: Puncture perpendicularly 0.5—1.0 cun (15—25mm). Moxibustion is applicable.

Neiguan (PC6, Luo—Connecting point, one of the Eight Confluence points)

Location: On the palmar side of the forearm and on the line conecting Quze (PC3) and Daling (PC7), 2 cun proximal to the transverse crease of the wrist, between the tendons of m. palmaris longus and m. flexor carpi radialis (See Fig. 1—56).

Indications: Cardiac pain, palpitation, oppressed feeling on the chest, vomiting, epilepsy, mania, febrile diseases.

Method: Puncture perpendicularly 0.5—1.0 cun (15—25mm). Moxibustion is applicable.

Daling (PC7, Shu—Stream and Yuan—Source point)

Location: At the midpoint of the transverse crease of the wrist, between the tendons of m. palmaris longus and m. flexor carpi radialis (See Fig. 1—56).

Indications: Cardiac pain, vomiting, epilepsy, skin carbuncle and ulcers.

Method: Puncture perpendicularly 0.3—0.5 cun (9—15mm). Moxibustion is applicable.

Laogong (PC8, Ying—Spring point)

Location: At the center of the palm, between the 2nd and 3rd metacarpal bones, but close to the latter, and in the part touching the tip of the middle finger when a fist is made (See Fig. 1—57).

Indications: Cardiac pain, epilepsy, mania, canker sore.

Method: Puncture perpendicularly 0.3—0.5 cun (9—15mm). Moxibustion is applicable.

Zhongchong (PC9, Jing—Well point).

Location: At the center of the tip of the middle finger (See Fig. 1—57).

Indications: Cardiac pain, loss of consciousness, febrile diseases.

Method: Puncture shallowly 0.1 cun (about 3mm), or prick with the three edged needle to cause bleeding. Moxibustion is applicable.

3. *An Outline of Indications of the Commonly Used Acupoints*

The points of this meridian are mainly used in treatment of disorders of the heart, chest, and stomach, and mental disorders, as well as disorders appearing at the pathway of the meridian, such as restlessness, palpitation, cardiac pain, oppressed feeling in the chest, epilepsy and mania, spasm of elbow and arm, palmar fever. In concrete, Quze (PC3), Ximen (PC4), Jianshi (PC5), Neiguan (PC6), Daling (PC7) and Laogong (PC8) are mainly used in treating cardiac pain, palpitation, epilepsy, mania. Additionally, Quze (PC3), Jianshi (PC5), Neiguan (PC6) and Daling (PC7) are also used to treat vomiting; and Zhongchong (PC9), to induce resuscitation for first aid.

十、手少阳三焦经（共 23 穴）

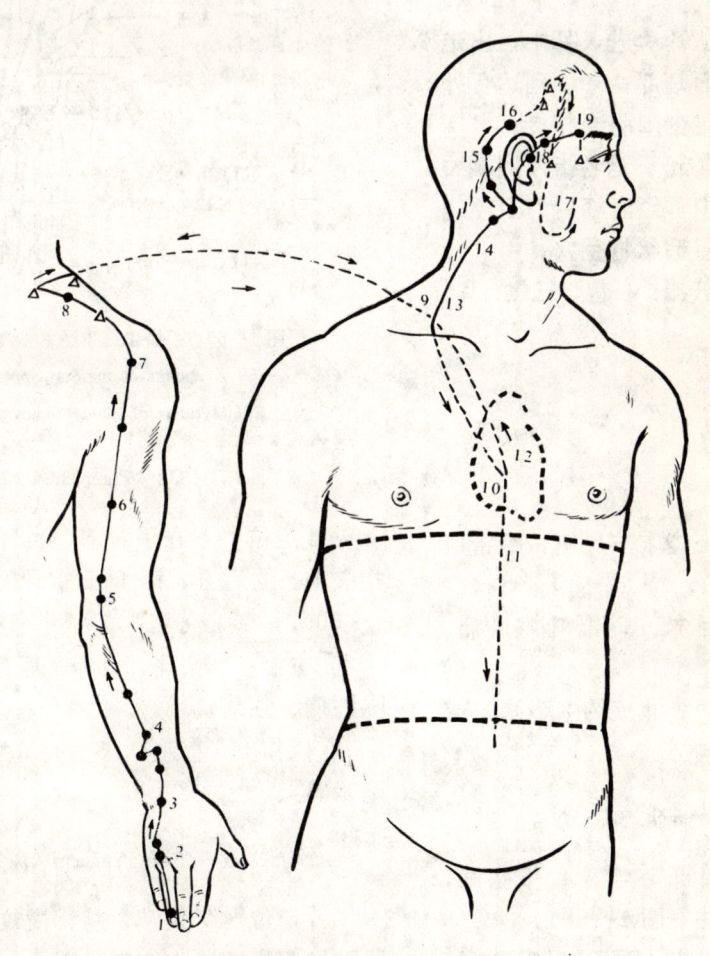

图 1—58 手少阳三焦经循行示意图

Fig. 1—58 The Running Course of the Sanjiao (Triple Energizer) Meridian of Hand—Shaoyang

（一）经脉循行

1. 起于无名指末端关冲穴；2. 向上出于第四、五掌骨间；3. 沿着腕背；4. 出于前臂外侧桡骨和尺骨之间；5. 向上通过肘尖；6. 沿着上臂外侧；7. 上行至肩部；8. 交出于足少阳经的后面；9. 向前进入缺盆部；10. 分布于胸中，联络心包；11. 向下通过横膈，从胸至腹，属于上、中、下三焦。

12. 胸中的支脉：从胸向上；13. 出于缺盆部；14. 上走项部；15. 沿耳后直上；16. 出于耳上部，行额角；17. 再屈而下行至面颊部，到达眼眶下部。

18. 耳部支脉：从耳后进入耳中，出走耳前，与前脉交叉于面颊部；19. 到达目外眦丝竹空穴之下，与足少阳胆经相接。

体表穴位分布线：起于无名指尺侧端关冲穴，上循臂外侧之中，经肩峰后、上项绕耳后、至耳后，止于眉毛丝竹空穴。

体内相关的组织脏器：心包、三焦、耳、目。

（二）本经常用腧穴

关冲 （SJ1 Guānchōng 井穴）

[定位] 在手环指末节尺侧，距指甲角 0.1 寸（图 1—60）。

[主治] 头痛、目赤、耳聋、咽喉肿痛、热病。

[操作] 浅刺 0.1 寸（约 3 毫米）或点刺出血。

液门 （SJ2 Yèmén 荥穴）

[定位] 在手背部，当第 4、5 指间，指蹼缘后方赤白肉际处（图 1—60）。

[主治] 头痛、目赤、耳聋、咽喉肿痛、疟疾。

[操作] 直刺 0.3～0.5 寸（约 9～15 毫米）。

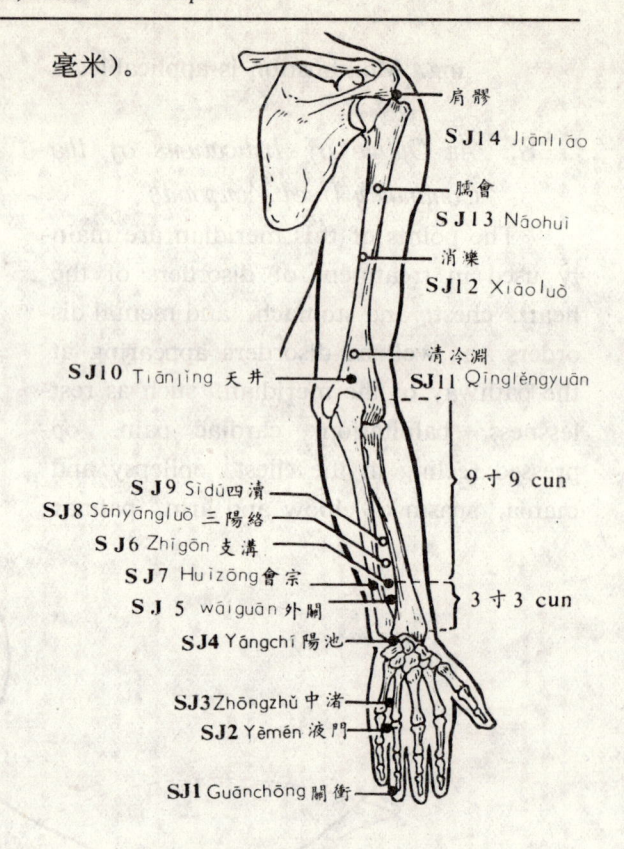

图 1—59 手少阳三焦经主要穴位图

Fig. 1—59 Acupoints of the Sanjiao (Triple Energizer) Meridian of Hand—Shaoyang

中渚 （SJ3 Zhōngzhǔ 输穴）

[定位] 在手背部，当环指本节（掌指关节）的后方，第 4、5 掌骨间凹陷处（图 1—60）。

[主治] 头痛、目赤、耳聋、耳鸣、咽喉肿痛、热病。

[操作] 直刺 0.3～0.5 寸（约 9～15 毫米）。

阳池 （SJ4 Yángchí 原穴）

[定位] 伏掌，腕背横纹中，当指伸肌腱尺侧缘凹陷中取穴（图 1—60、61）。

[主治] 腕痛、目赤、耳聋、咽喉肿痛、疟疾、消渴。

[操作]　直刺0.3～0.5寸（约9～15毫米）。

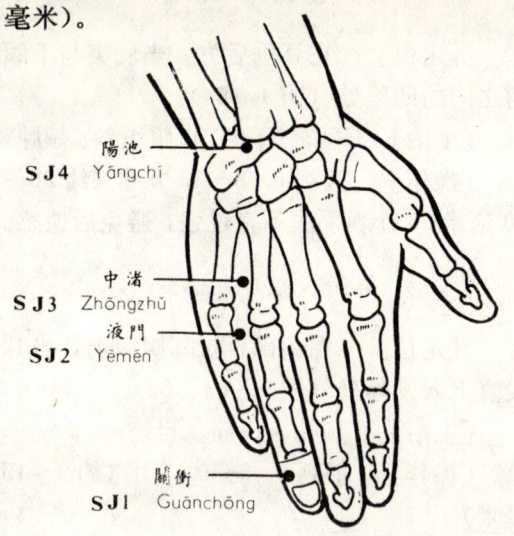

图1-60　关冲、液门、中渚、阳池

Fig. 1—60 Guanchong (SJ1), Yemen (SJ2), Zhongzhu (SJ3), and Yangchi (SJ4)

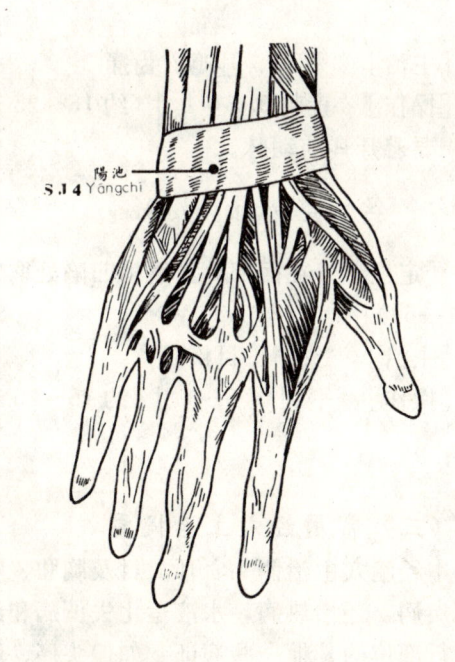

图1—61　阳池穴

Fig. 1—61 Yangchi (SJ4)

外关　(SJ5　Wàiguān　络穴)

[定位]　在前臂背侧，当阳池与肘尖的连线上，腕背横纹上2寸，尺骨与桡骨之间（图1—62）。

[主治]　头痛、目赤肿痛、耳鸣、耳聋、胁肋痛、上肢痹痛、热病。

[操作]　直刺0.5～1寸（约15～25毫米）。

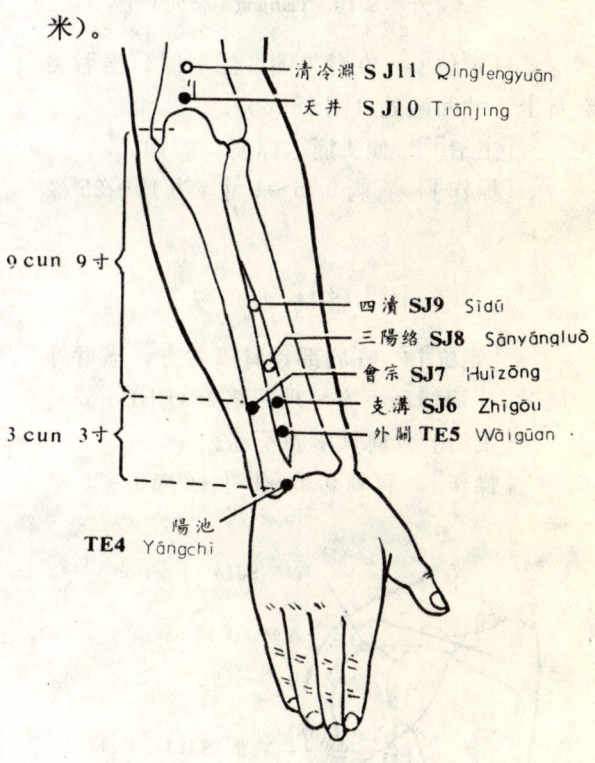

图1—62　手少阳三焦经上肢常用穴

Fig. 1—62 Commonly Used acupoints of the Triple Ehergizer Meridian at the upper Limb

支沟　(SJ6　Zhīgōu　经穴)

[定位]　在前臂背侧，当阳池与肘尖的连线上，腕背横纹上3寸，尺骨与桡骨之间（图1—62）

[主治]　暴喑、胁肋痛、便秘、热病。

[操作]　直刺0.5～1寸（约15～25毫米）。

会宗 (SJ7 Huìzōng 郄穴)

[定位] 在前臂背侧，当腕背横纹上3寸，支沟尺侧，尺骨的桡侧缘（图1—62）。

[主治] 耳聋、癫痫。

[操作] 直刺0.5~1寸（约15~25毫米）。

天井 (SJ10 Tiānjǐng 合穴)

[定位] 在臂外侧，屈肘时，当肘尖直上1寸凹陷处（图1—63）。

[主治] 偏头痛、瘰疬、癫痫。

[操作] 直刺0.5~1寸（约15~25毫米）。

肩髎 (SJ14 Jiānliáo)

[定位] 在肩部，肩髃后方，当臂外展时，于肩峰后下方呈现凹陷处（图1—63）。

[主治] 肩臂挛痛不遂。

[操作] 直刺0.5~1寸（约15~25毫米）。

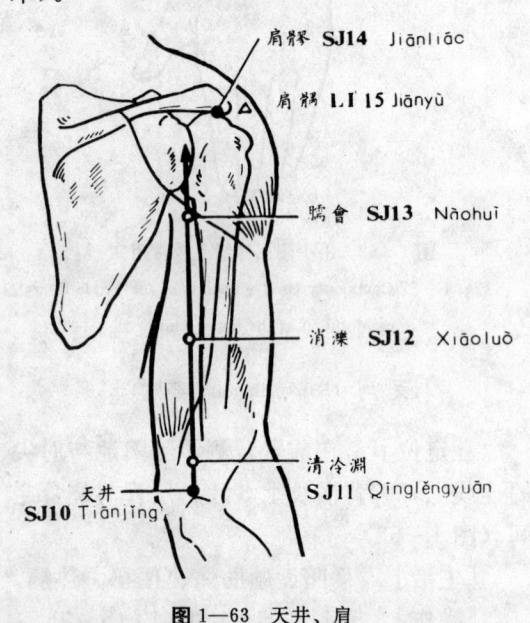

图1—63 天井、肩

Fig. 1—63 Tianjing (SJ10) and jianliao (SJ14)

翳风 (SJ17 Yìfēng)

[定位] 在耳垂后方，当乳突与下颌角之间的凹陷处（图1—64）。

[主治] 耳鸣、耳聋、口眼歪斜、颊肿。

[操作] 直刺0.8~1.2寸（约20~30毫米）。针刺手法不宜过强，避免后遗感。

角孙 (SJ20 Jiǎosūn)

[定位] 在头部，折耳廓向前，当耳尖直上入发际处（图1—64、65）。

[主治] 颊肿、齿痛、目翳。

[操作] 平刺0.3~0.5寸（约9~15毫米）。

耳门 (SJ21 ěrmén)

[定位] 在面部，耳屏上切迹前方，下颌骨髁状突后缘张口凹陷中取穴（图1—64）。

[主治] 耳聋、耳鸣、齿痛

[操作] 直刺0.5~1寸（约15~25毫米）。要避开耳前动脉。

丝竹空 (SJ23 Sīzhúkōng)

[定位] 在面部，当眉梢凹陷处取穴（图1—64）。

[主治] 头痛、目疾。

[操作] 平刺0.5~1寸（约15~25毫米）。

(三) 常用经穴主治提要

本经腧穴主治侧头、耳、目及胸胁、咽喉部疾病，还治热病，水液运化失调病和经脉循行部位的其他一些病证。如偏头痛、腹胀水肿、小便不利、耳聋、目赤肿痛、面颊肿痛、肘臂外侧中痛等。其中关冲、液门、中

经络腧穴概要

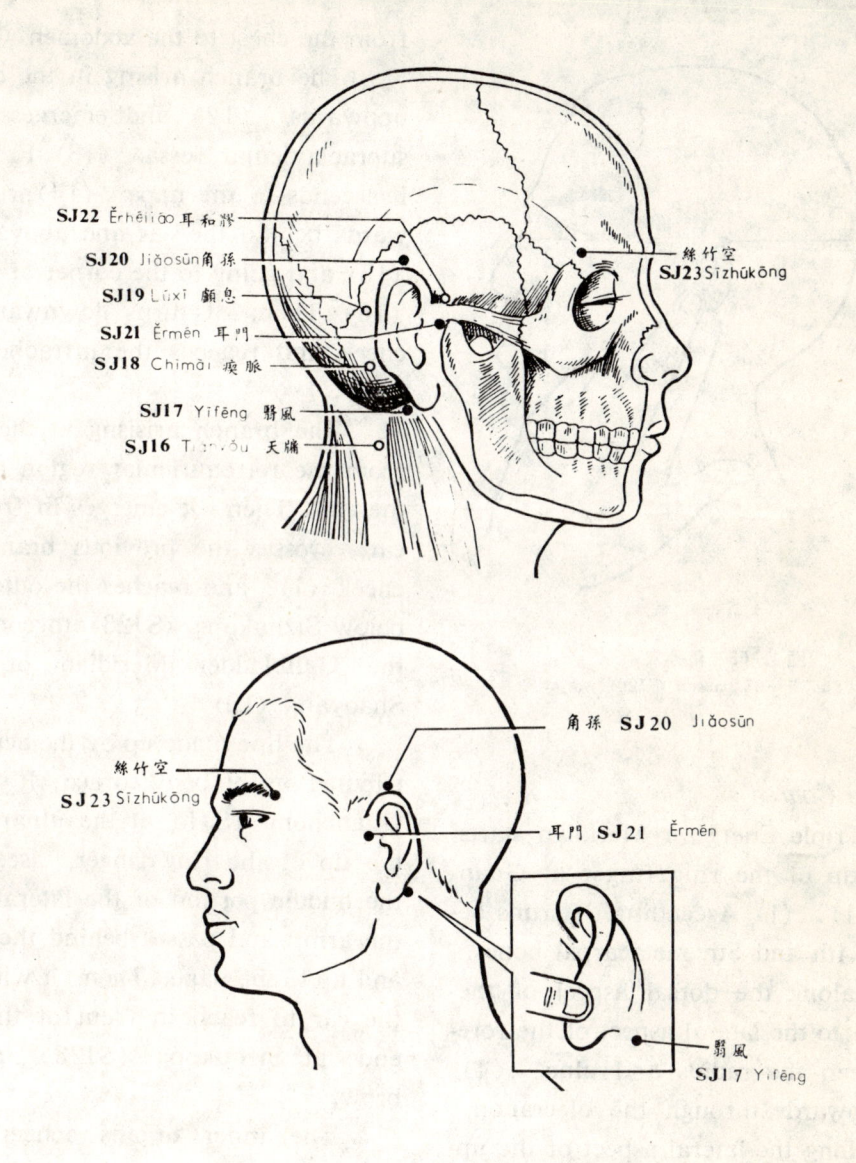

图 1—64 翳风、角孙、耳门、丝竹空
Fig. 1—64 Yifeng (SJ17), Jiaosun (SJ20), Ermen (SJ21) and Sizhukong (SJ23)

渚、外关、丝竹穴治头痛、目赤；阳池、关冲、液门、翳风、耳门治耳鸣、耳聋；关冲、液门、中渚还能治咽喉肿痛；肩髎治上肢痹痛，肩痛不遂；支沟治暴喑，胁肋痛；角孙治颊痛、齿痛等。

X. THE SANJIAO (TRIPLE ENERGIZER) MERIDIAN OF HAND — SHAOYANG (23 acupoints in total)

· 107 ·

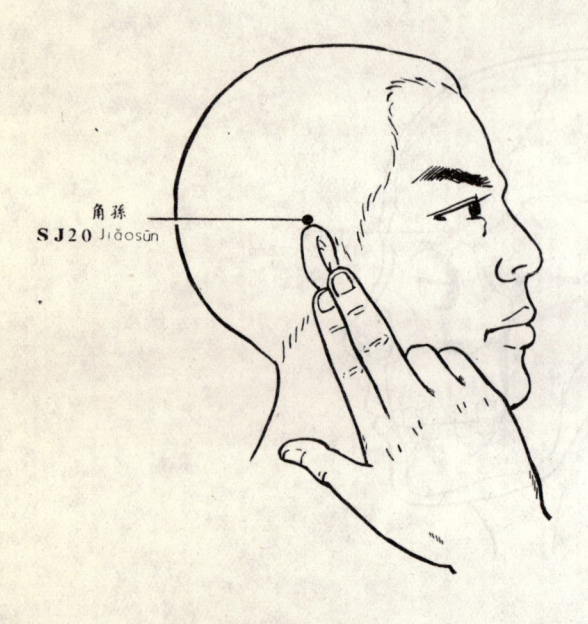

Fig. 1—65 Jiaosun (SJ20)

1. The Course

The Triple Energizer Meridian starts from the tip of the ring finger at Guanchong (SJ1). (1) Ascending, it runs between the 4th and 5th metacarpal bones, (2) and along the dorsal aspect of the wrist, (3) to the lateral aspect of the forearm between the radius and ulna, (4) Passing upwards through the olecranon, (5) and along the lateral aspect of the upper arm, (6) it reaches the shoulder region, (7) where it runs across and passes behind the Meridian of Foot—Shaoyang, (8) runs forward to enter the supraclavicular fossa, (9) and distributes in the chest to connect with the pericardium, (10) It then runs downwards throngh the diaphragm to the abdomen, and connects with the upper, middle and lower jiao (i.e. triple energizer), its pertaining organ, from the chest to the abdomen (11).

The branch arising in the chest runs uppwards, (12) and emerges from the supraclavicular fossa, (13) From there, it ascends to the nape, (14) running upwards behind the ear and above the ear, (15) and going to the corner of forehead, (16) Then, it turns downwards to the cheek and reaches the infraobital region (17).

The branch arisisng at the ear runs from the retroauricular region and enters the ear. Then, it emerges in front of the ear, crosses the previous branch at the cheek (1), and reaches the outer canthus below Sizhukong (SJ23) to connect with the Gallbladder Meridian of Foot—Shaoyang (19).

The line made up by the acupoints distributed on the body suface: It starts from Guanchong (SJ1) at the ulnar aspect of the tip of the ring finger, ascends along the middle portion of the lateral aspect of the arm, and passes behind the acromion and up to the nape. Then, it winds behind the ear to reach in front of the ear and ends at Sizhukong (SJ23) in the eyebrow.

The inner organs concerned: The pericardium, sanjiao, ear, eye.

2. The Commonly Used Acupoints

Guanchong (SJ1, Jing—Well point)

Location: At the ulnar side of the distal segment of the ring finger, about 0.1 cun posterior to the corner of the nail (See Fig. 1—60).

Indications: Headache, redness of the eye, deafness, sore and swelling throat, febrile diseases.
Method: Puncture shallowly 0.1 cun (about 3mm), or prick with the three edged needle to cause bleeding. Moxibustion is applicable.

Yemen (SJ2, Ying—Spring point)

Location: On the dorsum of the hand, between the 4th and 5th fingers, at the junction of the red and white skin, proximal to the margin of the web (See Fig. 1—60).
Indications: Headache, redness of eye, deafness, swelling and sore throat, malaria.
Method: Puncture perpendicularly 0.3—0.5 cun (9—15mm). Moxibustion is applicable.

Zhongzhu (SJ3, Shu—Stream point)

Location: On the dorsum of the hand, proximal to the 4th metacarpophalangeal joint, in the deprpession between the 4th and 5th metacarpal bones (See Fig. 1—60).
Indications: Headache, redness of the eye, deafness, tinnitus, swelling and sore throat, febrile diseases.
Method: Puncture perpendicularly 0.3—0.5 cun (9—15mm). Moxibustion is applicable.

Yangchi (SJ4, Yuan—Source point)

Location: At the midpoint of the dorsal transverse crease of the wrist, at the depression at the ulnar side of the tendon of m. extensor digitorum communis (See Fig. 1—60, 1—61).
Indications: Pain in the wrist, redness of the eye, deafness, swelling and sore throat, malaria, diadetes.
Method: Puncture perpendicularly 0.3—0.5 cun (9—15mm). Moxibustion is applicable.

Waiguan (SJ5, Luo—Connecting point, one of the Eignt Confluence points)

Location: On the dorsal side of the forearm and on the line connecting Yangchi (SJ4) and the tip of the olecranon, 2 cun proximal to the transverse crease of the dorsal wrist, between the radius and ulna (See Fig. 1—62).
Indications: Headache, redness, swelling and pain of the eye, tinnitus, deafness, hypochondriac pain, pain in the upper limb, febrile diseases.
Method: Puncture perpendicularly 0.5—1.0 cun (15—25mm). Moxibustion is applicable.

Zhigou (SJ6, Jing—River point)

Location: On the dorsal side of the forearm and on the line connecting Yangchi (SJ4) and the tip of the olecranon, 3 cun proximal to the transverse crease of the dorsal

wrist, between the radius and ulna (See Fig. 1—62).
Indications: Sudden aphonia, hypochondriac pain, constipation, febrile disease.
Method: Puncture perpendicularly 0.5—1.0 cun (15—25mm). Moxibustion is applicable.

Huizong (SJ7, Xi—Cleft point)

Location: On the dorsal side of the forearm, 3 cun proximal to the dorsal crease of the wrist, on the ulnar side of Zhigou (SJ6) and on the radial border of the ulna (See Fig. 1—62).
Indications: Deafness, epilepsy, mania.
Method: Puncture perpendicularly 0.5—1.0 cun (15—25mm). Moxibustion is applicable.

Tianjing (SJ10, He—Sea point)

Location: On the lateral side of the upper arm, with the elbow flexed, at the depression about 1 cun proximal to the tip of the olecranon of the ulna (See Fig. 1—62).
Indications: Migraine, tuberculous cervical lymphadenitis, epilepsy.
Method: Puncture perpendicularly 0.5—1.0 cun (15—25mm). Moxibustion is applicable.

Jianliao (SJ14)

Location: On the shoulder, posterior and inferior to the acromion, at the depression about 1 cun posterior to Jianyu (LI15) when the upper arm is horizontally abducted (See Fig. 1—63).
Indications: Pain and motor impairment of the shoulder and arm.
Method: Puncture perpendicularly 0.5—1.0 cun (15—25mm). Moxibustion is applicable.

Yifeng (SJ17)

Location: Posteior to the ear lobe, in the depression between the mastoid process and mandibular angle (See Fig. 1—64).
Indications: Tinnitus, deafness, deviation of the mouth and eye, swelling of the cheek.
Method: Puncture perpendicularly 0.8—1.2 cun (20—30mm). Too strong manipulation is not applicable, otherwise sequela may be caused. Moxibustion is applicable.

Jiaosun (SJ20)

Location: On the head, above the ear apex within the hairline (See Fig. 1-64, 1—65).
Indications: Swelling of the cheek, toothache, nebula of the cornea, parotitis.
Method: Puncture horizontally 0.3—0.5 cun (9—15mm). Moxibustion is applicable.

Ermen (SJ21)

Location: On the face, anterior to the supratragic notch of the auricle, at the depression behind the posterior border of the condyloid process of the mandible (See Fig. 1—64).

Indications: Tinnitus, deafness, toothache.
Method: Puncture perpendicularly 0.5—1.0 cun (15—25mm), avoiding the auriculotemporal artery. Moxibustion is applicable.

Sizhukong (SJ23)

Location: On the face, in the depression at the lateral end of the eyebrow (See Fig. 1—64).
Indications: Headache, eye disorders.
Method: Puncture horizontally 0.5—1.0 cun (15—25mm).

3. *An Outline of Indications of the Commonly Used Acupoints*

The points of this meridian are mainly indicated in disorders of the head, ear, eye, chest and hypochondriac region, and throat. Additionally, they are also indicated in febrile diseases, disorders of transportation and transformation of fluid, as well as other symptoms appearing on the pathway of the meridian, such as, migraine, abdominal distension, edema, dysuria, deafness, redness and pain and swelling of the eye, swelling and pain of the cheek, and pain in the lateral side of the elbow, arm and shoulder. In the concrete, Guanchong (SJ1), Yemen (SJ2), Zhongzhu (SJ3), Waiguan (SJ5), and Sizhukong (SJ23) are indicated in headache, redness of the eye; Yangchi (SJ4), Guanchong (SJ1), Yemen (SJ2), Yifeng (SJ11), and Ermen (SJ21), in tinnitus, deafness; Guanchong (SJ1), Zhongzhu (SJ3) and Yemen (SJ2), in swelling and sore throat; Jianliao (SJ14), in pain in the upper limb and shoulder with motor impairment; Zhigou (SJ6), in sudden aphonia, hypochondriac pain; and Jiaosun (SJ20), in swelling of the cheek, toothache.

十一、足少阳胆经（共44穴）

（一）经脉循行

1. 起于目外眦瞳子髎穴；2. 向上抵达额角部；3. 下行至耳后（风池）；4. 沿着颈部行于手少阳经之前，到肩上交出于手少阳经之后；5. 向下进入缺盆。

6. 耳部支脉：从耳后进入耳中；7. 出走耳前；8. 到达目外眦后方。

9. 外眦部的支脉：从目外眦分出；10. 向下走至大迎；11. 会合于手少阳经，抵达目眶下；12. 下行经颊车；13. 再由颈部向下会合前脉于缺盆；14. 然后再向下进入胸中，通过横膈；15. 联络肝脏；16. 属于胆；17. 循着胁肋内；18. 走出于少腹两侧腹股沟动脉部；19. 绕过外阴部毛际；20. 横行进入髋关节部。

21. 缺盆部直行的脉：下行到腋部；22. 沿着侧胸；23. 经过季胁；24. 下行会合前脉于髋关节部；25. 再向下沿着大腿外侧；26. 出于膝外侧；27. 下行经腓骨前面；28. 直下到达腓骨下端；29. 再向下出于外踝之前，沿着足背部；30. 进入第四趾外侧端。

31. 足背部支脉：从足临泣处分出，沿第一、二跖骨之间，出于大趾端，穿过趾甲，回过来到达趾甲后的毫毛部，与足厥阴肝经相接。

图 1—66 足少阳胆经循行示意图

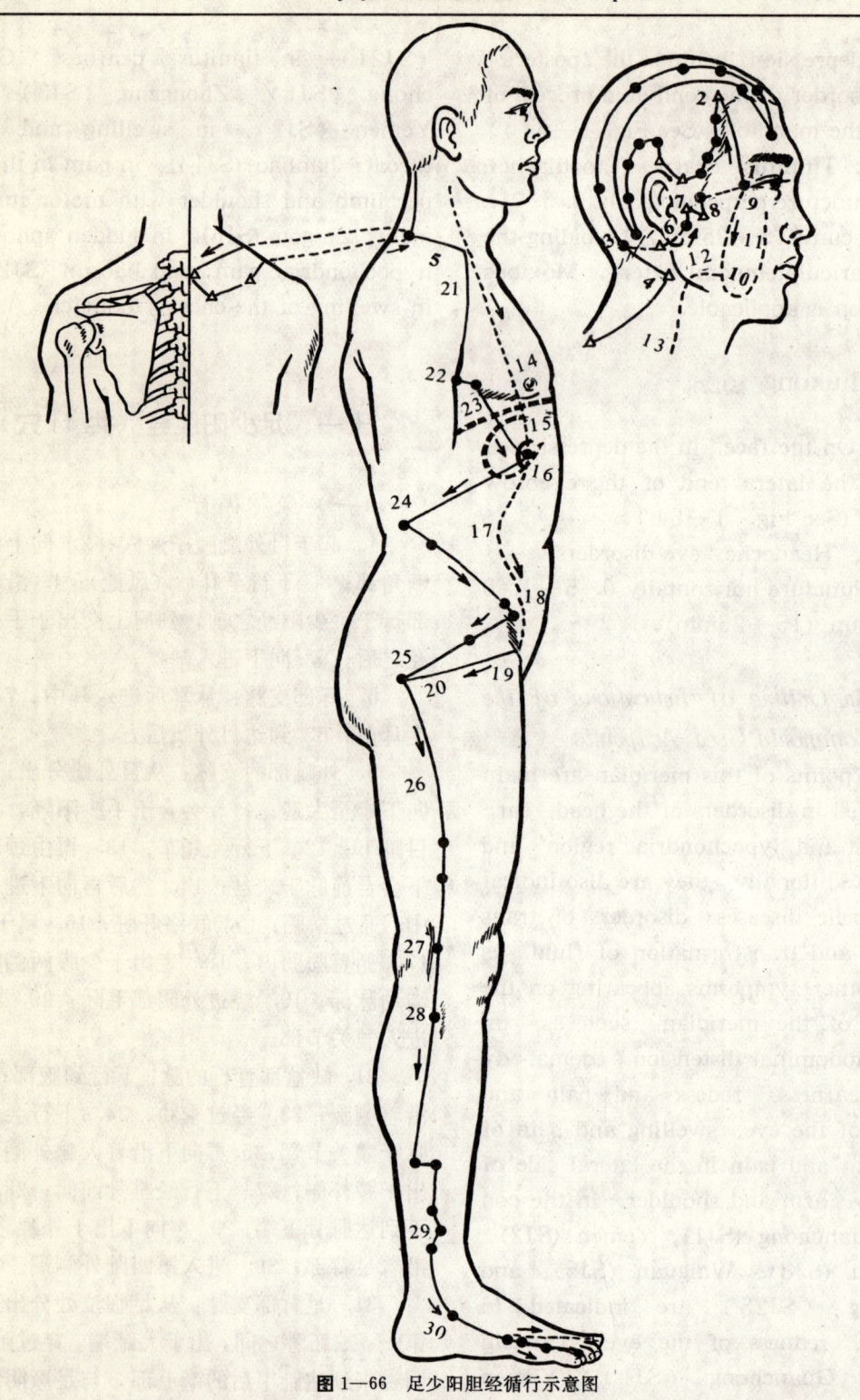

Fig. 1—66 The Running Course of the Gallbladder Meridian of Foot—Shaoyang

体表穴位分布线：起于目外眦瞳子髎穴，斜下耳前，上额角，绕耳后回折前额，向后行头颞侧面至枕后风池穴，经肩上，循胁肋腰间下行至臀，沿下肢外侧正中，过外踝前，止于第四趾外侧端足窍阴穴。

体内相关的组织脏器：肝、胆、目、耳。

（二）本经常用腧穴

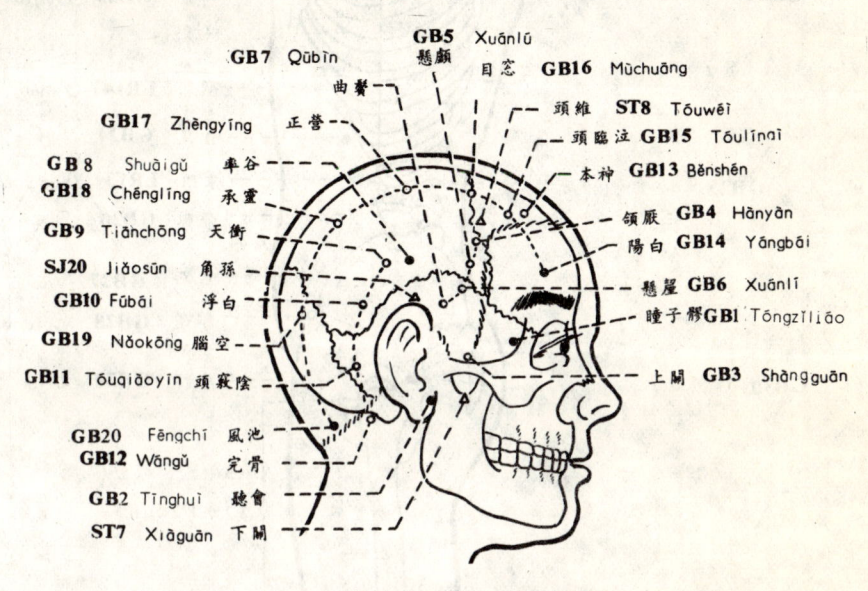

图 1—67① 足少阳胆经穴位图
Fig. 1—67① Acupoints of the Gallbladder Meridian of Foot—Shaoyang

瞳子髎（GB1 Tóngzǐliáo）

[定位] 在面部，目外眦旁，眶骨外侧缘凹陷处（图1—68）。

[主治] 头痛，目赤肿痛，青盲、目翳。

[操作] 向后平刺或斜刺0.3～0.5寸（约9～15毫米），或用三棱针点刺出血。

听会（GB2 Tīnghuì）

[定位] 在面部，耳屏间切迹前方，下颌骨髁状突后缘，张口有凹陷处取穴（图1—68、69）。

[主治] 耳聋、耳鸣、齿痛、口歪。

[操作] 张口，直刺0.5～1寸（约15～25毫米）。

率谷（GB8 Shuàigǔ）

[定位] 在头部，耳尖直上，入发际1.5寸，角孙直上方（图1—70）。

[主治] 偏头痛、眩晕、小儿惊风。

[操作] 平刺0.5～1寸（约15～25毫米）。

阳白（GB14 Yángbái）

[定位] 在前额部，当瞳孔直上，眉上1寸（图1—68）。

[主治] 头痛、目痛、眼睑瞤动。

[操作] 平刺0.3～0.5寸（约9～15毫米）。

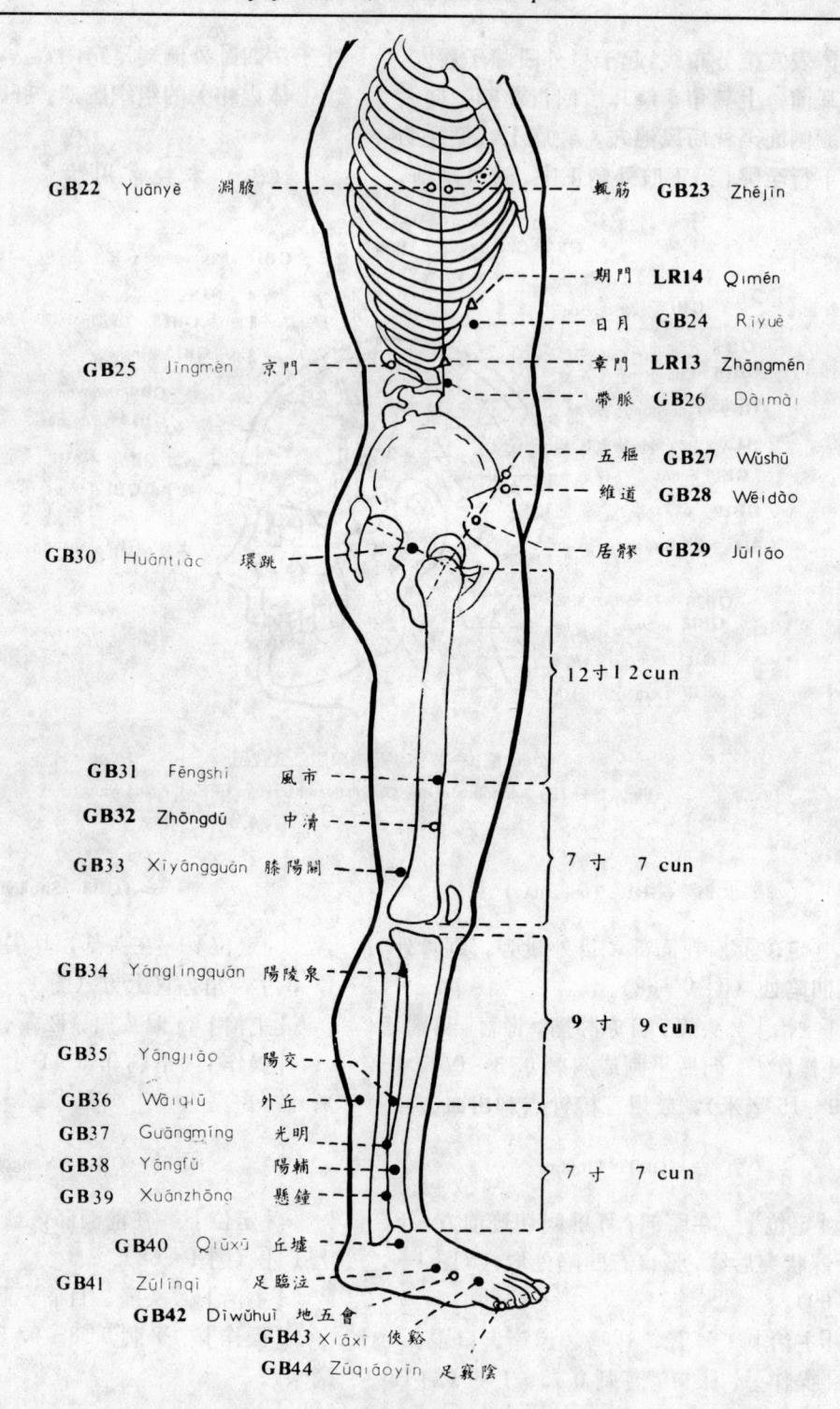

图 1—67② 足少阳胆经穴位图
Fig. 1—67② Acupoints of the Gallbladder Meridian of Foot—Shaoyang

图 1—68 瞳子髎、阳白、听会

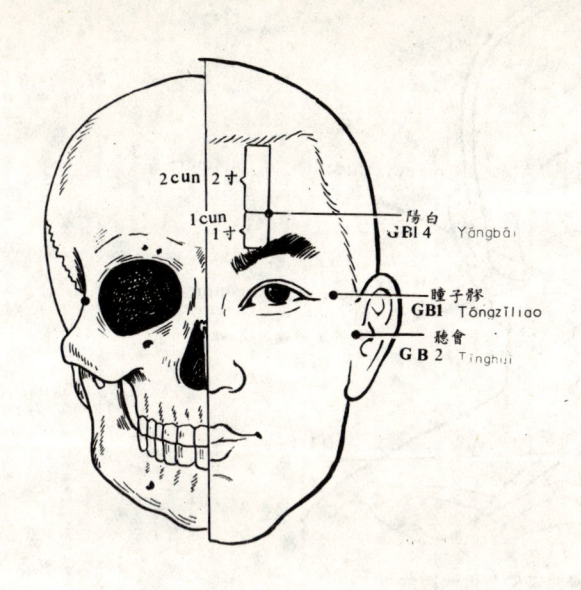

Fig. 1—68 Yangbai (GB14), Tongziliao (GB1) and Tinghui (GB2)

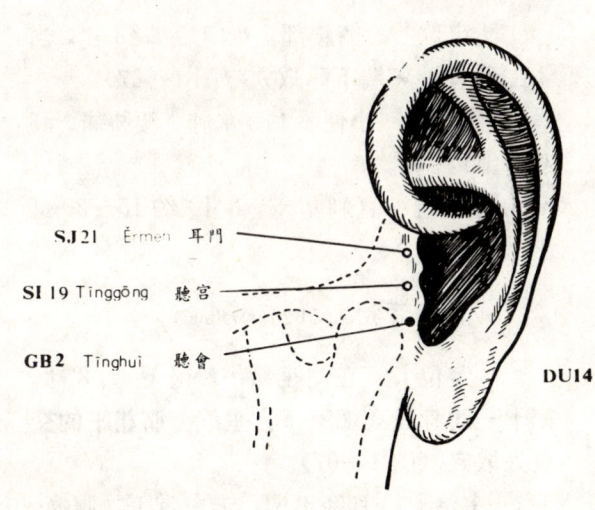

图 1—69 听会穴

Fig. 1—69 Tinghui (GB2)

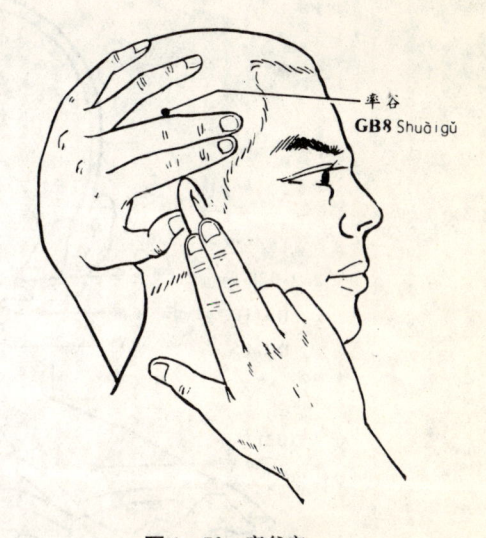

图 1—70 率谷穴

Fig. 1—70 Shuaigu (GB8)

风池（GB20 Fēngchí）

［定位］ 在项后枕骨下，与风府相平，当胸锁乳突肌与斜方肌上端之间的凹陷中取穴（图1—71）。

［主治］ 头痛、目赤痛、鼻渊、颈项强痛、感冒、癫痫。

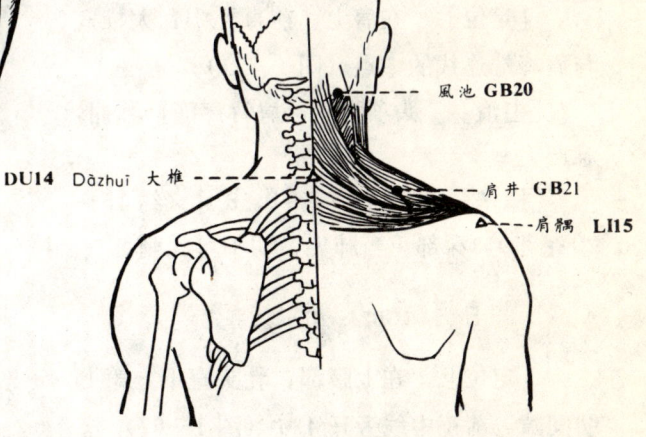

图 1—71① 风池、肩井定位与风池刺法

Fig. 1—71① Location of Fengchi (GB20) and Tianjing (GB21) and Needling of Fengchi (GB20)

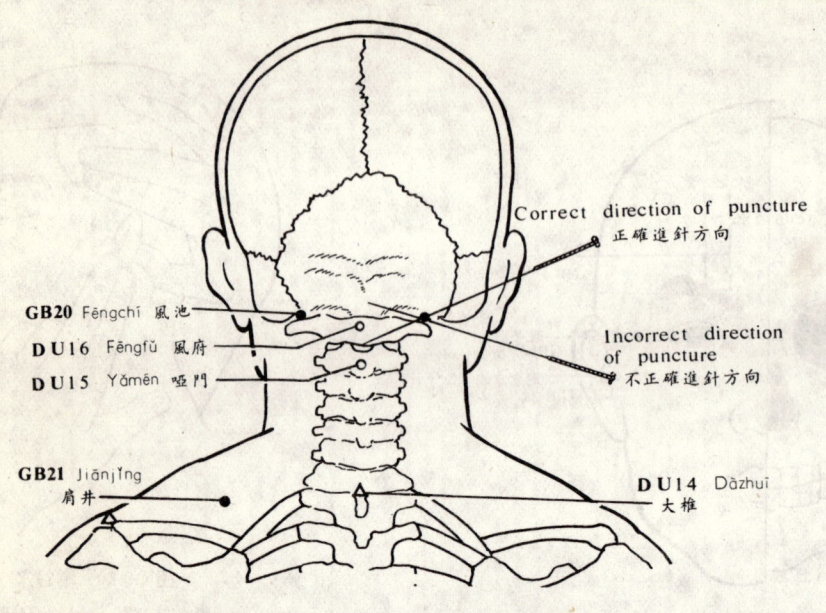

图 1—71② 风池、肩井定位与风池刺法
Fig. 1—71② Location of Fengchi (GB20) and Tianjing (GB21) and Needling of Fengchi (GB20)

［操作］ 针尖向下朝鼻尖方向斜刺 0.5～0.8寸（约15～20毫米），深部中间为延髓，必须严格掌握针刺的角度与深度（图1—71）。

肩井 (GB21 Jiānjǐng)

［定位］ 在肩上，前直乳中，大椎穴与肩峰端连线的中点（图1—71）。

［主治］ 头项强痛，肩背疼痛，乳痈，难产。

［操作］ 直刺 0.5～0.8寸（约15～20毫米），深部正当肺尖，切不可深刺。

日月 (GB24 Rìyuè 募穴)

［定位］ 在上腹部，乳头直下，第七肋间隙，前正中线旁开4寸（图1—67）。

［主治］ 胁肋疼痛，呕吐，呃逆，黄疸。

［操作］ 斜刺或平刺 0.5～0.8寸（约15～20毫米）。

京门 (GB25 Jīngmén 募穴)

［定位］ 侧腰部，章门后1.8寸，当十二肋骨游离端下际取穴（图1—67）。

［主治］ 小便不利、水肿、腰胁痛、肠鸣、泄泻。

［操作］ 直刺 0.5～1寸（约15～20毫米）。

带脉 (GB26 Dàimài)

［定位］ 在侧腹部，章门下1.8寸，第十一肋骨游离端直下方垂线与脐相平的交点处取穴（图1—67）。

［主治］ 月经不调，赤白带下，腹痛。

［操作］ 直刺 0.5～0.8寸（约15～20毫米）。

环跳 (GB30 Huántiào)

［定位］ 在股外侧部，侧卧屈股，在股骨大转子最凸点与骶管裂孔连线的外1/3

与中 1/3 交点处取穴（图 1—67、72）。

［主治］ 腰痛、下肢痿痹。

［操作］ 直刺 2～3 寸（约 50～75 毫米）。

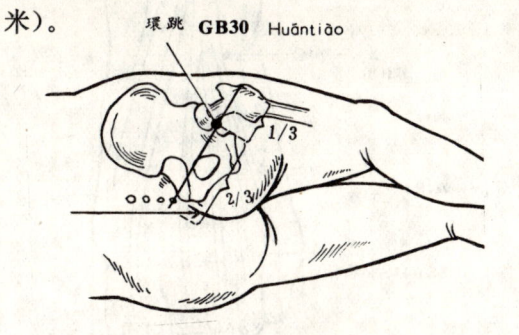

图 1—72 环跳穴
Fig. 1—72 Huantiao (GB34)

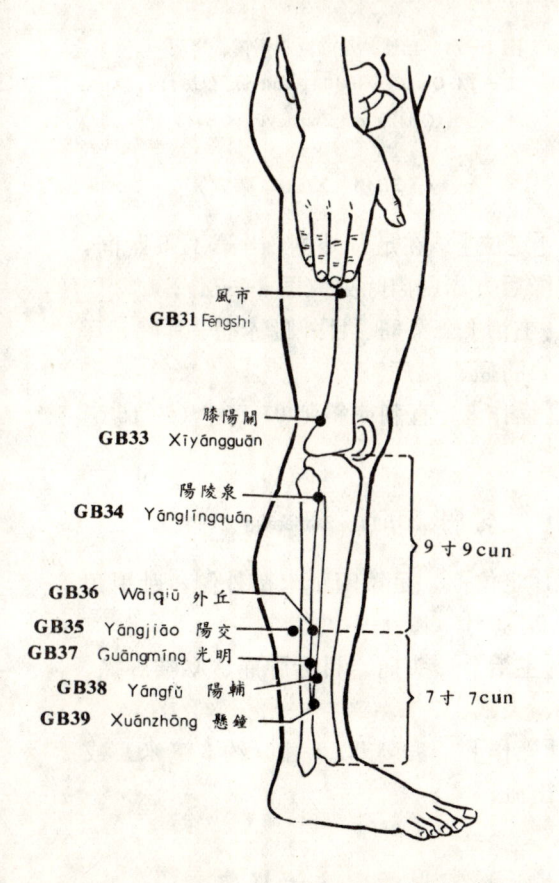

图 1—73 足少阳胆经下肢常用穴
Fig. 1—73 Commonly Used Acupoints of the Gallbladder Meridian at the Lower Limb

风市 (GB31 Fēngshì)

［定位］ 大腿外侧部的中线上，腘横纹上 7 寸处取穴；或直立垂手，中指尖处取之（图 1—73）。

［主治］ 下肢痿痹，遍身瘙痒。

［操作］ 直刺 1～2 寸（约 25～50 毫米）。

膝阳关 (GB33 Xīyángguān)

［定位］ 在膝外侧，阳陵泉穴上 3 寸，股骨外上髁的上方凹陷中取穴（图 1—73）。

［主治］ 膝肿痛

［操作］ 直刺 0.8～1 寸（约 20～25 毫米）。

阳陵泉 (GB34 Yánglíngquán)

［定位］ 在小腿外侧，腓骨小头前下方凹陷中取穴（图 1—73）。

［主治］ 胁痛、下肢痿痹、黄疸、小儿惊风。

［操作］ 直刺 1～1.5 寸（约 25～40 毫米）。

阳交 (GB35 Yángjiāo)

［定位］ 在小腿外侧，外踝尖上 7 寸，腓骨后缘取穴（图 1—73）。

［主治］ 胸胁胀痛、下肢痿痹、癫狂。

［操作］ 直刺 0.5～0.8 寸（约 15～20 毫米）。

外丘 (GB36 Wàiqiū 郄穴)

［定位］ 在小腿外侧，外踝尖上 7 寸，与阳交穴相平，腓骨前缘取之（图 1—73）。

［主治］ 胸胁胀痛，下肢痿痹，癫狂。

［操作］ 直刺 0.5～0.8 寸（约 15～20 毫米）。

光明（GB37 Guāngmíng 络穴）

［定位］ 在小腿外侧，外踝尖直上5寸，腓骨前缘取穴（图1—73）。

［主治］ 目痛、夜盲、下肢痿痹。

［操作］ 直刺0.5～0.8寸（约15～20毫米）。

阳辅（GB38 Yángfǔ 经穴）

［定位］ 在小腿外侧，外踝尖上4寸，腓骨前缘稍前方取穴（图1—73）。

［主治］ 偏头痛、下肢痿痹。

［操作］ 直刺0.5～0.8寸（约15～20毫米）。

悬钟（GB39 Xuánzhōng 髓会穴、又名绝骨）

［定位］ 在小腿外侧，足外踝尖上3寸，腓骨前缘取穴（图1—73）。

［主治］ 胁痛、下肢痿痹、颈项强。

［操作］ 直刺0.5～1寸（约15～25毫米）。

丘墟（GB40 Qiūxū 原穴）

［定位］ 在足外踝的前下方，当趾长伸肌腱的外侧凹陷处（图1—74）。

［主治］ 胸胁胀痛、下肢痿痹。

［操作］ 直刺0.5～0.8寸（约15～20毫米）。

足临泣（GB41 Zúlínqì 输穴）

［定位］ 在足背外侧，当足4趾本节（第4跖趾关节）的后方，小趾伸肌腱的外侧凹陷处（图1—74）。

［主治］ 目痛、目外眦痛、胁痛、乳痈、月经不调。

［操作］ 直刺0.5～0.8寸（约15～20毫米）。

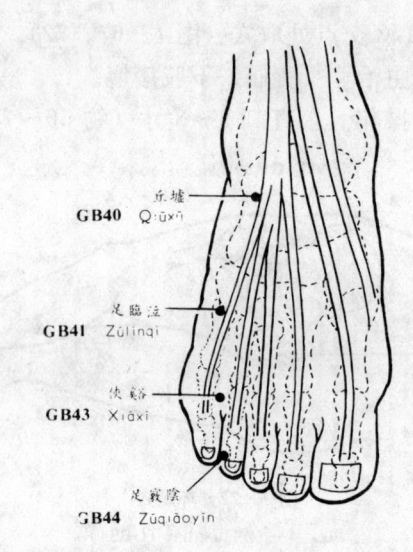

图1—74 丘墟、足临泣、侠溪、窍阴
Fig. 1—74 Qiuxu (GB40), Zulinqi (GB41), Xiaxi (GB43) and Zuqiaoyin (GB44)

侠溪（GB43 Xiáxī 荥穴）

［定位］ 在足背外侧，当第4、5趾间，趾蹼缘后方赤白肉际处（图1—74）。

［主治］ 头痛、目外眦赤痛、耳鸣、耳聋、胁肋痛、热病。

［操作］ 直刺或斜刺0.5寸（约15毫米）。

足窍阴（GB44 Zúqiàoyīn 井穴）

［定位］ 足第四趾末节外侧，趾甲角旁约0.1寸（图1—74）。

［主治］ 头痛、目赤肿痛、咽喉肿痛、热病、失眠。

［操作］ 浅刺0.1寸（约3毫米）或点刺出血。

（三）常用经穴主治提要

本经腧穴主治侧头、目、耳、咽喉病、神志病、热病，肝胆病及经脉循行部位的其他病证。如偏头痛、胸胁痛、口苦、咽干、目赤肿痛、耳鸣耳聋等病。其中瞳子髎、阳白、光明治目疾；听会，侠溪治耳病；风池疏风通络治外感头痛、鼻塞；率谷，足临泣治偏头痛、三叉神经痛；肩井治头项强痛、乳痈；日月、阳陵泉、丘墟治肝胆疾患之胸胁痛，口苦，黄疸；京门治水肿，小便不利；带脉治妇科疾患；足窍阴开窍泻热，治目赤咽喉肿痛；环跳，风市，阳交，阳辅，悬钟，外丘等穴主要治下肢痿痹。

XI. THE GALLBLADDER MERIDIAN OF FOOT — SHAOYANG (44 acupoints in tota).

1. The Course

The meridian orginates from Tongziliao (GB1) at the outer cantus (1) and descends to the corner of the forehead (2). Then, it curves downwards to the retroauricular region at Fengchi (GB20) (3), and runs along the neck in front of the Triple Energizer Meridian of Hand — Shaoyang to the shoulder at which it runs across and behind the Meridian of Hand—Shaoyang (4). Then, it goes downwards to the supraclavicular fossa (5).

The branch arising at the auricle runs from the retroauricular region to enter the ear (6). It then emerges and passes the preauricular region (7) to the posterior aspect of the outer canthus (8).

The branch arising at the outer canthus (9) runs downwards to Daying (ST5) (10) and meets the Meridian of Hand—Shaoyang. Then, it reaches the infraorbital region (11). From there, it descends through Jiache (ST6) (12) and through the neck to meet its trunk at the supraclavicular fossa (13). From there, it further descends into the chest, and passes through the diaphragm (14) to connect with the liver (15) and the gallbladder, its pertaining organ (16). Then, it descends inside the hypochondriac region (17) and emerges at the lateral side of the lower abdomen near the femoral artery at the inguinal region (18). From there, it curves around the margin of the pubic hair (19) and transverses to enter the hip region (20).

The straight branch arising at the supraclavicular fossa (21) descends to the axilla (22) and runs downwards along the lateral side of the chest (23) and through the hypochondriac region (24) to join the previous branch at the hip region (25). Then, it descends along the lateral side of the thigh (26) to the lateral side of the knee (27). Going further downwards along the anterior aspect of the fibula (28) to the lower end of the fibula (29), it descends in front of the extenal malleolus and runs along the dorsum of the foot (30) to terminate at the lateral side of the tip of the 4th toe (31).

The branch arising at the dorsum of the foot starts from Zulinqi (GB41), runs between the 1st and 2nd metatarsal bones to the distal portion of the big toe, passes through the nail, and turns back to the hairy region posterior to the toe — nail, where it connects with the Liver Meridian of Foot—Jueyin (31).

The line made up by the acupoints distributed on the body surface: It origintes from the outer canthus at Tongziliao (GB1), and descends obliquely in front of the auricle. Then, it ascends to the corner of the forehead, curves around the retroauricular region, and turns back to the forehead. From there, it runs backwards on the temple to reach Fengchi (GB20) at the back of the head, descends through the shoulder, hypochondrium and waist to the hip, runs along the middle portion of the lateral aspect of the lower limb, passing in front of the external malleolus, and terminates at Zuqiaoyin (GB44) at the lateral side of the tip of the 4th toe.

The inner organs conerned: The liver, gallbladder, eye, ear.

2. The Commonly Used Acupoints

Tongziliao (GB1)

Location: On the face, 0.5 cun lateral to the outer canthus, at the depression on the lateral border of the orbit (See Fig. 1—68).
Indications: Headache, redness, swelling and pain of the eye, glaucoma, nebulae of corna.
Method: Puncture horizontally of obliquely backward 0.3—0.5 cun (9—15mm). Or prick with the three edged needle to cause bleding.

Tinghui (GB2)

Location: On the face, anterior to the intertragic notch, at the depression porsterior to the condyloid process of the mandible when the mouth is open (See Fig. 1—68, 1—69).
Indications: Deafness, tinnitus, toothache, deviation of the mouth.
Method: Ask the patient to open his mouth and puncture perpendicularly 0.5—1.0 cun (15—25mm). Moxibustion is applicable.

Shuaigu (GB8)

Location: On the head and at the temple, directly above the auricular apex, 1.5 cun above the hairline, directly above Jiaosun (SJ20) (See Fig. 1—70).
Indications: Migraine, dizziness, infantile convulsion.
Method: Puncture horizontally 0.5—1.0 cun (15—25mm). Moxibustion is applicable.

Yangbai (GB14)

Location: At the forehead, 1 cun above the midpoint of the eyebrow, approximtely at the junction of the upper 2/3 and lower 1/3 of the line drawn from the anterior hairline to the eyebrow (See Fig. 1—68).
Indications: Headche, eye pain, flickering of the eyelids.
Method: Puncture horizontally 0.3—0.5 cun (9—15mm). Moxibustion is applicable.

Fengchi (GB20)

Location: In the posterior aspect of the

neck, below the occipital bone, on the level of Fengfu (DU16), at the depression between the upper ends of m. sternocleido — mastoideus and m. trapezus (See Fig. 1—71).

Indications: Headache, redness and pain of the eye, sinusitis, stiffness and pain of the neck, common cold, epilepsy.

Method: Puncture obliquely towards the nasal apex 0.5—0.8 cun (15—25mm), the angle and depth of acupuncture must be controlled precisely because the deeper part of this point is the medulla oblongata (See Fig. 1—71). Moxibustion is applicable.

Jianjing (GB21)

Location: On the shoulder, directlly above the nipple, at the midpoint of the line connecting Dazhui (DU14) and the acromion (See Fig. 1—71).

Indications: Stiffness and pain of the head and neck, pain in the shoulder and back, acute mastitis, difficult labour.

Method: Puncture perpendicularly 0.5—0.8 cun (15—20mm). Deep puncture is prohibited since its deeper area is the apex of the lung. Moxibustion is applicable.

Riyue (GB24, Front-Mu point of the Gallbladder)

Location: On the upper abdomen, directly below the nipple, at the 7th intercostal space, 4 cun lateral to the anterior midline (See Fig. 1—67).

Indications: Hypochondriac pain, vomiting, hiccup, jaundice.

Method: Punctre obliquely or horizontally 0.5—0.8 cun (15—20mm). Moxibustion is applicable.

Jingmen (GB25, Front—Mu point of the kidney)

Location: On the side of the waist, 1.8 cun posterior to Zhangmen (LR13), below the free end of the 12th rib (See Fig. 1—67).

Indications: Dysuria, edema, pain in the hypochondrium and waist, borborygmus, diarrhea.

Method: Puncture perpendicularly 0.5—1.0 cun. Moxibustion is applicable.

Daimai (GB26)

Location: On the lateral side of the abdomen, 1.8 cun below Zhangmen (LR13), at the crossing point of a vertical line through the free end of the 11th rid and a horizontal line through the umbilicus (See Fig. 1—67).

Indications: Abnormal menstruation, leukorrhea with the reddish discharge, abdominal pain.

Method: Puncture perpendicularly 0.5—0.8 cun (15—20mm). Moxibustion is applicable.

Huantiao (GB30)

Location: On the lateral side of the thigh, when the patient is in the lateral recumbent position with the thigh flexed, at the junction of the lateral 1/3 and medial 2/3 of the line connecting the highest point of the greater trochanter and the hiatus of the sacrum (See Fig. 1—67, 1—72).

Indications: Lumbago, flaccidity and arthralgia of the lower limbs.

Method: Puncture perpendicularly 2. 0—3. 0 cun (50—75mm). Moxibustion is applicable.

Fengshi (GB31)

Location: At the midline of the lateral aspect of the thigh, 7 cun proximal to the transverse popliteal crease. Or, when the patient is standing upright with the hands hanging by the sides of the body, the point is where the tip of the middle finger reaches (See Fig. 1—73).

Indications: Flaccidity and arthralgia of the lower limbs, general itching.

Method: Pumcture perpendicularly 1. 0— 2. 0 cun (25—50mm). Moxibustion is applicable.

Xiyangguan (GB33)

Location: On the lataral side of the knee, 3 cun directly proximal to Yanglingquan (GB34), at the depression superior to the lateral epicondyle of the femur (See Fig. 1 —73).

Indications: Swelling and pain in the knee.

Method: Puncture perpendicularly. 0. 8— 1. 0 cun (20—25mm).

Yanglingquan (GB34, He—Sea point, Influential point of the tendon)

Location: On the lateral side of the leg, at the depression inferior and anterior to the head of the fibula (See Fig. 1—73).

Indications: Hypochondriac pain, flaccidity and arthralgia of the lower limbs, jaundice, infantal convulsion.

Method: Puncture perpendicularly 1. 0—1. 5 cun (25—40mm). Moxibustion is applicable.

Yangjiao (GB35)

Location: On the lateral side of the leg, 7 cun proximal to the tip of the external malleolus, at the posterior border of the fibula (See Fig. 1 —73).

Indications: Pain and distension of the chest and hypochondrium, flaccidity and arthralgia of the lower limb, epilepsy and mania.

Method: Puncture perpendicularly 0. 5—0. 8 cun (15—20mm). Moxibustion is applicable.

Waiqiu (GB36, Xi—Cleft point)

Location: On the lateral side of the leg, 7 cun above the tip of the external malleolus, level to Yangjiao (GB

35), at the anterior border of the fibula (See Fig. 1—73).

Indications: Distension and pain in the chest and hypochondrium, flaccidity and arthralgia of the lower limbs, epilepsy and mania.

Method: Puncture perpendicularly 0.5—0.8 cun (15—20mm). Moxibustion is applicable.

Guangming (GB37, Luo—Connecting point)

Location: On the lateral side of the leg, 5 cun proximal to the tip of the external malleolus, at the anterior border of the fibula (See Fig. 1—73).

Indications: Pain in the eye, night blindness, flaccidity and arthralgia of the lower limb.

Method: Puncture perpendicularly 0.5—0.8 cun (15—20mm). Moxibustion is applicable.

Yangfu (GB38, Jing—River point)

Location: On the lateral side of the leg, 4 cun proximal to the tip of the external malleolus, a little anterior to the anterior border of the fibula (See Fig. 1—73).

Indications: Migraine, flaccidity and arthralgia of the lower limb.

Method: Punctaure perpendicularly 0.5—0.8 cun (15—20mm). Moxibustion is applicable.

Xuanzhong (GB39, Influential point dominating the marrow, also known as Juegu)

Location: On the lateral side of the leg, 3 cun proximal to the tip or the external malleolus, at the anterior border of the fibula (See Fig. 1—73).

Indications: Hypochondriac pain, flaccidity and arthralgia of the lower limb, stiff neck.

Method: Puncture perpendicularly 0.5—1.0 cun (15—25mm). Moxibustion is applicable.

Qiuxu (GB40, Yuan—Source point)

Location: At the depression inferoanterior to the lateral malleolus, lateral to the tendon of the long extensor muscle of the toes (See Fig 1—74).

Indications: Distension and pain in the chest, flaccidity and arthralgia of the lower limb.

Method: Puncture perpendicularly 0.5—0.8 cun (15—20mm). Moxibustion is applicable.

Zulinqi (GB41, Shu—Stream point, one of the Eight Confluence points)

Location: On the lateral side of the instep of the foot, posterior to the 4th metatarsophalangeal joint, in the depression lateral to the tendon of the extensor muscle of the little toe (See Fig, 1—74).

Indications: Pain in the eye, pain in the outer canthus, hypochondriac pain, acute mastitis, abnormal menstration.

Method: Puncture perpendicularly 0.5—0.8 cun (15—20mm). Moxibustion is applicable.

Xiaxi (GB43, Ying-Spring point)

Location: On the lateral side of the instep of the foot, at the 4th intermatatarsal space, proximal to the margin of the web, at the junction of the red and white skin (See Fig. 1-74).

Indications: Headache, redness and pain in the outer canthus, tinnitus, deafness, hypochondriac pain, febrile diseases.

Method: Puncture perpendicularly of obliquely 0.5 cun (about 15mm). Moxibustion is applicable.

Zuqiaoyin (GB44, Jing—Well point)

Location: On the lateral side of the distal segment of the 4th toe, 0.1 cun from the corner of the toenail (See Fig 1—74).

Indications: Headache, redness and swelling and pain of the eye, swelling and sore throat, febrile diseases, insomnia.

Method: Puncture shallowly 0.1 cun (about 3mm), of prick with the three — edged needle to cause bleeding. Moxibustion is applicable.

3. *An Outline of Indications of the Commonly Used Acupoints*

The points of this meridian are mainly indicated in disorders of the lateral side of the head, eye, ear, and throat, mental disorders, febrile dsieases, and diseases of liver and gallbladder, as well as some other symptoms appearing on the pathway of this meridian, such as migraine, pain in the chest and hypochondrium, bitter taste in the mouth, dry throat, redness, swelling and pain of the eye, tinnitus, deafness. In the concrete, Tongziliao (GB1), Yangbai (GB14) and Guangming (GB37) are indicated in disorders of the eye; Fengchi (GB20), in headache and stuffy nose due to attack by the exogenous pathogenic factor by expelling the wind and dredging the meridian; Shuaigu (GB8) and Zulinqi (GB41), in migraine, trigeminal neuralgia; Jianjing (GB21), in stiffness and pain in the neck, acute mastitis; Riyue (GB24), Yanglingquan (GB34) and Qiuxu (GB40), in pain in the chest and hypochondrium, bitter taste in the mouth, and jaundice in diseases of the liver and gallbladder; Jingmen (GB25), in edema, dysuria; Daimai (GB26), in diseases of the gynecology; Zuqiaoyin (GB44), in redness of the eye, swelling and sore throat by inducing resuscitation and expelling the heat; and Huantiao (GB30), Fengshi (GB31), Yangjiao (GB35), Waiguan (GB36), Yangfu (GB38) and Xuanzhong (GB39), in flaccidity and arthralgia of the lower limb.

十二、足厥阴肝经（共14穴）

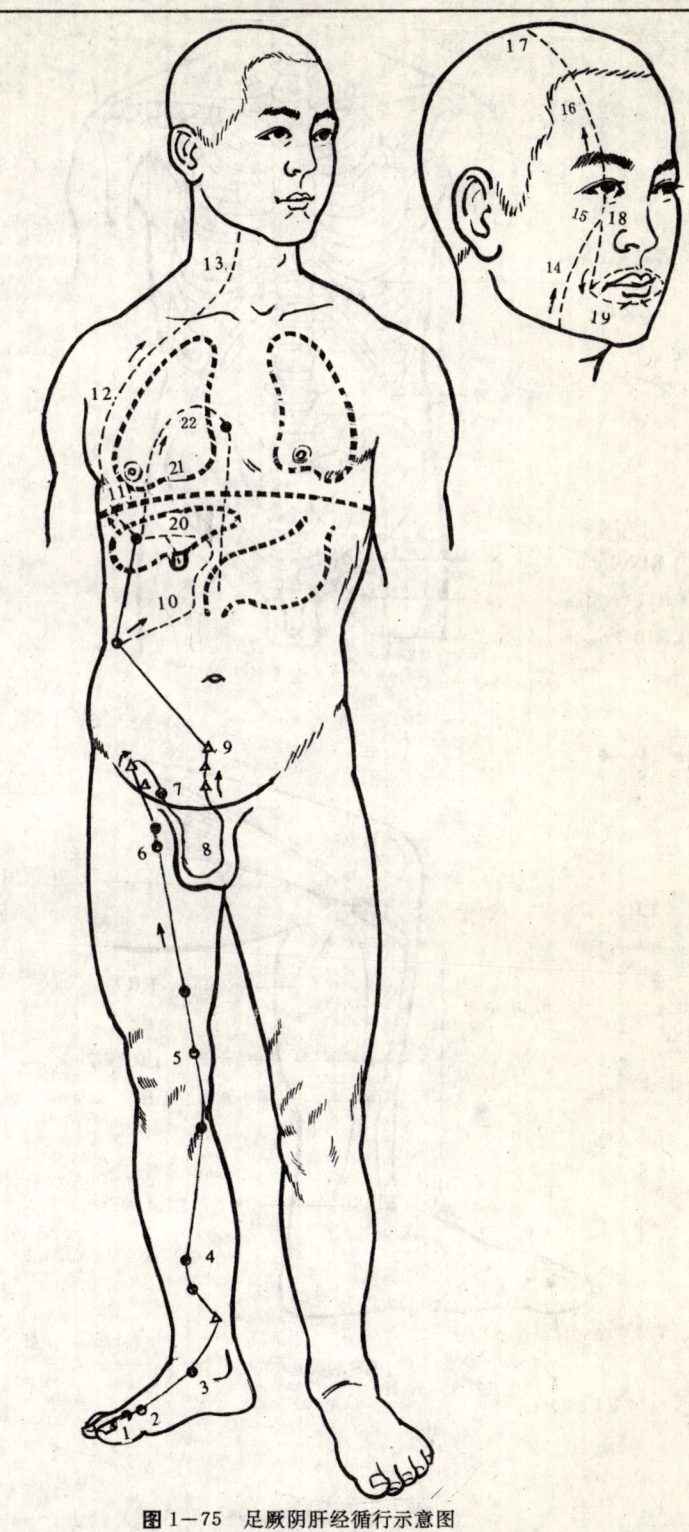

经络腧穴概要

图 1—75 足厥阴肝经循行示意图
Fig. 1—75 The Running Course of the Liver Meridian of Foot—Jueyin

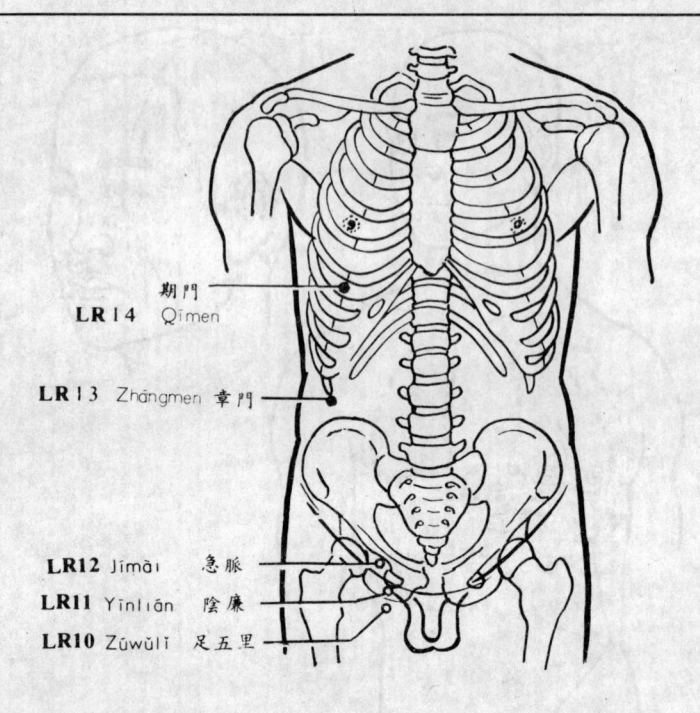

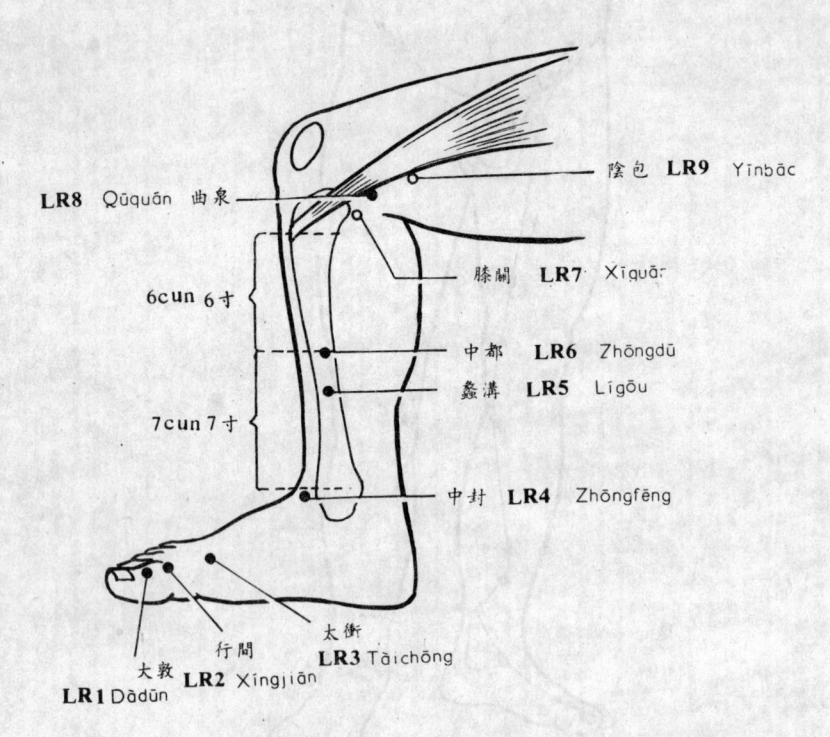

图 1—76 足厥阴肝经穴位图
Fig. 1—76 Acupoints of the Liver Meridian of Foot—Jueyin

（一）经脉循行

1. 起于足大趾上毫毛处大敦穴；2. 向上沿着足跗部上行；3. 经过内踝前1寸；4. 向上至内踝上八寸处，交出足太阴经之后；5. 上行膝之内侧；6. 沿着大腿内侧；7. 进入阴毛中；8. 绕过阴器；9. 抵达小腹；10. 挟着胃旁、属于肝脏，联络于胆；11. 向上通过横膈；12. 分布于胁肋；13. 沿着喉咙的后面；14. 向上进入鼻咽部；15. 连接于"目"系（眼球连系于脑的部位）；16. 向上出走于前额；17. 与督脉会合于巅顶；18. 其支脉从"目系"下行颊里；19. 环绕唇内；20. 另一支脉从肝分出；21. 通过横膈；22. 向上流注于肺与手太阴肺经相接。

体表穴位分布线：起于足大趾毫毛处大敦穴，沿足大趾，次趾之间，经内踝前上行，至内踝上八寸处交于足太阴经之后，循大腿内侧当中，绕阴部，经小腹，上季胁，止于乳下第六肋间期门穴。

体内相关的组织脏器：肝、胆、胃、肺、喉咙、鼻、咽、目。

（二）本经常用腧穴

大敦 (LR1 Dàdūn 井穴)

[定位] 在足大趾末节外侧，距趾甲角0.1寸（图1—77）。

[主治] 疝气、遗尿、崩漏、子宫脱垂、癫痫。

[操作] 针刺0.1～0.2寸（约3～6毫米）。

行间 (LR2 xíngjiān 荥穴)

[定位] 在足背侧，第一、二趾间，趾蹼缘的后方赤白肉际处取穴（图1—77）。

[主治] 崩漏、小便不利、头痛、目赤肿痛、口歪、胁痛、癫痫。

[操作] 直刺0.5～0.8寸（约15～20毫米）。

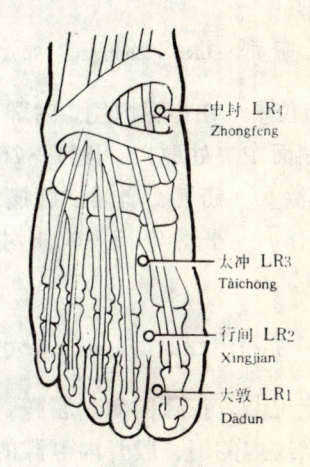

图1—77 大敦、行间、太冲、中封
Fig. 1—77 Dadun (LR 1), Xingjian (LR 2,) Taichong (LR 3) and Zhongfeng (LR 4)

太冲 (LR3 Tàichōng 输穴、原穴)

[定位] 在足背侧，当第1跖骨间隙的后方凹陷处（图1—77）。

[主治] 崩漏、遗尿、疝气、头痛、眩晕、口歪、胁痛、癫痫。

[操作] 直刺0.5～0.8寸（约15～20毫米）。

中封 (LR4 Zhōngfēng 经穴)

[定位] 在足背侧，内踝前，商丘与解溪连线之间，靠胫骨前肌腱的内侧凹陷中取穴（图1—77）。

[主治] 疝气、遗精、小便不利。

[操作] 直刺0.5～0.8寸（约15～20毫米）。

蠡沟 (LR5 Lígōu 络穴)

[定位] 在小腿内侧，内踝尖上5寸，

胫骨内侧面的中央处取穴（图1—76）。

［主治］ 月经不调、带下、小便不利。

［操作］ 平刺0.5～0.8寸（约15～20毫米）。

中都（LR6 Zhōngdū 郄穴）

［定位］ 在小腿内侧，内踝尖上7寸，胫骨内侧面中央处取穴（图1—76）。

［主治］ 疝气、崩漏、腹痛。

［操作］ 平刺0.5～0.8寸（约15～20毫米）。

曲泉（LR8 Qūquán 合穴）

［定位］ 在膝内侧，屈膝，当膝关节内侧面横纹内侧端、股骨内侧髁的后缘、半腱肌、半膜肌止端的前缘凹陷处（图1—78）。

［主治］ 腹痛、小便不利、疝气、遗精。

［操作］ 直刺1～1.5寸（约25～40毫米）。

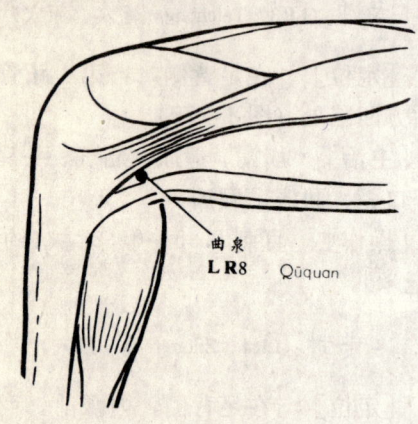

图1—78 曲泉穴
Fig. 1—78 Ququan (LR 8)

章门（LR13 Zhāngmén 募穴，脏会穴）

［定位］ 在侧腹部，第十一肋游离端的下方（图1—79）。

［主治］ 腹胀、泄泻、胁痛。

［操作］ 斜刺0.5～0.8寸（约15～20毫米）。不宜深刺，以免伤及内脏。

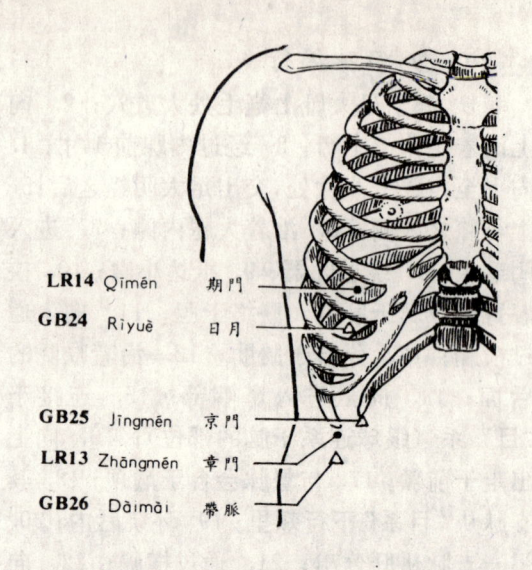

图1—79 章门、期门
Fig. 1—79 Zhangmen (LR 13) and Qimen (LR14)

期门（LR14 Qímén 募穴）

［定位］ 在胸部，当乳头直下，第6肋间隙，前正中线旁开4寸（图1—79）。

［主治］ 胸胁胀痛、呕吐。

［操作］ 斜刺或平刺0.5～0.8寸（约15～20毫米）。不宜深刺，以免伤及内脏。

（三）常用经穴主治提要

本经腧穴主要用于肝及与肝有密切关系的胆、肾、心、脾、肺等脏之病证。如头痛、眩晕、神志病、眼病、疝气、黄疸、胁痛及经脉循行部位的其他病证。其中行间、太冲疏理肝气、治头晕目眩、目赤肿痛、崩漏；此外，行间、太冲还能降血压；中封，蠡沟，中都，曲泉治疝气、腹痛、遗精、小便不利；章门、期门治胁痛、黄疸等肝胆疾患。

XⅡ. THE LIVER MERIDIAN OF FOOT

— JUEYIN (14 acupoints in total)

1. *The Course:* This meridian starts from Dadun (LR 1) at the hairy region of the dorsum of the big toe (1), ascends along the dorsum of the foot (2), passes through the point 1 cun in front of the medial malleolus (3), and reaches the area 8 cun proximal to the medial malleolus, where it crosses and then runs behind the Meridian of the Foot—Taiyin (4). Then, it ascends along the medial aspect of the knee (5) and along the medial aspect of the thigh (6) to the pubic hairy region (7), curves around the external genitalia (8), and reaches the lower abdomen (9). It then rums upwards and encircles the stomach to enter the liver, its pertaining organ, and connects with the gallbladder (10). From there, it continues to ascend, passing through the diaphragm (12) and distributing itself over the hypochondrium and costal region (12). Then, it ascends along the posterior aspect of the throat (13) to the nasopharynx (14) and connects with the brain (15). Running further upward, it emerges at the forehead (16) and meets the Governor Vessel at the vertex of the head (17).

The branch arising from the "eye system" (i. e. the connetion of the eyeball and brain) descends into the cheek (18) and curves around the inner surface of the lips (19).

Another branch arising from the liver (20) passes through the diaphragm (21), ascends into the lung, and connects with the Lung Meridian of Hand — Taiyin (22).

The line made up by the acupoints distributed over the body surface: It starts from Dadun (LR 1) at the hairy region of the dorsum of the big toe, runs along the interspace between the big and 2nd toes, passes in front of the internal malleolus, and ascends to the point 8 cun proximal to the medial malleolus where it crosses and then runs behind the Meridian of Foot—Taiyin. From there, it runs upwards along the middle portion of the medial aspect of the thigh, curves around the external genitalia, and ascends through the lower abdomen to hypochondrium. Then, it terminates at Qimen (LR 14) at the 6th intercostal space below the nipple.

The inner organs concerned: The liver, gallbladder, stomach, lung, throat, nose, eye.

2. *The Commonly Used Acupoints*

Dadun (LR 1, Jing—Well point)

Location: At the lateral aspect of the dorsum of the terminal phalanx of the big toe, 0. 1 cun from the corner of the nail (See Fig. 1—77).

Indications: Hernia, enuresis, metrorrhagia and metrostaxis, prolapse of the uterus, epilepsy and mania.

Method: Puncture obliquely 0. 1—0. 2 cun (3—6mm). Moxibustion is applicable.

Xingjian (LR 2, Ying—Spring point)

Location: On the instep of the foot, between the 1st and 2nd toes, at the junction of the red and white skin proximal to the margin of the web (See Fig 1—77).

Indications: Metrorrheagia and metrostaxis, dysuria, headache, redness and swelling and pain of the eye, deviation of the mouth, hypochondriac pain, epilepsy and mania.

Method: Puncture perpendicularly 0.5—08 cun (15—20mm). Moxibustion is applicable.

Taichong (LR 3, Shu—Stream and Yuan—Source point)

Location: At the dorsum of the foot, at the depression of the posterior end of the 1st interosseous metatarsal space (see Fig. 1—77).

Indications: Metrorrhagia and metrostaxis, enuresis, hernia, headache, dizziness, deviation of the mouth, hypochondriac pain, epilepsy and mania.

Method: Puncture perpendicularly 0.5—0.8 cun (15—20mm). Moxibustion is applicable.

Zhongfeng (LR 4, Jing—River point)

Location: On the instep of the foot, 1 cun anterior to the medial malleolus, at the depression medial to the tendon of m. tibialis anterior, on the line connecting Shangqiu (SP 5) and Jiexi (ST41) (See Fig. 1—77).

Indications: Hernia, emission, dysuria.

Method: Puncture perpendicularly 0.5—0.8 cun (15—20mm). Moxibustion is applicable.

Ligou (LR 5, Luo—Connecting point)

Location: On the medial side of the leg, 5 cun proximal to the tip of the medial aspect of the tibia (See Fig. 1—76).

Indications: Abnormal menstruation, leukorrhea, dysuria.

Method: Puncture horizontally 0.5—0.8 cun (15—20mm). Moxibustion is applicable.

Zhongdu (LR 6, Xin—Cleft point)

Location: On the medial side of the leg, 7 cun proximal to the tip of the medial malleolus, at the midline of the medial aspect of the tibia (See Fig. 1—76).

Indications: Hernia, metrorrhagia and metrostaxis, abdominal pain.

Method: Puncture horizontally 0.5—0.8 cun (15—20mm). Moxibustion is appplicable.

Ququan (LR 8, He—Sea point)

Location: On the medial side of the knee, when the knee is flexed, the point is at the depression proximal to the medial end of the transverse popliteal crease, posterior to the medial epicondyle of the tibia, on the anterior part of the insertions of m. semimembranosus and m. semitendinosus

(See Fig. 1—78).
Indications: Abdominal pain, dysuria, hernia, emission.
Method: Puncture perpendicularly 1.0—1.5 cun (25—40mm). Moxibustion is applicable.

Zhangmen (LR 13, Front—Mu point of the spleen, Influential point dominating the zang organs)

Location: Right below the free end of the 11th rib, at the lateral side of the chest (See Fig. 1—79).
Indications: Abdominal pain and distension, diarrhea, hypochondriac pain.
Method: Puncture obliquely 0.5—0.8un (15—20mm). Deep puncture is not advisable, otherwise the inner organ may be injured. Moxibustion is applicable.

Qimen (LR 14, Front—Mu point of the Liver)

Location: On the chest, when the patient lies supine, directly below the nipple, at the 6th intercostal space, 4 cun lateral to the anterior midline (See Fig. 1—79).
Indications: Hypochondriac pain and distension, vomiting.
Method: Puncture obliquely or horizontally 0.5—0.8cun (15—20mm). Deep puncture is not advisable, otherwlse the inner organ may be injured. Moxibustion is applicable.

3. *An Outline of the Commonly Used Acupoints of this Meridian*

The acupoints of this meridian are mainly indicated in the disorders of the liver and organs which closely related to the liver, including the gallbadder, kidney, heart, spleen, lung, etc, such as headache, dizziness, mental disorders, eye problems, hernia, jaundice, hypochondriac pain, and other disorders appearing on the pathway of this meridian. In the concrete, Xingjian (LR 2) and Taichong (LR 3) are indicated in dizziness, redness and swelling and pain of the eye, and metrorrhagia and metrostaxis by soothing the liver and regulating the circulation of qi. Additionally, they may be used to relieve hypertension. Zhongfeng (LR 14), Ligou (LR 5), Zhongdu (LR 6), and Ququan (LR 8) are indicated in hernia, abdominal pain, emission, dysuria; and Zhangmen (LR 13) and Qimen (LR 14), in the disorders of the liver and gallbladder, such as hypochondriac pain, jaundice.

十三、任脉（共24穴）

（一）经脉循行

1. 起于小腹内，下出会阴部；2. 向上行于阴毛部；3. 沿着腹内，向上行至关元等穴；4. 一直到达咽喉部；5. 再向上环绕口唇；6. 经过面部；7. 进入目眶下承泣穴。

体表穴位分布线：起于前后二阴间会阴穴，沿腹胸正中线上行颈喉部，止于颏下正中承浆穴。

体内相关的组织脏器：胞宫、咽喉、口唇、眼。

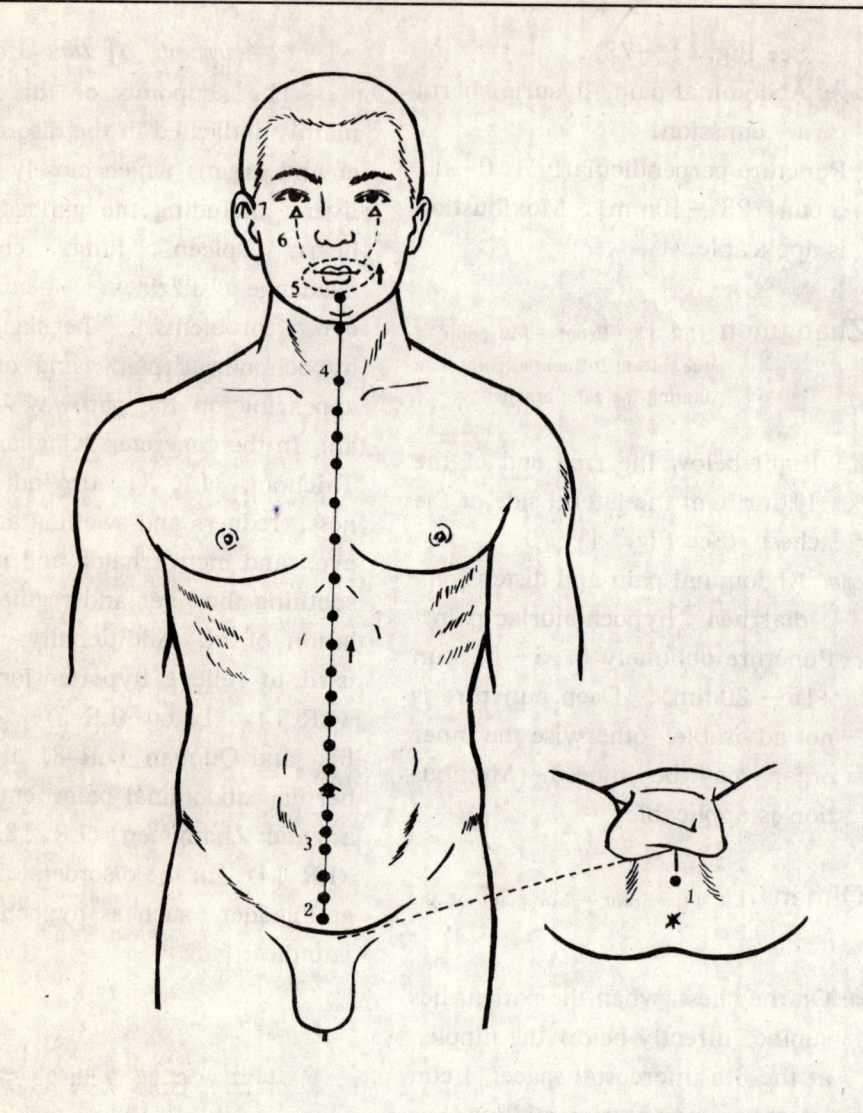

图 1—80 任脉循行示意图
Fig. 1—80 The Running Course of the Conception Vessel (Ren Meridian)

(二) 本经常用腧穴

会阴 (RN1 HuìYīn)

[定位] 在会阴部,男性在阴囊根部与肛门连线的中点;女性在大阴唇后联合与肛门连线的中点(图 1—81)。

[主治] 小便不利,遗精,月经不调,昏迷。

[操作] 直刺 0.5～1 寸(约 15～25 毫米)。

中极 (RN3 Zhōngjí 募穴)

[定位] 在下腹部,前正中线上,当脐中下 4 寸(图 1—81)。

· 132 ·

［主治］ 遗尿、小便不利、遗精、月经不调、子宫脱垂。

［操作］ 直刺0.5～1寸（约15～25毫米）。

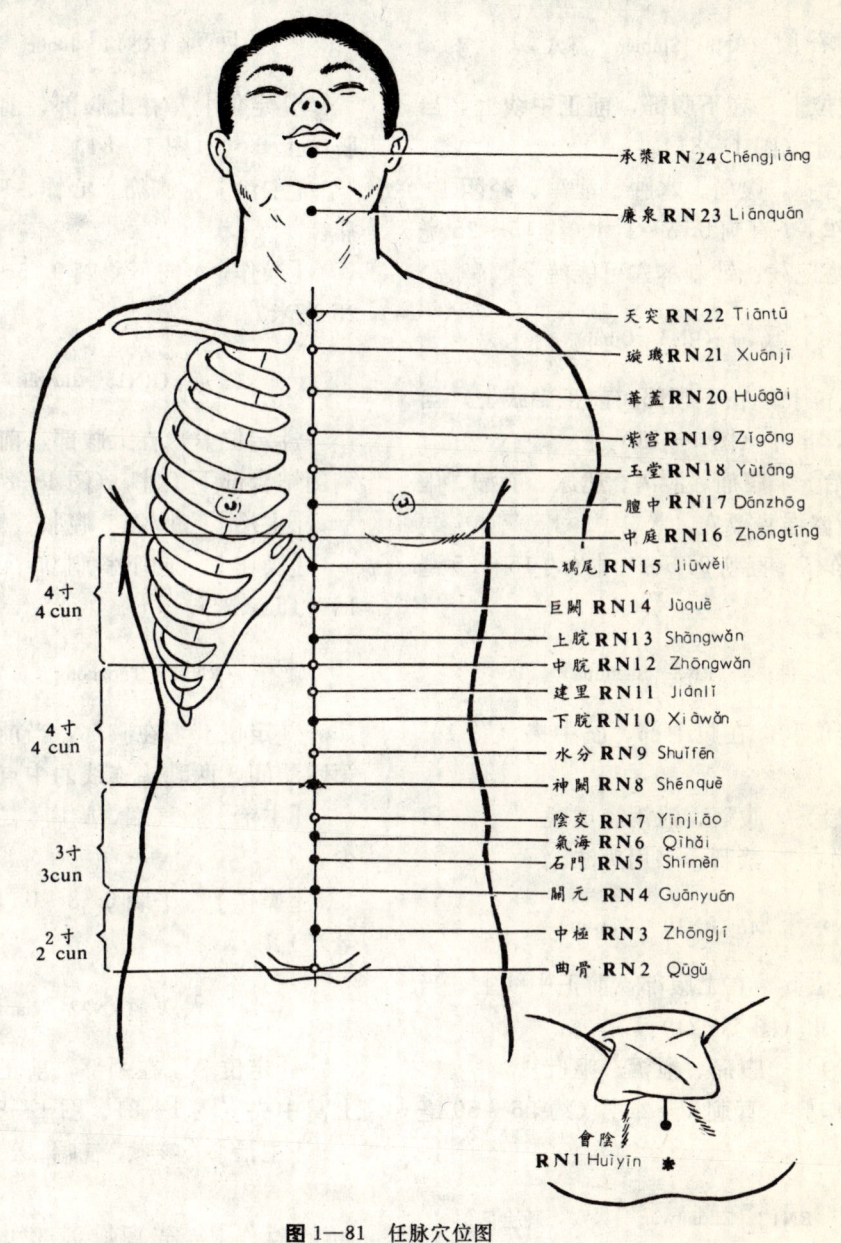

图1—81 任脉穴位图
Fig. 1—81 The Acupoints of the Ren Meridian (Conception Vessel)

关元 （RN4 Guānyuán 募穴）

［定位］ 在下腹部，前正中线上，当脐中下3寸（图1—81）。

［主治］ 遗尿、尿闭、泄泻、阳萎、月经不调、虚劳。为保健强身要穴。

［操作］ 直刺0.5～1寸（约15～25毫米）。

石门 (RN5 Shímén 募穴)

［定位］ 在下腹部，前正中线上，当脐中下2寸（图1—81）。

［主治］ 腹痛、水肿、泄泻、经闭。

［操作］ 直刺0.5～1寸（约15～25毫米）。古籍记载：针刺本穴可能绝孕。

气海 (RN6 Qìhǎi)

［定位］ 在下腹部，前正中线上，当脐中下1.5寸（图1—81）。

［主治］ 腹痛、泄泻、遗尿、崩漏、虚脱。为保健强身要穴。

［操作］ 直刺0.5～1寸（约15～25毫米）。

神阙 (RN8 Shénquè)

［定位］ 在腹中部，脐中央（图1—81）。

［主治］ 腹痛、泄泻、虚脱。

［操作］ 禁刺；多用灸法。

下脘 (RN10 Xiàwǎn)

［定位］ 在上腹部，前正中线上，当脐中上2寸（图1—81）。

［主治］ 腹痛、泄泻、呕吐。

［操作］ 直刺1～2寸（约25～50毫米）。

中脘 (RN12 Zhōngwǎn 募穴，腑会穴)

［定位］ 在上腹部，前正中线上，当脐中上4寸（图1—81）。

［主治］ 胃痛、呕吐、腹胀、泄泻、癫狂。

［操作］ 直刺1～1.5寸（约25～40毫米）。

巨阙 (RN14 Jùquè 募穴)

［定位］ 在上腹部，前正中线上，当脐中上6寸（图1—81）。

［主治］ 胸痛、心悸、呕吐、癫、狂、痫。

［操作］ 向下斜刺0.5～1寸（约15～25毫米）。

鸠尾 (RN15 Jiūwěi 络穴)

［定位］ 在上腹部，前正中线上，当胸剑结合部下1寸，（图1—81）。

［主治］ 胸痛、腹胀、癫、狂、痫。

［操作］ 向下斜刺0.4～0.6寸（约10～15毫米）。

膻中 (RN17 Tànzhōng 募穴，气会穴)

［定位］ 在胸部，当前正中线上，平第四肋间，两乳头连线的中点（图1—81）。

［主治］ 气喘，胸痛、心悸、呕吐、乳少。

［操作］ 平刺0.3～0.5寸（约9～15毫米）。

天突 (RN22 Tiāntù)

［定位］ 在颈部，前正中线上，胸骨上窝中央（图1—81、图1—82）。

［主治］ 咳嗽、气喘、暴喑、咽喉肿痛、噎膈。

［操作］ 先直刺0.2寸（约6毫米），然后将针尖转向下方，紧靠胸骨后方刺入1寸（约25毫米左右）（图1—83）；避免刺伤肺脏及有关动、静脉和气管。

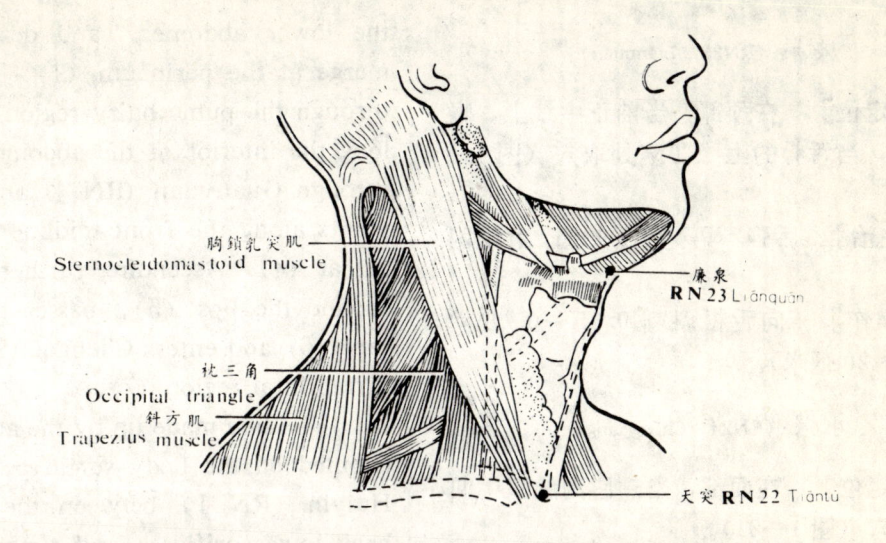

经络腧穴概要

图 1—82 天突、廉泉
Fig. 1—82 Tiantu (RN 22) and Lianquan (RN 23)

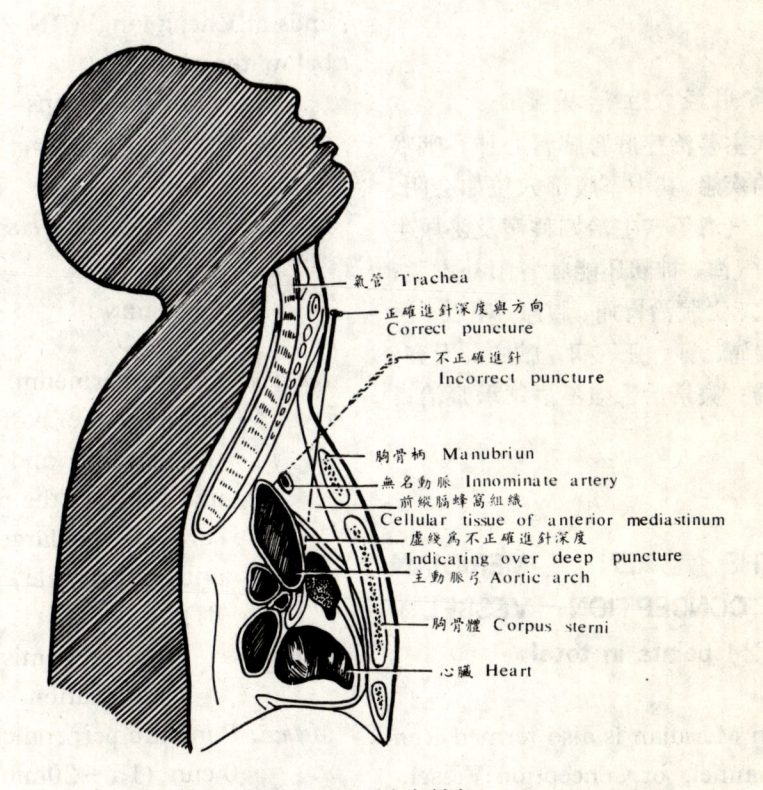

胸锁乳突肌 Sternocleidomastoid muscle
廉泉 RN 23 Liánquán
枕三角 Occipital triangle
斜方肌 Trapezius muscle
天突 RN 22 Tiāntū

图 1—83 天突穴刺法
Fig. 1—83 Needling at Tiantu (RN 22)

气管 Trachea
正确进针深度与方向 Correct puncture
不正确进针 Incorrect puncture
胸骨柄 Manubriun
无名动脉 Innominate artery
前纵膈蜂窝组织 Cellular tissue of anterior mediastinum
虚线为不正确进针深度 Indicating over deep puncture
主动脉弓 Aortic arch
胸骨体 Corpus sterni
心脏 Heart

廉泉 (RN23 Liánquán)

[定位] 在颈部，当前正中线上，喉结上方，当舌骨的上缘凹陷处取穴（图1—82）。

[主治] 舌强不语，舌下肿痛，吞咽困难。

[操作] 向舌根斜刺 0.5～0.8寸（约15～20毫米）。

承浆 (RN24 Chéngjiāng)

[定位] 在面部，当颏唇沟的正中凹陷处取穴（图1—81）。

[主治] 口歪、齿痛。

[操作] 斜刺 0.3～0.5寸（约9～15毫米）。

（三）常用经穴主治提要

本经经穴主要治疗肝肾脾胃心肺，咽喉及有关脏腑的疾患。其中下腹部穴位如会阴、中极、关元、气海等穴主治妇科病及泌尿生殖病；关元、气海、神阙还能壮肾阳补虚脱；上腹穴位中脘、上脘治胃痛、腹胀、呕吐；巨阙、鸠尾治胸痛、癫、狂、痫；膻中、天突治咳嗽、气喘；廉泉治舌强不语；承浆治口齿疾患。

XIII. THE REN MERIDIAN (CONCEPTION VESSEL)
(24 points in total)

The Ren Meridian is also termed Renmai, Ren Channel, or Conception Vessel.

1. The Course

The channel starts from the inside of the lower abdomen, and descends to emerge at the perineum (1). It ascennds through the pubic hairy region (2) and along the interior of the abdomen, passing through Guanyuan (RN 4) and the other points along the front midline (3) to the throat (4). Ascending further, it curves around the lips (5), passes through the face (6) and enters Chengqi (ST1) at the infraorbital region (7).

The line made up by the acupoints distributed on the body surface: It starts at Huiyin (RN 1) between the front and back lower orifices, and runs upwards along the midline of the abdomen and chest and through the neck and throat. Then, it ends at Chengjiang (RN 24) at the center below the chin.

The inner organs concernd: The uterus, throat, lip, eye.

2. The Commonly Used Acupoints

Huiyin (RN 1)

Location: On the perineum, at the midpoint between the posterior border of the scrotum and anus in male, and between the posterior commissure of the large labia and the anus in female (See Fig. 1—81).

Indications: Dysuria, emission, abnormal menstruation, coma.

Method: Puncture perpendicularly 0.5—1.0 cun (15—20mm). Moxibustion is applicable.

Zhongji (RN 3, Front—Mu point of the

bladder)

Location: On the lower abdomen, 4 cun below the center of the umbilicus, at the midline of the abdomen (See Fig. 1—81).

Indications: Enuresis, dysuria, emission, abnormal menstruation, prolpse of the uterus.

Method: Puncture perpendicularly 0.5—1.0 cun (15—25mm). Moxibustion is applicable.

Guanyuan (RN 4, Front—Mu point of the small intestine)

Location: On the lower abdomen, 3 cun below the center of the umbilicus, at the midline of the abdomen (See Fig. 1—81).

Indications: Enuresis, retention of urine, diarrhea, impotence, abnormal menstruation, consumptive diseases.

Note: the point is one of the important acupoints for tonification.

Method: Puncture perpendicularly 0.5—1.0 cun (15—25mm). Moxibustion is applicable.

Shimen (RN 5, Front — Mu point of Sanjiao)

Location: On the lower abdomen, 2 cun below the center of the umbilicus, at the midline of the abdomen (See Fig. 1—81).

Indications: Abdominal pain, edema, diarrhea, amenorrhea.

Method: Punture perpendicularly 0.5—1.0 cun (15—25mm). Moxibustion is applicable.

Note: it is recorded in ancient books that puncturing this point might cause sterility.

Qihai (RN 6)

Location: On the lower abdomen, 1.5 cun below the center of the umbilicus, at the midline of the abdomen. (See Fig. 1—81).

Indications: Abdominal pain, diarrhea, enuresis, metrorrhagia and metrostaxis, collapse. It is an important acupoint for tonification.

Method: Puncture perpendicularly 0.5—1.0 cun (15—25mm). Moxibustion is applicable.

Shenque (RN 8)

Location: On the middle abdomen and at the center of the umbilicus (See Fig. 1—81).

Indications: Abdominal pain, diarrhea, collapse.

Method: Puncture is prohibited. Moxibustion is applicable.

Xiawan (RN 10)

Location: On the upper abdomen, 2 cun above the center of the umbilicus, at the midline of the abdomen (See Fig. 1—81).

Indications: Abdominal pain, diarrhea, vomiting.

Method: Puncture perpendicularly 1.0—2.

0 cun (25—50mm). Moxibustion is applicable.

Zhongwan (RN 12, Front—Mu point of the stomach, Influential point dominating fu organs)

Location: On the upper abdomen, 4 cun above the center of the umbilicus, at the midline of the abdomen (See Fig. 1—81).
Indications: Stomachache, vomiting, abdominal distension, diarrhea, epilepsy and mania.
Method: Puncture perpendicularly 1.0—1.5 cun (25—40mm). Moxibustion is applicable.

Juque (RN 14, Front—Mu point of the heart)

Location: On the upper abdomen, 6 cun above the center of the umbilicus, at the midline of the abdomen (See Fig. 1—81).
Indications: Pain in the chest, palpitation, vomiting, epilepsy and mania.
Method: Puncture obliquely 0.5—1.0 cun (15—25mm). Moxibustion is applicable.

Jiuwei (RN 15, Luo—Connecting point)

Location: On the upper abdomen, 7 cun above the center of the umbilicus, at the midline of the abdomen, 1 cun below the xiphisternal synchondrosis (See Fig. 1—81).
Indications: Pain in the chest, abdominal distension, epilepsy and mania.
Method: Puncture obliquely downward 0.4—0.6 cun (10—15mm). Moxibustion is applicable.

Danzhong (RN 17, Front—Mu point of the pericardium, Influential point dominating qi)

Location: On the chest, midway between the nipples, at the midline of the chest, parallel to the 4th intercostal space (See Fig. 1—81).
Indications: Asthma, pain in the chest, palpitation, vomiting, lack of lactation.
Method: Puncture horizontally 0.3—0.5 cun (9—15mm). Moxibustion is applicable.

Tiantu (RN 22)

Location: On the neck and on the anterior midline, at the center of the suprasternal fossa (See Fig. 1—81, 1—82).
Indications: Cough, asthma, sudden aphonia, swelling and sore throat, dysphagia.
Method: First puncture perpendicularly 0.2 cun (about 6mm) and then insert the needle tip downward along the posterior border of the sternum about 1.0 cun (15mm) (See Fig. 1—83). Avoid wounding the lung and conerned artery, vein and trachea. Moxibustion is applicable.

Lianquan (RN 23)

Location: On the neck and on the anterior midline, above the Adam's apple, at the depression above the upper of the hyoid bone (See Fig. 1—82).
Indications: Aphonia with stiffness of tongue, swelling and pain of the subglossal region, difficulty in swallowing.
Method: Puncture obliquely 0.5—0.8cun (15—20mm) towards the root of the tongue. Moxibustion is applicable.

Chengjiang (RN 24)

Location: On the face, at the depression in the center of the mentolabial groove (See Flg. 1—81).
Indications: Deviation of the mouth, toothache.
Method: Puncture obliquely 0.3—0.5 cun (9—15mm). Moxibustion is applicable.

3. *An Outline of Indications of the Commonly Used Acupoints*

The points of this channel are mainly used to treat disorders of liver, kidney, spleen, stomach, heart, lung, throat, and some other organs. In the concrete, among the points at the lower abdomen, Huiyin (RN 1), Zhongji (RN 3), Guanyuan (RN 4) and Qihai (RW 6) are indicated in diseases of gynecology and urogenital system; and Guanyuan (RN 4), Qihai (RN 6) and Shenque (RN 8), in collapase by reinforcing yang of kidney. While among the points at the upper abdomen or above it, Zhongwan (RN 12) and Shangwan (RN 13) are indicated in stomachache, abdominal distension, and vomiting; Juque (EN 14) and Juwei (RN 15), in pain of the chest, epilepsy and mania; Dangzhong (RN 17) and Tiantu (RN 22) in cough, asthma; Lianquan (RN 23), in aphasia with stiffness of tongue; and Chengjiang (RN 24) in disorders of the mouth and toothache.

十四、督脉（共13穴）

（一）经脉循行

1. 起于小腹内，向下出于会阴部；2. 向后循行于脊柱内部；3. 向上到达项后风府，进入脑内；4. 再上行巅顶；5. 沿着前额下行至鼻柱。

体表穴位分布线：起于尾骨下端长强穴，沿腰背正中线上行至头顶正中，向前下行鼻柱，止于上唇内龈交穴。

体内相关的组织脏器：胞宫、脑、脊柱。

（二）本经常用腧穴

长强（DU1 Chángqiáng 络穴）

［定位］ 尾骨端下，尾骨端与肛门连线之中点取穴（图1—86）。

［主治］ 便血、痔疾、癫狂。

［操作］ 斜刺，针尖向上，与骶骨平行刺入0.5～1寸（约15～25毫米），（图1—87）直刺易伤直肠。

腰阳关（DU3 Yāoyángguán）

［定位］ 在腰部，当后正中线上，第

图 1—84 督脉循行示意图
Fig. 1—84 The Running Course of the Governor Vessel (Du Meridian)

四腰椎棘突下凹陷中（图 1—85）。

［主治］ 月经不调，遗精，腰骶痛，下肢痿痹。

［操作］ 向上斜刺 0.5～0.8 寸（约 15～20 毫米）。

命门 (DU4 Mìngmén)

［定位］ 在腰部，当后正中线上，第

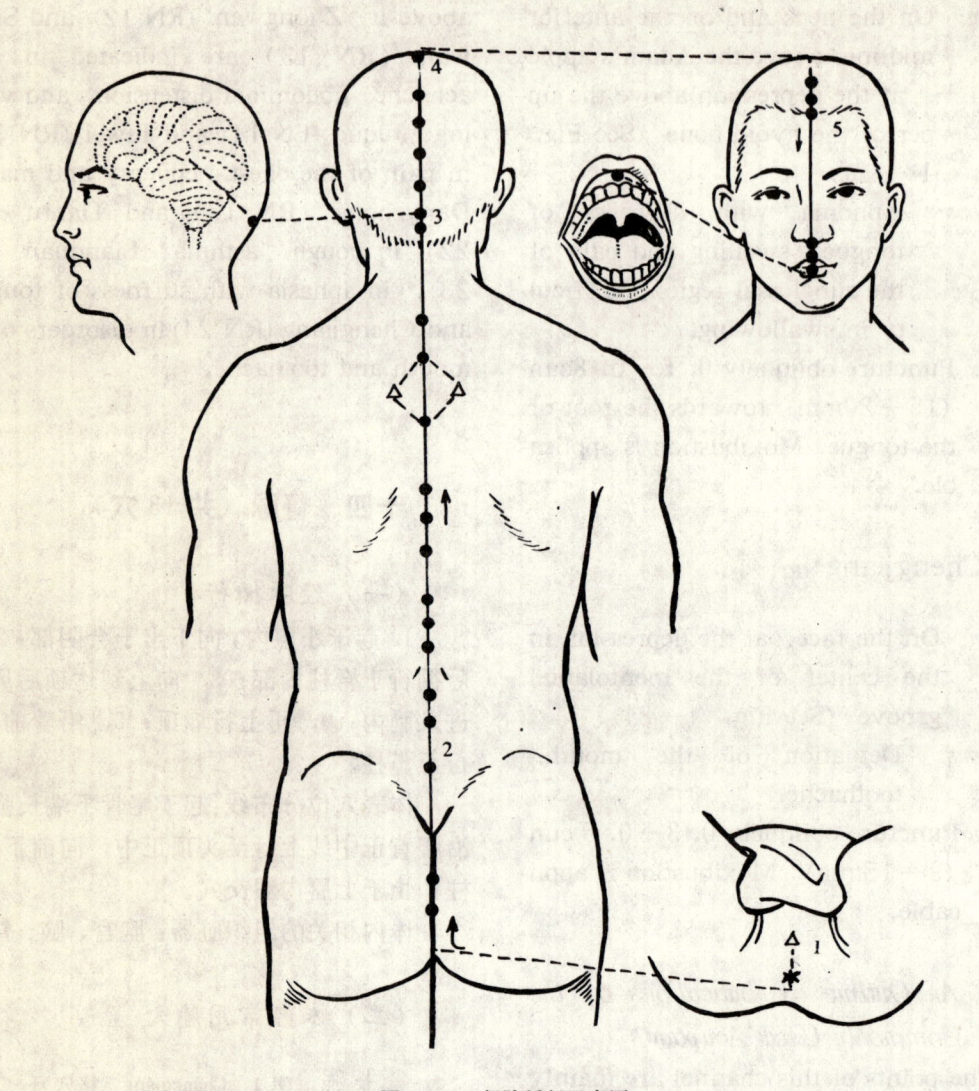

二腰椎棘突下凹陷中取穴（图 1—85）。

［主治］ 阳萎、遗精、带下、腰痛、泄泻、月经不调。

［操作］ 向上斜刺 0.5～0.8 寸（约 15～20 毫米）。

至阳 (DU9 Zhìyáng)

［定位］ 在背部，当后正中线上，第

七胸椎棘突下凹陷处取穴。(图 1—85)。

[主治] 黄疸、咳喘、脊强、背痛。

[操作] 向上斜刺 0.5～0.8 寸（约 15～20 毫米）。

陶道 (DU13 Táodào)

[定位] 在背部，当后正中线上，第一胸椎棘突下凹陷中取穴（图 1—85）。

[主治] 头痛、疟疾、热病。

[操作] 向上斜刺 0.5～0.8 寸（约 15～20 毫米）。

大椎 (DU14 Dàzhuī)

[定位] 在后正中线上，第七颈椎棘突下凹陷中取穴（图 1—85）。

[主治] 咳嗽、气喘、头痛、项强、热病、疟疾、癫痫。

[操作] 向上斜刺 0.5～0.8 寸9约 15～20 毫米）。

哑门 (DU15 Yǎmén)

[定位] 在项部，当后发际正中直上 0.5 寸，第一颈椎下（图 1—88）。

[主治] 暴喑、舌强不语、癫、狂、痫。

[操作] 缓慢向下颌方向斜刺入 0.5 寸（约 15 毫米），不可深刺或向上斜刺（图 1—89），以免误伤延髓。

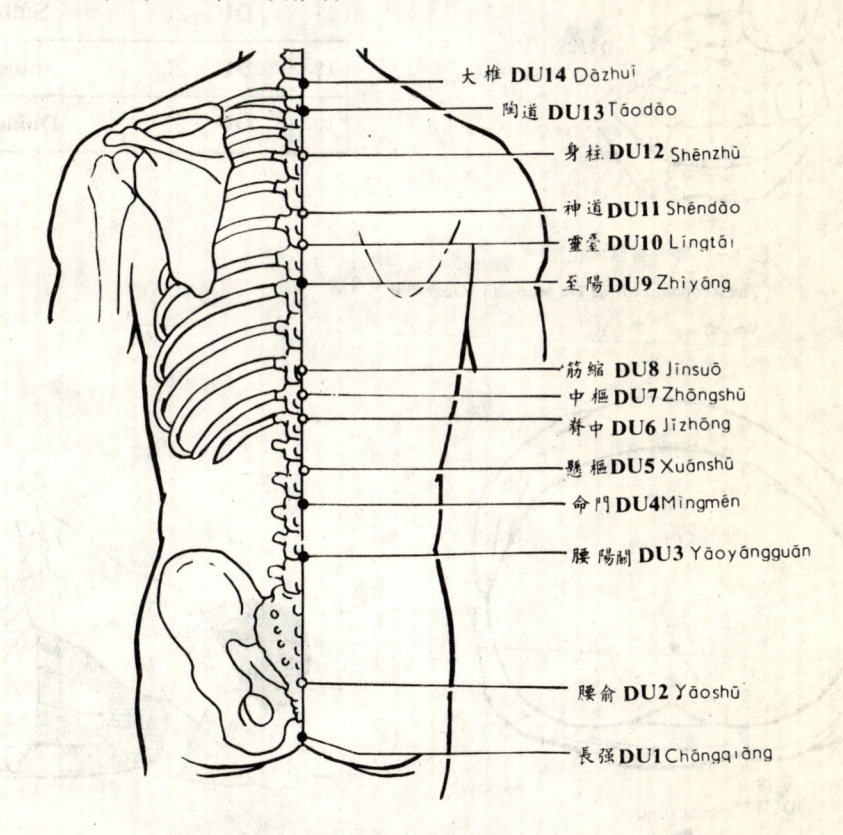

图 1—85① 督脉穴位图

Fig. 1—85① The Acupoints of the Du Meridian (Governor Vessel)

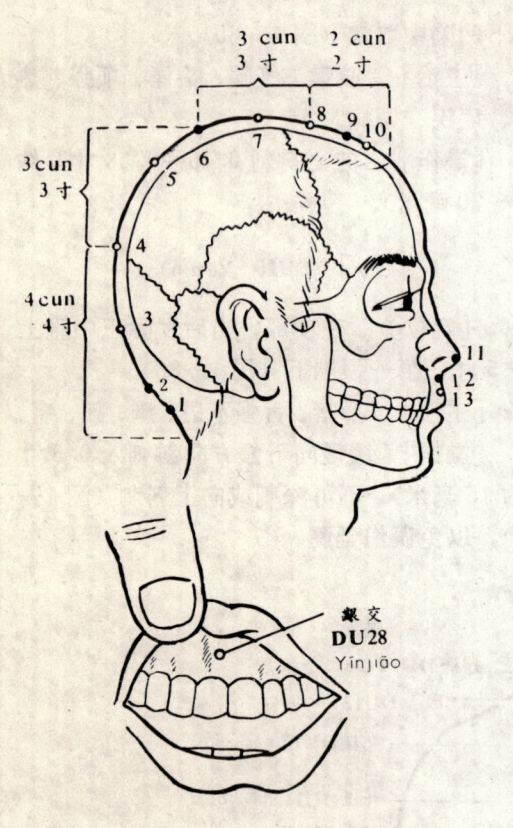

Summary of Meridians, Collaterals and Acupoints

1.	DU	15	Yǎmén	哑门
2.	DU	16	Fēngfǔ	风府
3.	DU	17	Nǎohù	脑户
4.	DU	18	Qiángjiān	强间
5.	DU	19	Hòudǐng	后顶
6.	DU	20	Bǎihuì	百会
7.	DU	21	Qiándǐng	前顶
8.	DU	22	Xìnhuì	囟会
9.	DU	23	Shàngxīng	上星
10.	DU	24	Shéntíng	神庭
11.	DU	25	Sùliáo	素髎
12.	DU	26	Shuǐgōu	水沟
13.	DU	27	Duìduān	兑端

图 1—85② 督脉穴位图

Fig. 1—85② The Acupoints of the Du Meridian (Governor Vessel)

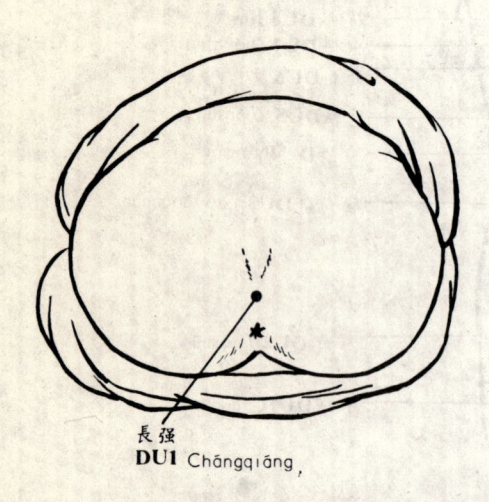

图 1—86 长强穴

Fig. 1—86 Changqiang (DU 1)

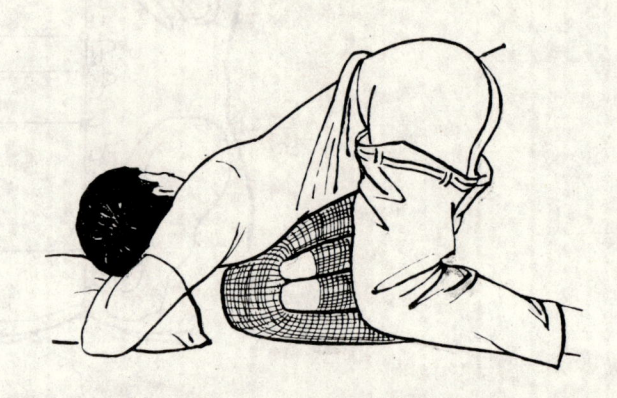

图 1—87 长强穴针刺姿式

Fig. 1—87 Patient's Posture in Needling at Changqiang (DU 1)

经络腧穴概要

［主治］ 头痛、项强、眩晕、咽喉肿痛、癫狂。

［操作］ 向下颌方向缓慢刺入0.5寸（约15毫米），不可深刺或向上斜刺，以免误伤延髓。

百会 (DU20 Bǎihuì)

［定位］ 在头部，当前发际正中直上5寸，或两耳尖连线的中点处（图1—90）。

［主治］ 头痛、眩晕、中风、癫狂、脱肛、阴挺。

［操作］ 平刺0.5～0.8寸（约15～20毫米）。

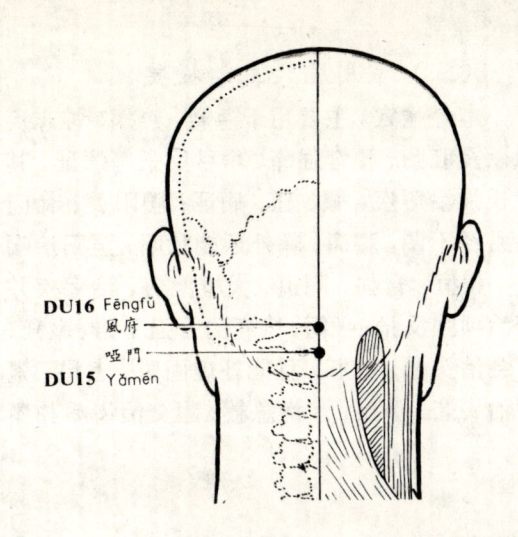

图1—88 哑门、风府
Fig. 1—88 Yanmen (DU 15) and Fengfu (DU 16)

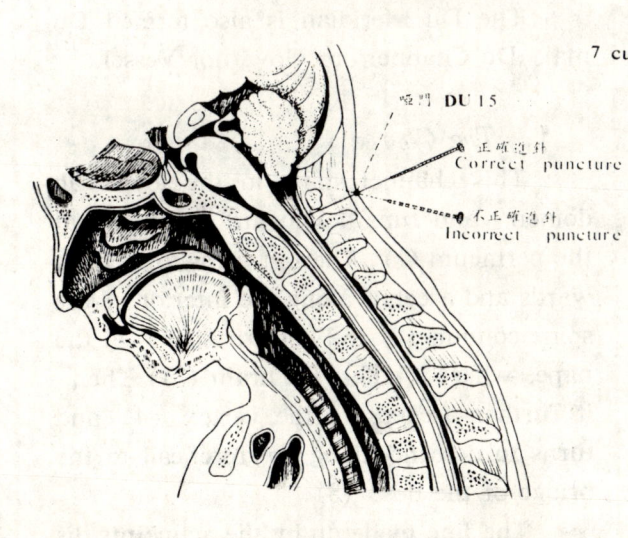

图1—89 哑门穴刺法
Fig. 1—89 Needling at Yamen (DU15)

风府 (DU16 Fēngfǔ)

［定位］ 在项部，枕外隆凸直下，两侧斜方肌之间的凹陷中，或于后发际正中直上1寸处取穴（图1—88）。

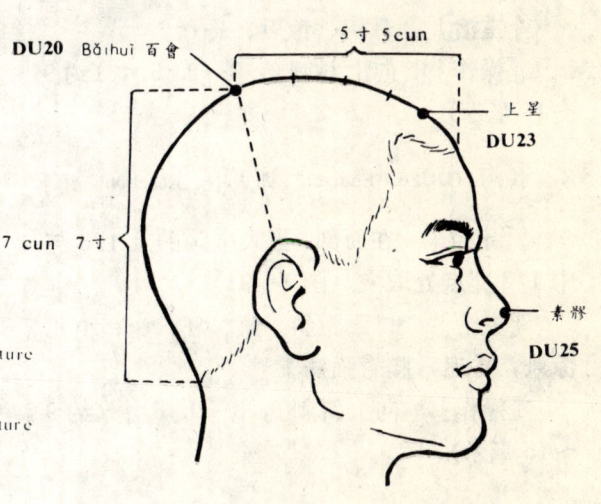

图1—90 百会、上星、素髎
Fig. 1—90 Baihui (DU 20), Shangxin (DU 23) and Suliao (DU 25)

上星 (DU23 Shàngxīng)

［定位］ 在头部，当前发际正中直上1寸（图1—90、91）。

［主治］ 头痛、鼻渊、鼻衄、癫狂。

［操作］ 平刺0.5～1寸（约15～25毫米）。

素髎 (DU25 Sùliáo)

［定位］ 在面部，当鼻尖的正中央处

· 143 ·

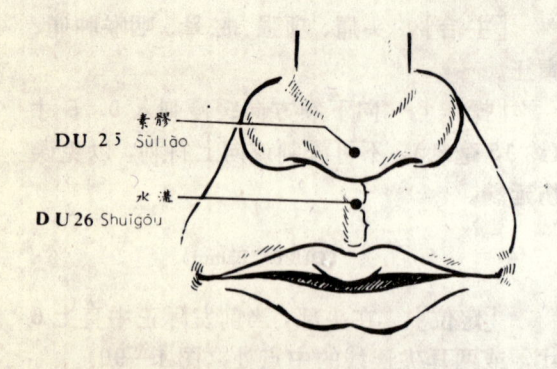

图 1—91 素髎、水沟（人中）
Fig. 1—91 Suliao (DU 25) and Shuigou (DU 26)

取穴（图 1—90、91）。

[主治] 鼻疾、惊厥、昏迷。

[操作] 向上斜刺 0.3～0.5 寸（约 9～15 毫米）。

水沟（DU26 Shuǐgōu 即人中 Rénzhōng）

[定位] 在面部，当人中沟的上 1/3 与中 1/3 交点处取穴（图 1—91）。

[主治] 口眼歪斜、癫、狂、痫，小儿惊风，昏迷，腰脊强痛。

[操作] 向上斜刺 0.3～0.5 寸（约 9～15 毫米）。

龈交（DU28 Yínjiāo）

[定位] 在上唇内，唇系带与上齿龈的相接处（图 1—92）。

[主治] 齿龈肿痛、癫狂。

[操作] 向上斜刺 0.2～0.3 寸（约

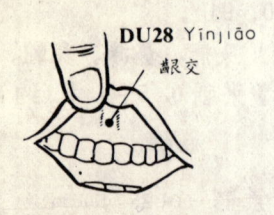

图 1—92 龈交穴
Fig. 1—92 Yinjiao (DU 28)

6～9 毫米），或点刺出血。

（三）常用腧穴主治提要

本经腧穴，主要用于急救、热病、神志疾患以及肛肠、腰脊强痛、角弓反张等病证。其中长强治痔疾、癫、狂、痫证；腰阳关、命门治月经不调，腰痛，除外还能壮阳；至阳治喘咳，黄疸，脊强；陶道、大椎泄热，治疟疾并兼治项强反张；哑门、风府治舌强不语、癫狂；百会治头晕、脱肛，且能补虚固脱；上星、素髎治头痛、鼻疾；水沟急救；龈交治齿龈肿痛等。

XIV. THE DU MERIDIAN (GOVERNOR VESSEL) (28 points in total)

The Du Meridian is also termed Dumai, Du Channel, or Governor Vessel.

1. *The Course*

This channel starts in the lower abdomen, and runs downward to emerge at the perineum (1). Then, it turns to go backwards and ascends along the interior of the spine column (2) to Fengfu (Du 16) at the nape, where it enters the brain (3). Then, it further ascends to the vertex (4) and turns to descend along the forehead to the bridge of the nose (5).

The line made up by the acupoints distributed on the body surface: It starts at Changqiang (DU 1) at the lower end of the coccyx, and ascends along the midline of the waist and back to the vertex. Then, it descends anteriorly to the bridge of the nose and ends at Yinjiao (28) inside the upper lip.

The inner organs concerned: The uterus, brain, spinal column.

2. The Commonly Used Acupoints

Changqiang (DU 1, Luo—Connectig point)

Location: Below the tip of the coccyx, at the midpoint of the line connecting the tip of the coccyx and the anus (See Fig. 1—86).
Indications: Bloody stool, hemorrhoids, epilepsy and mania.
Method: Puncture obliquely upwards 0.5—1.0 cun (15—25mm) closely along the anterior border of the coccyx (See Fig. 1—87). The rectum may be easily injured if puncturing perpendicularly. Moxibustion is applicable.

Yaoyangguan (DU 3)

Location: On the lower back and on the posterior midline, at the depression below the spinous process of the 4th lumbar vertebra, parallel to the iliac crest (See Fig. 1—85).
Indications: Abnormal menstruation, emission, pain in the lumbo—sacral region, flaccidity and arthralgia of the lower limb.
Method: Puncture obliquely upwards 0.5—0.8 cun (15—20mm). Moxibustion is applicable.

Mingmen (DU 4)

Location: On the lower back and on the posterior midline, at the depression below the spinous process of the 2nd lumbar vertebra (See Fig. 1—85).
Indications: Impotence, emission, leukorrhea, lumbago, diarrhea, abnormal menstruation.
Method: Pucture obliquely upwards 0.5—0.98 cun (15—20mm). Moxibustion is applicable.

Zhiyang (DU 9)

Location: On the back and on the posterior midline, at the depression below the spinous process of the 7th thoracic vertebra, parallel to the inferior angle of the scapula (See Fig. 1—85).
Indications: Jaundice, cough and asthma, stiffness of the spinous column, pain in the back.
Method: Puncture obliquely upwards 0.5—0.8 cun (15—20mm). Moxibustion is applicable.

Taodao (DU 13)

Location: On the back and on the posterior line, at the depression below the spinous process of the 1st thoracic vertebra (See Fig. 1—85).
Indications: Headache, malaria, febrile diseases.
Method: Puncture obliquely upwards 0.5—0.8 cun (15—20mm). Moxibustion is applicable.

Dazhui (DU 14)

Location: On the pasterior midline, at the depression below the spinous process of the 7th cervical vertebra (See Fig. 1—85.

Indications: Cough, asthma, headache, stiff neck, febrile diseases, malaria, epilepsy.

Method: Puncture obliquely upwards 0. 5—0. 8 cun (15—20mm). Moxibustion is applicable.

Yamen (DU 15)

Location: On the nape and at the midline of the back of the head, at the depression 0. 5 cun below Fengfu (RN 16) and 0. 5 cun above the hairline, below the lst cervical vertebra (See Fig. 1—88).

Indications: Sudden hoarseness of voice, aphasia with stiffness of the tongue, insanity and epilepsy.

Method: Puncture slowly and obliquely 0. 5 cun (about 15mm). Either deep or upward puncture is prohibited, otherwise the medullary bulb may be injured (See Fig. 1—89).

Fengfu (DU 16)

Location: On the nape, at the depression between m. trapezius of the two sides, directy below the external occipital protuberance, or at the midline of the back of the head, 1 cun above tne posterior hairline (See Fig. 1—88).

Indications: Headache, stiff neck, dizziness, swelling and sore throat, epilepsy.

Method: Puncture slowly obliquely towards the lower jaw 0. 5 cun (about 15mm). Deep or upward puncturing is prohibited, otherwise the medullary bulb may be injured.

Baihui (DU 20)

Location: On the head, 5 cun directly above the midpoint of the anterior hairline, at the midpoint of the line connecting the apexes of both ears. Or, at the cross point of the line connecting the apexes of the two auricles and the midline of the head (See Fig. 1—90).

Indications: Headache, dizziness, apoplexy, epilepsy and mania, prolapse of rectum, prolapse of uterus.

Method: Puncture horizontally 0. 5—0. 8 cun (15—20mm). Moxibustion is applicable.

Shangxing (DU 23)

Location: 1 cun directly above the midpoint of the anterior hairline, at the midline of the head (See Fig. 1—90, 1—91).

Indications: Headache, sinusitis, epilepsy and mania, epistaxis.

Method: Puncture horizontally 0. 5—1. 0 cun (15—25mm). Moxibustion is applicable.

Suliao (Du 25)

Location: On the face, at the center of the nose apex (See Fig. 1—90, 1-91).

Indications: Nasal disorders, convulsion, loss of consciousness.
Method: Puncture obliquely 0. 3—0. 5cun (9—15mm).

Shuigou (DU 26, also known as Renzhong)

Location: On the face, at the junction of the upper third and the middle third the philtrum (See Fig. 1—91).
Indications: Deviation of the mouth and eye, epilepsy and mania, infantile convulsion, loss of consciousness, stiffness and pain in the spinous column.
Method: Puncture obliquely upward 0. 3—0. 5 cun (9—15mm).

Yinjiao (Du 28)

Location: Inside of the upper lip, when the upper lip is lifed, the point is at the junction of the labial frenum of the upper lip and the upper gum (See Fig. 1—92).
Indications: Swelling and pain in the gum, epilepsy and mania.
Method: Puncture obliquely upward 0. 2—0. 3 cun (6—9mm), or prick with the three edged needle to cause bleeding.

3. *An Outline of Indications of the Commonly Used Acupoints*

The points of this channel are mainly used in first aid, febrile diseases, mental disorders, problems of the anus and rectum, stiffness and pain in the lower back, opisthotonos. In concrete, Changqiang (DU1) is indicated in hemorrhoids, epilepsy and mania; Yaoyangguan (DU 3) and Mingmen (DU 4), in abnormal menstruation, lumbago (these two points can te used to reinforce yang); Zhiyang (DU 9), in asthma and cough, jaundice, stiffness of the spinous column; Taodao (DU 13) and Dazhui (DU 14), in malaria, opisthotonos by reducing heat; Yamen (DU 15) and Fengfu (DU 16), in aphasia with stiffness of the tongue, epilepsy; Baihui (DU 20), in dizziness, prolapse of the rectum, which is also used to restore vital energy and strengthen astringency; Shangxing (DU 23) and Suliao (DU 25), in headache, nasal disorders; Shuigou (Du 26), for fisrt aid; and Yinjiao (DU 28), in swelling and pain of the gum.

第四节　常用经外奇穴

一、头颈部

四神聪 (EX—HN Sìshéncōng)

［定位］　在头顶部、百会穴前后左右各1寸处，共四穴（图1—93）。

［主治］　头痛、眩晕、失眠、健忘、癫、狂、痫证、偏瘫、脑积水。

［操作］　平刺0.5～0.8寸（约15～20毫米）。

印堂 (EX—HN Yìntáng)

［定位］　在额部，当两眉头之中间（图1—94）。

［主治］　头痛、头晕、鼻渊、鼻衄、小

儿急慢惊风，目赤肿痛、三叉神经痛。

［操作］　提捏局部皮肤，向下平刺 0.3～0.5 寸（约 9～15 毫米）；亦可用三棱针点刺出血。

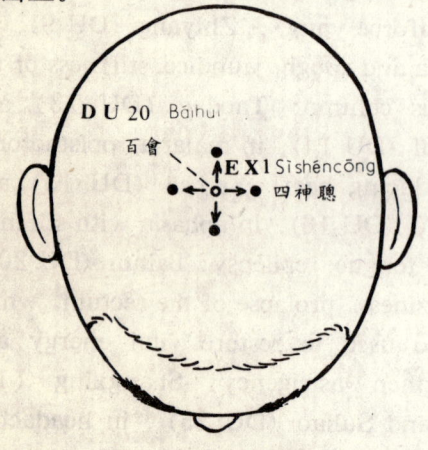

图 1—93　四神聪
Fig. 1—93 Sishencong (EX—HN1)

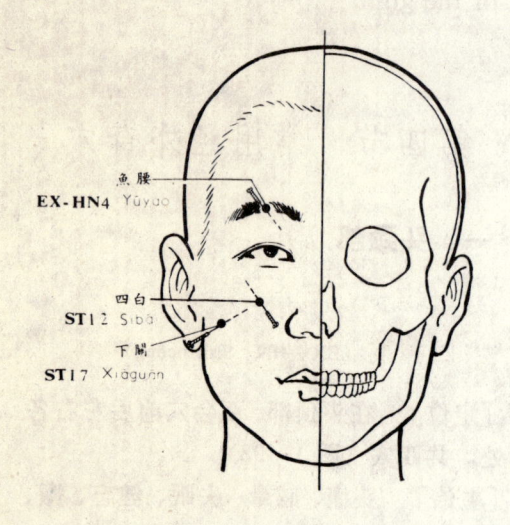

图 1—94　印堂、鱼腰、球后
Fig. 1—94 Yintang (EX—HN3), Yuyan (EX—HN4) and Qiuhou (EX—HN7)

太阳（EX—HN　Tàiyáng）

［定位］　在颞部，当眉梢与目外眦之间，向后约一横指的凹处（图 1—96）。

［主治］　偏正头痛、目赤肿痛、三叉神经痛。

［操作］　直刺或斜刺 0.3～0.5 寸（约 9～15 毫米）。

鱼腰（EX—HN　Yúyào）

［定位］　在额部，瞳孔直上，眉毛中（图 94、95）。

［主治］　目赤肿痛，眉棱骨痛，目翳，眶上神经痛。

［操作］　平刺 0.3～0.5 寸（约 9～15 毫米）。

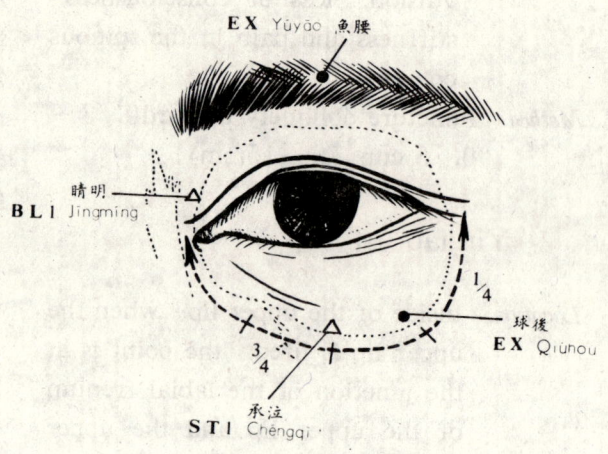

图 1—95　鱼腰、球后
Fig. 1—95 Yuyao (EX—HN4) and Qiuhou (EX—HN7)

球后（EX—HN　Qiúhòu）

［定位］　在面部，眶下缘外 1/4 与内 3/4 交界处取穴（图 1—94、1—95）。

［主治］　目疾。

［操作］　轻拨眼球向上，沿眶下缘缓慢直刺 0.5～1.5 寸（约 15～40 毫米），不提插。

牵正（EX—HN　Qiānzhèng）

［定位］　耳垂前 0.5～1 寸（图 1—96）。

经络腧穴概要

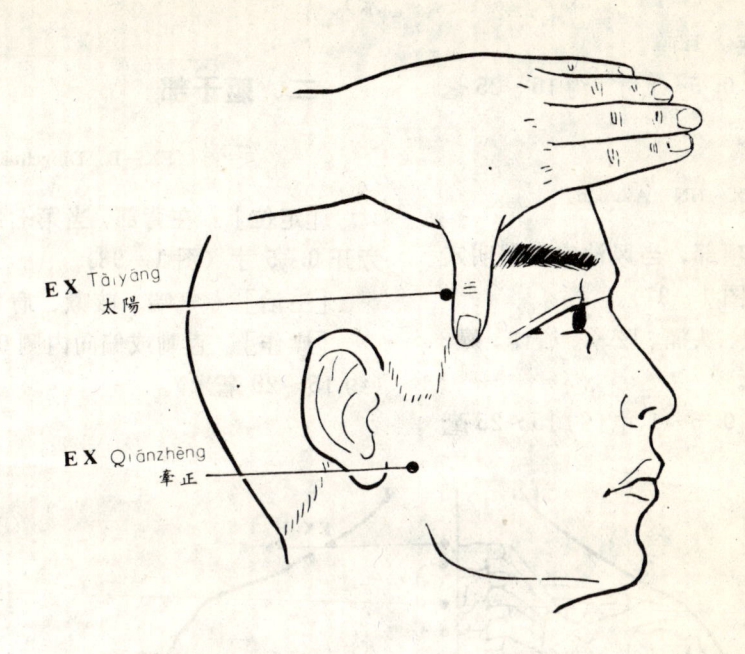

图 1—96 太阳、牵正
Fig. 1—96 Taiyang (EX—HN5) and Qianzheng (EX—HN16)

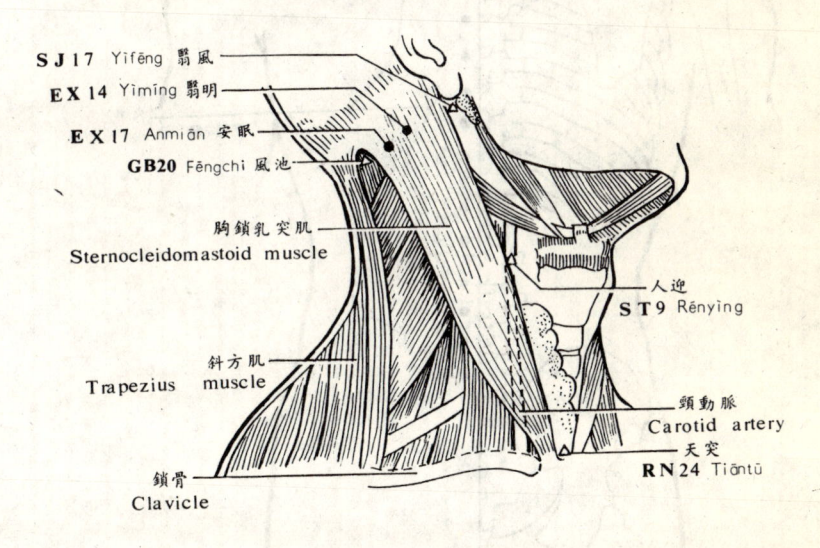

图 1—97 翳明、安眠
Fig. 1—97 Yiming (EX—HN14) and Anmian (EX—HN17)

[主治] 口眼歪斜、口疮、下牙痛。

[操作] 向前斜刺或平刺 0.5～0.8 寸（约 15～20 毫米）。

翳明（EX—HN Yìmíng）

[定位] 在项部，当翳风后 1 寸（图

· 149 ·

1—97)。

［主治］ 目疾、耳鸣。

［操作］ 直刺 0.5～1 寸（约 15～25 毫米）。

安眠（EX—HN Anmián）

［定位］ 在项部，当风池穴与翳明穴连线的中点取穴（图 1—97）。

［主治］ 失眠、头痛、眩晕、心悸、癫、狂、痫证、高血压。

［操作］ 直刺 0.5～1 寸（约 15～25 毫米）。

二、躯干部

定喘（EX—B Dìngchuǎn）

［定位］ 在背部，当第七颈椎棘突下，旁开 0.5 寸（图 1—98）。

［主治］ 气喘、咳嗽、肩背痛。

［操作］ 直刺或偏向内侧 0.5～0.8 寸（约 15～20 毫米）。

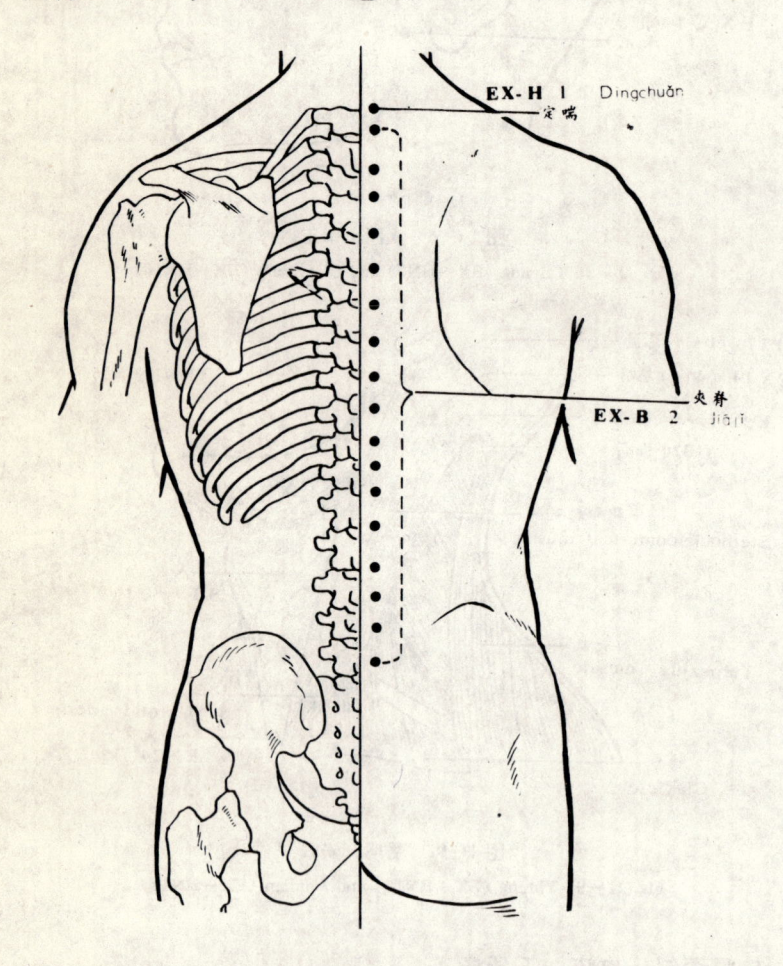

图 1—98 定喘、夹脊
Fig. 1—98 Dingchuan (EX—B1) and Jiaji (EX—B2)

夹脊 (EX—B Jiájǐ)

[定位] 在背腰部，当第1胸椎至第5腰椎棘突下两侧，后正中线旁开0.5寸，一侧17穴（图1—98）。

[主治] 第一胸椎至第三胸椎治上肢疾患；第一胸椎至第八胸椎治胸部疾患；第六胸椎至第五腰椎治腹部疾患；第一腰椎至第五腰椎治下肢疾患。

[操作] 斜刺0.5～1寸（约15～25毫米）。

三、四肢部

十宣 (EX—UE Shíxuān)

[定位] 手十指尖端距指甲游离缘0.1寸处，左右共十穴（图1—99）。

[主治] 昏迷、癫痫、高热、咽喉肿痛。

[操作] 浅刺0.1～0.2寸（约3～6毫米）或点刺出血。

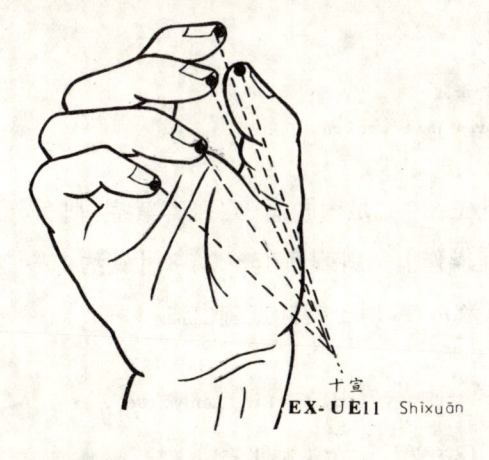

图1—99 十宣穴
Fig. 1—99 Shixuan (EX—UE 11)

八邪 (EX—UE Bāxié)

[定位] 在手背侧，微握拳，第1～5指间，指蹼缘后方赤白肉际处，左右共八穴（图1—100）。

[主治] 手背肿痛，手指麻木，目痛，烦热。

[操作] 向上斜刺0.5～0.8寸（15～20毫米）；或点刺出血。

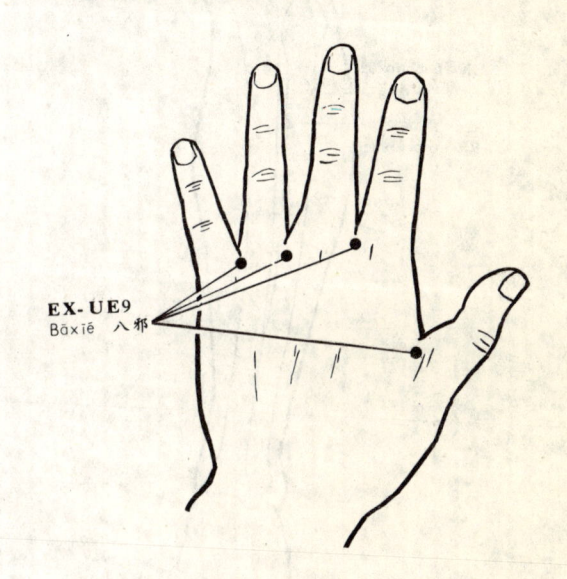

图1—100 八邪穴
Fig. 1—100 Baxie (EX—UE9)

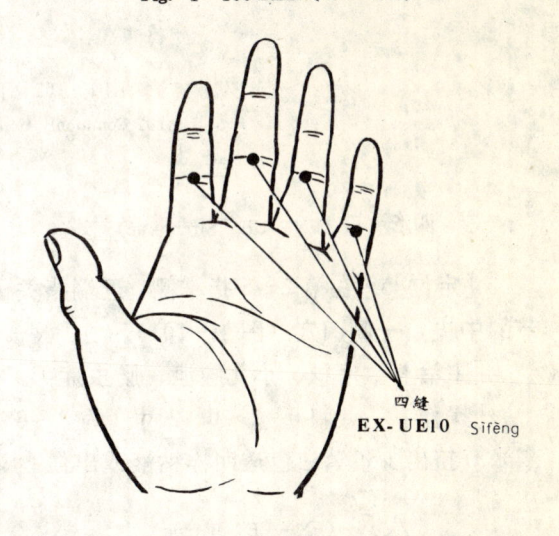

图1—101 四缝穴
Fig. 1—101 Sifeng (EX—UE10)

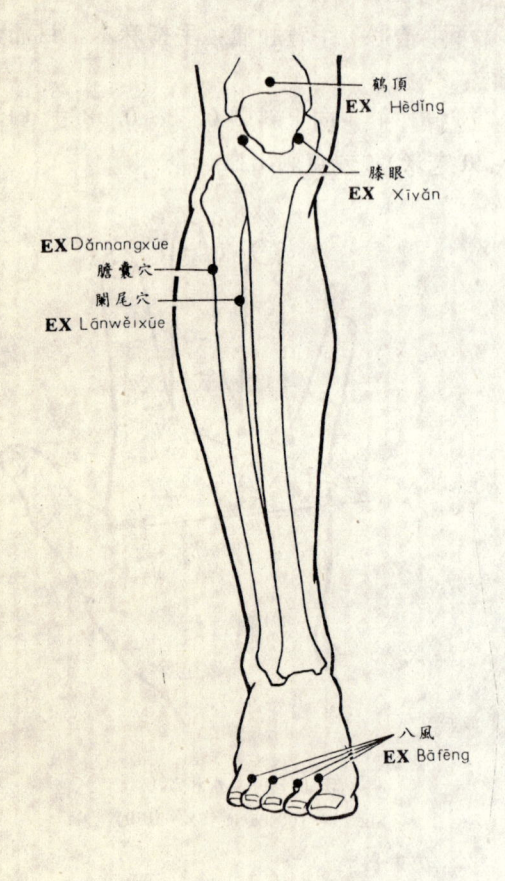

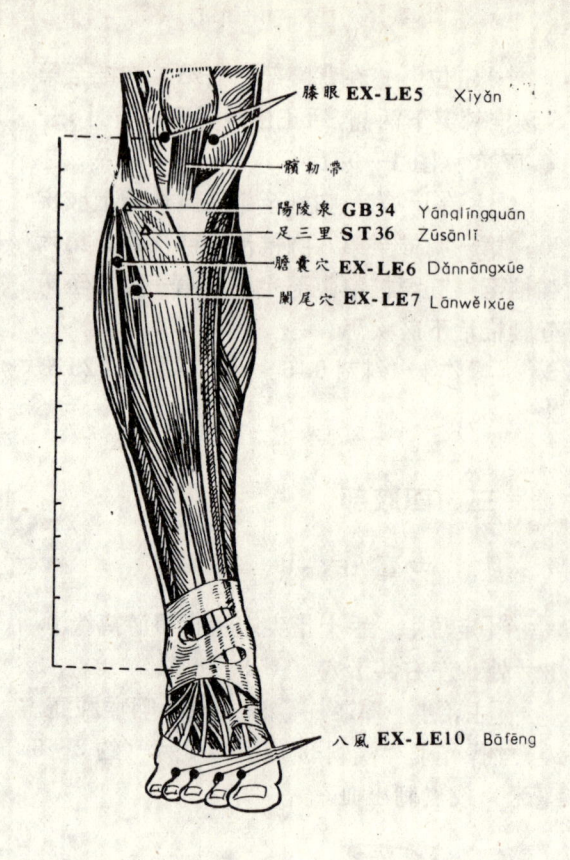

图 1—102 下肢常用经外奇穴
Fig. 1—102 Commonly Used Extra Points at the Lower Limb

四缝穴（EX—UE Sìfèngxué）

［定位］ 在第2～5指掌侧，近端指关节的中央，一侧四穴（图1—101）。

［主治］ 疳积、小儿腹泄、肠虫症。

［操作］ 点刺0.1～0.2寸（约3～6毫米）挤出少量黄白色透明样粘液或出血。

八风（EX—LE Bāfēng）

［定位］ 在足背侧，第1～5趾间，趾蹼缘后方赤白肉际处，一侧四穴，左右共八穴（图1—102）。

［主治］ 足跗肿痛、足趾青紫症，脚气。

［操作］ 斜刺0.5～0.8寸（约15～20毫米），或用三棱针点刺出血。

阑尾穴（EX—LE Lánwěixué）

［定位］ 在小腿前侧上部，当犊鼻下5寸，胫骨前缘旁开一横指（图1—102）。

［主治］ 急、慢性阑尾炎、胃痛。

［操作］ 直刺0.5～1寸（约15～25毫米）。

胆囊穴（EX—LE Dǎnnángxué）

［定位］ 在小腿外侧上部，当腓骨小头前下方凹陷处（阳陵泉）直下2寸（图1—102）。

［主治］ 急、慢性胆囊炎，胆石症，胆道蛔虫症，胆绞痛，胁痛。

［操作］ 直刺1～1.5寸（约25～40毫米）。

膝眼（EX—LE Xíyǎn）

［定位］ 屈膝在髌韧带两侧凹陷处，在内侧的称内膝眼，在外侧的称外膝眼（图1—102）。

［主治］ 膝关节酸痛、鹤膝风。

［操作］ 向膝中斜刺0.5～1寸（约15～25毫米）或向对侧膝眼透刺。

鹤顶（EX—LE Hédǐng）

［定位］ 在膝上部，髌底的中点上方凹陷处（图1—102）。

［主治］ 膝痛、瘫痪。

［操作］ 直刺1～1.5寸（约25～40毫米）。

SECTION 4 THE COMMONLY USED EXTRA — ORDINARY POINTS

1. *The Points on the Head and Neck Regions*

(1) Sishencong (EX—HN1)

Location: Four points, at the vertex of the head, 1.0 cun anterior, posterior, and lateral to Baihui (DU 20) (See Fig. 1—93).

Indications: Headache, dizziness, insomnea, poor memory, epilepsy and mania, hemiplegia, hydrocephalus.

Method: Puncture horizontally 0.5—0.8 cun (15—20mm). Moxibustion is applicable.

(2) Yintang (EX—HN3)

Location: On the forehead, midway between the medial ends of the two eyebrows (See Fig. 1—94).

Indications: Headache, dizziness, sinusitis, epilepsy, acute or chronic infantile convulsion, swelling and redness and pain in the eye, trigeminal neuralgia.

Method: Lift and pinch the local skin, then puncture horizontally downwards 0.3—0.5 cun (9—15mm), or prick with the three — edged needle to cause bleeding. Moxibustion is applicable.

(3) Taiyang (EX—HN5)

Location: At the temporal part of the head and on the depression 1.0 cun posterior to the midpoint between the lateral end of the eyebrow and the outer canthus (See Fig. 1—96).

Indications: Headache and migraine, redness and swelling and pain of the eye, trigerminal neuralgia.

Method: Puncture perpendicularly of horizontally 0.3—0.5 cun (9—15mm), or prick with the three

— edged needle to cause bleeding.

(4) Yuyao (EX—HN 4)

Location: On the forehead, directly above the pupil, in the eyebrow (See Fig. 1—94, 1—95).
Indications: Redness and swelling and pain of the eye, pain of the supercillary arch, nebula of the cornea supraorbital neuralgia.
Method: Puncture horizontally 0. 3—05 cun (9—15mm).

(5) Qiuhou (EX—HN7).

Location: On the face, at the junction of the lateral fourth and medial three fourths of the infraorbital margin (See Fig. 1—90, 1—95).
Indications: Eye troubles.
Method: Gently push the eyeball upward, then slowly puncture perpendicularly 0. 5—1. 5 cun (15—25mm) along the infraorbital margin without movements of thrusting, lifting and twisting.

(6) Qianzheng (EX—HN16)

Location: On the face, 0. 5—1. 0 cun anterior to the earlobe. (See Fig. 1—96).
Indications: Deviation of the mouth and eye, ulcer in the mouth, pain in the lower tooth.
Method: Puncture obliquely of horizontally anteriorly 0. 5—0. 8 cun (15—20mm).

(7) Yiming (EX—HN14)

Location: On the nape, 1 cun posterior to Yifeng (SJ 17), at the midpoint of the line connecting Yifeng (SJ 17) and Fengchi (GB 20) (See Fig. 1—97).
Indications: Eye troubles, tinnitus.
Method: Puncture perpendicularly 0. 5—1. 0 cun (15—25mm).

(8) Anmian (EX—HN17)

Location: At the midpoint of the line connecting Fengchi (GB20) and Yiming (EX—HN 14) (See Fig. 1—97).
Indications: Insomnia, headache, dizziness, palpitation, epilepsy and mania, hypertension.
Method: Puncture perpendicularly 0. 5—1. 0 cun (15—25mm).

2. The Points on the Trunk

(1) Dingchuan (EX—B1)

Location: On the back, below the spinous process of the 7th cervical vertebra, 0. 5 cun lateral to the posterior midline (See Fig. 1—98).
Indications: Asthma, cough, pain in the shoulder and back.
Method: Puncture perpendicularly or obliquely toward the inside 0. 5—0. 8 cun (15—20mm). Moxibustion is applicable.

(2) Jiaji (EX—B2, also known as Huatuojia-

ji)

Location: On the back and low back, a group of 34 points on both sides of the spinal column, below the spinous processes from the 1st thoracic vertebra to the 5th lumbar vertebra, 0.5 cun lateral to the posterior midline (See Fig. 1-98).

Indications: The points respectively lateral to each of the spinous processes of the 1st — 3rd thoracic vertebrae are indicated in upper limb troubles; while those of the 1st — 8th thoracic vertebra, in disorders of the chest; those of the 6th thoracic vertebra to the 5th lumbar vertebra, in disorders of abdomen; and those of the 1st — 5th lumbar vertebrae, in disorders of the lower limbs.

Method: Puncture obliquely 0.5—1.0 cun (15—25mm). Moxibustion is applicable.

3. Points on the Four Extremities

(1) Shixuan (EX—UE 11)

Location: Ten points on both hands, at the tips of the ten fingers, 0.1 cun from the free margin of the nails (See Fig. 1—99).

Indications: Coma, epilepsy, high fever, swelling and sore throat.

Method: Puncture shallowly 0.1—0.2 cun (3—6mm) or prick with the three —edged needle to cause bleeding.

(2) Baxie (EX—UE 9)

Location: Four points on the dorsum of each hand, at the junction of the red and white skin proximal to the margin of the webs between each two of the five fingers of a hand (See Fig. 1—100).

Indications: Swelling and pain in the dorsum of the hand, numbness of the fingers, pain in the eye, restlessness with fever.

Method: Puncture obliquely upwards 0.5 — 0.8 cun (15—20mm), or prick with the three — edged needle to cause bleeding. Moxibustion is applicable.

(3) Sifeng (EX—UE 10)

Location: Four points on each hand, on the palmar side of the 2nd to 5th fingers and at the center of the proximal interphalangeal joints (See Fig. 1—101).

Indications: Malnutriton and indigestion syndrome in children, infantile diarrhea, helminth.

Method: Prick 0.1—0.2 cun (3—6mm) and squeeze out a small amount of yellow — white transparent fluid or to cause bleeding.

(4) Bafeng (EX—LE 10)

Location: Eight points on the instep of both feet, at the junction of the red and white skin proximal to the margin of the webs between each two neighbouring toes (See Fig.

1—102).

Indications: Pain and swelling in the dorsum of foot, blue — purple toes, beriberi.

Method: Punctrue obliquely 0.5—0.8 cun (15—20mm) or prick whth the three—edged needle to cause bleeding. Moxibustion is applicable.

(5) Lanwei (EX—LE 7)

Location: At the upper part of the anterior surface of the leg, 5 cun below Dubi (ST 35), one finger breadth lateral to the anterior crest of the tibia (See Fig. 1—102).

Indications: Acute or chronic appendicitis, stomachache.

Method: Puncture perpendicularly 0.5—1.0 cun (15—25mm).

(6) Dannang (EX—LE 6)

Location: At the upper part of the lateral surface of the leg, 2 cun directly below the depression anterior and inferior to the head of the fibula (Yanglingquan, GB 34) (See Fig. 1—102).

Indications: Acute or chronic cholecystitis, cholelithiasis, biliary ascaridiasis, colic of gallbadder, hypochondriac pain.

Method: Puncture perpendicularly 1.0—1.5 cun (25—40mm).

(7) Xiyan (EX—LE 5)

Location: In the depression on both sides of the patellar ligament when the knee is flexed. The medial and lateral points are named "Neixiyan" and "Waixiyan" respectively (See Fig. 1—102).

Indications: Aching in the knee joint, arthralgia of knee or arthroncus of knee.

Method: Punctrure obliquely 0.5—1.0 cun (15—25mm) toward the center of the knee, or toward the opposite Xiyan (EX—LE 5). Moxibustion is applicable.

(8) Heding (EX—LE 2)

Location: Above the knee, at the depression of the midpoint of the upper border of the patella (See Fig. 1—102).

Indications: Pain in the knee, paralysis.

Method: Puncture perpendicularly 1.0—1.5 cun (25—40mm). Moxibustion is applicable.

第二章
耳针、头针、腕踝针分区与穴位定位

CHAPTER TWO
LOCATION AND INDICATIONS OF OTOPOINTS, SCALP ACUPUNCTURE LINES AND WRIST—ANKLE ACUPUNCTURE POINTS

第一节 耳廓表面解剖及耳穴定位

一、耳廓表面的解剖（图2—1）

1. 耳轮：耳廓最外缘的卷曲部分
2. 耳轮脚：耳轮深入至耳腔内的横行突起处。
3. 耳轮结节：耳轮后上方稍突起处。
4. 耳轮尾：耳轮末端与耳垂的交界处。
5. 对耳轮：在耳轮的内侧，与耳轮相对的隆起部；其上方有两分叉，向上分叉的一双叫"对耳轮上脚"，向下分叉的一双叫"对耳轮下脚"。
6. 三角窝：对耳轮上、下脚之间的三角形凹窝。
7. 耳舟：耳轮与对耳轮之间的凹窝，又称舟状窝。
8. 耳屏：耳廓前面的瓣状突起，又称耳珠。
9. 屏上切迹：耳屏上缘与耳轮脚之间的凹陷。
10. 对耳屏：对耳轮下方与耳屏相对的隆起部。
11. 屏间切迹：耳屏与对耳屏之间的凹陷。
12. 屏轮切迹：对耳屏与对耳轮之间的稍凹陷处。
13. 耳垂：耳廓下部无软骨的皮垂。

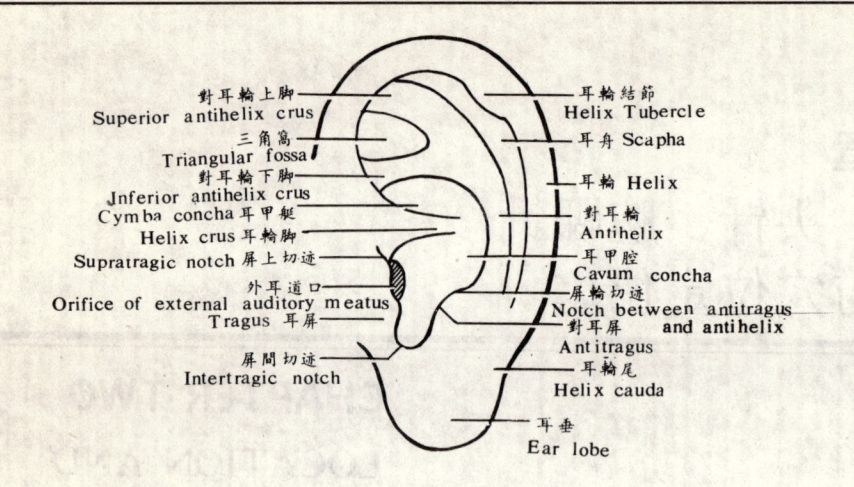

Fig. 2-1 Anatomical Structure of the Auricle Surface

Fig. 2-2 Regularity of Distribution of Otopoints

14. 耳甲腔：耳轮脚以下的耳腔部分。
15. 耳甲艇：耳轮脚以上的耳腔部分。
16. 外耳道开口：耳甲腔内，为耳屏所遮盖着的孔窍。

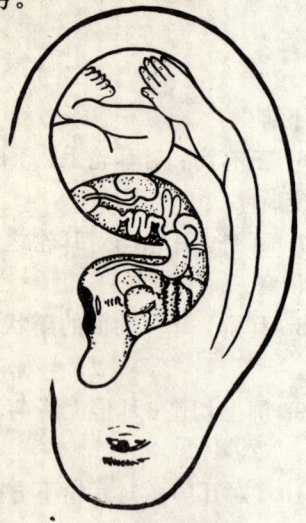

AURICULAR SURFACE AND LOCATION AND INDICATIONS OF OTOPINTS

I. ANATOMICAL TERMINOLOGY OF THE AURICULAR SURFACE (See Fig. 2-1)

1. **Helix**: The prominent rim of the auricle.
2. **Helix Crus**: A part of the helix, which transverses in the auricular cavity.
3. **Auricular Tubercle**: The small tubercle on the posterior—superior aspect of the helix.
4. **Helix Cauda**: The lower end of the helix, at the junction of the helix and earlobe.
5. **Antihelix**: The inner ridge opposite to the helix, which divides above into two branches, the superior and inferior crura of the antihelix.

SECTION 1 ANATOMICAL TERMINOLOGY OF THE

6. Triangular Fossa: The triangulr depression between the two crura of the antihelix.
7. Scapha: The depression between the helix and the antihelix.
8. Tragus: The valviform prominence in front of the auricle.
9. Supratragus Notch: The notch between the superior border of the tragus and the crus of the helix.
10. Antitragus: The prominence on the lower part of the antihelix and opposite to the tragus.
11. Intertragic Notch: The notch between the tragus and antitragus.
12. Notch between Antitragus and Antihelix: The depression between the antitragus and antihelix.
13. Earlobe: The lower and soft part of the auricle.
14. Cavum Concha: The part of the auricular cavity, which is below the helix crus.
15. Cymba Concha: The part of the auricicular cavity, which is above the helix crus.
16. Orifice of the External Auditary Meatus: The orifice lying in the cavity of the conchae and covered by the tragus.

二、耳穴分布规律、定位及适应症

耳穴在耳廓的分布有一定的规律，一般说，它好像在子宫内倒置的胎儿，头部向下，臀部朝上（图2—2）。其常用耳穴分布的基本规律，定位（图2—3）及适应症如下：

II. DISTRIBUTION, LOCATION AND INDICATIONS OF THE OTOPOINTS

There is a certain regularity of the distribution of the otopoints (i. e. the acupoints on the auricle) on the auricle. Most otopoints are named according to their function on body organs, and after the names of the body organs. "Stomach", for example, is a name of one body organ, meanwhile it is the name of an otopoint as the point has the function on the stomach. Generally, the otopoints seem to distribute in the position like that of a fetus lying in inverse site in the uterus, with its head downwards and the buttock upwards (See Fig. 2—2). The basic regularity of the distribution, location, and indications of the commonly used otopoints (See Fig. 2—3) are seen in Table 2—1.

表2—1 常用耳穴分布的基本规律、定位、适应症

解剖名称与分布规律	穴 名	定 位	主 治 病 证
耳轮内上方相当于二阴	直肠下端	在与大肠穴同水平的耳轮处	便秘、脱肛、痔疮
	尿道	在与膀胱穴同水平的耳轮处	遗尿、尿频、尿潴留
	外生殖器	在与下脚端穴同水平的耳轮处	阴道炎、阳萎、睾丸炎
	耳尖	将耳轮向耳屏对折时，耳廓上尖端处	放血数滴有退热消炎、降血压功能

解剖名称与分布规律	穴名	定位	主治病证
耳轮脚相当于膈	耳中（膈）	耳轮脚上	呃逆、黄疸、皮肤病
耳轮脚周围相当于消化系统	口	在耳甲腔、紧靠外耳道的后壁	面瘫、口腔溃疡、流涎
	食道	耳轮脚下方内2/3处	呕吐、吞咽困难
	贲门	耳轮脚下方外1/3处	恶心、呕吐、贲门痉挛
	胃	耳轮脚消失处	胃痛、呕吐、消化不良等消化系统病
	十二指肠	耳轮脚上方后1/3处	十二指肠溃疡、幽门痉挛
	小肠	耳轮脚上方中1/3处	消化不良
	大肠	耳轮脚上方内1/3处	痢疾、便秘、腹泻等胃肠疾病
	阑尾	大肠与小肠穴之间	阑尾炎等肠道疾病
耳舟相当于上肢	指	耳轮结节上方的耳舟部	相应部位疾病
	腕	平耳轮结节突起处的耳舟部	
	肘	腕与肩穴之间	
	肩	与屏上切迹同水平的耳舟部	
	肩关节	在肩穴与锁骨穴之间	
	锁骨	与屏轮切迹同水平，偏耳轮尾侧	
对耳轮相当于躯干	腹	对耳轮上，与对耳轮下脚下缘同水平处	腹腔疾患、妇科病
	胸	对耳轮上，与屏上切迹同水平处	胸胁痛、乳腺炎
	颈	屏轮切迹偏耳舟侧处	落枕、单纯性甲状腺肿
	脊椎	对耳轮的耳腔缘，从上自下分成三段．上1/3为腰骶椎．中1/3为胸椎．下1/3为颈椎	相应部位疾病
对耳轮上脚相当于下肢	趾	对耳轮上脚的外角	相应部位疾病
	踝	对耳轮上脚的内上角	
	膝	对耳轮上脚的起始部，与对耳轮下脚上缘同水平	
对耳轮下脚相当于臀	臀	对耳轮下脚外1/2处	坐骨神经痛
	坐骨	对耳轮下脚内1/2处	
	下脚端（交感）	对耳轮下脚与耳轮内侧交界处	相当交感与副交感神经功能的综合，主治消化、呼吸、循环等内脏病

解剖名称与分布规律	穴 名	定 位	主治病证
三角窝相当于盆腔	子宫(精宫)	三角窝耳轮内侧缘的中点	月经不调、痛经、各类妇科炎症及男子性功能减退、障碍等.
	神门	三角窝外1/3处,对耳轮上、下脚交叉之前	有镇静、镇痛、消炎功能.主治失眠、各种痛症皮肤搔痒症
耳屏相当于鼻咽部	外鼻	耳屏外侧面中央	鼻疖、鼻炎、酒齄鼻
	咽喉	耳屏内侧面的上1/2	咽喉、扁桃体肿痛
	内鼻	耳屏内侧面的下1/2,咽喉的下方	鼻炎、感冒
	上屏尖	耳屏上部隆起的尖端	各种炎症、痛症
	下屏尖(肾上腺)	耳屏下部隆起的尖端	有升压、止血、退热、抗过敏等作用.主治低血压、昏厥、哮喘、各种皮肤病,中暑
	外耳	耳屏上切迹微前凹陷中	耳鸣、耳聋、内耳性眩晕
对耳屏相当于头枕	缘中(脑点)	对耳屏尖与屏轮切迹的中点	相当脑垂体的作用,主治妇产科病、尿崩症、侏儒症
	平喘(腮腺)	对耳屏的尖端	哮喘、咳嗽、腮腺炎
	脑(皮质下)	对耳屏的内侧面	有镇静、镇痛、消炎功能.主治失眠、多梦、各种痛症、炎症
	睾丸(卵巢)	对耳屏内侧面前下方,是脑穴内的一部分	生殖系统疾病
	枕	对耳屏外侧面的后上方	神经系统病、皮肤病、昏厥
	额	对耳屏外侧面的前下方	头额痛、头晕
	颞(太阳)	对耳屏外侧面、枕与额穴之间	偏头痛
屏轮切迹相当于脑干	脑干	屏轮切迹正中处	有镇静熄风功能.主治角弓反张、抽搐、头痛、脑病后遗症
屏间切迹相当于内分泌	屏间(内分泌)	屏间切迹底部	有调节内分泌功能主治妇科疾病,生殖系统疾病
	目₁	屏间切迹前下方	各种眼病
	目₂	屏间切迹后下方	

解剖名称与分布规律	穴 名	定 位	主 治 病 证
耳甲艇相当于腹腔	膀胱	对耳轮下脚下缘,大肠穴直上方	泌尿系统病
	肾	对耳轮下脚下缘、小肠穴直上方	泌尿、生殖系统病、妇科病、耳病
	胰(胆)	肝、肾穴之间,左耳为胰、右耳为胆	胰腺炎、胆道疾患
	肝	胃、十二指肠穴的后方	肝病、眼病、胁痛
	脾	肝穴的下方,耳甲腔的外上方	消化系统病、血液病
耳甲腔相当于胸腔	心	耳甲腔中心最凹陷处	有强心、抗休克、升压、降压功能,主治心悸、昏厥、心痛
	肺	心穴的上、下、外三面	呼吸系统病、皮肤病、鼻病
	气管	口与心穴之间	咳嗽、哮喘
	三焦	外耳道口、屏间穴的上方	有利尿消肿功能,治便秘、水肿
耳垂相当于面部	眼	耳垂5区的中央	各种眼病
	舌	耳垂2区中央	舌肿痛、舌强
	扁桃体	耳垂8区正中	扁桃体炎
	齿$_1$	耳垂1区外下角	牙病
	齿$_2$	耳垂4区正中	
	升压点	屏间切迹下方	低血压、虚脱
	上颌	耳垂3区正中	牙痛、下颌关节炎
	下颌	耳垂3区上部横线中点	
	内耳	耳垂6区正中稍上方	耳病、眩晕、耳鸣
耳背	降压沟	耳廓背面,由上方斜向下方行走的凹沟	高血压
	上耳背	耳背上方的软骨隆起处	皮肤病、背痛
	中耳背	耳背上、下方之间最高处	
	下耳背	耳背下方的软骨隆起处	
	耳迷根	耳廓背与乳突交界处的耳根部	胃痛、胆道蛔虫痛、腹泻、哮喘

Table 2—1 Distribution, Location, Action and Indications of Commonly Used Otopoints

Area with organ *	Name of otopoint	Location	Action and chief indications
Hellix — Two lower orifices	Lower Portion of Rectum	At helix, Level with Ot (otopoint) Large Intestine	Constipation, prolapse of anus, hemorrhoids
	Urethra	At helix, level with Ot. Bladder	Enuresis, frequent urination, retension of urine
	External Genitalia	At helix, Level with Ot. End of Inferior Antihelix Crus	Vaginitis impotence, orchitis
	Ear Apex	At the tip of the auricle when the helix is folded towards tragus	Removing heat, anti—inflammation, lowering blood pressure for fever, hypertension, inflammation
Helix crus --Diaphragm	Diaphragm (Middle Ear)	On helix curs	Hiccup, jaundice, skin disorders
Periphery helix crus-- Digestive system	Mouth	At concha, close to the posterior border of orifice of external auditary meatus	Facial paralysis, canker sore, sialosis
	Esophagus	At medial 2/3 of inferior aspect of helix crus	Vomiting, dysphagia
	Cardiac Orifice	At lateral 1/3 of inferior aspect of helix crus	Nausea, vomiting, cardiospasm
	Stomach	At area where helix crus terminates	Disorders of digestive system such as stomachache, vomiting, dyspesia
	Duodenum	At lateral 1/3 of superior aspect of helix crus	Duodenal ulcer, pylorospasm
	Small Intestine	At middle 1/3 of superior aspect of helix crus	Dyspepsia
	Large Intestine	At medial 1/3 of superior aspect of helix crus	Intestinal diseases such as dysentery, constipation, abdominal pain
	Appendix	Between Ot. Large Intestine and Ot. Small Intestine	Intestinal diseases such as appendicitis

Area with organ *	Name of otopoint	Location	Action and chief indications
Scapha-- Upper limb	Finger	At scapha, above the auricular tubercle	Disorders of the corresponding areas
	Wrist	At scapha, level with auricular tubercle	
	Elbow	Between Ot. Wrist and Ot. Shoulder	
	Shoulder	At scapha, level with supratragic notch	
	Shoulder Joint	Between Ot. Shoulder and Ot. Clavicle	
	Clavicle	Level with notch between antitragus and antihelix, near helix cauda	
Antihelix ——Trunk	Abdomen	On antihelix, Level with lower margin of inferior crus of antihelix	Abdoninal or gynecological diseases
	Chest	On antihelix, level with supratragic notch	Pain in chest and hytpochondrium, mastitis
	Neck	At notch between antihelix and antitragus, near scapha	Strained neck, simple goiter
	Spinal Column	On a curved line of margin of antihelix, near auditary cavity. The line is divided equally into three segments. The upper 1/3 is Ot. Lumbosacral Vertebrae; the middle 1/3, Ot. Thoracic Vertebrae and the low 1/3, Ot. Cervical Vertebrae	Disorders at the corresponding areas of the body
Superior crus of antihelix --Lower limbs	Toe	At supero-lateral angle of superior antihelix crus	Disorders of the corresponding areas
	Ankle	At supero — medial angle of superior antihelix crus	
	Knee	At the beginning area of superior antihelix crus, level with superior border of inferior antihelix crus	

Area with organ *	Name of otopoint	Location	Action and chief indications
Inferior crus of antihelix --Buttock	Buttocks	At the lateral half of inferior antihelix crus	Sciatica
	Sciatic Nerve (Ischium)	At medial half of inferior antihelix crus	
	Sympathetic (End of Inferior Antihelix Curs)	At junction of inferior antihelix crus and meidal margin of helix	Acts as sympathetic and parasympathetic nerves for internal organ diseases such as disorders of digestive, circulating and respiratory systems
Triangular Fossa--Pelvic cavity	Uterus (Seminal Palace, Tiankui)	Medial to the triangular fossa and near the midpoint of medial border of helix	Irregular menstruation, dysmenorrhea, inflammations in gynopathy, decrease or disorder of sexual function in man
	Shenmen	At lateral 1/3 of triangular fossa, in the bifurcating point between superior and inferior crura of antihelix	Insomnia, pain, skin itching. Action to ease mind, relieve pain, and subdue antiinflammation.
Tragus--Nasopharynx	External Nose	At the center of lateral aspect of tragus	Nasal carbuncle, rhinitis, rosacea
	Pharynx and Larynx	At upper half of medial aspect of tragus	Pain and swelling of throat and tonsil
	Internal Nose	At the lower half of medial aspect of tragus, below Ot. Pharynx—Larynx	Rhintis, common cold
	Supratragic Apex (Tragic Apex)	At the tip of prominence at the upper tragus	Pain, inflammation
	Infratragic Apex (Adrenal Gland)	At the tip of prominence at lower tragus	Elevating blood pressure, stopping bleeding, removing heat and lowering hypersensitivity for hypertension, coma, asthma, skin disease, sunstriking
	External Ear	At the depression slightly anterior to the supratragic notch	Tinnitus, deafness, auditary vertigo

Area with organ *	Name of otopoint	Location	Action and chief indications
Antitragus ——Head	Brain Point (Yuanzhong)	Midpoint between antitragic apex and the notch of antitragus and antihelix	Gynopathy, diabetes, dwarfism
	Soothing Asthma (Ear—Asthma, Parotid Gland, Antitragic Apex)	At the antitragus apex	Asthma, cough, parotitis
	Brain (Subcortex)	At the medial apsect of antitragus	Easing mind, stopping pain, and eliminating inflammation, for insomnia, dreaminess, inflammation
	Testis (Ovary)	A part of Ot. Brain, antero—inferior to the medial aspect of antitragus	Disorders of genital system
	Occiput	Posterosuperior to the lateral aspect of antitragus	Disorders of nerve system, skin problem, faintness
	Forehead	Antero—inferior to the lateral aspect of antitragus	Headache, light—Headness
	Temporal (Taiyang)	On lateral apsect of antitragus, between Ot. Occiput and Forehead	Migraine
Notch between antitragus and antihelix ——Brain stem	Brain Stem	At the center of the notch	Opisthotonos, spasm, headache, sequela of encephalopathy
Intertragic notch—— Endocrine	Endocrine (Pingjian)	At the bottom of the notch	Regulating endocrine, for gynopathy, disorders of genital system
	Eye I	Anterior—inferior to the notch	Eye disorders
	Eye II	Posterior—inferior to the notch	

Area with organ *	Name of otopoint	Location	Action and chief indications
Cymba concha ——Abdominal cavity	Bladder	At the lower margin of inferior antihelix crus, directly above Ot. Larger Intestine	Disorders of urinary system
	Kidney	At lower border of inferior antihelix crus, directly above Ot. Small Intestine	Disorders of urogenital system, gynopathy, ear disorders
	Pancreas, Gallbladder	Between Ot. Liver and Kidney, that in the left ear termed Pancreas, and right one, Gallbladder	Pancreatitis, biliary diseases
	Liver	Posterior to Ot. Stomach and Duodenum	Diseases of liver and eye, hypochondriac pain
	Spleen	Below Ot. Liver, superolateral to Cavum concha	Diseases of digestive system and blood
Cavum concha ——Thoracic cavity	Heart	At the central depression of cavum concha	Improving heart function, anti—shock and regulating blood pressure, for palpitation, coma, cardialgia
	Lung	At the areas superior, inferior, and lateral to Ot. Heart	Disorders of respiratory system, skin and nose
	Trachea	Between Ot. Mouth and Heart	Cough, asthma
	Sanjiao	At the orifice of external auditary meatus, above Ot. Endocrine	Constipation, edema

Area with organ *	Name of otopoint	Location	Action and chief indications
Earlobe ——Face	Eye	At the center of zone 5 of earlobe	Disorders of eye
	Tongue	At the center of zone 2 earlobe	Swelling, pain, stiffness of tongue
	Tonsil	At the center of zone 8 of earlobe	Tonsillitis
	Tooth I	At inferolateral angle of zone 1 of earlobe	Tooth disorders
	Tooth II	At the center of zone 4 of earlobe	
	Spot for Elevating Blood Pressure	Below the intertragic notch	Hypotension, prostration syndrome
	Maxilla	At the center of zone 3 of earlobe	Toothache, inflammation of mandibular articulation
	Mandibule	At the midpoint of the upper transverse line of zone 3 of earlobe	
	Internal Ear	Slightly above the center of zone 6 of earlobe	Ear disorders, vertigo, tinnitus
Back of auricle	Groove for Lowering Blood Bressure	At the groove on retroauricle, running from the upper to the lower obliquely	Hypertension
	Upper Portion of Auricle	At the upper chondral prominence on retroauricle	Skin diseases, back pain
	Middle Portion of Back of Auricle	At the highest spot, between the upper and lower chondral prominences	
	Lower Portion of Back of Auricle	At the lower chondral prominence of retroauricle	
	Root of Auricular Vagus Nerve	At the junction of retroauricle and mastoid, level with helix crus	Stomachache, bitiary ascariasis, diarrhea, asthma

"✷": *Auricular area with its corresponding organ or system of the body.*

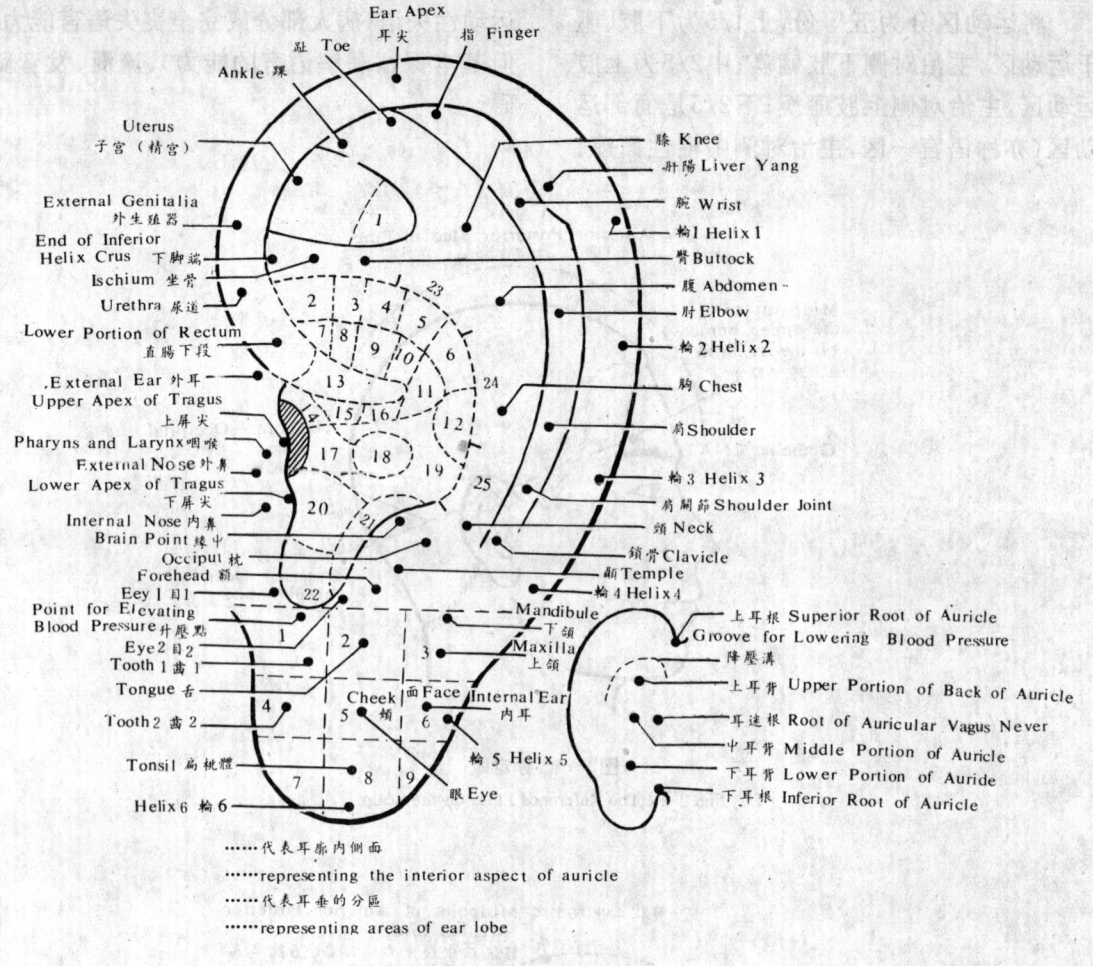

图2-3 常用耳穴分布图
Fig. 2-3 The Commonly Used Otopoints

第二节 常用头针刺激区定位与主治病证

为了便于刺激区的定位,在头部有两条标定线;

前后正中线:从两眉间中点至枕外粗隆下缘的头部正中线(图2-4)

眉枕线:从眉毛上缘中点至枕外粗隆尖的头侧水平连线(图2-4)。

一、运动区

上点在前后正中线中点向后移0.5厘米处;下点在眉枕线和鬓角发际前缘相交处(若鬓角发际不明显者,可从颧弓中点向上引一垂直线,将此线与眉枕线交点前移0.5厘米处作为下点)。上下两点间连线即为运动区(图2-5)。

将运动区分为五等份,上1/5为下肢、躯干运动区,主治对侧下肢瘫痪;中2/5为上肢运动区,主治对侧上肢瘫痪;下2/5是面部运动区(亦称语言一区,主治对侧中枢性面瘫、运动性失语(病人部分或完全丧失语言能力,但基本保留理解语言的能力)、流涎、发音障碍。

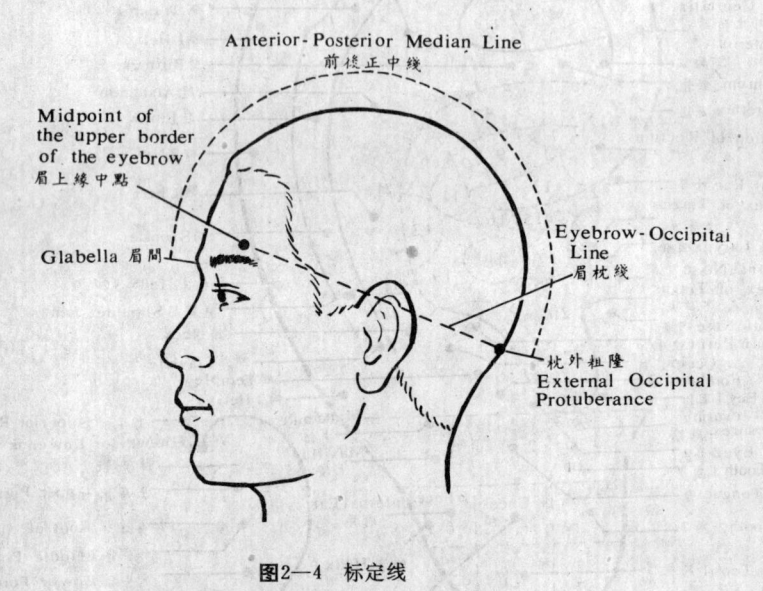

图2—4 标定线

Fig. 2—4 The Reference Lines on the Scalp

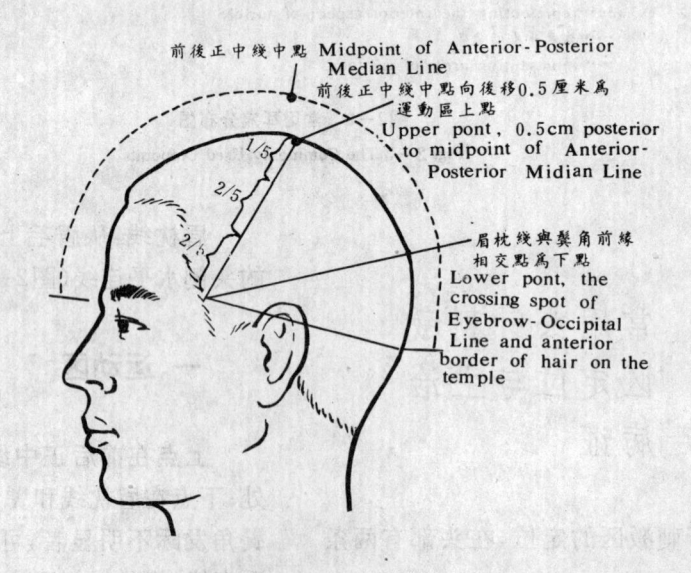

图2—5 运动区

Fig. 2—5 The Motor Area

SECTION 2 LOCATION AND INDICATIONS OF COMMONLY USED SCALP ACUPUNCTURE LINES

In order to locate the stimulation areas on the scalp precisely, the following two reference lines on the scalp have been determined:

The anterior—posterior median line: The vertical line connecting the center of the glabella and the midpoint of the lower border of the external occipital protuberance (See Fig. 2—4).

And the eyebrow—occipital line: The horizontal line connecting the midpoint of the upper border of the eyebrow and the highest prominence of the external occipital protuberance (See Fig. 2—4).

I. MOTOR AREA

Its upper point is 0.5 cm posterior to the midpoint of the anteroposterior median line, and its lower point at the junction of the eyebrow-occipital line and the temporal hair line (if the temporal hair line is not obvious, the point 0.5 cm anterior to the Junction of the eyebow—occipital line and the line ascending vertically from the midpoint of the zygomatic arch is taken as the lower point). The line connecting these two points represents the motor area (See Fig. 2—5).

The motor area is epually divided into five parts: the upper 1/5 of the line, which represents the motor area of the lower limbs and trunk and is indicated in paralysis of the lower limb; the middle 2/5, which represent the motor area of the upper limbs and are indicated in paralysis of the upper limb; and the lower 2/5, which represent the motor area of the face (also termed Speech Area 1) and are indicated in central contralateral facial paralysis, aphasia (partly of whole losting speech ability, but remaining the ability to understand the language), salivation, and dysphonia.

二、感觉区

运动区后移1.5厘米的平行线即为感觉区(图2—6)。

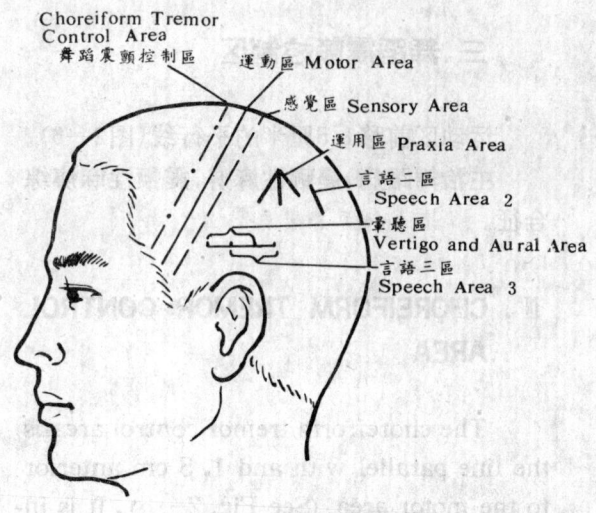

图2—6 侧面刺激区

Fig. 2—6 In lateral View

上1/5是下肢、头、躯干感觉区,主治对侧腰腿痛,麻木,感觉异常,及头顶疼痛;中2/5是上肢的感觉区,主治上肢疼痛,麻木,感觉异常;下2/5是面感觉区,主治对侧面部麻木、偏头痛、三叉神经痛、颞颌关节炎等。

II. SENSORY AREA

The sensory area refers to the line parallel with and 1.5 cm posterior to the motor area (See Fig. 2—6). The upper 1/5 represents the sensory area of the lower limbs, head and trunk, and is indicated in pain and numbness and paresthesia of the contralateral loin and legs, and vertex pain; the middle 2/5 represent the sensory area of the upper limbs and are indicated in pain, numbness and paresthesia of the upper limbs; and the lower 2/5, represent the sensory areas of the face and are indicated in numbness of the opposite side of the face, and migraine and trigeminal neuralgia and arthritis of the temporomandibular joint at the opposite side.

三、舞蹈震颤控制区

运动区前移1.5厘米的平行线(图2—6)。

主治舞蹈病,震颤性麻痹,震颤性麻痹综合征。

III. CHOREIFORM TREMOR CONTROL AREA

The choreiform tremor control area is the line parallel with and 1.5 cm anterior to the motor area (See Fig. 2—6). It is indicated in chorea, Parkinson's disease.

四、晕听区

耳尖直上1.5厘米处,向前后各引2厘米(共4厘米)的水平线(图2—6)。

主治眩晕、耳鸣、听力减退。

IV. VERTIGO AND AURAL AREA

The vertigo and aural area is the line with its midpoint 1.5cm above the apex of the auricle, extending horizontally 2.0 cm forward and backward (See Fig. 2—6). It is indicated in vertigo, tinnitus, decrease of the hearing ability.

五、言语二区

顶骨结节后下方2厘米处为起点,向后引一条平行于前后正中线、长3厘米的直线(图2—6)。

主治命名性失语(又称健忘性失语。病人称呼"名称"的能力障碍)。

V. SPEECH AREA 2

The speech area 2 refers to the straight line beginning at the point 2 cm inferoposterior to the parietal eminence and extending 3 cm backward, parallel with the antero—posterior median line (See Fig. 2—6). It is indicated in anomic aphasia.

六、言语三区

晕听区的中点向后引4厘米长的水平线(图2—6)。

主治感觉性失语(病人理解语言的能力障碍,往往答非所问)。

VI. SPEECH AREA 3

The speech area 3 refers to the line extending from the midpoint of the vertigo and aural area horizontally 4 cm backward (See Fig. 2—6). It is indicated in sensory aphasia (disorder in comprehension of speech).

七、运用区

从顶骨结节起,向下引一垂直线和与该线夹角为40度的前后两线,三线长度均为3厘米(图2—6)。

主治失用症(又称运用不能症。病人肌力、肌张力及基本运动正常,但技巧能力障碍,如不能解扣,系带等)。

Ⅶ. PRAXIA AREA

The praxia area refers to the three lines beginning from parietal eminence, one of them extending vertically downward 3 cm and the others extending respectively anteriorly and posteriorly 3 cm at the 40° angle with the former line (See Fig. 2—6). It is indicated in apraxia (the

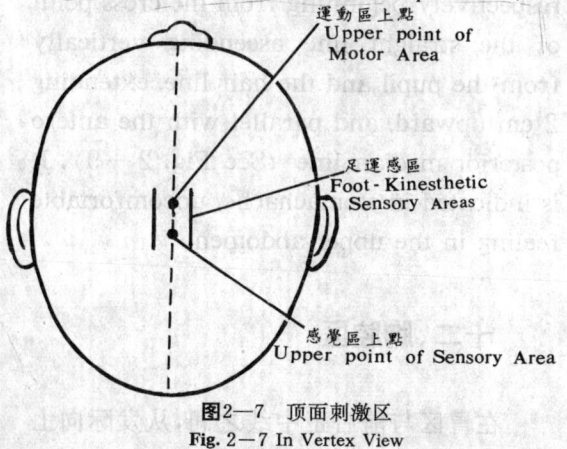

图2—7 顶面刺激区
Fig. 2—7 In Vertex View

muscular power and tension and basic motor are normal but there is disturbane in skill ability such as disability to undo a button and tie abootlac).

八、足运感区

前后正中线的中点左右旁开1厘米,向后各引一条平行于正中线长3厘米的直线(图2—7)。

主治对侧下肢瘫痪、疼痛、麻木、急性腰扭伤、夜尿、子宫脱垂、皮层性多尿等。

Ⅷ. FOOT — KINESTHETIC SENSORY AREA

The foot kinesthetic sensory area refers to two straight lines, beginning from the points 1 cm respectively lateral to the midpoint of the anteroposterior median line, extending 3 cm backward, parallel with the antero — posterior median line (See Fig. 2—7). It is indicated in paralysis, pain and numbness of the contralateral lower limb, acute sprain in the lumbar repion, nocturnal enuresis, prolapse of the uterus, cortical polyuria, etc.

九、视区

枕骨粗隆顶端旁开1厘米处,向上引平行于前后正中线长4厘米的直线(图2—8)。

主治皮层性视力障碍。

Ⅸ. VISUAL AREA

The visual area refers to two straiight lines beginning from the point 1 cm lateral to the external occipital protuberance and extending 4 cm upward, parallel with the anteroposterior median line (See Fig. 2-8). It is indicated in cortical disturbance of vision.

行于前后正中线2厘米长的直线(图2-9)。
主治胃痛、上腹部不适等症。

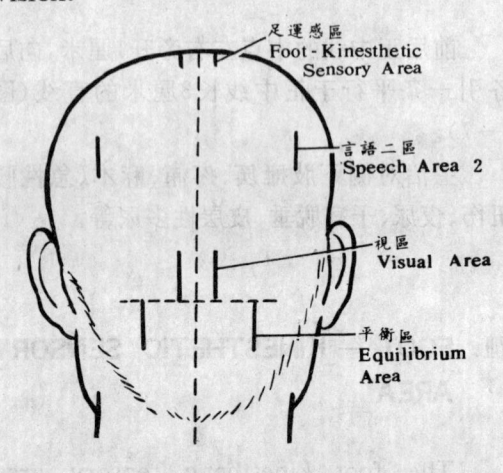

图2-8 后面刺激区
Fig. 2-8 In Posterior View

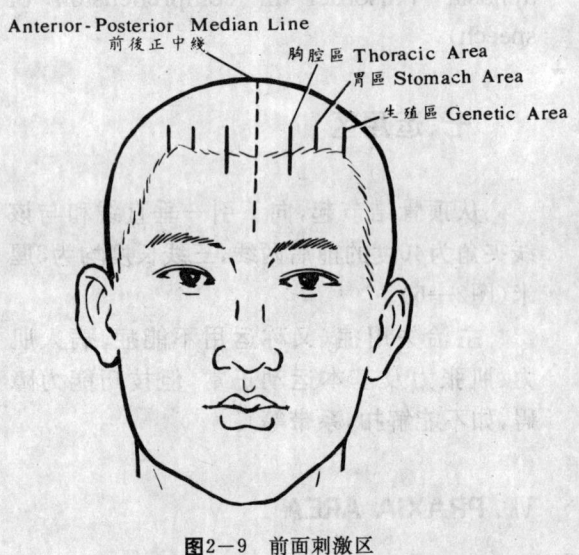

图2-9 前面刺激区
Fig. 2-9 In Anterior View

十、平衡区

枕骨粗隆顶端旁开3.5厘米处,向下引平行于前后正中线长4厘米的直线(2-8)。
主治小脑性平衡障碍。

X. EQUILIBRIUM AREA

The equilibrium area refers to two straight lines beginning from the point 3.5 cm lateral to the occipital protuberance and extending 4 cm downward, parallel with the anteroposterior median line (See Fig. 2-8). It is indicated in cerebellar disturbance of equilibrium.

十一、胃区

从瞳孔直上的发际处为起点,向上引平

XI. STOMACH AREA

The stomach area refers to two lines, respectively beginning from the cross point of the straight line ascending vertically from the pupil and the hair line, extending 2 cm upward, and parallel with the anteroposterior median line (See Fig. 2-9). It is indicated in stomachache, uncomfortable feeling in the upper abdomen.

十二、胸腔区

在胃区与前后正中线之间,从发际向上下各引2厘米长,平行于前后正中线的直线(图2-9)。
主治支气管哮喘,胸闷,胸痛,心悸不适等症。

XII. THORACIC AREA

The thoracic area refers to two lines, respectively, between the stomach area and anteroposterior medcian line, extending from the hair line upward 2 cm and downward 2 cm, parallel with the anteroposterior median line (See Fig. 2-9). It is indicated in bronchial asthma, oppressed feeling in the chest, pain in the chest, palpitation.

十三、生殖区

从额角处向上引平行于前后正中线的2厘米长直线(图2-9)。

主治功能性子宫出血、盆腔炎、白带多、子宫脱垂等。

XIII. GENETIC AREA

The genetic area refers to two lines, respectively beginning from the corner of the forehead and extending upward 2 cm, parallel with the anteroposterior median line (See Fig. 2-9). It is indicated in functional metrorrhagia, pelvic inflammation, leukorrhagia, prolapse of uterus.

[附]《中国头皮针施术部位标准化方案》(王雪苔等:《中国针灸大全》)。

一、额区

1. 额中线

[定位] 在额部正中发际内,自发际上0.5寸,即神庭穴(前发际正中直上0.5寸)向下针1寸。属督脉经。(图2-10)。

[主治] 神志病,头、鼻、舌、咽喉病等。

2. 额旁1线

[定位] 在额部额中线外侧,直对目内眦角自发际上0.5寸,即眉冲穴(攒竹穴直上,入发际0.5寸)沿经向下针1寸。属足太阳膀胱经。(图2-10)。

[主治] 肺、支气管、心脏等上焦病证。

3. 额旁2线

[定位] 在额部额旁1线的外侧,直对瞳孔,自发际上0.5寸,即头临泣穴(阳白穴直上,入发际0.5寸)沿经向下针1寸。属足少阳胆经。(图2-10)

[主治] 脾、胃、肝、胆、胰等中焦病证。

4. 额旁3线

[定位] 在额部额旁2线的外侧,直对目外眦角,自头维穴内侧0.75寸处,即本神穴(神庭穴旁3寸,当神庭穴与头维穴连线的内2/3与外1/3连接点处)与头维穴之间发际上0.5寸,向下针1寸。属足少阳胆经和足阳明胃经(图2-10)。

[主治] 肾、膀胱、生殖系统等下焦病证。

APPENDIX: STANDARD NOMENCLATURE OF CHINESE SCALP ACUPUNCTURE LINES

(Put forward in The Complete Works on Chinese Acupuncture and Moxibustion, compiled by Wang Xuetiai, et al)

I. FOREHEAD REGION

1. Middle Line of Forehead

Location: 1 cun long from Shenting (DU 24, on the anterior median line, 0.5 cun above the hair line) straightly downward along the Governor Vessel (Du Meridian) (See Fig. 2—10), belonging to the Governor vessel.

Indications: Mental disorders, diseases of head, nose, tongue and throat.

2. Line 1 Lateral to Forehead

Location: 1 cun long from Meichong (BL 3, directly superior to Cuanzhu, BL 2, 0.5 cun above the hair line) straightly downward along the Bladder Meridian, Belonging to the Bladder Meridian (See Fig. 2—10).

Indications: Disorders of lung, bronchus, and heart which are located in upper —jiao (i.e. Shang—jiao).

3. Line 2 Lateral to Foreshead

Location: 1 cun long from Toulinqi (GB 41) straightiy downward along the Gallbladder Meridian, belonging to the Gallbladder Meridian of Foot—Shaoyang (See Fig. 2—10).

Indications: Dicorders of spleen, stomach, liver, gallbladder and pancreas which are located in the middle —jiao (I.e. Zhong—jiao).

4. Line 3 Lateral to Forehead

Location: 1 cun long from the point 0.75 cun medial to Touwei (ST8) straightly downward, belonging to the Gallbladder Meridian of Foot —Shaoyang and the Stomach meridian of Foot — Yangming (See Fig. 2—10).

Indications: Disorders of kidney, urinary bladder, and genetic system, which are located in the lower —jiao (i.e. Xia—Jiao).

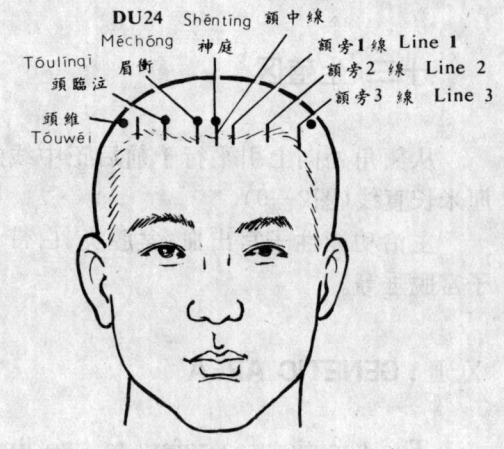

图2—10 前面图
Fig. 2—10 In Anterior View

二、顶区

5. 顶中线

［定位］ 在头顶部正中线,自百会穴向前至前顶穴(百会穴前1.5寸)。属督脉经。(图2—11)。

［主治］ 腰腿足病证,如瘫痪,麻木,疼痛及皮层性多尿,脱肛,小儿夜尿,高血压、头顶痛等。

6. 顶颞前斜线

［定位］ 在头部侧面,即自前顶穴起,止于悬厘穴(头维穴至曲鬓穴即耳前鬓发后缘直上平角孙穴连线的下1/4与上3/4交界处)。贯穿督脉,足太阳膀胱经和足少阳胆经(图2—12)。

［主治］ 可将全线分五等分,上1/5治下肢运动异常,如瘫痪、无力、关节痛等;中2/5治上肢运动异常,如瘫痪、无力、关节痛等;下2/5治头面部病证,如中枢性面瘫,运动性失语,流涎,脑动脉硬化等。

7. 顶颞后斜线

［定位］ 在头部侧面,位于顶颞前斜线之后,与之相距1寸,即自百会穴起,止于曲鬓穴。贯穿督脉,足太阳膀胱经和足少阳胆经(图2—12)。

［主治］ 可将全线分五等分,上1/5治下肢感觉异常,中2/5治上肢感觉异常,下2/5治头面部感觉异常。

8. 顶旁1线

［定位］ 在头顶部,顶中线外侧,两线相距1.5寸,即自承光穴(五处穴后1.5寸)起沿经往后针1.5寸。属足太阳膀胱经。(图2—13)。

［主治］ 腰腿病症,如瘫痪,麻木,疼痛等。

［注］ 五处穴——曲差穴上0.5寸,距头部正中线1.5寸。

曲差穴——神庭穴旁1.5寸,当神庭穴与头维穴连线的内1/3与2/3连接点取之。

9. 顶旁2线

［定位］ 在头顶部,顶旁1线外侧,两线相距0.75寸,即自正营穴(头临泣穴后2寸)起沿经往后针1.5寸。属足少阳胆经(图2—13)。

［主治］ 肩、臂、手病证,如瘫痪、麻木、疼痛等。

II. VERTEX REGION

5. *Middle Line of Vertex*

Location: From Baihui (DU 20) to Qianding (DU 21) along the Governor Vessel belonging to the Governor Vessel (Du Meridian) (See Fig. 2—11).

Indications: Disorders of waist and lower limb such as paralysis, numbness and pain, cortical po— lyuria, prolapse of anus, infantile nocturnal enuresis, hypertension, and pain in the vertex.

6. *Anterior Oblique Line of Vertex— Temporal*

Location: From Qianding (DU 21) obliquely to Xuanli (GB6, at the junction of the lower 1/4 and upper 3/4 of the line connecting Touwei, ST8, and Qubin GB 7), passing across the Governor vessel (Du Meridian), the Bladder Meridian of Foot — Taiyang and the Gallbladder Meridian of Foot — Shaoyang (See Fig. 2—12).

Indications: when the line is divided equally into five portions, the upper 1/5 is indicated in dyskinesia of the lower limb such as paralysis, and arthralgia; the middle 2/5 in dyskinesia of the upper limb such as paralysis, asthenia and arthralgia; and the lower 2/5 in disorders of head and face such as cortical paralysis, aphasis, salivation and cerebral arteriosclerosis.

7. Posterior Oblique Line of Vertex—Temporal

Location: From Baihui (DU 20) obliquely to Qubin (GB 7), 1 cun posterior to and parallel with the Anterior Oblique Line of Vertex — Temporal, passing across the Governor Vessel (Du, Meridian) the bladder Meridian of Foot — Taiyang and the Gallbladder Meridian of Foot — Shaoyang (See Fig. 2—12).

Indications: When the line is divided equally into five portions, the upper 1/5 is indicated in sensory disorders of lower limb, the middle 2/5 in sensory problems of upper limb, and the lower 2/5 in sensory troubles of face.

8. Line 1 Lateral vertex

Location: 1.5 cun lateral to Middle Line of Vertex, 1.5 cun long from Chengguang (BL6) backward along the Foot — Taiyang, belonging to the Bladder Meridian of Foot — Taiyang (See Fig. 2—13).

Indications: Disorders of waist and leg such as paralysis, numbness, and pain.

Note: Chengguang (BL6) is located at 1.5 cun posterlor to Wuchu (GB5) which is at the area 0.5 cun above Quchai (BL4), Quchai (BL 4) being the point 1.5 cun lateral to Shenting (DU 24) and at the junction of the medial 1/3 and the lateral 2/3 of the line connecting Shenting (DU 24) and Touwei (ST8).

9. Line 2 Lateral to Vertex

Locatlon: 0.75 cun lateral to the Line 1 Lateral to Vertex, 1.5 cun long from zhengying (GB 17) backward along the Foot —Shaoyang, belonging to the Gallbladder Meridian of Foot — Shaoyang (See Fig. 2—13).

Indications: Disorders in shoulder, upper arm, and hand, including paralysis, numbness and pain.

三、颞区

10. 颞前线

[定位] 在头部侧面,颞部两鬓内,即自颔厌穴(头维穴至曲鬓穴弧形线的上1/4与下3/4交界处)起,止于悬厘穴。属足少阳胆经(图2—13)。

[主治] 偏头痛,运动性失语,周围性面神经麻痹及口腔疾病等。

11. 颞后线

[定位] 在头部侧面,颞部耳尖直上方,即自率谷穴起,止于曲鬓穴。归属足少阳胆经(图2—13)。

[主治] 偏头痛,眩晕,耳聋,耳鸣等疾病。

III. TEMPORAL REGION

10. Anterior Temporal Line:

Location: From Hanyan (GB4, at the junction of upper 1/4 and lower 3/4 of the line connecting Touwei, ST8, and Qubin, GB7) to Xuanli (GB 6), beonging to the Gallbladder Meridian of Foot—Shaoyang (See Fig. 2—13).

Indications: Migraine, aphasia, Bell's palsy, disorders of the mouth.

11. Posterior Temporal Line:
Location: From Shuaigu (GB8) to Qubin (GB7), belonging to the Gallbladder Meridian of Foot—Shaoyang (See Fig. 2—13).
Indications: Migraine, vertigo, deafness, tinnitus.

四、枕区

12. 枕上正中线

［定位］ 在枕部，为枕外粗隆上方正中的垂直线，即自强间穴（风府穴直上3寸）起，止于脑户穴（风府穴直上1.5寸）。属督脉（图2—14）。

［主治］ 眼病、腰脊痛等疾病。

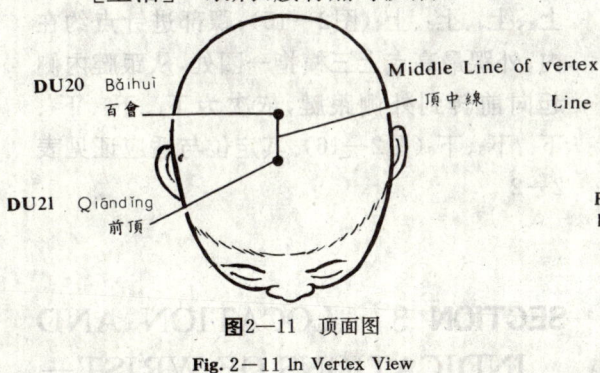

图2—11 顶面图
Fig. 2—11 In Vertex View

13. 枕上旁线

［定位］ 在枕部，与枕上正中线平行往外0.5寸，属足太阳膀胱经（图1—14）。

［主治］皮层性视力障碍，白内障，近视等，眼病及足癣，腰肌劳损等疾病。

14. 枕下旁线

［定位］ 在枕部，为枕外粗隆下方两侧2.6寸的垂直线，即自玉枕穴（后发际正中直上2.5寸，旁开1.3寸）起，止于天柱穴。属足太阳膀胱经（图2—14）。

［主治］ 小脑疾病引起的平衡障碍，后头痛等疾病。

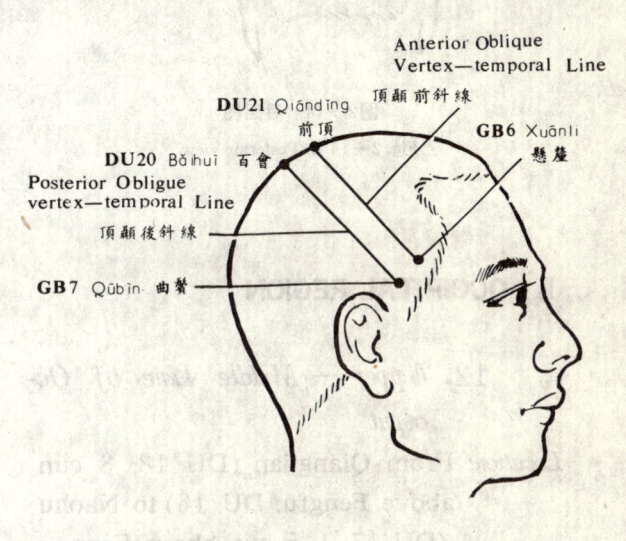

图2—12 侧面图（一）
Fig. 2—12 In Lateral View A

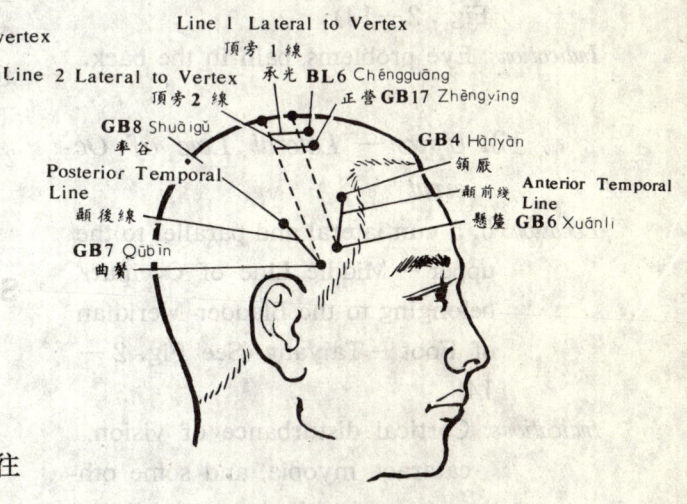

图2—13 侧面图（二）
Fig. 2—13 In Lateral View B

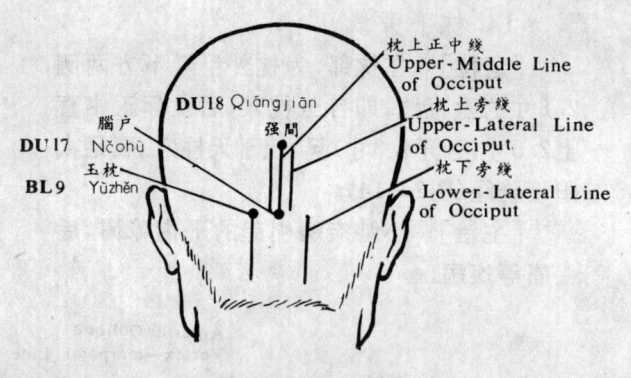

Fig. 2—14 In Posterior view

IV. OCCIPITAL REGION

12. Upper — Middle Line of Occiput

Location: From Qiangjian (DU 18, 3 cun above Fengfu, DU 16) to Naohu (DU 17, 1.5 cun above Fengfu, DU 16), belonging to the Governor Vessel (Du Meridian) (See Fig. 2—14).

Indications: Eye problems, pain in the back.

13. Upper — Lateral Line of Occiput

Location: 0.5 cun lateral and parallel to the upper — Middle Line of Occiput, belonging to the Bladder Meridian of Foot — Taiyang (See Fig. 2—14).

Indications: Cortical disturbance of vision, cataract, myopia, and some other eye problems, as well as Hongkong foot, lumbar muscle strain.

14. Lower — Lateral Line of Occiput

Location: 2.6 cun long line from Yuzhen (BL9, 2.5 cun above the posterior hairy line and 1.3 cun lateral to the posterior median line) to Tianzhu (BL10), belonging to the Bladder Meridian of Foot — Taiyang (See Fig. 2—14).

Indications: Disorders due to problem of cerebellum such as disequilibrium, and pain of the back of head.

SECTION 3 LOCATION AND INDICATIONS OF WRIST—ANKLE ACUPUNCTURE POINTS

There are 12 stimulating points by needle in the wrist—ankle acupuncture in total. The points of the wrist acupuncture are located at the circle about two finger—breadths proximal to the transverse crease of the wrist, which are, in order, termed upper 1—6 from the ulnar side to the radial side of the palmar surface and then from the radial side to the ulnar side of the dorsal surface (See Fig 2—15); the points of the ankel acupuncture are located at the circle about 3 finger—breadths proximal to the highest points of the internal and external condyles, which are termed lower 1—6 in the order circling the ankel from he internal side of the Achilles tendon to the external side of the Achilles tendon (See Fig. 2—16).

The location and indications of the wrist—ankle acuduncture points are as the following table:

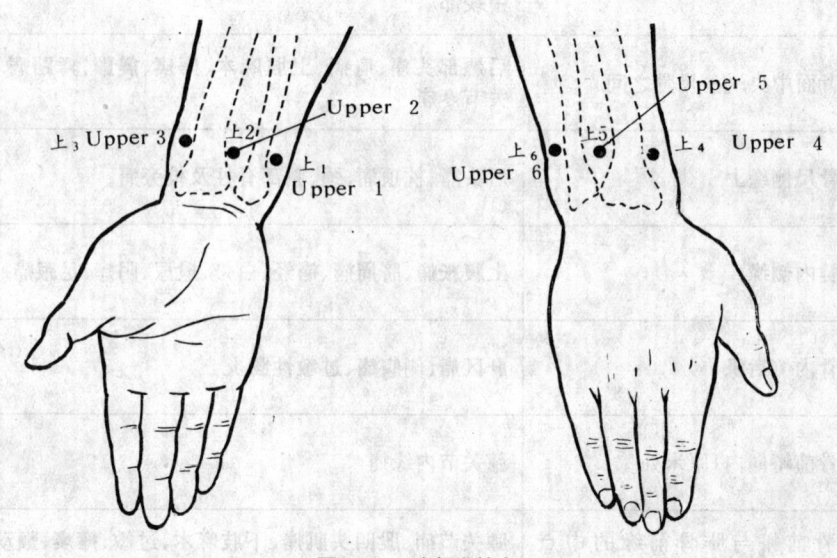

Fig. 2—15 Stimulating Points of Wrist—Puncture

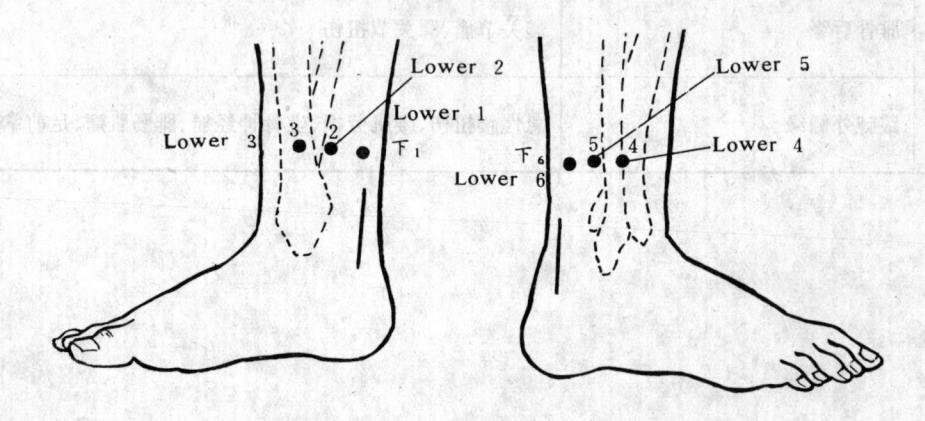

Fig. 2—16 Stimulating Points of Ankle—Acupuncture

表2—2　刺激点定位及主治病证

刺激点	定　位	主　治　病　证
上₁	尺骨内侧（尺侧）缘与尺侧腕屈肌腱间	前额头痛、眼病、鼻病、面肿、前牙痛、三叉神经痛、气管炎、胃病、心脏病、眩晕、失眠、高血压、癔病
上₂	掌长肌腱与桡侧腕屈肌腱之间	前颞头痛、后牙痛、颌下肿痛、胸闷、胸痛、哮喘、手心痛、指端麻木
上₃	掌面、桡动脉桡侧	高血压、胸痛（腋前线部）
上₄	手掌向内，拇指侧的桡骨缘上	头顶痛、耳病、下颌关节功能紊乱、肩周炎（肩前痛）、胸痛（腋中线部）
上₅	腕背面中央，桡、尺骨之间	后颞部头痛、肩痛、上肢麻木、瘫痪、震颤、舞蹈病，肘、腕、指关节疼痛
上₆	尺骨尺侧缘上	后头痛、枕顶痛、颈、胸部脊柱及椎旁痛
下₁	跟腱内侧缘	上腹胀痛、脐周痛、痛经、白带、遗尿、阴痒、足跟痛
下₂	胫骨内侧后缘	肝区痛、侧腹痛、过敏性肠炎
下₃	胫骨前嵴向内1厘米处	膝关节内缘痛
下₄	胫骨前嵴与腓骨前缘的中点（胫、腓骨之间）	膝关节痛、股四头肌痛、下肢麻木、过敏、瘫痪、颤动、舞蹈病，趾关节痛
下₅	腓骨后缘	髋关节痛、踝关节扭伤
下₆	跟腱外侧缘	急性腰扭伤、腰肌劳损、坐骨神经痛、腓肠肌痛、足前掌痛

Table 2—2 Location and Indications of Wrist—Ankle Acupuncture Points

Stimulation points	Location	Indication
Upper 1	Between the internal side (ulnar side) of the ulna and the tendon of ulnar flexor muscle of wrist	Foreheadache, eye disorders, nasal disorder, facial swelling, pain of anterior teeth, trigeminal neuralgia, bronchitis, gastronal disorders, heart disease, dizziness, insomnia, hypertension
Upper 2	Between tendon palmaris longus and tendon of radial flexor muscle of wrist	Pain of anterior temple, pain of posterior teeth, submandibular swelling and pain, chest distress and pain, asthma, pain in the center of palm, numbness of finger—tip.
Uppper 3	At palmar surface, radial to radial artery	Hypertension, chest pain (region around the anterior line of axilla)
Upper 4	With palm facing inward, at redial border of radius	Parietal headache, ear disorder, functional disorder of mandibular articulation, periathritis of shoulder joint (pain in the anterior area of shoulder), pain in chest (at the middle line of axilla)
Upper 5	At center of dorsal wrist, between radius and ulna	Pain of posterior temple, shoulder pain, numbness of upper limb, paralysis, tremble, chorea, pain of joints of elbow, wrist and finger
Upper 6	At lateral border of ulna	Pain of back of head, occipital pain and vertex pain, pain of neck, chest, spinal column and the area near it
Lower 1	At interior border of Achiles tendon	Pain and distension of upper abdomen, pain around umbilicus, dysmeorrhea, leukorrhagia, enuresis, pruritus vulvae, pain in heel
Lower 2	At posterior border of interior side of shin—bone	Hepatalgia, pain in lateral side of abdomen, allergic enteritis
Lower 3	1cm medial to anterior spine of tibia	Pain in medial border of knee joint
Lower 4	At posterior border of tibia and anterior border of fibula	Pain in knee joint, pain of quadriceps femoris, numbness of lower limb, hypersensitivity, paralysis, tremor, chorea, pain of toe joint
Lower 5	At posterior border of fibula	Pain of hip joint, sprain of ankle joint
Lower 6	At lateral border of Achiles tendon	Acute lumbar sprain, lumbar muscle strain, sciatic neuralgia, pain of gastrocnemius, pain of anterior plantas

第三章
常用针具、器械及消毒法

CHAPTER THREE
COMMONLY USED INSTRUMENTS IN ACUPUNCTURE AND MOXIBUSTION AND STERILIZATION

第一节 常用针具

一、毫针

毫针是针刺治病的主要针具，临床应用最为广泛，一般以不锈钢所制者为佳。

1. 毫针结构：毫针结构可分为针尖、针身、针根、针柄、针尾五个部分（图3—1）。

针尖 针的前端锋锐部分，是接触腧穴刺入机体的前锋，又称针芒。

针身 针尖与针柄之间的主体部分。宜光滑、挺直、富有弹性、便于刺进机体行使手法，又称针体。

针柄 针身之后，一般以金属丝缠绕，便于手持针着力的部分。

针根 针身与针柄连接处。

针尾 针柄的末端。

2. 毫针的规格：毫针规格主要指针身的粗细和长短，常用规格如下

表3—1 长短规格

寸	0.5	1.0	1.5	2.0	3	4	5
毫米	15	25	40	50	75	100	125
用途	多用于头面、肌肉浅表处穴位及耳穴刺激		多用于躯干、四肢肌肉较丰满处		多用于臀部、大腿肌肉丰满处及透穴，如阳陵泉透阴陵泉和皮下透刺		

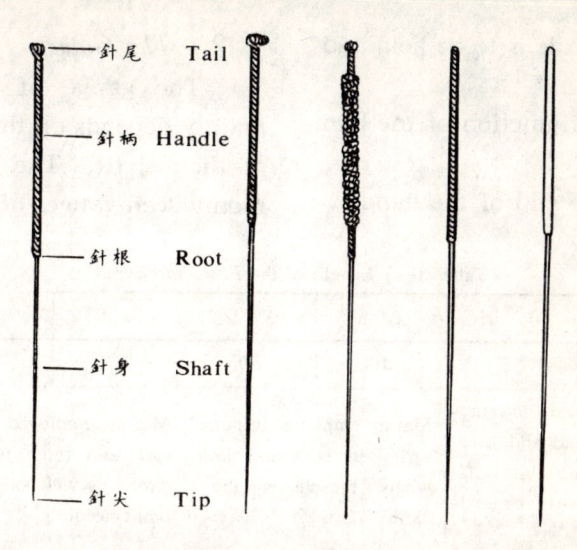

Fig. 3—1 The Structure of the Filiform Needle

(Labels: Tail 针尾, Handle 针柄, Root 针根, Shaft 针身, Tip 针尖)

表 3—2 粗细规格

号数	26	27	28	30	31	32
直径（毫米）	0.45	0.42	0.38	0.32	0.30	0.28
用途	多用于体质壮实成人，及头针刺激		常用于各种不同体质的病人，刺激四肢、躯干部穴位		多用于体质虚弱患者、儿童，及有重要脏器的部位如眼和面部等	

SECTION 1 COMMONLY USED NEEDLE APPARATUSES

I. FILIFORM NEEDLE

The filiform needle is the main needle apparatus in treating diseases by acupuncture, whlch is widely used in clinilc. A good filiform needle is generally made up of stainless steel.

1. *The Structure*

A filiform needle may be divided into five parts (See Fig 3—1):

The tip: the front sharp part of the needle, which is the vanguard of the needle to touch and puncture into the point on tne body, also named needle awn;

The shaft: the main part of the needle between the tip and the handle, which should be smooth, uprignt and flexible, so as to make it easier to puncture into the body and perform the manipulation, also termed needle body;

The handle: the part behind the shaft of the needle, generally, circuited with metal wire, where the needle is to be held and the force is acted on ;

The root: the conjunction of tne handle and shaft;

And the tail: the end of the handle.

2. The Gauge

The gauge of the filiform needles mainly depends on the length and diameter of their shaft. The following is the commonly seen gauges of the filiform needles.

Tab. 3−1 Length of the Filiform Needle

cun	0.5	1.0	1.5	2.0	3.0	4.0	5.0
mm	15	25	40	50	75	100	125
Usage	Mainly employed in puncturing on head and face and area with thin soft tissues, as well as auricle		Mainly employed in puncturing on trunk and limb where muscle is abundant		Mainly employed in puncturing on buttock and thigh where muscle is abundant, as well as for point—through—point needling		

Tab. 3−2 Diameter of the Filiform Needle

No	26	27	28	30	31	32
dia. (mm)	0.45	0.42	0.38	0.32	0.30	0.28
Usage	Mainly employed in puncturing on adults with strong physical constitution, and for scalp acupuncture			Mainly used in puncturing on limb and trunk	Mainly used in puncturing on children with poor physical constitution and on points around which important organ is located	

二、三棱针

三棱针即古代"九针"中的锋针，是用来点刺放血的针具。为不锈钢制成，针柄粗呈圆柱型，针身长约6厘米，呈三棱型，尖端三面有刃，针尖锋利（图3—2）。有大、中、小三个型号，规格见表8。

表3—3 三棱针常用规格（毫米）

类别	针长	柄粗	针身长	针身宽
大号	60.5	3.0	18.0	3.0
中号	60.5	2.0	12.0	2.0
小号	60.5	1.0	6.0	1.0

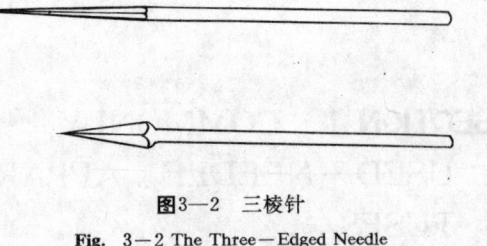

图3—2 三棱针

Fig. 3−2 The Three−Edged Needle

II. THREE—EDGED NEEDLE

The three—edged (triangular prismatic) needle, called the sharp needle in ancient times, is a needling apparatus to be used to prick to cause bleeding. It is made up of stainless steel with a big round handle, a triangular prismatic shaft about 6 cm long, and a sharp tip (See Fig 3—2). It is classified into the big, middle and small gauges. The gauge of the three—edged needle is shown in the following table.

Tab. 3—3 The Commonly Seen Gauges of the Three —Edged Needle (mm)

Classification	needle length	handle diameter	shaft length	shaft diameter
big	60.5	3.0	18.0	3.0
middle	60.5	2.0	12.0	2.0
small	60.5	1.0	6.0	1.0

三、皮内针

皮内针又称"埋针"。是久留针的一种发展。针具为一种粗细30号（直径0.32毫米）或32号（直径0.28毫米）合金丝制成。临床常用如下两种。

1. 麦粒型或环型：麦粒型针柄约为米粒大小，针身长0.5～1厘米（图3—3）。由于操作不便，留针时易对皮肤有压损，故改为针柄呈圆环状，直径约0.3厘米，针身长0.5厘米左右并与针柄成直线的环型皮内针（图3—3）。用于四肢躯干部埋针。

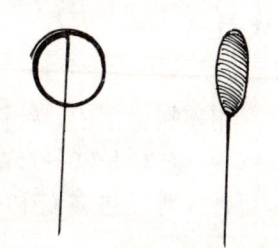

图3—3 麦粒型、环型皮内针
Fig. 3—3 The wheat—Granule—Shaped and Circle—Shaped Needle

2. 揿钉型：揿钉型皮内针针柄呈圆环状，直径约0.3厘米，针身长0.2～0.3厘米与针柄垂直形似图钉（图3—4）。用于耳穴埋针。

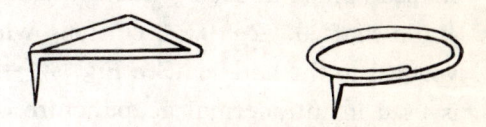

图3—4 揿针
Fig. 3—4 The Thumb—Pin—Shaped Needle

III. INTRADERMAL NEEDLE

The intradermal needle, also termed embedment needle, is the result of development of the technique of retaining the needle in the body. It is made up of the alloy steel wire 0.32 mm or 0.28 mm in diameter. The following two kinds of the intradermal needle are usually used in clinic.

1. The Wheat—Granule—Shaped or Circle—Shaped Needle

The wheat—granule—shaped needle has its handle at about a rice size and its shaft at 0.5—1.0 cm long (See Fig. 3—3). As causing difficulty in the operation and easily resulting in impairment of the skin by its pressure on the skin, it is improved by changing it into the circle—shaped needle, which has a circle—shaped handle with 0.3 cm in diameter, and a shaft about 0.5 cm at length (See Fig. 3—3). The circle—shaped or wheat—granule—shaped needle is usually used in intradermal acupuncture on the limb and trunk.

2. The Thumb—Pin—Shaped Needle

The thumb—pin—shaped needle, also termed thumb—tack—shaped needle, is like a thumb tack in shape with a circle—shaped handle about 0.3 cm in diameter, and a shaft 0.2—0.3 cm long which is vertical to the handle (See Fig. 3—4). It is used in intradermal acupuncture on the points.

四、皮肤针

皮肤针亦称梅花针,七星针。结构可分三部分。

针柄（杆）：是手握部分,用塑料、有机玻璃、胶木或电木等材料制成,长约18～25厘米富有弹性（图3—5）。

针头：是嵌装针组的部分。有单用与双用两种（图3—5）。头端直径0.2～1厘米。

针组（束）：是刺激皮肤的部分。有用七根钢针捆在一起的圆柱形,亦有用七根钢针等距散在成梅花形（图3—5）。

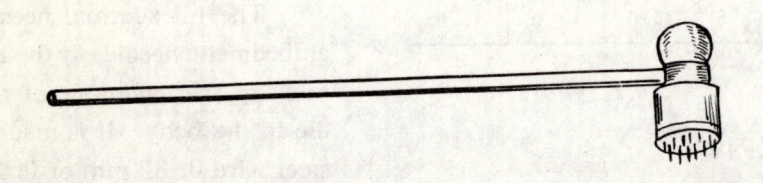

Fig. 3—5 The Skin Needle

IV. SKIN NEEDLE

The skin needle, also termed plum—blossom needle or seven—star needle, consists of the following three parts:

The handle: the part to be held by the hand, made up of plastics, plexiglass, or bakelite, which is 18—25 cm long and rich in elasticity (See Fig. 3—5).

The head: the part where the needle are inlaid, which is 0.2-1.0 cm at diameter. It may be inlaid with needles on its one bottom or both bottoms (See Fig. 3-5).

The bundle of the needles: the part to sever to puncture on the skin. In the bundle, seven steel needles may be inlaid with a round column shape, or with a plum—blossom shape (See Fig. 3—5).

五、火针

火针多采用不锈钢制成,针体较粗,直径一般为0.5～1毫米。长50～75毫米（2～3寸）。针柄多用竹或骨质包裹（图3—6）,以免烫手。

V. HOT NEEDLE

常用针具、器械及消毒法

The hot needle is usually made up of the stainless steel, which has a comparatively thick shaft, generally with 0.5—1.0 mm diameter and 50—75mm (2.0—3.0 cun) length, and a handle usually wrapped with the material of bamboo or bone so as to avoid burning the hand (See Fig. 3—6).

六、鍉针

鍉针为古代九针之一。以不锈钢粗钢丝制成，也有采用骨质或硬木材料制成的，针头钝圆，形似黍粟，不致刺入皮肤，针身长约75～100毫米（3～4寸），针柄部或用铝丝缠绕（图3—7）。

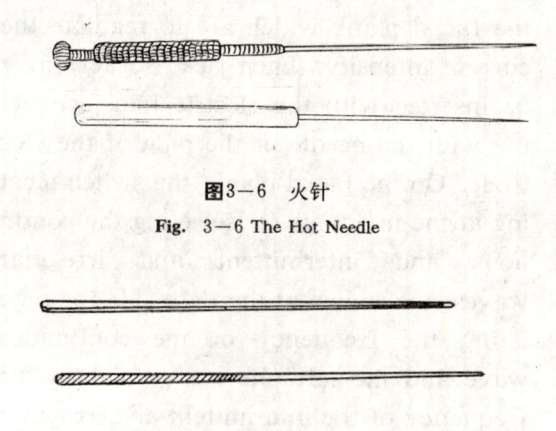

图3—6 火针
Fig. 3—6 The Hot Needle

图3—7 鍉针
Fig. 3—7 The Dull Needle

Ⅵ. DULL NEEDLE

The dull needle, one of the ancient nine needles, is made up of the stainless steel wire, or material of the bone or hard wood, with a dull and broomcorn—millet—shaped tip, which can not puncture through the skin, a 3.0—4.0 cun (75—100 mm) long shaft, and a handle which may be circuited with the aluminium wire (See Fig 3—7).

第二节 常用器械及材料

一、电针器

电针器种类很多，有蜂鸣式电针器，电子管电针器，半导体电针器等，只要能控制输出电压，电流到所需强度的器械，均可作电针器。但应注意最大输出电压和电流量的关系。例如最大输出电压在40V以上者，最大输出电流应限制在1mA以内，以免发生触电危险。由于半导体电针器具有体积小，重量轻、携带方便、安全耐用故临床使用广泛，目前针灸医师最常用的为G6805电针治疗仪（图3—8）。性能稳定，可交直流两用，输出波型有连续波，疏密波，断续波等。连续波频率为160～5000次/min，疏密波和断续波为14～26次/min。正脉冲峰值为50V，波宽为500μS，负脉冲峰值为35V，波宽为250μS。

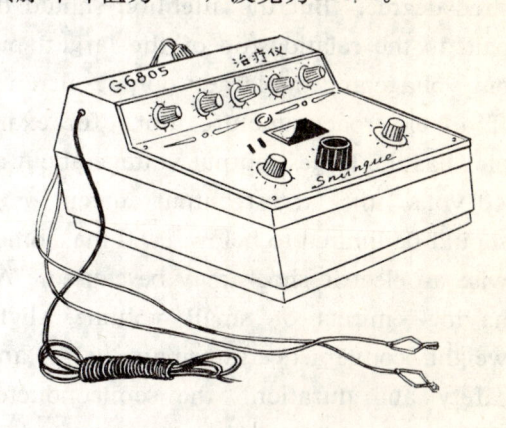

图3—8 G6805电针治疗仪
Fig. 3—8 The G 6805 Electroacupuncture Therapeutic Unit

· 189 ·

仪器顶部有五个输出插孔，对应于面板上五个电流强度调控旋钮。各插孔可插入针夹电极插头或电极板插头。面板上：位于中间指示灯下的旋钮，用以选择连续波，疏密波，断续波三种不同输出波型。右侧的旋钮用作连续波频率的调节，左侧旋钮用作疏密波及断续波频率的调节。

SECTON 2　COMMONLY USED OTHER INSTRUMENTS AND MATERIALS

Ⅰ. ELECTROACUPUNCTURE APPARATUS

There are many kinds of the electric acupuncture apparatuses, including the buzzing electroacupuncture unit, transistor electroacupuncture unit, semiconductor electroacupuncture unit, etc. Any electric apparatus can be used as an electroacupuncture unit if its output voltage and current can be controlled at the desired degree. But the attention should be paid to the relationship of the largest output voltage and the largest output current. If an electroacupuncture unit, for example, has the largest output voltage about at 40 volts, the largest output current of it should be limited to below 1. 0 ma, otherwise an electric shock may be caused. As having emirets of small volume, light weight, convenience in bringing with, and safety and duration, the semiconductor electroacupuncture unit is widely used in clinic. At present, of many semiconductor electroacupuncture units, the most—frequently used one by the doctors of acupuncture and moxibustion is the G 6805 electroacupuncture therapeutic unit (See Fig. 3—8) with steady function, dual—purposes in connecting with either direct or indirect current, and various forms of output waves, including continuous wave, intermittent wave and irregular wave. The frequency of the continuous wave is 160—500 turns per minute; the irregular and intermittent wave is 14—26 turns per minute. In the positive pulse, the peak value is 50 volt and amplitude 500 μs; and in the negative pulse, the peak value 35 volt and the amplitude 250 μs. There are five jacks on the vertex of the unit, which are in corresponding with the five switches on the facial plank which are to regulate the current intensity. Each jack (socket) may be inserted with the electric plug connecting with the needle or the plug of the electrode. On the facial plank, the switch locating at the middle is for selecting the continuous and intermittent and irregular waves, the switch at the right side for regulating the frequency of the continuous wave and the left one for regulating the frequency of the intermittent and irregular waves.

二、耳穴探测器

耳穴探测器品种颇多，大都可作探穴，治疗两用。常用有WQ－10C型多用电子穴位测定治疗仪（图3－9）、HB－EDT－1型袖珍穴位诊断治疗仪（图3－9），均有探穴及治疗等功能，其WQ－10H型多用电子穴位测定治疗仪，尚可作电兴奋治疗及经络敏感测定。

常用针具、器械及消毒法

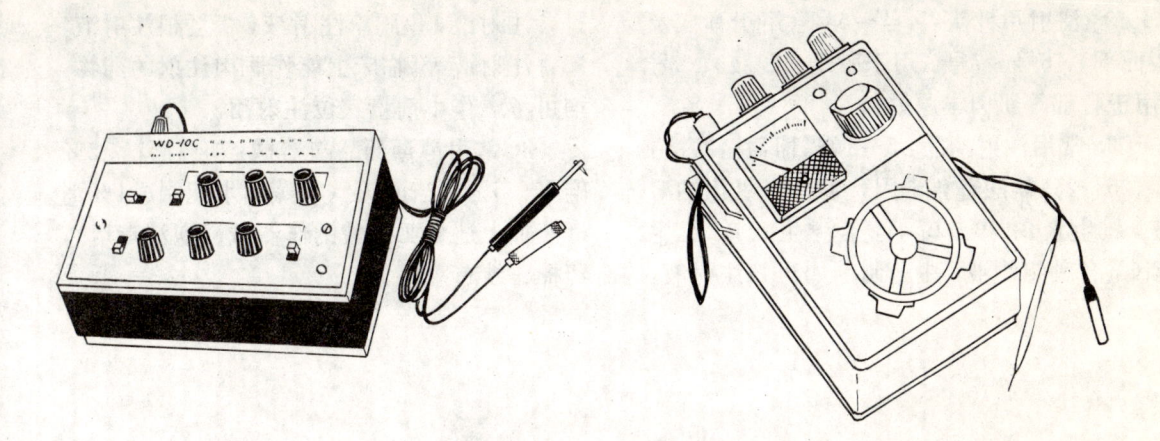

图3—9 耳穴探测仪
Fig. 3—9 Electric Unit for Probing Otopoint

II. ELECTRLC UNIT FOR PROBING THE OTOPOINTS

There are many kinds of the electric units for probing otopoints, most of them being of dual purposes——for probing otopoints and for treating diseases, of which WQ—10 A type electronic multi—purpose therapeutic unit (See Fig. 3—9) and HB—EDT—1 diagnostic and therapeutic unit (See Fig. 3—9) are most frequently used in clinic.

三、其他器械

1. 注射器：1毫升（用于耳穴注射），2毫升，5毫升，10毫升，20毫升。

表3—4 消毒用器械

品　名	规　　格	用　途
有盖方盘	15cm×23cm 或 30cm×20cm 大小不等	存放消毒针具
无盖方盘	43cm×29cm，大小不等	存入各种针灸用器械与材料
敷料缸	口径12.5cm 左右	存放消毒棉球与纱布敷料等
普通止血钳 敷料镊	16cm（全直齿） 16cm（无齿）	钳夹消毒棉球、针具
海绵钳	25cm	钳夹消毒注射器等
广口瓶	250ml 500ml	存放消毒酒精棉球 存放消毒钳镊等

2. 注射用针头：4号～5号（用于耳穴及头面部），6号～7号（用于躯干、四肢）、9号（用于臀部等肌肉丰厚处）。

3. 常用注射药品：5～10%葡萄糖溶液，0.25～2%盐酸普鲁卡因，0.9%氯化钠溶液，维生素B_1、B_2、B_{12}，复合维生素B、维生素C，各种组织液，中药制剂如当归注射液，丹参注射液，鱼腥草注射液，板兰根注射液，麝香注射液等。临床上能作肌肉注射的药物，均可考虑作小剂量穴位注射用。

4. 常用消毒药品与器械：75%酒精、2%碘酊、5%新洁而灭（与蒸馏水配制成1%消毒液加上适量亚硝酸钠作器械浸泡消毒用），药棉、纱布敷料。

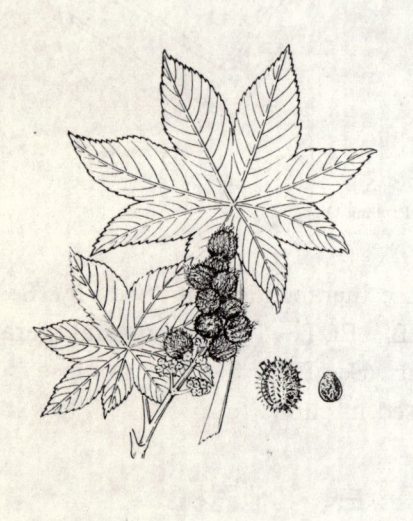

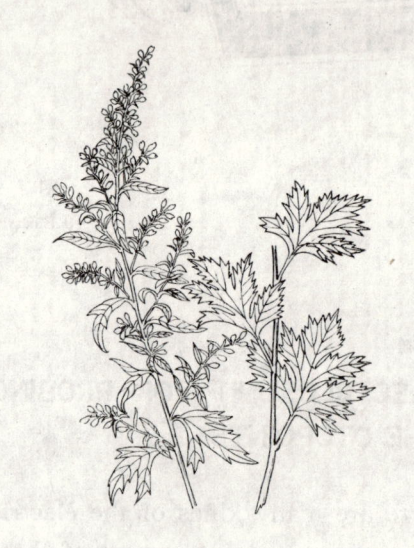

艾叶 Moxa Leave　　　　　　蓖麻 Ricini

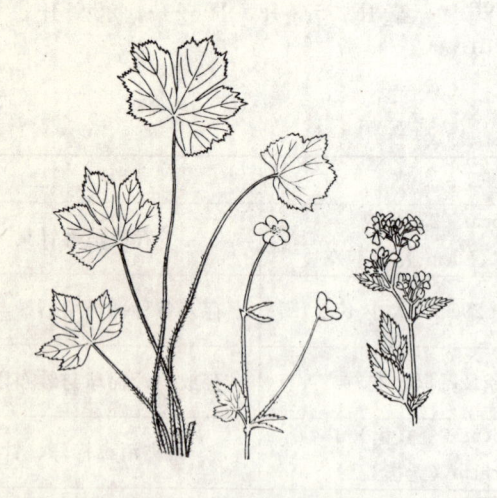

白芥子 Semen Sinapis Albae　　　大蒜 Garlic

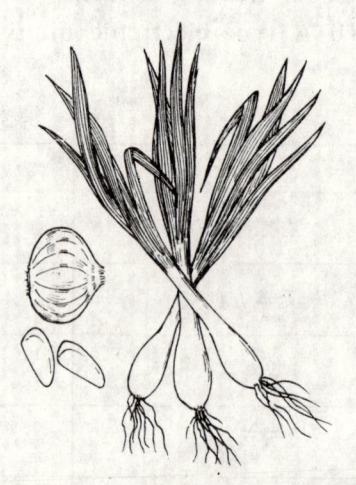

图3—10① 常用灸用材料
Fig. 3—10① Materials for Moxibustion

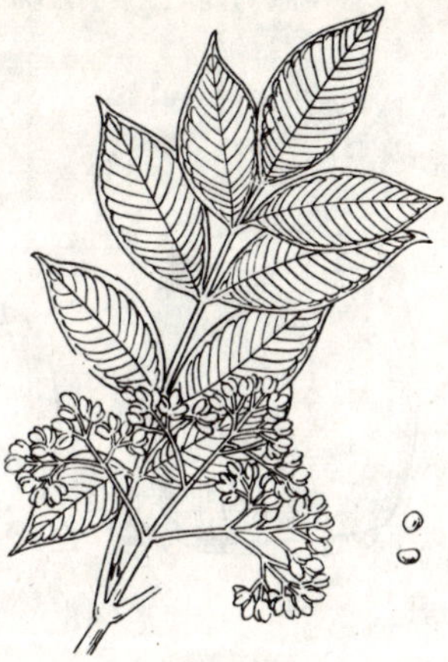

常用针具、器械及消毒法

吴茱萸　Euodia Rulaecarpa

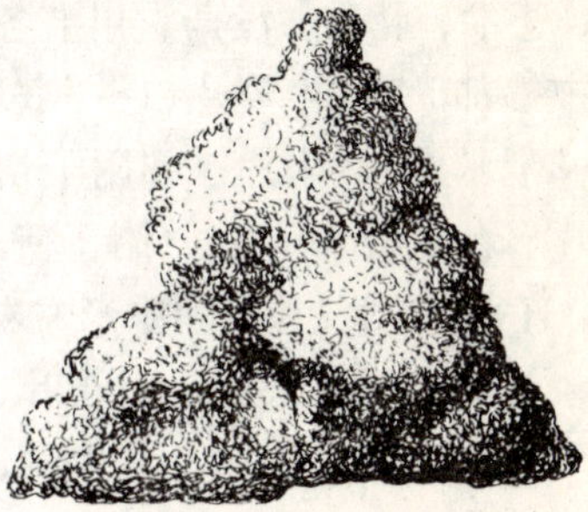

艾绒　Moxa Wool

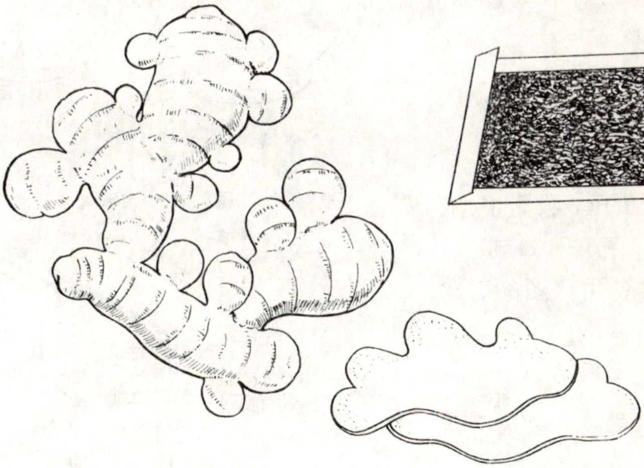

生姜　Ginger

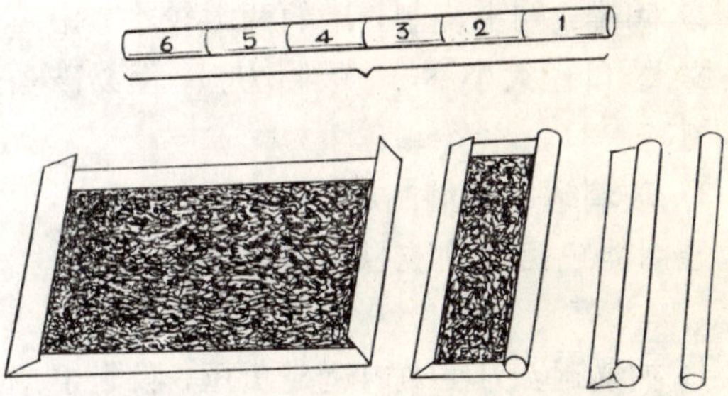

艾条　Moxa Stick

图3—10②　常用灸用材料
Fig. 3—10②　Materials for Moxibustion

5. 灸用材料（图3—10）：艾绒（艾叶加工制作），纯艾条（常用为直径1.5厘米，长20厘米）、药条（即艾绒中掺入药物粉末。常用药末：肉桂、干姜、丁香、独活、细辛、白芷、雄黄、苍术、乳香、没药、川椒各等分，每双艾条中掺加6克）。生姜片（1～3毫米厚），蒜片（1～2毫米厚）、附片（熟附子切成3毫米左右厚片、水浸透）、附饼（附子研末、酒调和作饼，直径3厘米、厚0.8厘米左右）、食盐、灯草、蓖麻子、吴茱萸、毛茛叶、白芥子、灸用清油（麻油、菜油、花生油、花生油均可）、酒精灯。

6. 罐具：1) 竹罐：坚固细毛竹所制长6～9厘米，口径3厘米，4.5厘米，6厘米不等，平正光滑。（图3—11）。不易跌碎，但易爆裂漏气。

2) 陶罐：陶土烧制，罐的两端较小，中间略膨大。口径大小不一，吸附力强，但易破碎（图3—12）。

3) 玻璃罐：玻璃制成，口径大小不一，质地透明能窥测罐内皮肤瘀血程度（图3—13）。

4) 抽气罐：为使罐内造成负压，吸附于皮肤上的，大小不一的特制罐（图3—14）亦有用青、链霉素瓶磨去底制成备用（图3—14）

7. 耳穴贴敷材料：绿豆、中药王不留行籽、1000高斯以上的磁珠、胶布等。

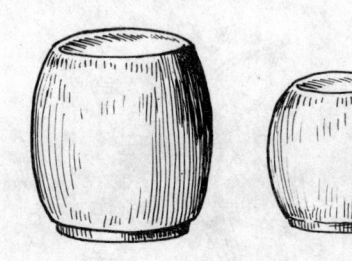

图3—12 陶罐
Fig. 3—12 Pottery Jar

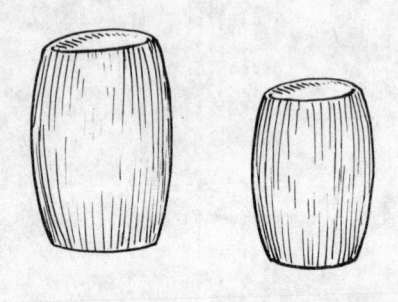

图3—13 玻璃罐
Fig. 3—13 Glass Jar

图3—11 竹罐
Fig. 3—11 Bamboo Jar

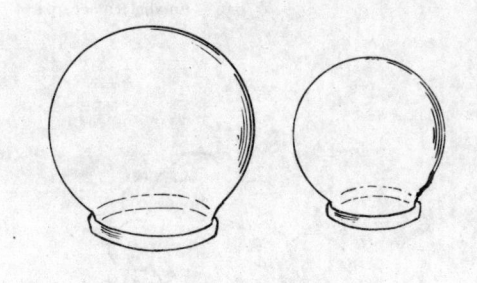

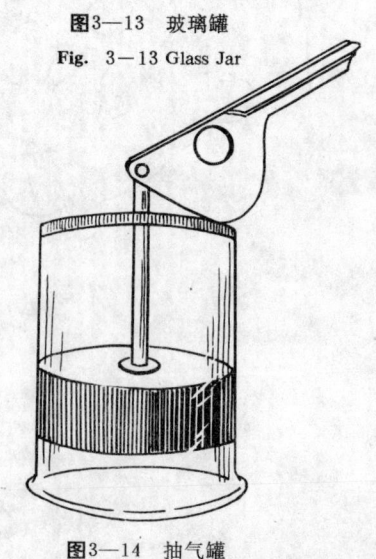

图3—14 抽气罐
Fig. 3—14 Aspirating Jar

III. OTHER INSTRUMENTS AND MATERIALS

1. Syringe

1 ml syringe used in otopoint injection, and 2—20 ml syringes used in body point injection.

2. Syringe Needle

No. 4—5 needles used for injection at otopoints, head and face; No. 6—7 needle for injection at trunk and extremities; No. 9 for injection at buttock as well as other regions with rich muscle.

3. Commonly Used Injections

5—10 % of glucose solution, 0.25—2% of procaine hydrochloride, 0.9% of sodium chloride solution, Vitamin B_1, B_2, B_{12} and C, compound Vitamin B, various kinds of tissue fluid, some herb medicine injections such as radix angelicae injection, radix salviae miltiorrhizae injection, herba houttuyniae injection, radix isatidis injection and moschus injection, and other drugs which can be used for intramuscular injection.

4. Equipments and Drugs for Sterilization

(1). Drugs: 75% of alcohol, 2% of iodine tincture, 5% of bromogeramine which is mixed with distilled water into 1% of disinfectant for disinfection of equipment.

(2). Equipment: See Tab. 3—4.

5. Materials for Moxibustion (See Fig. 3—10)

They may inclucde the follows:

Moxa wool made of dry moxa leaves, moxa stick (usually 1.5 cm in diameter and 20 cm in length), moxa-and-

Tab. 3—4 Equipments for Sterilization

Name	gauge	usage
Square dish with lid	various size, but usually at 15×23 cm	container for sterilized needle
Square dish without lid	various size, but usually at 43×29 cm	container for acubustion equipment and materials
Dressing drum	12.5 cm in diameter	container for sterilized dressing
Hemostatic forceps or dressing clamps	16 cm long	hold sterilized cotton ball and needle
Sponge forceps	25 cm long	hold sterilized syringe, etc
Wide mouth bottle	250 ml in content 500 ml in content	container for alcohol cotton ball container for sterilized forceps or clamps

drug stick made of moxa wool and drug powders (the commonly used powders are made of Cortex Cinnamomi, Dried Ginger, Flos Caryophylli, Radix Angelicae Pubescentis, Herba Asari, Radix Angelicae Dahuricae, Realgar, Rhizome Atractylodis, Resina, Boswelliae Carterii, Myrrha, Pericarpium Zanthoxyli, each of them being equal, and 6 g of these powders for each stick), slice of ginger about 1—3 mm thick, slice of garlic 1—2 mm thick, slice of Radix Aconiti Praeparata about 3 mm thick and soaked by water, Radix Aconiti Praeparata cake made from a paste of monkshood and white wine, about 3 cm in diameter and 0.8 cm thick, salt, rush, Semen Ricini, Fructus Euodiae, Semen Sinapis Albae, Vegetable oil, and alcohol lamp.

6. Jars

Bamboo jar: Cut down a Section of bamboo 6—9 cm in length and 3—6 cm in diameter, forming a cylinder shaped as a drum. One end is used as the bottom, and the other as the opening. The rim of the jar should be made smoothly (See Fig. 3—11). The bamboo jar is not easily broken by falling down but eaisly broken by playing fire in it.

Pottery jar: There are various pottery jars in different diameters. The jar is easily broken by falling down (See Fig. 3—12).

Glass jar: Since a glass jar is transparent, the local congestion can be seen so as to control the treatment (See Fig. 3—13).

Aspirating jar: As an aspirating jar is easy for pumping the air in the jar out, it is availabe in many places. It is in different size (See Fig. 3—14). or made from penicillin or streptomycin injection bottle (See Fig. 3—14).

7. Materials for Sticking and Pressing Method on Otopoimts

They include mung bean, semen vaccariae (vaccaria seed), over 1000 abt. magnetic ball, adhesive plaster, etc.

Fig. 3—5 Sterilization by the Autoclave

第三节 常用消毒方法

针前必须将针具，施术部位及医生手指进行消毒，常用消毒法如下：

一、针具消毒

1. 高压蒸气灭菌法：将针具用布包好，放在高压蒸气锅内灭菌消毒（图3—15），一

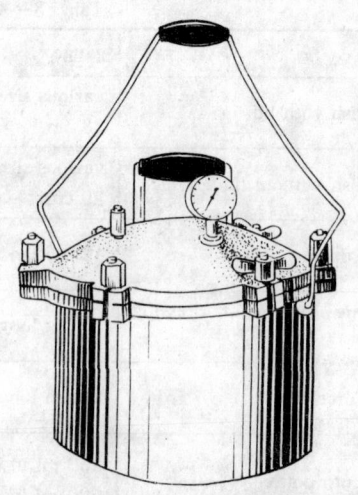

图3—15 高压灭菌锅消毒

Fig. 3—15 Sterilization by the Autoclave

SECTION 3 COMMON METHODS OF STERILIZATION

Prior to treatment, the needle apparatuses, the area of the patient's body to be punctured, and the operator's fingers should be sterilized. Commonly used methods of sterilization are as follows.

I. STERILIZATION OF THE NEEDLE APPARATUSES

1. *By Autoclave*

The needles are wrapped in a piece of cloth and put into the autoclave for sterilization (See Fig 3—15). Generally, the needle apparatuses can be sterilized under 15 pounds of air pressure and high termperature of 120°c for 15 minutes.

2. *By Soaking in the Drug Fluid*

The needles are soaked in 75% of alcohol for 30—60 minutes, then they are taken out and wiped off the liquid from them with the sterilized dry cotton ball, being ready to be used. Or they are soaked in 0.1% of bromogeramini which is added with 0.5% of sodium nitrite for 1—2 hours, and then dried with the sterilized dressing or cotton ball. They, then, are ready to be used. All equipments which will get in touch with the filiform needle directly, such as needle box and plate, forceps and tube, should be sterilized and kept aseptic.

II. STERILIZATION OF THE SKIN AREAS TO BE PUNCTURED

The skin area selected for needling is swabbed round and outward with 75% of alcohol cotton ball from the needling point to its round areas (See Fig. 3—16). Or the area is swabbed first with 2% of iodine, and then it is cleaned with 15% of alcohol.

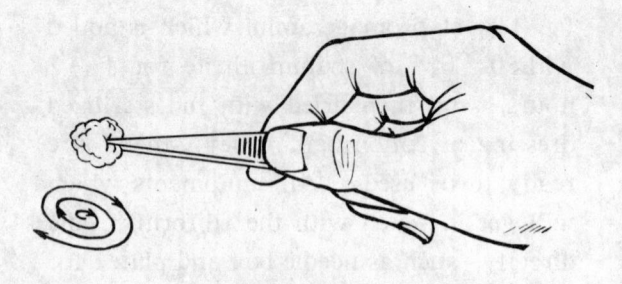

图3—16 施术部位消毒
Fig. 3—16 Sterilization of the Skin to Be Punctured

Prior to needling, the operator's fingers should be first washed clearly with soap, and then swabbed with 75% of alcohol cotton ball.

Generally, in an operation, one needle is only for one point. The needle having been used should be kept in another box in order to be sterilized for next time use. A strict sterilization should be given to the needle having been used for the patient with infectious disease, and if the condition permitting, the needle is only used once for ever.

III. STERILIZATION OF THE OPERATOR'S FINGERS

下 篇
针灸技法

PART TWO
SKILL OF
ACUPUNCTRUE
AND
MOXIBUSTION

第四章
针灸技法述要

CHAPTER FOUR
A GENERAL DISCUSSION ON THE SKILL OF ACUPUNCTURE AND MOXIBUSTION

针灸治病获得临床效果的关键，在于取穴的准确、配穴的恰当及操作技能的熟练三个方面。其中，尤其与医者技法的熟练程度密切相关。

针灸技法包括针法与灸法两大类。本章着重介绍临床常用针法中的毫针、三棱针、皮内针、皮肤针、锟针、火针、电针、水针、耳针、头针、腕踝针及灸法、拔罐等的操作技法与适用范围。

第一节 毫 针

毫针技法临床运用最为广泛，它以毫针为治病的工具。为了进针顺利，行针自如，减少病人痛苦，操作前必须选择好针具。一般要求针尖端正无钩，尖带圆形如松针。锐利适度，针身光滑挺直，坚韧而富有弹性。针根处无剥蚀伤痕。针柄牢固而无松动。

除外尚须根据病人性别、年龄、形体胖瘦、身材高矮、体质强弱、病情虚实、病变部位深浅、所取穴位的具体部位，选择长短、粗细适宜的针具。

针具用完后要注意收藏，针尖处不能碰撞硬物，一旦发现针尖带钩、弯曲、剥蚀等，当剔除不用。

一、针刺练习

（一）常用持针法

1. 两指持针法：用拇、食二指指腹捏拿针柄（图4—1①），或以拇、食二指捏拿消毒棉球裹住针身，露出针尖3~5毫米（图4—1②）。前者适于操持0.5~1寸的短毫针（毫针长短指针身的长度与公制的比例见第三章第一节，以下均同），后者宜于操持2~3寸毫针速刺进针。

2. 三指持针法：拇指在内，食、中二指在外固定针柄（图4—2①），或拇、中指挟持针

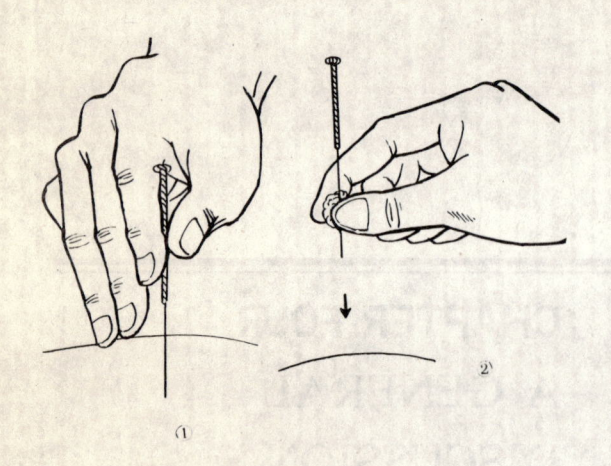

图 4—1 两指持针法
Fig. 4—1 Holding The Neeale With Two Fingers

柄，食指顶压针尾（图 4—2②），适宜 1～1.5寸长毫针捻转进针。也有用拇指、中指指腹捏挟针身，食指指腹紧附中指之后，端固针身，露出针尖 3～5 毫米（图 4—2③），本法宜于1.5～3 寸长毫针速刺进针。

3. 四指持针法：拇、食、中三指捏拿针柄，无名指抵住针身（图 4—3），适于 1.5～2 寸毫针捻转进针。

（二）指力与手法的练习

由于毫针的针身细软，如果没有一定的指力，就很难随意进针，并进行各种手法操作。这样不仅影响治疗效果，亦不能使病人乐

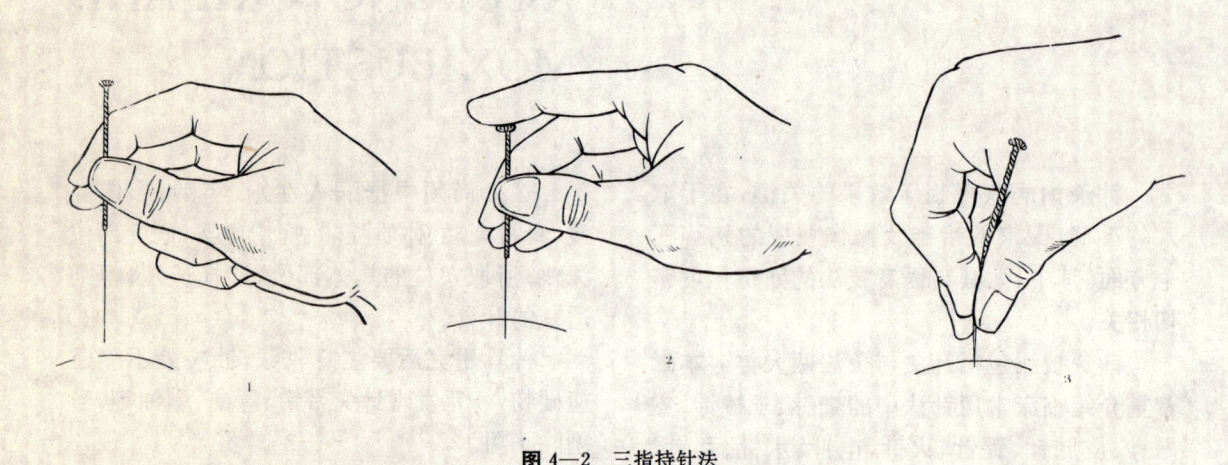

图 4—2 三指持针法
Fig. 4—2 Holding the Needle with Three Fingers

于接受。故练好指力和手法，是初学针刺者必不可少的基本技能训练。

1. 指力练习：这是练针的第一步，即用松软纸张折叠成长 7～8 厘米，宽 4～5 厘米见方，厚约 2～3 厘米的纸垫，外用线如"井"字扎紧。左手捏住纸垫，右手拇、食、中三指，或拇、食、中、无名指持针柄（见"常用持针法"2、3），针尖抵于纸垫，手指渐加压力前后交替来回捻动针柄（图 4—4①），在捻转时应尽量使针体保持垂直，待针穿透纸垫后另换一处。或左手固握纸垫，右手持捏针身（见"常用持针法"1、2），利用腕力快速进针，直到一刺即入（图 4—4②），撒手后不见针倒、歪斜或针弯。如此反复练习，先用短针，继用长针。前者练习捻转进针指力，后者练习速刺进针指力。

2. 手法练习：这是练针的第二步，即用棉花一团，外用白布将棉花包裹，以线封口扎紧做成直径约 6～7 厘米的圆球。练针方法同纸垫练针法，因棉团松软，还可进行捻转、提插等基本手法的练习。

针灸技法述要

(1) 捻转练习：在配合练好指力的基础上，练习捻转的速度。要求由慢到快，幅度由小到大，并保持针体不可前后上下滑动（图4—5①），进而练习头针捻针法，即右手拇指指腹贴于针柄，食指内屈以桡侧与拇指指腹相合挟持针柄，利用食指的快速屈伸活动使针体转动（图4—5②），至每分钟达150～200次以上。

(2) 提插练习：左手持棉团，右手拇、食二指挟持针柄，中指扶持针根或针身，无名指、小指贴在棉团上作支点，拇、食二指上提下插（图4—6），达到针身不偏不斜，不弯，继而取消支

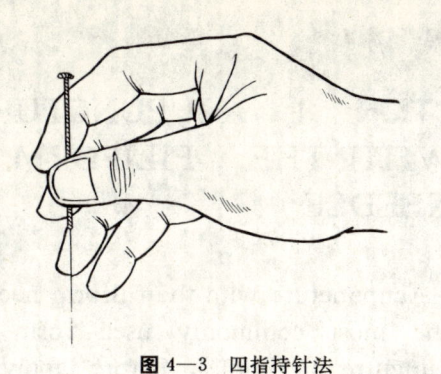

图 4—3 四指持针法
Fig. 4—3 Holding the Needle with Four Fingers

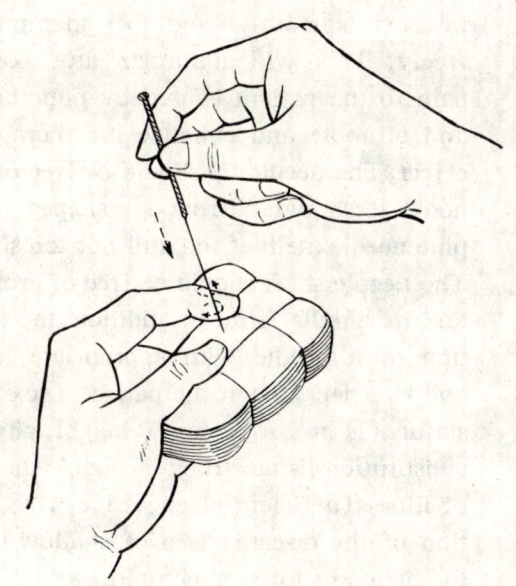

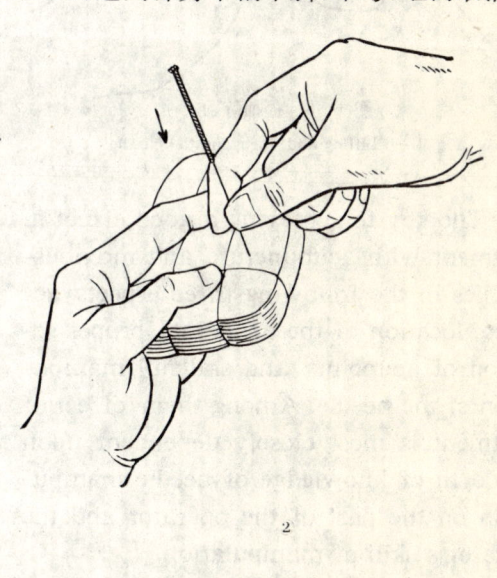

图 4—4 指力练习
Fig. 4—4 Practicing the Finger Force

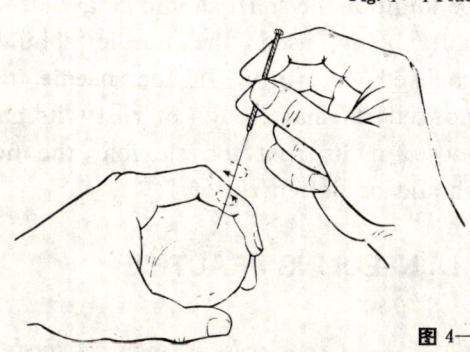

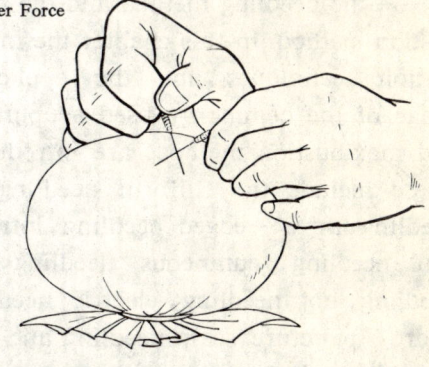

图 4—5 捻转练习
Fig. 4—5 Twirling and Rotating Needle

点，如此反复练习。

通过纸垫、棉团练针有了一定的指力，并掌握了行针的基本手法后，可在自身肌肉丰厚处的四肢穴位上（如足三里、阳陵泉等）消毒试针，以便体会进针的指力与手法掌握的程度，使得操作者在临床针刺时心中有数。

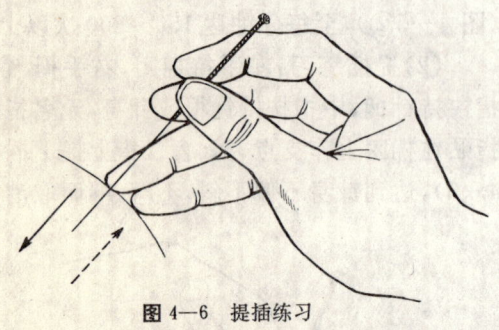

图 4—6 提插练习
Fig. 4—6 Lifting and Thrusting the Needle

The key to achieving a good effect in treatment with acupuncture and moxibustion lies in the following three aspects: accurate location of the acupoints, proper selection of acupoints, and skillfull manipulation of the needle. Among them, effect of treatment is most closely dependent upon the depth of knowledge of needle manipulation on the part of the operator and the operator's skill at manipulation.

The techniques of acupuncture and moxibustion include two big classifications ———the needling method and the moxibustion method. In this chapter the manipulation techniques and the application range of the commonly used acupuncture and moxibustion methods are introduced. These include the filiform needling, ear needling, three—edged needling, intradermal needling, cutaneous needling, dull needling, hot needling, electric needling, hydro—puncture, scalp needling and wrist—ankle needling. The moxibustion method and the cupping method are also introduced.

SECTION 1 ACUPUNCTURE WITH THE FILIFORM NEEDLE

Acupuncture with the filiform needle is the most commonly used form of acupuncture in clinics. Before applying puncture, one should select a needle which is in good condition in order that it can be inserted smoothly and be manipulated freely. This will minimize any possible pain to the patient caused by puncturing, and promote and enhance the therapeutic effect. The needle tip should be free of any hook. It should be round — shaped like a pine needle, neither too dull nor too sharp. The needle shaft should be free of erosion, and its handle firm. In addition, the selection of a needle with appropriate length and size depends on the patient's sex, age, stature (is he fat or thin), height, physical constitution (is he strong or poor), the state of illness (deficient or excessive), the location of the disease (deep of shallow), and the acupoint to be punctured.

The needle apparatus should be preserved carefully. Hooks on the tip and bending of the shaft should be avoided. Before being used, the needle should be checked carefully. If the needle tip is hooked, its shaft rough or rusty, its handle loose, or its root too flexible, the needle should be gotten rid of.

I. NEEDLING PRACTICE

1. *Commonly Used Methods of Holding the Needle*

(1) Holding the Needle with Two Fingers:

The needle handle is held with the thumb and index finger, their bellies pinching the handle (See Fig. 4—1A). Or the needle shaft is held with the thumb and index finger with a sterilized cotton ball wrapped around the shaft, exposing the tip for 3—5mm (See Fig. 4—1B). The former method is suitable for holding a short filiform needle 0.5—1.0 cun long and the latter suitable for holding a needle 2.0—3.0 cun long, to make a swift insertion. Note: The Length of a filiform needle refers to that of the needle shaft, see Section I of Chapter III in detail.

(2) Holding the Needle with Three Fingers

The needle handle is held with the thumb, index and middle fingers, with the thumb opposite to the others (See. Fig. 4—2A). Or the needle is held with the thumb, index and middle fingers, the thumb and middle finger holding the handle and the index finger pressing the tail (See Fig. 4—2B.) These two methods are suitable for insertion of a needle 1—1.5 cun long in a twirling and rotating manner. A needle shaft can also be held with the thumb, index and middle fingers, with the bellies of the thumb, index and middle finger holding the shaft, and the index finger belly closely attached to the dorsum of the middle finger to fix the shaft, exposing the tip for 3—5 mm (See Fig. 4—3C). This method is suitable for swift insertion of a needle 1.5—3 cun long.

(3) Holding the Needle with Four Fingers

The thumb, index and middle fingers hold the handle of the needle, and the ring finger steadies the shaft of the needle (See Fig. 4—3). This method is suitable for insertion of a 2 cun long needle in a twirling and rotating technique.

2. *The Practice of the Finger Force and Manipulations*

As the filiform needle is very slender and flexible, one cannot insert and manipulate it properly without adequate finger force. Under inadequate finger force, the therapeutic effect can not be achieved, and the patient would not willingly accept this therapy. So, it is indispensable that a beginner practices his or her finger force and manipulation well as part of his or her training in basic skills.

(1) Practising the Finger Force

This is the first step in practising needling. Fold a piece of soft paper into a pad about 7—8 cm long, 5 cm wide and 2—3 cm thick. Tie its sides up with thread. Then, hold the paper pad with the left hand and the needle handle with the thumb, index, middle and ring fingers of the right hand. Bring the tip of the needle to the pad, insert the needle into the pad, and rotate its handle back and forth with the force gradually getting stronger (See Fig. 4—4A). The needle must be kept upright as far as possible while rotating. After completely piercing through the paper pad, change to another place on the pad to practise. It is advisable to practise with a short needle in the beginning, and then with longer ones. Another practice is, while holding the paper pad with the left hand and the needle shaft with the right (See "commonly used methods of holding the needle"), quickly insert the needle with the wrist force. Continue the practice of insertion in this way until that the needle is inserted freely, does not fall down or incline, and is not bent after the hand lets go of it (See Fig. 4—4B). It is advisable to start practising with shorter needles, and then with longer ones. The former practice is designed mainly to train the finger force of insertion with the twirling and rotating manner, and the latter to train the finger force of swift insertion.

(2) Practising the Manipulations

This is the second step for practising needling. Make a small cotton ball by wrapping cotton with a piece of white cloth, and tying it with thread, forming a ball 6—7 cm in diameter. When practising needling on the cotton ball, one can train his finger force in the same way as on the paper pad. Moreover, one can practise various basic manipulations, including rotating, lifting and thrusting, etc. (See Fig. 4—5).

a. Twirling and rotating the needle: Based on the practice of twirling and rotating in cooperation with finger force traing, twirling and rotating manipulation can be further trained, especially as to its speed. In practice, first rotate and twirl the needle slowly and within a small range, and then gradually quicken the pace and widen the range, keeping the needle shaft from sliding up and down, or back and forth (See Fig. 4—5A). Based on this, practise the twirling manner on scalp puncture. The needle handle is held with the thumb and index finger of the right hand, with the bellies of the thumb and index finger cooperating in twirling the needle handle, making the needle shaft rotate at over 150—200 turns per minute by quick movements of extension and flexion of the index finger (See Fig. 4—5B).

b. Lifting and thrusting the needle: Hold the cotton ball with the left hand, and hold the needle handle with the thumb and index finger of the right hand and the needle root or shaft with the middle finger. The ring finger and small finger of the right hand touch the cotton ball for support. Then, the needle is thrust and lifted with an up—and—down movement of the thumb and index finger (See Fig. 4—6). Repeat this practice until the needle shaft does not incline or bend while thrusting or lifting the needle and the support point is no longer needed.

After having acquired a certain finger force and mastering the basic manipulation through the practices on the paper pad and the cotton ball, a learner is advised to puncture at acupoints on his own limbs where muscle is abundant, such as Zusanli (ST36) and Yanglingquan (GB34), afer sterilization of the area to be punctured. With this way the learner will realize the level of his or her skill at manipulation and the condition of his or her finger force, so as to have a better idea of how he or she will perform in future clinical practice.

二、体位选择

针前选择好适当的体位,有利于正确取穴施术,病人体位舒适还有利于持久留针,防止晕针。常用的体位有如下几种:

1. 仰卧位:适于取前头、颜面、颈、胸、腹和上、下肢部位腧穴(图4—7)。

2. 俯卧位:适于取后头项、背、腰骶、下肢后侧及上肢部分腧穴(图4—8)。

图4—7 仰卧位
Fig. 4—7 The Supine Posture

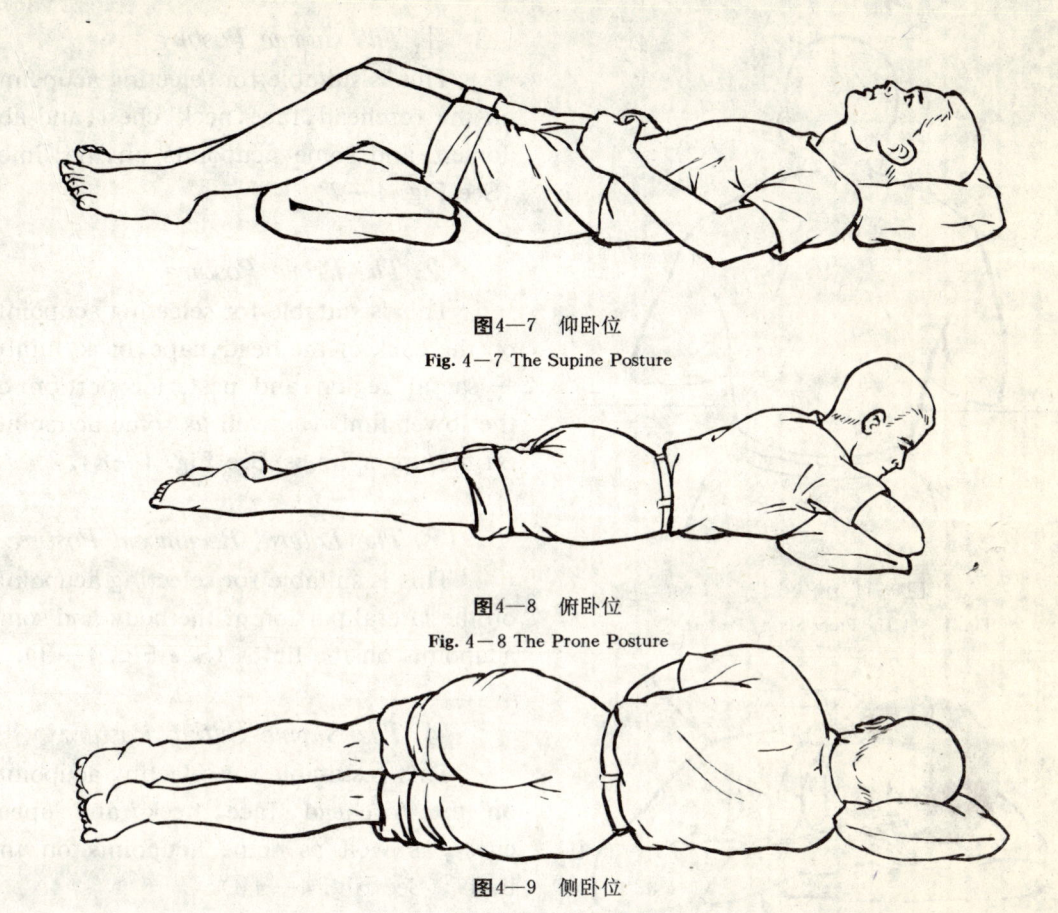

图4—8 俯卧位
Fig. 4—8 The Prone Posture

图4—9 侧卧位
Fig. 4—9 The Lateral Recumbent Posture

3. 侧卧位：适于取身体侧面和上、下肢部分腧穴（图4—9）。

4. 仰靠坐位：适于取前头、颜面、颈、上胸、上下肢部分腧穴（图4—10）。

5. 俯伏坐位：适于取后头、项背及上肢部分腧穴（图4—11）。

6. 侧伏坐位：适于取头侧、面颊、耳部及上肢部分腧穴（图4—12）。

临床上对于初诊、精神紧张或年老、体弱病重患者，应当尽量采取卧位，以防病人感到疲劳不适或晕针。

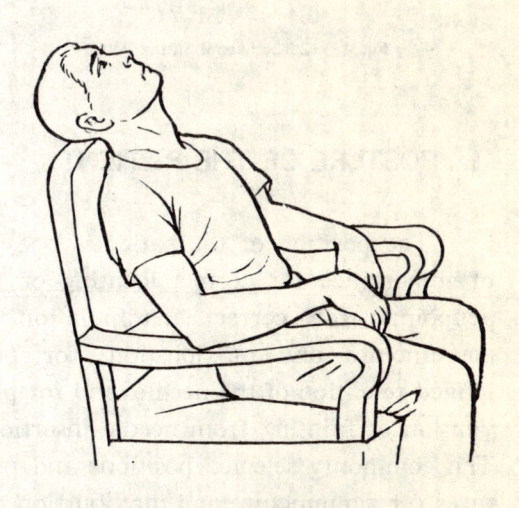

图4—10 仰靠坐位
Fig. 4—10 The Supine Sitting Posture

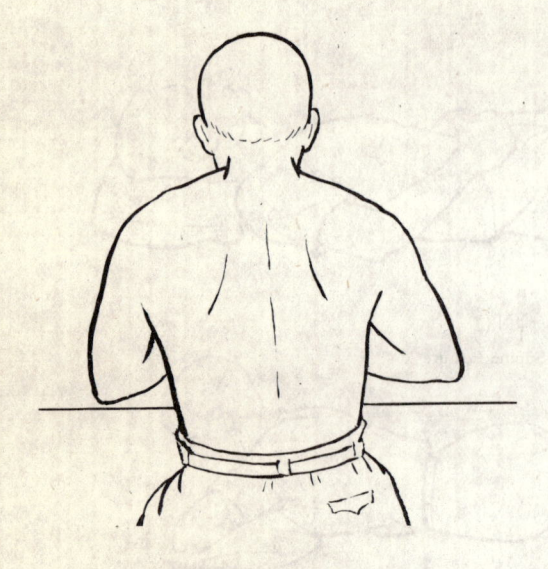

Fig. 4—11 The Prone Sitting Posture

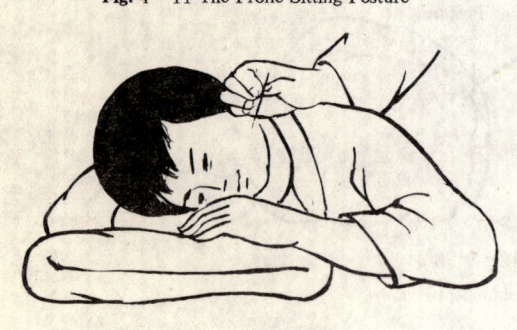

Fig. 4—12 The Lateral Sitting Posture

II. POSTURE OF THE PATIENT

The position of the patient's body is of importance for correct locating of the acupoints, for correct manipulation in acupuncture and moxibustion, for prolonged retention of the needle, and for prevention of fainting from needle insertion. The commonly selected positions and postures for acupuncture and moxibustion are as follows:

1. *The Supine Posture*

This is suitable for selecting acupoints on the forehead, face, neck, chest, and abdomen, and some acupoints on the limbs (See Fig. 4—7).

2. *The Prone Posture*

This is suitable for selecting acupoints on the back of the head, nape, back, lumbo—sacral region and posterior portion of the lower limbs, as well as some acupoints on the upper limbs (See Fig. 4—8).

3. *The Lateral Recumbent Posture*

This is suitable for selecting acupoints on the lateral portion of the body and some acupoints on the limbs (See Fig. 4—9).

4. *The Supine Sitting Posture*

This is suitable for selecting acupoints on the forehead, face, neck, and upper chest, as well as some acupoints on the limbs (See FIg. 4—10).

5. *The Prone Sitting Posture*

This is suitable for selecting acupoints on the back of the head, nape and back, as well as some acupoints on the upper limbs (See Fig. 4—11).

6. *The Lateral Sitting Posture*

This is suitable for selecting acupoints on the lateral aspect of the head, cheek, and auricle, as well as some acupoints on the upper limbs (See Fig. 4—12).

In the clinic, the lying postion should be selected as far as possible for a patient who is on the first visit, or in a state of nervous tension, or who is weak, aged, or seriously ill, in order to prevent the patient from discomfort, fatigue, or fainting from needle insertion.

三、进针法

是将针刺入穴位的方法。要求迅速、准确、无痛或少痛,它是检验针灸医师基本技能的第一关。

在进行针刺操作时,一般双手协同紧密配合。常将持针的右手称为"刺手",压按穴位辅助进针的左手称为"押手"。刺手的作用在于持针操作,进针时运用指力于针尖,以便使针快速刺透皮肤,并施行一定手法;押手的作用主要是固定腧穴位置,或使针身有所依附,帮助刺手顺利进针,减少疼痛。临床施术时,刺手(右手)和押手(左手)常配合使用。进针时一边以左手按压或提捏穴位周围皮下组织,一边以右手持针着力刺透皮肤,并协同施行手法。常用进针法有如下两类:

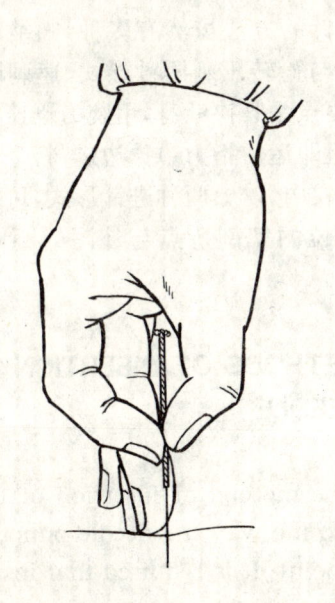

图4—13 单手进针

Fig. 4—13 Inserting the Needle with One Hand

1. 单手进针:即以右手拇、食二指捏持针柄,中指端紧靠穴位指腹抵住针身下端,当食指运用指力向下按压时,中指随之屈曲将针垂直刺入到所需深度(图4—13)。也可先用中指端在应针腧穴上揣摩片刻,待患者有酸、麻或舒适感后,再如前法刺入。本法适于0.5~1寸毫针进针。

2. 双手进针:即以左右两手配合进针。

(1)指切进针法:又称爪切进针法。即以左手拇指或食指的指甲切按在腧穴上,右手持针将针紧靠左手指甲缘刺入皮下(图4—14)。此法适于短针进针。

(2)舒张进针法:即左手拇、食二指将所刺腧穴部位的皮肤向两侧撑开,使皮肤绷紧,右手持针从左手拇、食指间快速刺入(图4—15)。此法适于皮肤松弛部位的进针。

(3)提捏进针法:即左手拇、食指将针刺腧穴部位的皮肤捏起,右手从捏起处的上端将针刺入(图4—16)。此法适于皮肉浅薄部位的进针,如印堂、列缺等。

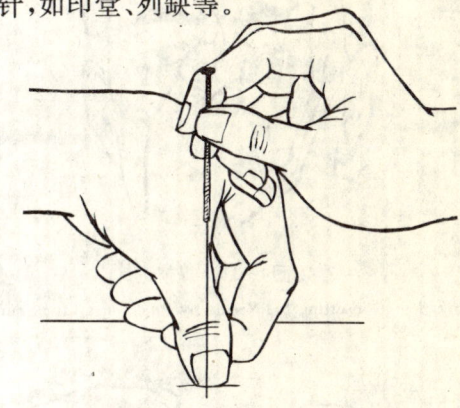

图4—14 指切进针

Fig. 4—14 Inserting the Needle Alded by the Pressure From the Finger of the Pressing Hand

(4)挟持进针法:即左手拇、食二指以酒精擦拭消毒后,捏住针身下端,或以左手将消毒棉球挟住针身下端露出针尖3~5毫米,右手采用执笔式(三指或四指持针法)持针,将针尖对准穴位,双手配合加压,迅速把针刺入皮下直至一定深度(图4—17)。此法适于3寸以上长针及肌肉丰厚处的四肢进针。

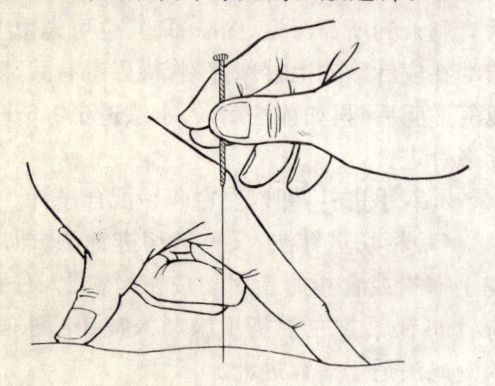

图4—15 舒张进针
Fig. 4—15 Inserting the Needle with Fingers Stretching the Skin

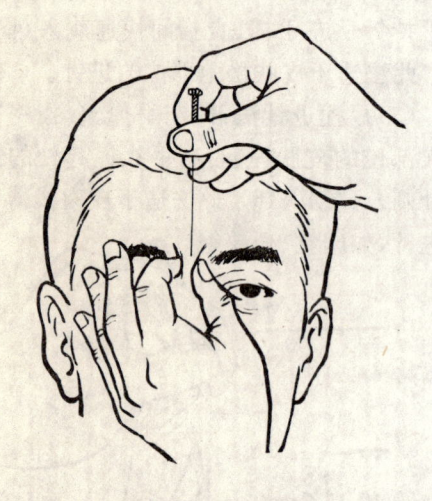

图4—16 提捏进针
Fig. 4—16 Inserting the Needle by Pinching up the Skin

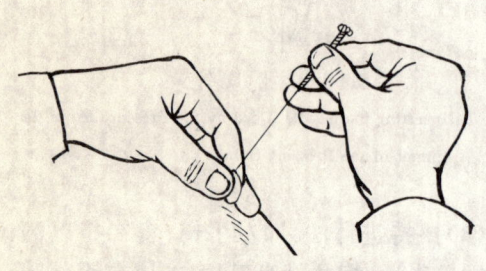

图4—17 挟持进针
Fig. 4—17 Inserting the Needle by Gripping It

(5)套管进针法：用直径2～3毫米(孔径)，或大小适中的，长4～5公分(厘米)消毒后的金属管或玻璃管，代替押手置于应刺的穴位上，选用平柄毫针套于管中，右手食指对准针尾，利用腕力将针弹扣入穴位，然后将套管抽出(图4—18)。此法进针快，易于掌握。

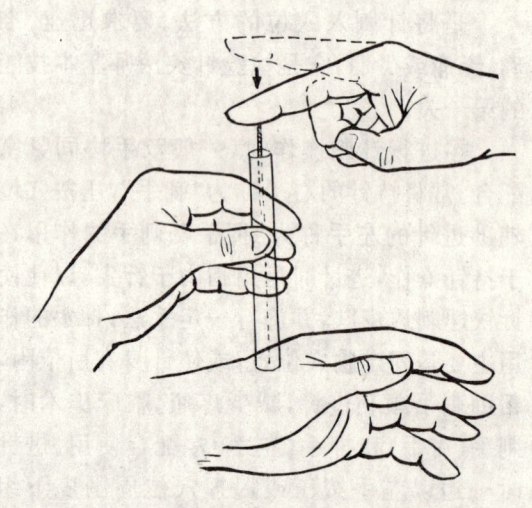

图4—18 套管进针
Fig. 4—18 Inserting the Needle with the Help of the Tube

进针的方法虽然有多种，归纳起来无非为速刺与捻转压刺两种形式。速刺即快速进针，其要点是紧挟针身，用腕力迅速叩针入穴内；捻压即运用指力边捻边进，将毫针如旋刀刺压于穴内。以上两种进针形式，可根据穴位所在部位的解剖特点与补泻的不同合理选用。

Ⅲ. METHODS OF INSERTION OF THE NEEDLE

The method of insertion of th needle refers to the way the needle punctures into an acupoint。It is required that insertion be swift and accurate , causing no or little pain. When examining a doctor of acupuncture and moxibustion, this is the first hurdle he or she must pass.

A doctor generally uses his or her two hands in coordination in the acupuncture operation. The right hand holding the needle is termed as the "puncturing hand", while the left hand which assists in insertion by pressing upon the area close to the acupoint is called the "pressing hand". The puncturing hand plays the role of holding and manipulating the needle, making finger force reach the tip of the needle so as to pierce quickly, and performing designed manipulations. The pressing hand plays the role of fixing the acupoint location, helping the puncturing hand to facilitate the insertion of the needle by surpporting the needle shaft, and minimizing possible pain to the patient during insertion. In clinical operations, the puncturing hand (right hand) and the pressing hand (left hand) usually work in coordination. In insertion, press or pinch up the subcutaneous tissue round the acupoint with the left hand, and at the same time hold and insert the needle through the skin with the right hand. The two hands cooperate in the performance of manipulation. The commonly used methods of insertion of the needle are as follows:

1. *Insertion with One Hand*

The needle handle is held with the thumb and index finger of the right hand, and the lower portion of the shaft is held by the tip of the middle finger of the right hand. The needle is inserted into the acupoint to the designed depth by downward pressure of the index finger and the flexing movement of the middle finger (See Fig. 4—13). This method may be performed after the acupoint to be punctured is massaged by the tip of the middle finger of the right hand for a few seconds and the patient experiences numbness, soreness or a comfortable feeling. This method is suitable for insertion of a filiform needle 0.5—1 cun long.

2. *Insertion with Both Hands*

The needle is inserted with both hands acting in coordination.

(1) Inserting the Needle Aided by the Pressure from the Finger of the Pressing Hand

It is also termed inserting the needle by pressure of the nails. Press the acupoint with the nail of the thumb or the index finger of the left hand, hold the needle with the right hand, and insert it into the acupoint close to the edge of the nail of the left hand (See Fig. 4—14). This is suitable for puncturing with short needles.

(2) Inserting the Needle with Fingers Stretching the Skin

Stretch the skin where the acupoint is located with the thumb and the index finger of the left hand to cause local tension, hold the needle with the right hand, and insert it into the skin quickly between the thumb and the index finger of the left hand (See Fig. 4—15).

This is suitable for inserting the needle into an acupoint around which the skin is loose.

(3) Inserting the Needle by Pinching up the Skin

Pinch up the skin around the acupoint with the thumb and index finger of the left hand, hold the needle with the right hand and insert it into the upper area of the pinched skin (See Fig. 4—16). This is suitable for inserting the needle into an acupoint around which the skin and muscle are thin, such as Yintang (EX 27), Lieque (LU 7), etc.

(4) Inserting the Needle by Gripping It

Grip the lower portion of the needle shaft with the thumb and index finger of the left hand which have been sterilized by swabbing them with the sterilized cotton ball. Or wrap the lower portion of the needle shaft by the sterilized cotton ball with the left hand, exposing the needle tip for 3—5 mm, hold the needle with the right hand like holding a pen (holding the needle with three or four fingers), and fix it directly over the acupoint. Then, quickly insert the needle into the skin to a required depth with the pressure on the needle given by the force from the two hands acting coordinately (See Fig. 4—17). This is suitable for puncturing with a 3—cun—long needle, as well as insering a needle into the acupoints at the extremities where the muscle is abundant.

(5) Inserting the Needle with the Help of the Tube

Select a sterilized metal or glass tube 2—3 mm in diameter or in proper size, and 4—5 cm in length, which plays the role to replace the pressing hand, put it on the selected acupoint, and place a needle having a flat handle into the tube. Then, direct the index finger of the right hand at the needle tail and quickly press the needle tail with the wrist force to insert the needle into the acupoint. Finally, draw the tube away (See Fig. 4—18). This method makes the insertion quick and is easily grasped.

Although there are various methods of insertion of the needle, all of them can be classified into two types, i.e. the swift insertion and the insertion with twirling, rotating and pressing the needle. In the swift insertion, the key point in operation is that the needle shaft is tightly held and the needle is quickly inserted into the acupoint with the wrist force. In the insertion with twirling, rotating and pressing manner, the needle is twisted as it being inserted into the acupoint with the pressure. The two types of insertion mentioned above should be selected according to the anatomic feature of the area where the acupoint is located and the reinforcing or reducing manipulation repuired

四、针刺角度与深度

针刺过程中,掌握正确的针刺角度、方向与深度,是获得针感,提高疗效,防止意外事故发生的重要环节。临床上同一腧穴,如果针刺的方向、角度与深度不同,所达的组织结构、产生的针感、治疗的效果,也会有明显的差异。临床上应根据施针部位、治疗需要以及病人体质等,灵活掌握针刺的角度与深度。

1. 针刺的角度:是指进针时针身与皮肤表面所形成的夹角。一般分成直刺、斜刺、横刺三类(图4—19)。

(1)直刺:针身与皮肤表面呈90°角,垂直刺入。适宜于四肢腹腰等全身大多数腧穴的针刺操作。

(2)斜刺:针身与皮肤表面约呈45°角,倾斜刺入。适宜于头面颈项等肌肉浅薄处,或内有重要脏器不宜直刺、深刺的腧穴。

（3）横刺：又称平刺，沿皮刺。针身与皮肤表面约呈15°角。适宜于皮肉浅薄处及透穴。

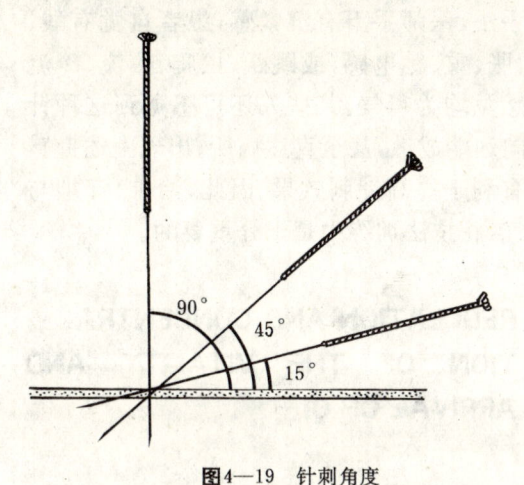

图4—19 针刺角度
Fig. 4—19 The Angle of the Insertion

2. 针刺深度：是指针身刺入腧穴内的深浅度，一般以既有针感而又不伤及脏器为原则。临床操作时要根据施术部位肌肉的厚薄，脏器所在位置，患者体质的强弱、肥瘦、年龄大小，病情轻重等决定针刺的深浅。

Ⅳ. ANGLE AND DEPTH OF INSERTION

In the process of puncture, correct angle and depth of insertion of the needle are very important, which help to induce the needling sensation, to enhance the therapeutic effect and to guarantee safety. Clinically, in needling the same acupoint, the tissure reached, needle senstion produced and therapeutic result achieved vary greatly with the change of the angle and depth of insertion. In clinical practice, the angle and depth of insertion should be designed according to the body area to be punctured, therapeutic purpose, and the patient's constitution.

1. *Angle of Needle Insertion*

It refers to the angle formed by the shaft of the needle inserted and the skin surface punctured. Generally, there are three kinds: the perpendicular puncture, the oblique puncture and the horizontal puncture (See Fig. 4—19).

(1) Perpendicular Puncture

The needle is inserted perpendicularly, forming a 90° angle with the skin surface. It is suitable for most points on the body, such as points at the limbs, abdomen and loin.

(2) Oblique Puncture

The needle is inserted obliquely, forming an angle of approximately 45° with the skin surface. This is suitable for points on the body where the muscle is thinner, such as points at the head, face, neck and nape, or for puncturing at points where the important viscera underly, which are not suitable to be punctured with perpendicular or deep puncture.

(3) Horizontal Puncture

Also called level puncture along the skin, or transverse insertion. The needle is inserted at about 15°angle with the skin surface. This is suitable for points at the parts of the body where the muscle is thinner or for point—through—point puncturre (i. e. penetration needling, a needling method performed by piercing two or more adjoining meridians or points simultaneously in one insertion, usually used for a strong stimulation).

2. Depth of Needle Insertion

It refers to the depth of insertion of the shaft of the needle into the acupoint. Generally, it is taken as the principle that the needle should be inserted to a certain depth where the needling sensation will be induced but the important organs or structures will not be injured. In clinical practice, it depends on the thickness of the soft tissue at the area to be punctured, location of the viscera, the patient's physical constitution (is he strong or weak), type of figure (is he fat or thin), age, and the pathological condition.

五、治神、守神与得气

治神、守神与得气,是针灸治病取得疗效的又一关键。

所谓"神",泛指人体生命活动的表现。即精神意识、思维活动、脏腑气血功能的外在表现等。治神与守神,是对医、患双方精神高度集中的要求。针灸施术前,医师要对病人做好耐心的解释工作,讲明针灸治病的特点,消除患者惧针的紧张心理,并充满治愈信心,使之心神安定、主动配合。针刺施行技法过程中,医师要全神贯注,集中精力于针下,以便细心体会针刺时的手感,患者也要配合体会施术部位的自我感觉,并随时告诉医师,以便调气治疗。中国医学早期文献《素问·针解论》中曾记载:"手如握虎者,欲其壮也;神无营于万物者,静观病人,无左右视也……"。即强调施术过程中医师必须要将全部注意力集中于针上,持针坚实就像抓住老虎一样,不能分心,要静心地观察病人神色及反应,以判断得气与否,切勿左顾右盼。

针刺腧穴的主要目的,在于激发人体的经气的正常运行,致使气血通畅,脏腑功能协调,阴阳平衡,从而能防治疾病。针刺能否发挥作用关键是得气。若针刺入穴位,通过一定的手法,医师手下有沉紧感,患者自觉有酸、麻、胀、重、触电感,或跳跃、虫爬、热流、冷流等感觉均为得气。某些人还可感觉到这种针感向远端放散,甚至直达病所。出现上述针感将有利于提高针刺效果。因此,治神、守神与得气,在技法训练中是十分重要的。

V. REGULATION AND CONCENTRATION OF THE VITALITY AND ARRIVAL OF QI

Regulation and concentration of the vitality (治神, 守神, Zhishen, Shoushen) and arrival of qi (得气 Deqi, inducing of needling sensation) concern greatly with the therapeutic result of treatment with acupuncture and moxibustion.

The vitality (神 Shen) is the general manifestation of the vital activities of the human body, namely, the outward signs of the mental activities and functions of qi, blood and zang—fu organs. Regulating the vitality and concentrating the vitality are required to both of the doctor and the patient. Both of them should concentrate their mental activities during the process of acupuncture and moxiustion. Prior to the operation of acupuncture and moxibustion, a doctor should give the patient a detail explanation ablout the characteristics of treatment with acupuncture and moxibustion in order to make the patient relieve possible psychological tension due to fear of being punctured and have confidence of curing disease, being calm and active to cooperate with the doctor. During the process of acupuncture, the doctor should be deeply absorbed in operation and concentrate his or her energy to understand the feeling around the needle carefully. On the other hand, the patient is asked to realize the self—feelings around the operated area in cooperation and tell them to the doctor at all times, so that the doctor can adjust treatment method. In Essay on Explanation of Acupuncture, one chapter of Plain Questions, it says;"In order to hold the needle firmly, a doctor should hold it like holding a tiger tail, and should pay attention to nothing but the patient , without looking other places, ……"It means that during the operation with acupuncture, a doctor should be engrossed in the needle and , as if he or she held a tiger tail, he or she should hold the needle firmly and concentrate his or her energy, and she or he should observe the patient's expression and reaction in order to judge whether the qi arrives or not.

The main purpose of puncturing at the acupoints is to induce the regular circulation of qi of the meridian, making qi and blood circulate freely without meeting any obstruction, functions of zang—fu organs be coordinated in each other, and yin and yang be in equilibrium, through which diseases can be prevented and treated. The factor which decides whether the acupuncture can exert its function or not is arrival of qi. If the needling sensation is present after the insertion of the needle into the acupoint and through some manipulations of the needle , the operator feels tenseness and heaviness around the needle; meanwhile the patient feels soreness, numbness, heaviness, distension, electrifying sensation, sensation of that something springs or an insect crawls, or cold flow or hot flow around the acupoint. These feelings, in some patients, may spread to some area of the body far from the punctured area or even to the diseased area. Inducing of these feelings, i. e. arrival of qi, will help in enhancing the effect of treatment with acupuncture. For these reasons, regulation and concentration of the vitality and arrival of qi are very important in manipulation.

六、行针法

进针后施以一定的手法,称为"行针"。行针的目的是促使针下得气,综合《医学入门》、《金针赋》、《针灸大成》、《针灸问对》、《神应经》等中国传统医学文献中所述的行针方法,并参考近、现代针灸名家的手法,可归纳为基本手法、辅助手法、补泻手法、其他手法等四类。

(一)基本手法

1. 提插法:针刺进腧穴一定深度后,使针在穴内进行上下、进退的操作方法。针由浅(上)层向下刺入深层为插;由深层(下)向上退到浅层为提(图4—20)。如此反复上提下插,称之"提插法",提插幅度大小、频率快慢,操作时间长短,可根据病人的体质、病情、腧穴的部位,医师要达到的治疗目的而定。若提插幅度大、频率慢、着力重,又称"捣动法",适宜于体质壮,针感差、病程短的病人;提插幅度小、频率快、着力轻,又称为"震颤法",适宜于体质差、针感弱的病人催气用。

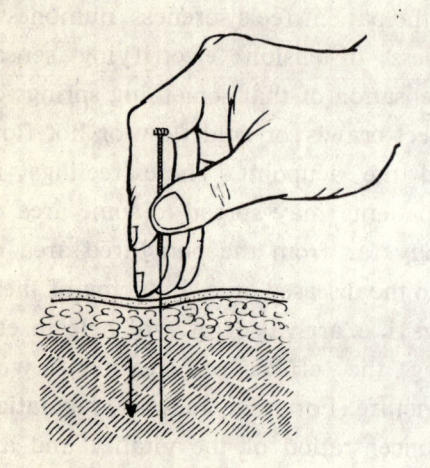

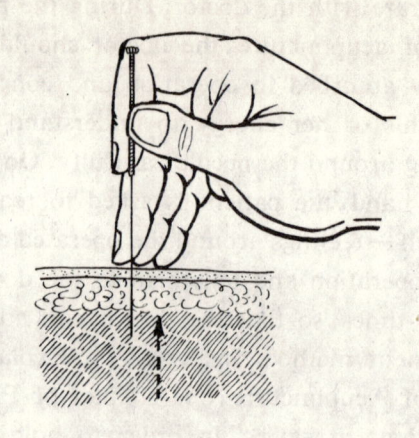

图4—20 提插法
Fig. 4—20 Thrusting and Lifting

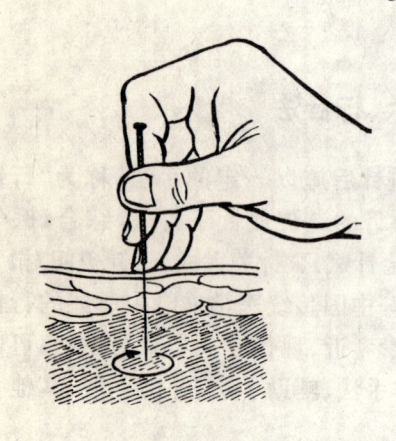

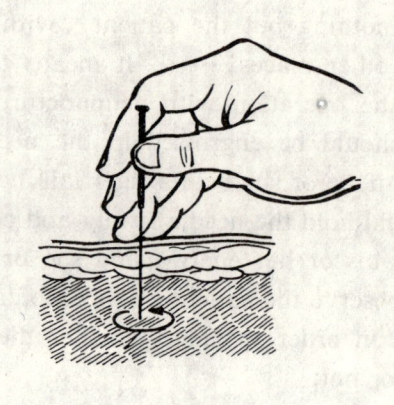

图4—21 捻转法
Fig. 4—21 Twirling and Rotating

2.捻转法：针刺入腧穴一定深度后，将针柄向前后左右来回旋转捻动的操作方法（图4—21）。

捻转角度的大小、频率的快慢、操作时间的长短，也应根据病人的体质、病情、医师要达到的治疗目的而定。

（二）辅助手法

1.循法：针刺入腧穴一定深度后，用手指的指腹顺着所在腧穴的经脉循行经络，或穴位上下、左右轻柔地循按（图4—22①）、或扣打（图4—22②），此法有助于激发经气的运行，探察经络的虚实，使气血和顺，有偏于补益的作用。

2.摄法：针刺入腧穴一定深度后，用大指指甲，或大指、食指、中指三指指甲，顺着所在腧穴经脉的循行经路上下来往切按或掐按（图4—23）。此法可使气血流行，邪气疏泻，但手法较重，偏于泻法范畴。

· 216 ·

开如飞鸟展翅之状一捻一放（图 4—26），亦可拇、食二指在针柄搓捻，一搓一放，一合一张（图 4—26），连续搓捻数次如飞鸟展翅之状，此法有行气、催气的作用，促使针感加强与传导。

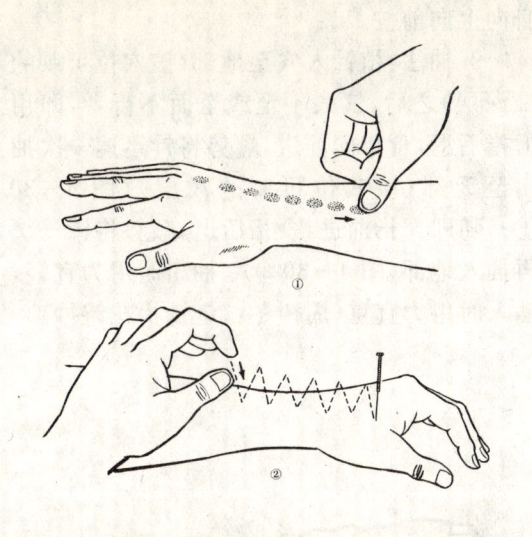

图 4—22 循法
Fig. 4—22 Massaging along the Meridian

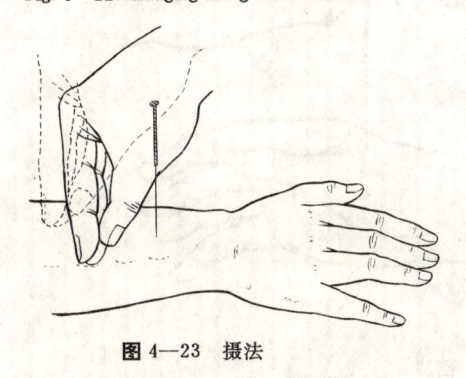

图 4—23 摄法
Fig. 4—23 Pinching along the Meridian

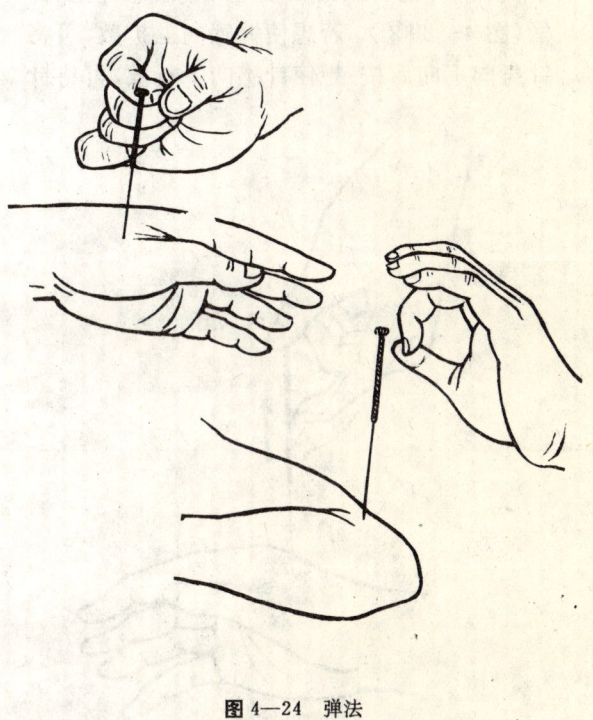

图 4—24 弹法
Fig. 4—24 Flicking Method

3. 弹法：针刺入腧穴一定深度后，用食指或中指轻弹针尾，使针体微微震动而使经气运行的一种方法（图 4—24）。

4. 刮法：针刺入腧穴一定深度后，用拇指指腹抵住针尾，以食指或中指的指甲，由下至上频频轻刮针柄，或以食指指腹抵住针尾，拇指指甲由下至上频频轻刮针柄（图 4—25）。

5. 飞法：针刺入腧穴一定深度后，拇指与食、中指相对捏持针柄，将针作较大幅度捻转，捻时中指内屈使针顺（左）转，放时食、中指外伸搓动针柄使针逆（右）转，手指顺势放

6. 盘法：针刺入腧穴一定深度后，手持针尾以 36°的盘转为特征（图 4—27①），亦可在行针得气后，将针提至浅部搬倒，使针身倾斜于 15～40°盘旋针体，盘旋的角度可在 180°～360°之间（图 4—27②）。且可配合补泻，常以左盘插针为补，右盘插针为泻。该法宜于在腹部腧穴施术。

7. 摇法：针刺入腧穴一定深度后，手持针柄左右摇动。若针身直立而摇（图 4—28①），可加强针感；若针身朝一定方向斜刺卧倒左右摇摆（图 4—28②），可促使针感向一定方向传导。

8. 按法：按法与弩法相似，即针刺入腧穴一定深度得气后，以手将针捻紧不进不退，中指抵住并按压针身，使针身弯曲如弩弓之状（图4—29①）。有守气、催气、保持及加强针感的作用。亦有将针柄用手指按紧，拇指在下，食、中、无名三指如切寸口脉那样按切针柄（图4—29②）。若想使针感向上扩散，可将针身向下向后按；想使针感向下行散，可将针身向上向前按。

9. 抽法：植针入穴至地部（该穴位可刺的最深层）之后，气久不至或至而不行者，即用拇指后退，食指向前进，顺势将针迅速一次抽出至天部（该穴位可刺的浅层）（图4—30①），随即拇指前进，食指后退，顺势将针一次再插入地部（图4—30②）。抽出时用力宜轻，插入时用力宜重（周树冬：《金针梅花诗抄》）

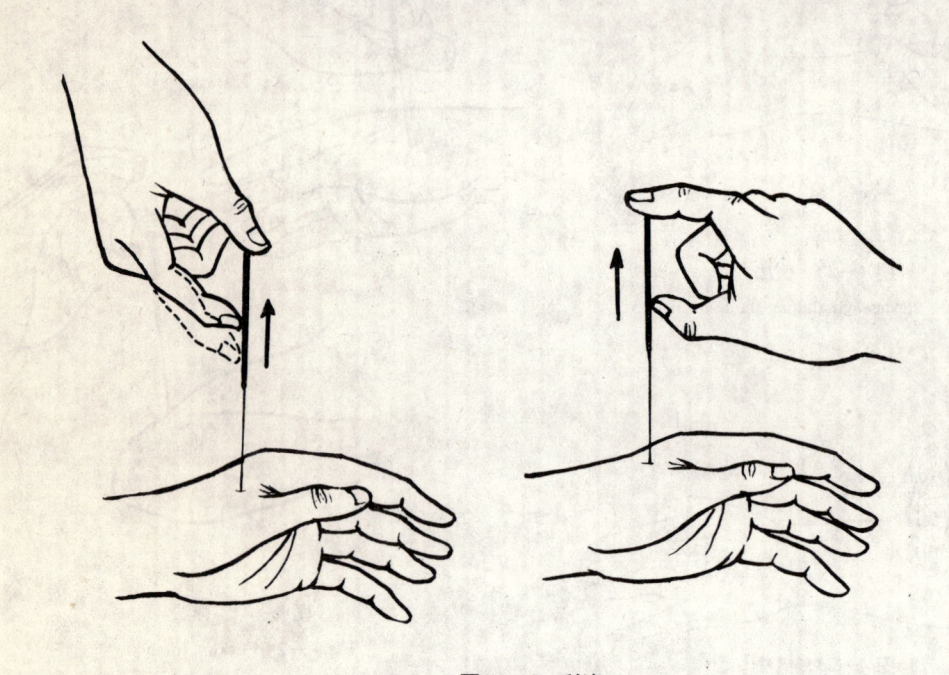

图 4—25 刮法
Fig. 4—25 Scraping Method

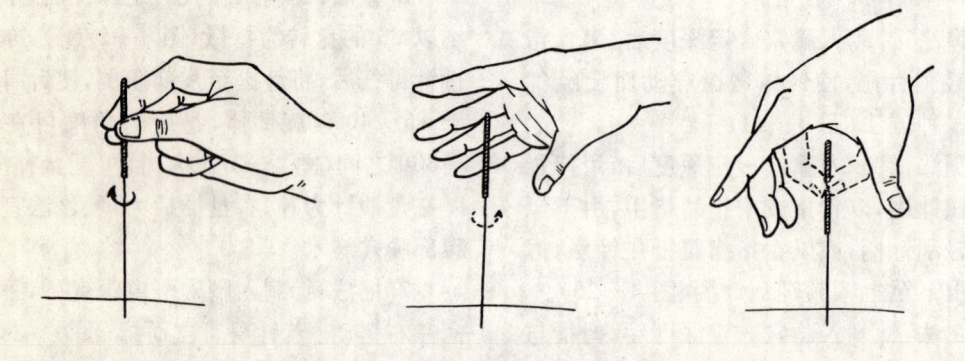

图 4—26 飞法
Fig. 4—26 Flying Method

图 4—27 盘法
Fig. 4—27 Circling Method

次,直至针感反应到远处为止。推捻针柄时,必须徐缓,匀整有力。(刘冠军:《中医针法集锦》·任作田氏论刺法)。

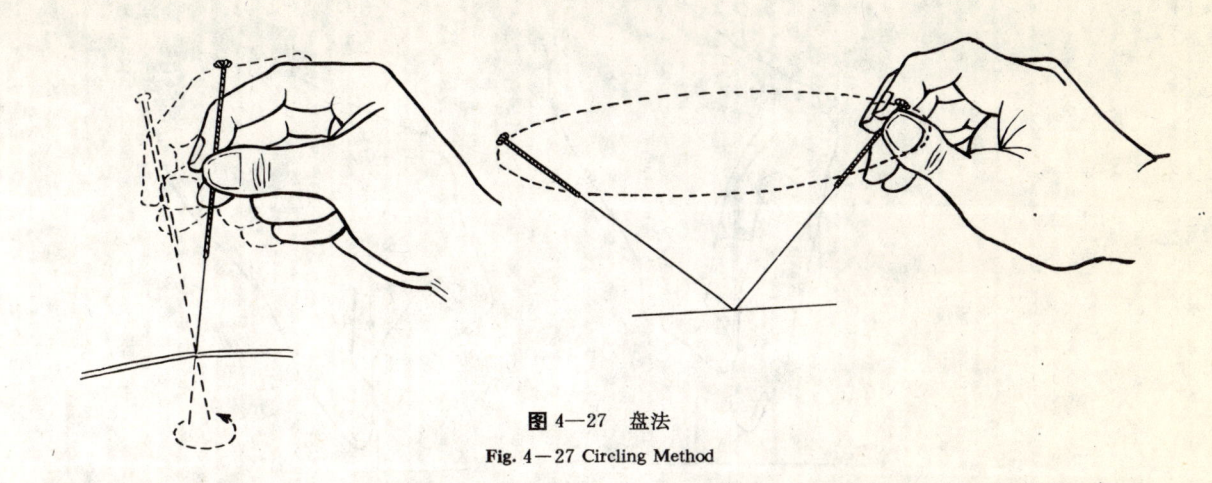

图 4—28 摇法
Fig. 4—28 Shaking Method

10. 敲法:行针得气后,停针之时为防止针下之气中辍,及催气前进时,可垂直频频敲其针尾,使针逐步深入(图 4—31),待达到一定深度后,再将针外提寸许重新敲击,如此反复数次。(周树冬:《金针梅花诗抄》)

11. 推法:气行不远时,用拇、食指将针由得气位轻轻提起,针尖面向意欲行气的方向,拇指向前均匀而有力地捻推针柄,拇指达到指腹后横纹时即轻轻退回(图 4—32),然后再用力向前推第二次,如此连推数次或 10 数

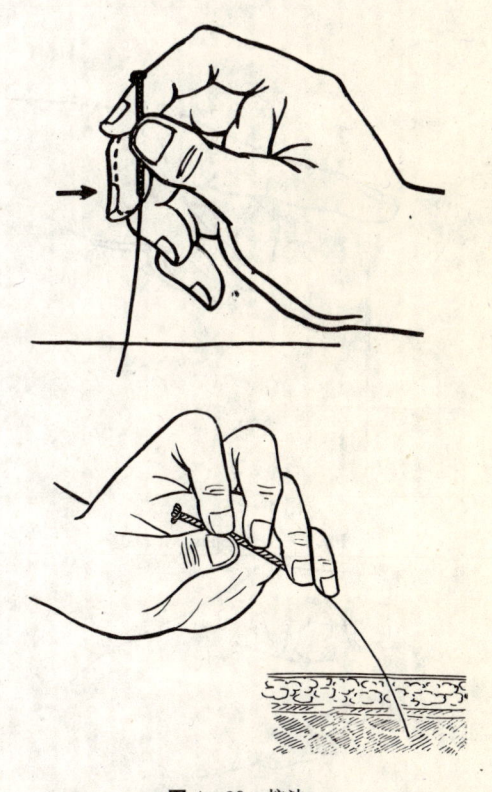

图 4—29 按法
Fig. 4—29 Pressing Method

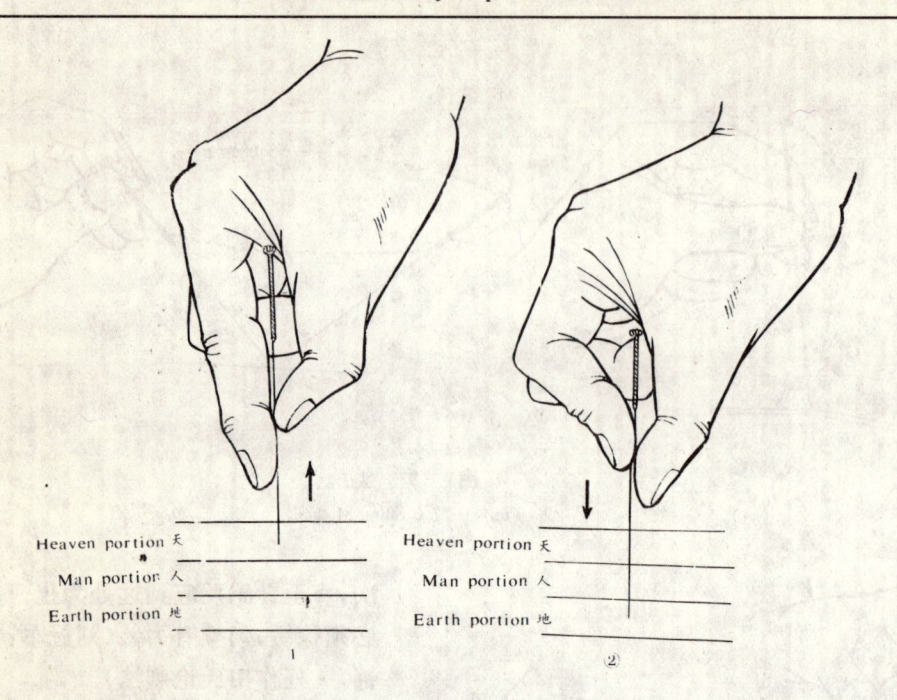

图 4—30 抽法
Fig. 4—30 Withdrawing Method

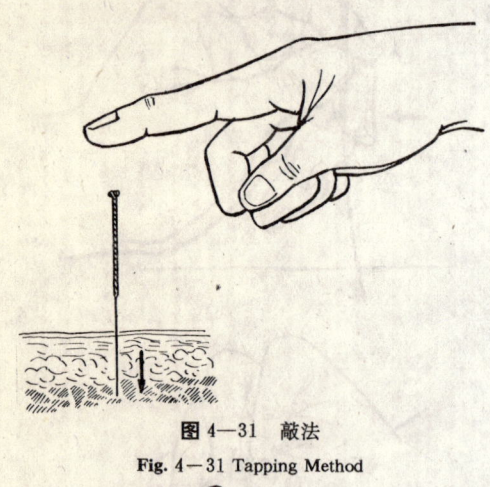

图 4—31 敲法
Fig. 4—31 Tapping Method

图 4—32 推法
Fig. 4—32 Pushing Method

(三) 补泻手法

通过行针使之得气后,就要根据病人本身的功能状况及疾病的表里、阴阳、寒热虚实状况施行补泻手法,以遵循"虚则补之"、"实则泻之"的治疗原则,提高临床疗效。

1. 常用补泻手法:

(1) 捻转补泻:针下得气后,拇指向前,食指退后左转为补;拇指退后,食指向前右转为泻(图 4—33)。此法是捻转与迎随互为结合的手法。有从经脉循行之逆顺以为施术的依据,即手三阳、足三阴及任脉右转为补;手三阴、足三阳及督脉左转为补;反之则为泻。

近些年来,某些针灸医师结合刺激量的大小,提出捻转角度小、用力轻、频率慢、操作时间短为"补";反之,捻转角度大、用力重、频率快、操作时间长为泻。如方基庆氏采取捻转角度小、刺激感应弱、捻转不超过180°,频率在60~80次/分左右为补法;捻转角度大、刺激感应强、捻转角度在360°左右,频率在100次/左右则为泻法(刘冠军:《中医针法集锦》)。

(2)提插补泻:针下得气后,先浅部后深部,重插轻提,提插幅度小、频率慢为补;先深部后浅部,轻插重提,提插幅度大,频率快为泻(图4—34)。

近年来,还有人提出,提插深浅度2~3分,频率60~80次/分左右,刺激感应弱为补

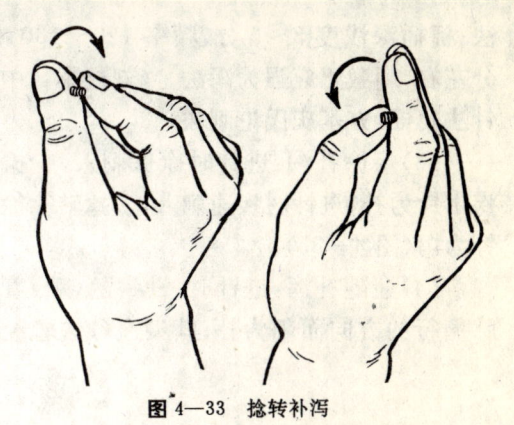

图4—33 捻转补泻
Fig. 4—33 Reinforcing and Reducing by Twirling and Rotating the Needle

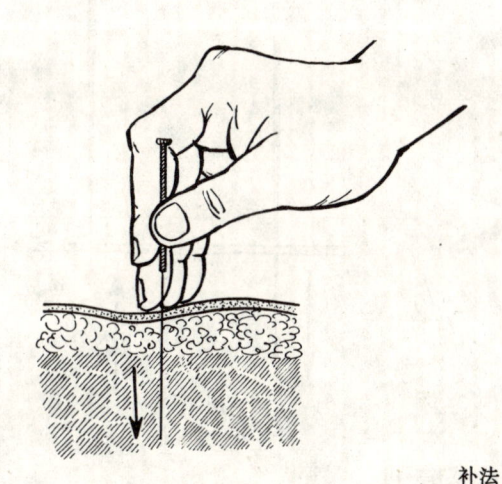

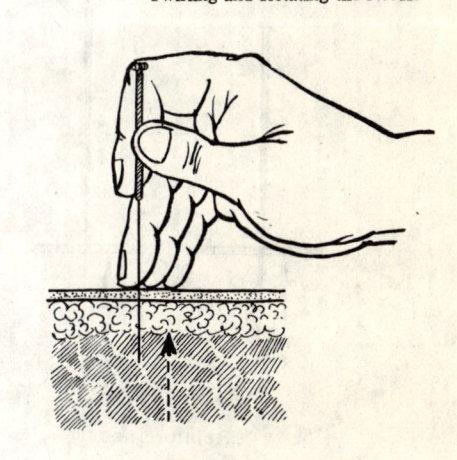

补法
Reinforcing

泻法
Reducing

图4—34 提插补泻
Fig. 4—34 Reinforcing and Reducing by Lifting and Thrusting the Needle

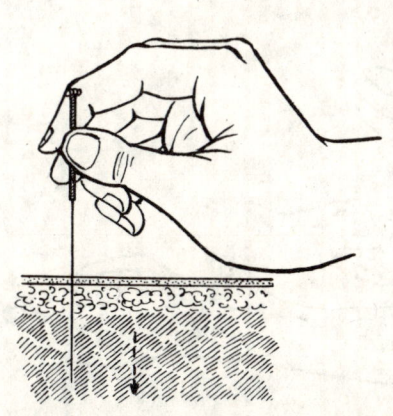

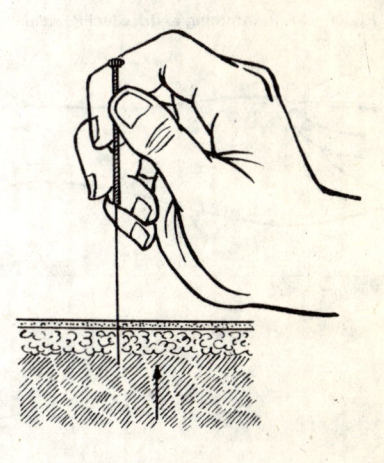

法；提插深浅度 3～5 分，频率 120～160 次/分左右，刺激感应强为泻法。（刘冠军：《中医针法集锦》方基庆氏论刺法）。

(3)疾徐补泻：进针时徐徐刺入，少捻转疾出针为补；进针时疾速刺入，多捻转徐徐出针为泻（图 4—35）。

(4)迎随补泻：进针时，针尖随（顺）着经脉循行的方向而刺为补；针尖迎（逆）着经脉循行的方向而刺为泻（图 4—36）。

(5)呼吸补泻：病人呼气时进针，吸气时出针为补；吸气时进针，呼气时出针为泻（图 4—37）。

(6)开阖补泻：出针时迅速揉按针孔为补；出针时摇大针孔而不揉按为泻（图 4—38）。

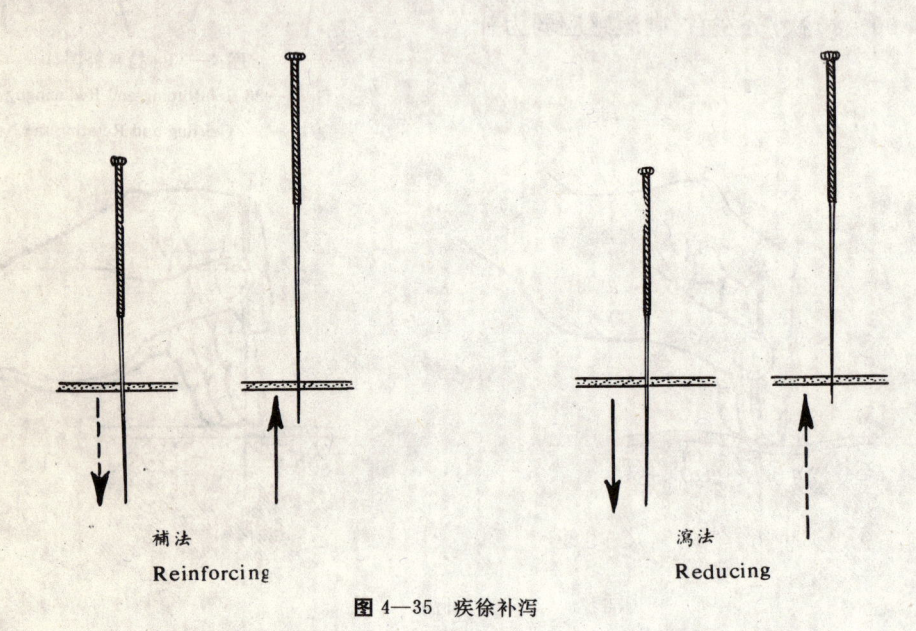

图 4—35 疾徐补泻

FIg. 4—35 Reinforcing and Reducing Achieved by Rapid and Slow Insertion and Withdrawal of the Needle

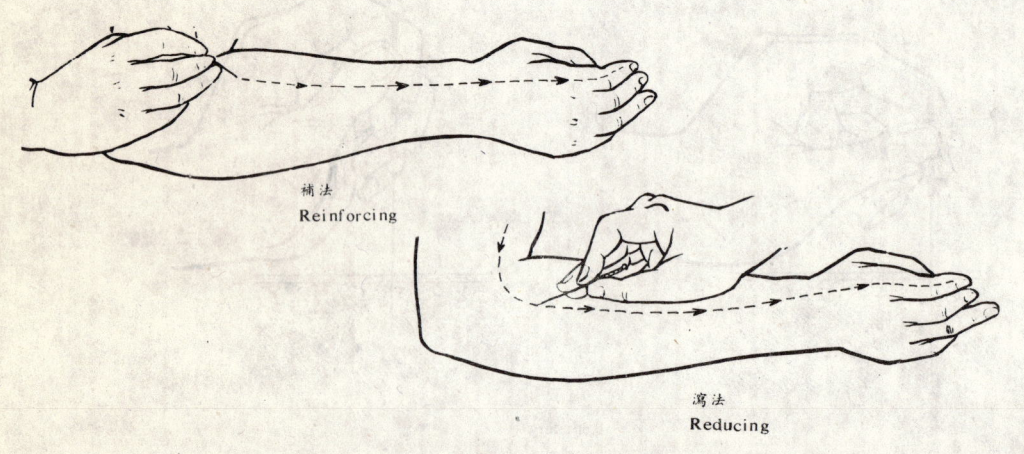

图 4—36 迎随补泻

Fig. 4—36 Reinforcing and Reducing Achieved by Puncturing along and against the Running Direction of the Meridian

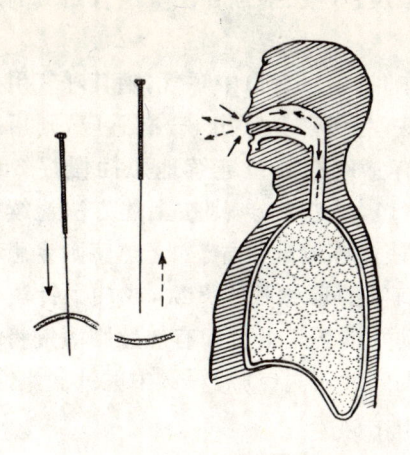

补法
Reinforcing

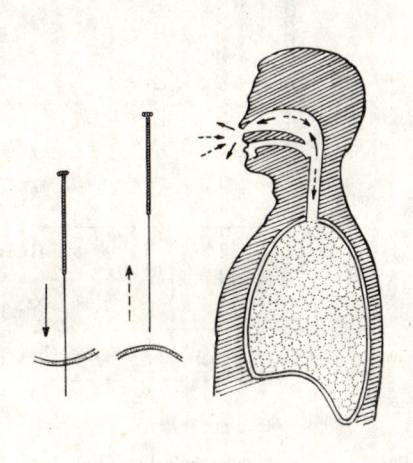

泻法
Reducing

图 4—37 呼吸补泻

Fig. 4—37 Reinforcing and Reducing Achieved by Manipulating the Needle in Cooperation with the Patient's Respiration

(7)平补平泻：针刺得气后，均匀地左右捻转提插为平补平泻。

近些年来有人提出，捻转 180°～360°，频率 100 次/分左右为平补平泻。（刘冠军：《中医外法集锦》.方基庆论刺法）临床中提插与捻转常合并使用。

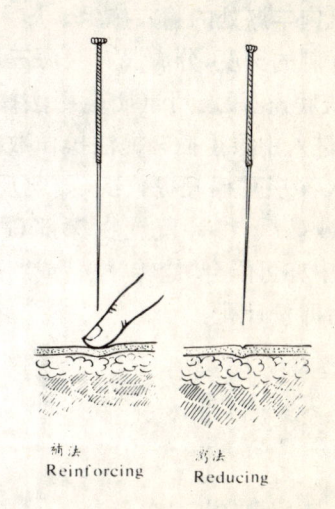

补法   泻法
Reinforcing   Reducing

图 4—38 开阖补泻

Fig. 4—38 Reinforcing and Reducing Achieved by Keeping the Needle Hole Open or Close

2. 常用复式补泻手法：复式补泻手法，是几种补泻手法相互配合运用的行针手法，常用的有如下几种：

(1)烧山火与透天凉：

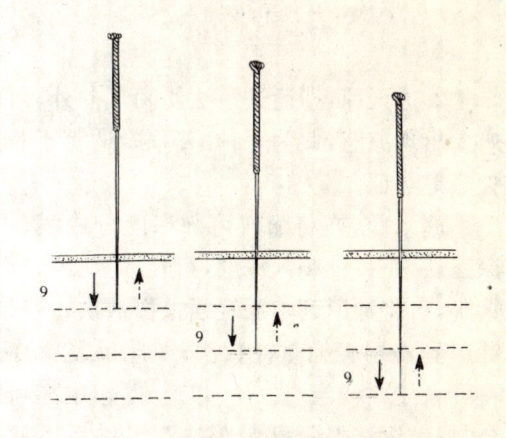

图 4—39 烧山火

Fig. 4—39 Heat—producing Needling

1)烧山火：即通过手法使阳气入内，病人在局部或全身出现温热感，此为一种温补法。

· 223 ·

适宜于肢体顽固麻痹、冷痹等虚寒证。这种手法宜于在肌肉丰厚处的腧穴施术。施术前先确定腧穴针刺的深度，分成浅、中、深三层，当针刺入皮肤后，在浅层用重插轻提法操作数次，再将针进入中层重插轻提法操作数次，最后将针进入深层重插轻提数次，如此反复操作至针下热感后，将针留置在深部（图4—39）。操作中亦可配合"捻转补法"或"呼吸补法"，出针后即按针孔。

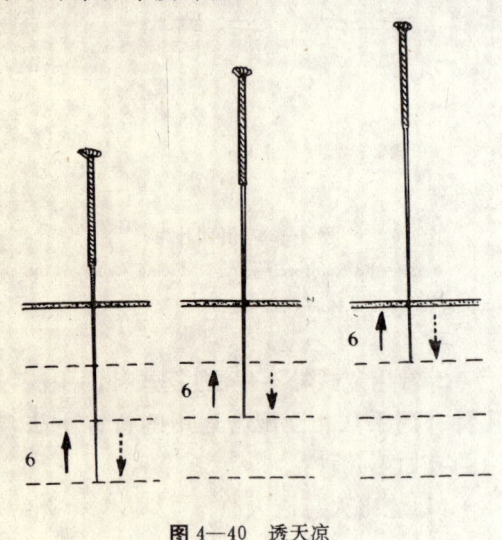

图4—40 透天凉

Fig. 4—40 Cool—producing Needling

2）透天凉：即通过手法使阴气向外，可使病人出现凉感，此为一种凉泻法，适宜于肌热骨蒸等热证。

施术前，亦将腧穴可刺深度分成浅、中、深三层，先将针刺入深层，用轻插重提法操作数次，再将针退到中层轻插重提数次，最后将针退到浅层轻插重提数次，如此反复操作后将针留置在浅层（图4—40）。操作中亦可配合"捻转泻法"或"呼吸泻法"，出针后不揉按针孔。

（2）进火与进水：

1）进火补法：是在烧山火手法基础上简化发展而成的一种热补法。首见于《针灸大成》，由徐疾、呼吸、提插补法等组合而成的复式手法。

操作时，令患者口中呼气，随其呼气用指切速刺法，将针刺入1分，一有感应，则用针尖向着有感应的部位连续地急插慢提3次（图4—41），每进1分，则按上述方法连续操作3次，使热感放散传导。如无热感则令患者做鼻吸口呼的自然呼吸3次，或加刮针法使针尖颤动并催其气至。如有热感则缓慢将针拔去急扪闭针穴。（刘冠军：《中医针法集锦》·郑魁山论刺法）。

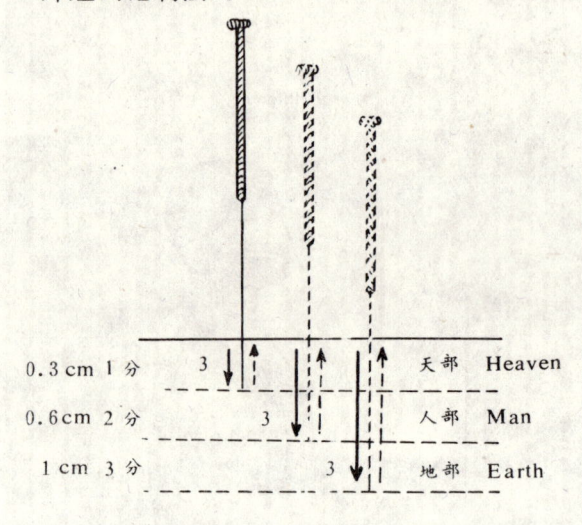

图4—41 进火补法

Fig. 4—41 Reinforcing Method by Fire(Yang)—Producing Needling

2）进水泻法：是在透天凉手法基础上简化发展而成的。亦首见于《针灸大成》，由徐疾、呼吸、提插泻法等组合而成的复式手法。

操作时，令患者口中吸气，随其吸气，用舒张押手法缓慢的不捻转地将针进至地部，待有感应，将针提退1分，在1分上下的范围内连续慢插急提3次（图4—42），每提退1分则按上述方法连续操作3次，使凉感放散传导，如无凉感，则令患者做鼻呼口吸的自然呼吸3次，或加摇法而催其气至，如有麻凉或

触电感觉则将针急速拔出,不扪闭针穴。(刘冠军:《中医针法集锦》·郑魁山论刺法)

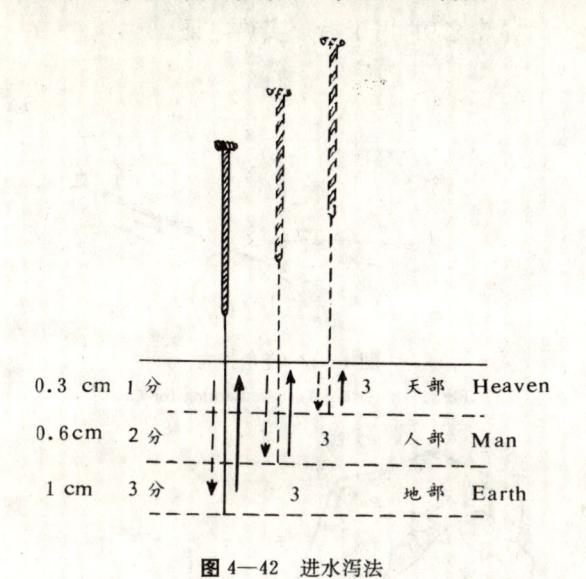

图 4—42 进水泻法
Fig. 4—42 Reducing Method by Water(Yin)-Producing Needling

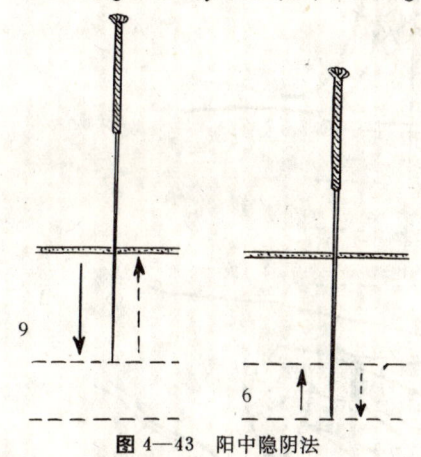

图 4—43 阳中隐阴法
Fig. 4—43 Yin Occluding in Yang

处,即将针插入深层后轻插重提6次,继将针退入浅层再重插轻提9次,如此反复数次后出针(图4—44)。

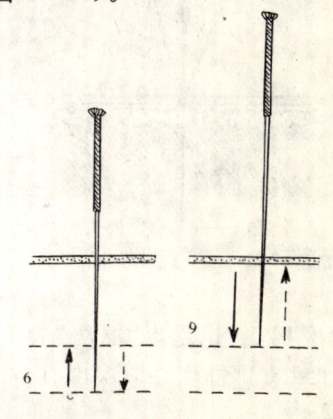

图 4—44 阴中隐阳法
Fig. 4—44 Yang Occluding in Yin

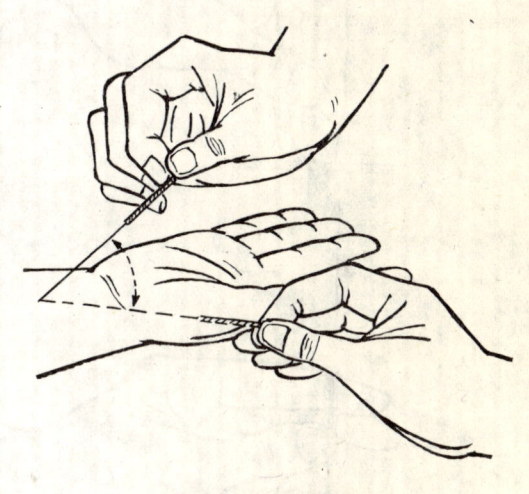

图 4—45 青龙摆尾
Fig. 4—45 Green Dragon Shaking Tail

(3)阳中隐阴与阴中隐阳:

1)阳中隐阴法:为先补后泻法。用于先寒后热或虚中夹实证。该法与烧山火有相似之处,即将针刺深度分两层,先将针纳入浅层后重插轻提9次,继将针进入深层再重提轻插6次,如此反复数次出针(图4—43)。

2)阴中隐阳法:为先泻后补法。用于先热后寒或实中有虚证。该法与透天凉有相似之

(四)其他手法

1.青龙摆尾:又名"苍龙摆尾",是以"摇"法为主的一种针法。即进针得气后向病所斜刺,不进不退持之不转,一左一右如船夫扶船舵一样将针柄缓缓摆动(图4—45)。本法宜于控制和加强针感传导,属飞经走气四法之一。能接通经气,调达气血,治疗各种痛症。

· 225 ·

动并结合上提动作(图 4—46)。本法宜加强针感,属飞经走气四法之一。有疏导经气,清泻邪热之功,用于治疗实热之证。

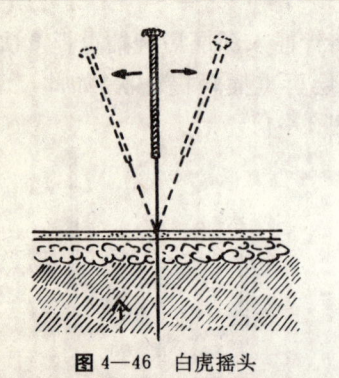

图 4—46 白虎摇头
Fig. 4—46 White Tiger Shaking Head

2. 白虎摇头:也是以"摇法"为主的另一种针法。即垂直进针到一定深度,将针左右摆

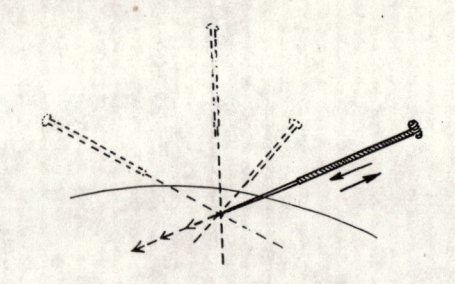

图 4—47 苍龟探穴
Fig. 4—47 Green Tortoise Seeking for Cave

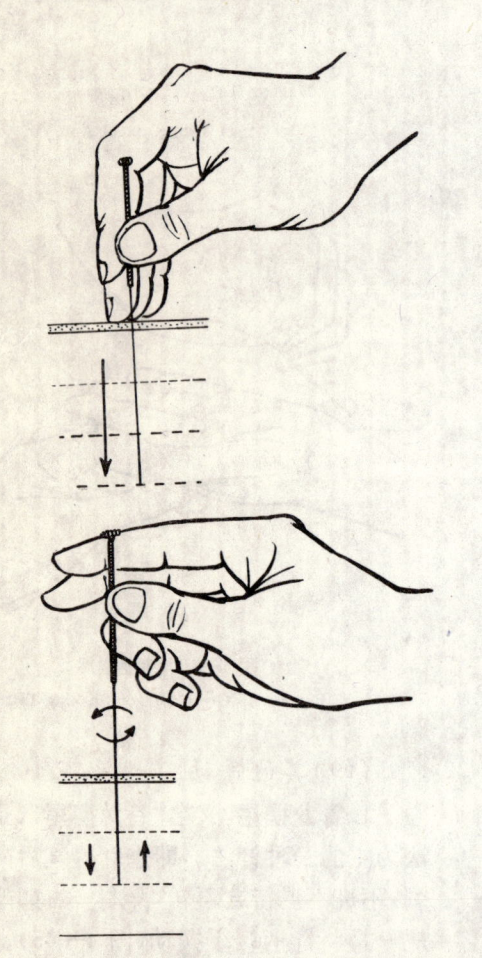

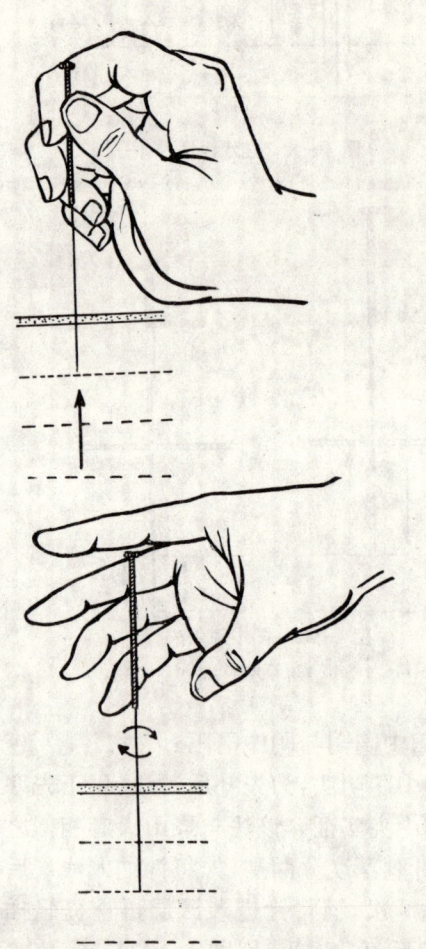

图 4—48 赤凤迎源
Fig. 4—48 Red Phenix Meeting Resource

针灸技法述要

5. 子午捣臼：是以"捻转"、"提插"相结合的一种针法。"子午"指左右捻转，"捣臼"指上下提插，即进针得气后先紧按慢提9次，再紧提慢按6次，同时结合左右捻转，反复施行（图4—49）。本法宜于补泻兼施，消肿利水。

6. 龙虎交战：是以"捻转"为主的一种针法。"龙"指左转，"虎"指右转，"交战"指左右交替。即进针后以左转为主，大指向前用力捻转9次，再以右转为主，大指向后用力捻转6次，如此反复施行（图4—50）。本法宜于镇痛。

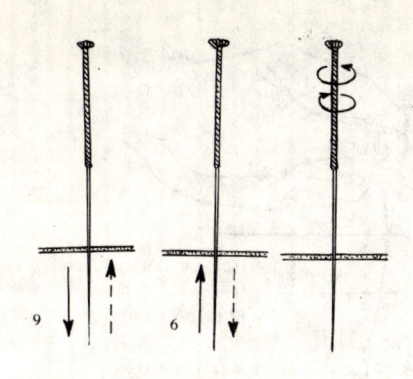

图4—49 子午捣臼
Fig. 4—49 Zi Wu Dao Jiu Needling

3. 苍龟探穴：是以"提插"为主的一种针法，针刺入穴位得气后退至浅层，然后向上下左右四方透刺，由浅入深一退三进，如龟入土探穴四方钻剔（图4—47）。本法宜通行多方经气，使针感扩散，属飞经走气四法之一。治疗各种痛症与痹症。

4. 赤凤迎源：是以"捻转"、"提插"、"飞"法相结合的一种针法。先将针刺入深层（地部），后上提至浅层（天部），待针得气自摇再插入中层（人部），如此上下左右提插、捻转、一捻一放，有如凤凰展翅飞旋（图4—48）。本法宜于通行络脉，属飞经走气四法之一。多用于治疗肌肉、关节的酸重、游走、疼痛。

7. 龙虎升降：是一种行气的手法。先进针到天部（浅层），左盘一转，紧按至人部（中层）慢提至天部（浅层），右盘一转再紧按至人部（中层）慢提至天部（浅层）。如此反复9次（图4—51①），然后插针入于地部（深层），右盘一转紧提慢按，左盘一转亦紧提慢按，如此6次（图4—51②）。（陆瘦燕等《刺灸法汇论》）。亦可先进针天部（浅层），持针向左捻转一圈，指力偏重于拇指顺势按针至人部（中层），复将针向右捻转一圈，指力偏重于食指，复乘势将针慢提至天部（浅层），随用中指扶住针腰，复按至人部（中层）如此施行9次是为龙降。然后插针至地部（深层）左转捻针1圈，右转捻针1圈，乘势紧提至人部（中层）慢按至

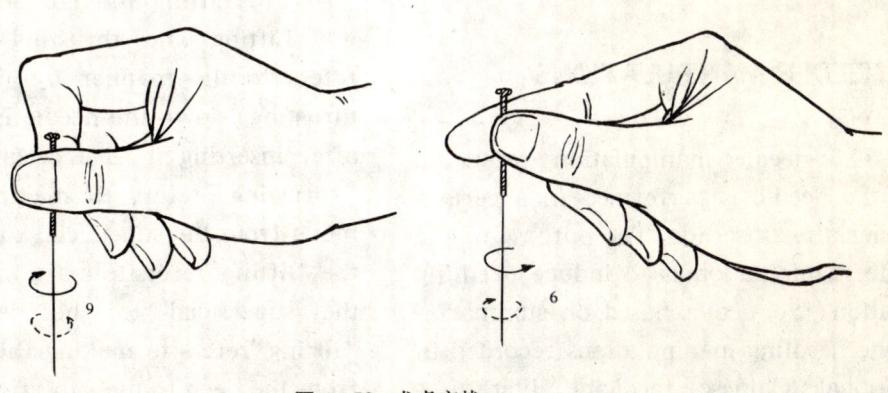

图4—50 龙虎交战
Fig. 4—50 Dragon—Tiger Fighting

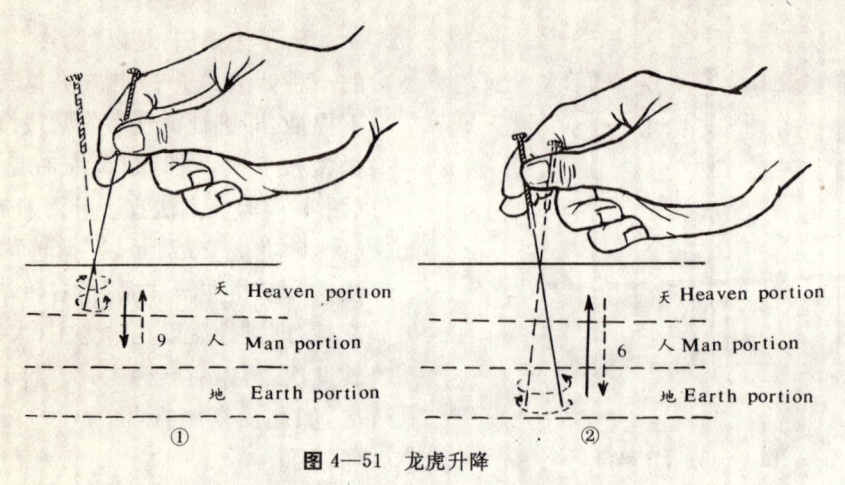

Fig. 4−51 Dragon−Tiger Ascending−Descending Method

地部（深层），如此反复6次，是为虎升。（陆寺康等《针刺手法一百种》）。

8. 进气法：是以"提插"、"呼吸"相结合的一种针法。即进针后刺入腧穴深层施行补法，如紧按慢提9次，然后将针斜向病所卧针深刺，嘱其吸气5或7次。本法宜于行气止痛。

9. 留气法：是以"提插"为主的一种针法。即进针后刺入中层（7分深），施行补法，如紧按慢提9次，然后将针直插至深层，再提回至原处。本法宜于行气消积。

10. 抽添法：是以"提插"为主的一种针法。即进针后先使得气，再向四周作多向提插，然后向下直刺按纳。本法宜于通经活络，治疗瘫痪、疮癞。

VI. NEEDLE MANIPULATIONS

The needle manipulation refers to that the needle is performed in a certain manner after insertion. The purpose of the needle manipulation is to induce needling sensation (i. e. deqi). Based on summarizing the needling manipulations recorded in traditional Chinese medicine literatures such as Elementary Coures for Medicine, The Rhymes for Golden Needle, Compendium of Acupuncture and Moxibustion, The Questions and Answers on Acupuncture and Moxibustion, and The Classic of Miraculous Cure, and on referring to the manipulations of some famous acupuncture — moxibustion doctors in modern times, the needle manipulations may be classified into four types: the basic manipulation, the reinforcing — reducing manipulation, the auxillary manipulation and the other manipulation.

1. *Basic Manipulations*

(1) Lifting and Thrusting

Lifting and thrusting manipulation refers to the manner by lifting up and thrustingg down the needle in the acupoint after inserting it to a certain depth. The "thrusting" refers to making the needle move from the superficial to the deep; and the "lifting" refers to make the needle from the superficial to the deep; and the "lifting" refers to making the needle move from the deep to the superficial (See Fig. 4 − 20). Repeating thrusting and lifting movements is taken as lifting — thrusting manipulation. The amplitude, frequency and duration of this movement depend on the patient's physical constitution, pathological condition, location of the acupoint, and therapeutic purpose. Generally, lifting and thrusting the needle with a great amplitude, slow frequency and strong force, also termed "pounding method", is suitable for the patient with strong physical constitution, poor needling sensation and short course of the disease; while that with less amplitude, quicker frequency and milder force, also termed "vibrating method", for the patient with weak physical constitution, and lower needling sensation, which functions to promote qi.

(2) Twirling and Rotating

Twirling and rotating manipulation refers to the manner by rotating the needle handle clockwise and anti — clockwise alternately after the needle is inserted to a certain depth (See Fig. 4—21). The amplitude, duration and frequency of twirling movement should depend on the patient's physical constitution, pathological condition and therapeutic purpose.

2. *Auxillary Manipulations*

(1) Massaging along the Meridian

After inserting the needle into the acupoint to a certain depth, gently press or tap the skin along the course of the meridian where the acupoint is located at or around the acupoint with the finger — bellies moving upward and downward, or left and right (See Fig. 4—22 A and B). This method may be conductive to induce the circulation of the channel qi, to understand the meridian condition (is it deficient or excessive), and to make qi and blood regular and circulated. It exerts reinforcing effect (i.e., an effect of reinforcing and nourishing the deficiency of Qi, blood, Yin and Yang) in domination.

(2) Pinching along the Meridian

After inserting a needle into an acupoint to a certain depth, pinch and press the body tissue with the nails of the thumb, index and middle fingers upwards and downwards along the meridian where the acupoint is located at (See Fig. 4—23). This method may promote the circulation of qi and blood and expulsion of the pathogenic factor, which is with a comparatively heavy manipulation and with reducing effect (i.e., an effect of purging and dispelling pathogenic factors) in domination.

(3) Flicking Method

After inserting a needle into an acupoint to a certain depth, gently flick the needle tail with the thumb or index finger, causing mild vibration of the needle so as to quicken the circulation of channel qi (See Fig. 4—24).

(4) Scraping Method

After inserting a needle into an acupoint to a certain depth, resist the needle tail with the thumb-belly, and scrape the needle handle from the lower to the upper with the nail of the index finger or middle finger, or resist the needle tail with the belly of the index finger and scrape the needle handle from the lower to the upper with the nail of the thumb frequently and gently (See Fig. 4—25).

(5) Flying Method

After inserting a needle into an acupoint to a certain depth, hold the needle handle with the index finger, middle finger and thumb, which is opposite to the formers, of the left hand, and rotate the needle in a great amplitude. Twirl the needle clockwise by the movement of the introflexion of the index and middle fingers on it, and release the needle with moving it anti—clockwise by the movement of abduction of the index and middle fingers on it. The alternate movements of twirling and releasing of the fingers make the fingers be like the spreading wings of a flying bird (See Fig. 4—26A). So the "flying" is termed for this method. Or twist and release the needle handle with the thumb and middle finger, the fingers with twirling and releasing movements are like the spreading wings of a flying bird (See Fig. 4—26B). This method has the function to promote circulation of qi and induce qi so as to make the needling sensation stronger and spread.

(6) Shaking Method

After inserting a needle into an acupoint to a certain depth, hold the needle tail with the hand and shake it left and right. If the needle shaft at a perpendicular posture is shaked, the needle sensation may be enhanced (See Fig. 4—27A); if with horizontal or oblique posture, the needling sensation may spread toward a certain direction (See Fig. 4—27B).

(7) Circling Method

After inserting a needle into an acupoint to a certain depth, hold the needle tail with the hand to move it in a circle (See Fig. 4—28A). Or after arrival of qi, lift the needle to the superficial portion of the acupoint to make the needle shaft inclined, then move it in a circle or a half circle at the angle of 15—40° formed by the needle shaft with the skin surface (See Fig. 4—28). This method may be in cooperation with some other reinforcing and reducing methods. As a rule, circling the needle clockwise with thrusting it is taken as reinforcing, while anti—clockise circling with lifting as reducing. This method is suitable for acupoints on the abdomen.

(8) Pressing Method

After arrival of qi by inserting a needle into an acupoint to a certain depth, hold the needle with the hand tightly without inserting or withdrawing, and steady and press the needle shaft with the middle finger, making the needle shaft bent like a bow (See Fig. 4—29A). This method has the function of keeping qi, inducing qi, retaining and enhancing the needling sensation. Another manner of this method in operation may be seen in clinic. That is, hold and press a needle handle tightly with the fingers, the thumb being below, and the index, middle and ring finngers feeling and pressing the needle handle like feeling the cunkou pulse (i. e. the locaton at both wrists, medial to the head of the radius, where the pulse diagnosis is performed in TCM, See Fig. 4—29B). If the needling sensation is required to spread upward, press the needle shaft downward and backward. Otherwise, press the needle shaft upward and forward to make the needling sensation propagated downward.

(9) Withdrawing Method

If qi does mot arrive or qi arrives but does not circulate further, but a comparatively long time having passed after inserting a needle into an acupoint to the "earth portion" of the acupoint (i. e. the deep portion of the acupoint), withdraw the needle quickly to the "heaven portion" of the acupoint (i. e. the shallow portion of the acupoint) with the thumb moving backward and the index finger moving forward (See Fig. 4—30A). Then, insert the needle to the earth portion again with the thumb moving forward and the index finger backward (See Fig. 4—30B). When withdrawing, the milder force should be given, and when inserting, the heavy force be given.

(10) Tapping Method

After arrival of qi by manipulating a needle, tap the needle tail vertically, and frequently, making the needle move gradually deeper until it reaches a certain depth (See Fig. 4—21). Then, withdraw the needle up for about 1 cun and tap the needle tail again. Repeat this course for several times. This manipulation can serve to prevent qi around the needle from being interrupted or to promote qi to flow forward.

(11) Pushing Method

When a needling sensation does not spread far enough, gently lift the needle from where the needling sensation is induced with the thumb and index finger, direct the needle tip towards the area the operator wants the needling sensation to spread to, evenly and forcefully twist and push the needle handle forward with the thumb and index finger until the distal transverse crease of the thumb touches the needle. Then gently withdraw the needle to the original place (See Fig. 4—32). Repeat this coures for several times or even several tens until the needling sensation reaches the designed far area. Note: during the operation, the needle handle should be twisted and pushed slowly and evenly and forcefully.

3. *Reinforcing and Reducing Manipulations*

After appearance of needling sensation through manipulating the needle, some reinforcing or reducing manipulations should be carried out according to the patient's physical constitution and pathological condition (does it belong to exterior or interior, yin or yang, coldness or heat, and deficiency or excess), which is known by differentiation of syndrome[①], so as to accord with the therapeutic principle that "the deficiency syndrome (referring to the morbid condition showing deficiency of genuine qi, lowered body resistance, and declining of function, such as yin—deficiency and yang—deficiency) should be treated with reinforcing and the excess syndrome[②] should be treated by reducing",

---

[①] Syndrome refers to symptom complex, a term to summarize collectively certain symptoms and signs according to the theories of TCM. For example, concurrent presence of chills, fever, headache, thin coating of the tongue, and superficial pulse constitutes the exterior syndrome.

[②] Excess syndrome is characterized by presence of excessive pathogenic factors which lead to intense body reaction, or by the presence of the pathologic products due to dysfunction of the internal organs, such as stagnant qi and blood, excessive fluid, retained phlegm and undigested food.

and to enhance the therapeutic effect. What we seek to reinforce by needling manipulation is the constructive qi of the body. That is the inborn resistance, the defensive mechanisms, and the adaptive capability of the body. And what we seek to reduce by needling manipulation is the evil qi, that includes such pathogenic factors as the six excessive atmospheric interferences, stagnancy of indigested food in gastrointestinal tract, blood stagnation, retention of phlegm, etc. Therefore, reinforcing manipulation is to reinforce bodily resistance, and reducing manipulation is to dispel the pathogenic factors. Moreover, the meaning of reinforcement and reduce is the same as above in the other branches of TCM.

(1) The Basic Reinforcing and Reducing Methods

a. Reinforcing and reducing by twirling and rotating the needle: Afftter presence of the needling sensation, if the needle is twisted clockwise, this manipulation is taken as reinforcing; on the contrary, the needle twisted anti—clockwise, it is taken as reducing (See Fig. 4—33). In fact, reinforcing or reducing by twirling and rotating the needle is a comprehensive method in which twirling and rotating manipulaions and puncturing along or against the running direction of the meridain are in combination.

It is said that reducing or reinforcing effect in this method depends on whether the needle tip twisting along or against the channel course, namely, reinforcing method is distinguished by right rotation (clockwise rotation) of the needle in puncturing at the acupoints of the three Yang meridians of hand, three yin meridians of foot and the Conception Vessel (the Ren Meridian) and by left rotation (anti—clockwise rotation) of the needle in puncturing at the three yin meridlans of hand, three yang meridians of foot and the Governor Vessel (the Du Meridian), vice versa.

In recent years, some doctors suggest that twirling the needle with a small extent, at lower frequency, with milder force, and for a short time be taken as reinforcing, on the contrary, twirling it with a greater extent and force, in higher frequency and for a comparatively long time as reducing. Dr. Fang Jiging, a famous acupuncturist, for example, thinks that twirling the needle in a small extent, with a mild stimulation, at an angle of less than 180°, and with a frequency of 60—80 turns per minute is taken as reinforcing; on the contrary, rotating the needle in a great amplitude and a strong stimulation, at an angle about 360° and a frequency of about 100 turns per minute as reducing.

b. Reinforcing and reducing by lifting and thrusting the needle: After arrival of qi, the reinforcing effect is obtained by thrusting and lifting the needle at the shallow portion first and then at the deep portion, thrusting the needle heavily and lifting it gently, thrusting and lifting in a small amplitude and lower frequency. On the contrary, a reducing effect is obtained by thrusting the needle gently and lifting it heavily, in a great amplitude and qucik frequency, and thrusting and lifting the needle first at the deep portion and then at the shallow portion (See Fig. 4—34).

In recent years it is said that a manner by lifting and thrusting the needle in 0.2—0.3 cun extent, at 60—80 turns per minute, and with mild stimulation is taken as reinforcingg, while the manner by lifting and thrusting the needle in 0.3—0.5 cun extent, at 120—160 turns per minute, and with strong stimulation as reducing.

c. Reinforcing and reducing achieved by rapid and slow insertion and withdrawal of the needle: Reinforcing is achieved by inserting the needle slowly, with less rotaion of the needle, and withdrawing the needle swiftly; while reducing achieved by inserting the needle rapidly, with frequent rotation, and withdrawing it slowly (See Fig. 4—35).

d. Reinforcing and reducing achieved by puncturing along and against the direction of the meridian: when inserting a needle, the tip of the needle pointing to the running direction of the course of the meridian is taken as reinforcing; while puncturing with the needle tip against the running direction of the meridian as reducing method (See Fig. 4—36). when needling the three yang meridians which run from the hand upward to the head, for example, a manner with the needle tip pointing downward, i.e against the meridian courses, is known as the reducing method, and a manner with the needle tip pointing to the opposite direction, i.e. following the running course of the meridians, is known as the reinforcing method.

e. Reinforcing and reducing achieved by manipulating the needle in cooperation with the patient's respiration: Reinforcing effect is achieved by inserting the needle during the patient's expiration and withdrawing it during the patient's inspiration; on the contrary, reducing effect is achieved by inserting the needle during the patient's inspiration and withdrawing it during the patient's expiration (See Fig. 4—37)

f. Reinforcing and reducing achieved by keeping the needle hole open or close: For reinforcing, the punctured hole is kneaded immediately the needle is withdrawn; on the contrary, for reducing the punctured hole is enlarged by shaking the needle as it is being withdrawn (See Fig. 4—38)

g. Uniform reinforcing and reducing: It is a method by twirling, lifting and thrusting the needle evenly after arrival of qi. In recent years, it is pointed out that manipulation by twirling and rotating the needle in 180—360° angle and about 100 turns per minute is taken as the uniform reinforcing and reducing. Generally, lifting and thrusting method and twirling and rotaing method are usually combined to achieve the uniform reinforcing and reducing effect.

(2) The commonly Used Comprehensive Reinforcing and Reducing Methods

The comprehensive reinforcing — reducing manipulation refers to that two or more reinforcing and reducing manipulations are used in coordination. The commonly used ones are as follows:

a. Heat—producing needling and cool—producing needling:

Heat—producing needling is a warm reinforcing methed to make yang—qi enter into the body, and to induce the warmer sensation at the local area or at the whole body to the patient. This method is suitable for treatment of cold disorders of deficiency type[①], such as intractable numbness, coldness and pain of the limbs. It is usually employed to the acupoints locating at the area with rich and thick muscle. For its operation, first determine the designed puncture depth, then divide it into the shallow, middle and deep portion. After inserting a needle into the skin, thrust it forcefully and lift it gently for several times at the shallow portion. Then, insert the needle deep to the middle portion, thrust it forcefully and lift it gently at this layer for several times. Finally, insert the needle to the deep portion and thrust it forcefully and lift it gently at this layer for several times. Repeat this course until the patient complains of hot sensation at the punctured area. Then, retain the needle at the deep portion until the needle is withdrawn (See Fig. 4—39). During the operation, the reinforcing manner by twirling and rotating needle or by manipulating the needle in cooperation with the patient's respiration can be applied in coordination. In this operation the puncture hole should be pressed as soon as the needle is withdrawn.

Cool—producing needling is a reducing and cooling method which makes yin—qi go outward and induces cool sensation to the patient. This method is applied to heat syndromes[②]. For its operation, following dividing the depth of the acupoint to be punctured into the shallow, middle and deep portions, insert the needle to the deep portion, gently thrust and forcefully lift it for several times at this layer. Then, withdraw the needle upward to the middle portion, gently thrust and forcefully lift it at this portion for several times. Finally, withdraw the needle upwards to the shallow portion, gently thrust and forcefully lift it at this portion for several time. After thos course for some times, retain the needle at the shallow portion before withdrawal of it (See Fig. 4—40). During the operation, the reducing method by twirling the needle or by manipulating the needle in cooperation with the patient's respiration may be combined. The puncture hole should not be pressed after withdrawing the needle.

b. Fire (yang) — producing needling and water (yin) —producing needling:

Reinforcing method by fire (yang) — producing needling is a comprehensive warm — reinforcing manipulation formed from simplifying and developing the heat —producing needling, first recorded in the

---

[①] A cold syndrome or disorder of deficiency type refers to a morbid condition resulting from insufficiency of genuine qi with endogenous cold, marked by pale complexion, loss of appetite, chillness and aversion to cold, abdominal distension and pain; or in women thin leukorrhagia, lumbago, loose stools, pale tongue with whitish coating, deep, slow and weak pulse.

[②] Heat syndrome refers a morbid condition due to attack of pathogenic heat or hyperactivity of yang—qi, usually seen in infectious disease and those caused by abnormal hyperactivity of the body, with manifestations such as fever, fidgets, flushed face, congested eyes, dry mouth and throat, red and dry lips, thirst with preference for cold drink, constipation, scanty dark urine, reddened tongue with dry brownish or black coating, and rapid pulse.

Compendium of Acupuncture and Moxibustion. In this needling manipulation the reinforcing method by rapid—slow insertion and withdrawal of the needle, the reinforcing method by manipulating the needle in cooperation with patient's respiration and the reinforcing method by lifting and thrusting the needle are combined. To the operation, ask the patient to breathe out with the mouth and, during his or her expiration, quickly insert the needle 0.1 cun deep, aided by the pressure of the fingers of the pressing hand. When the needling sensation being induced, continuously and rapidly thrust and slowly lift the needle with the needle tip towards the area at which the needling sensation is felt by the patient for 3 times (See Fig. 4—41). Insert the needle deep 0.1 cun by 0.1 cun until the needle tip reaches the designed depth, and repeat this course for three times after every insertion for 0.1 cun, making the hot sensation spread. If there is no hot sensation induced to the patient, ask the patient to breathe in with the nose and breathe out with the mouth naturally for 3 times, or scrape the needle handle to make the needle tip tremble, so as to promote arrival of qi. When the hot sensation being induced to the patient, slowly pull out the needle and immediately press the puncture hole.

Reducing method by water (yin) — producing needling is a comprehensive needling method formed from simplifying and developing the cool — producing needling, first recorded in Compendium of Acupuncture and Moxibustion. In this method, the reducing method by rapid and slow insertion and withdrawal of the needle, the reducing method by manipulating the needle in cooperation of the patient's respiration, and the reducing method by lifting and thrusting the needle are combined. To the operation, ask the patient to breathe in with the mouth and, when the patient does so, slowly insert the needle into the acupoint to the earth portion (deep portion) with the fingers stretching the skin, without twirling or rotating the needle. After presence of the needling sensation, withdraw the needle for 0.1 cun. Then, in a 0.1—cun extent, continuously slowly thrust and reapidly lift the needle for 3 times (See Fig. 4—42). Withdraw the needle upward 0.1 cun by 0.1 cun and repeat this course after every time of withdrawing the needle for 0.1 cun for three times, making the cool feeling spread. If there is no cool sensation induced, ask the patient to breathe out with the nose and breathe in with the mouth naturally for 3 times, or shake the needle handle to promote the needling sensation. When numbness, coldness, or electrifying sensation being induced to the patient, pull out the needle quickly and give no pressure over the puncture hole.

c. Yin occluding in yang and yang oocluding in yin:

Yin oocluding in yang: It refers to the needling method beginning with reinforcing needling manner followed by reducing manipulation. This method is applicable to syndromes of cold followed by heat[①], or deficiency complicated with excess[②]. To its operation, it has something like the hot — producing method, namely, divide the puncture depth into the shallow and the deep portions at first, then, insert the needle to the shallow portion. At this layer, forcefully thrust and gently lift the needle for 9 times. Then, insert the needle to the deep portion, and forcefully lift and gently thrust it for 6 times at this portion. Repeat this course for several times before withdrawal of the needle (See Fig. 4—43).

Yang oocluding in yin: It refers to the needling method beginning with reducing manner followed by reinforcing manipulation. This method is applicable to syndromes of heat followed by cold[③] or excess complicated by deifciency[④]. To its operation, it has something like cool—producing method, i.e., first insert the needle to the deep portion of the point, and gently thrust and forcefully lift it at this portion for 6 times. Then, withdraw the needle to the shallow portion, and forcefully thrust and gently lift it for 9 times at this portion. Repeat this course for several times before withdrawal of the needle (See Fig. 4—44).

4. Other Manipulations
(1) Green Dragon Shaking Tail

It is a needle manipulation in which "shaking method" plays the main role. To its operation, following insertion of the needle and arrival of qi, the needle is moved obliquely toward the diseased area without being thrust, lifted or rotated, and the needle is gently and slowly moved left and right like rowing a rudder (See Fig. 4—45). This method is appicable for controlling and strengthening propagation of needling sensation, belonging to one of the four methods of flying the meridian and circulating qi (Feijingzouqi 飞经走气, referring to needling manipulations for promoting circulation of meridian qi). As promoting flow of meridian—qi and regulating qi and blood, this method can be used in treating various syndromes characterized by pain.

(2) White Tiger Shaking Head

It is a needle manipulation in which "shaking method" plays the main role. To its operation, insert the needle perpendicularly to a designed depth, then shake it left and right as lifting it in coordination (See Fig. 4—46). This method is applicable for strengthening the needling sensation, belonging to one of the four methods of flying the channel and circulating qi. As promoting flow of meridian—qi and clearing and purging heat, this method is applied in

---

① A syndrome of cold followed by heat refers to a morbid condition beginning with symptoms and signs belonging to cold syndrome followed by manifestations belonging to heat syndrome.

② A syndrome of deficiency complicated with excess refers to a morbid condition of deficiency manifestations complicated with excess symptoms while the former is dominant.

③ A syndrome of heat followed by cold refers to a morbid conditoion beginning with symptoms and signs belonging to heat syndrome followed by manifestations belonging to cold syndrome.

④ A syndrome of excess complicated by deficiency refers to a morbid condition of excess manifestations complicated with deficiency symptoms while the former is dominant.

treatment of heat syndrome of excess type, which is due to affection by excessive exogenous pathogens which enter the interior of the body, transform into heat and lead to a fierce struggle with the undiminished body resistance, manifested as high fever, fidgets, thirst, constipation, abdominal pain and tenderness, deep—coloured urine, yellowish dry coating of the tongue, full and rapid palse.

(3) Green Tortoise Seeking for Cave

It is a manipulation of needle in which "lifting and thrusting manners" play the main role. To its operation, following that a needle is inserted into an acupoint and the needling sensation is inducd to the patient, the needle is withdrawn to the shallow portion of the acupoint and then thrust four directions — — upwards, downwards, leftwards and rightwards — — — from the shallow to the deep portions with the needle withdrawing once then thrusting three times, like a tortoise going into earth to search for a cave in various directions (See Fig. 4—47). This method is suitable for promoting circulation of meridian qi and making the needling sensation spread, belonging to one of the four methods of flying the channel and circulatint qi, and used in treatment of various syndromes characterized by pain, and arthralgia — syndrome or bi — syndrome which is marked by arthralgia, numbness and dyskinesia of the limbs and caused by attack of the meridians of the limbs by wind, cold and dampness pathogens.

(4) Red Phenix Meeting Resource

It is manipulation of needle in which "rotating, lifting, and thrusting and flying methods" are combined. That is, first, a needle is inserted into the deep portion (earh portion) of the acupoint. Then, it is lifted to the shallow portion (heaven portion) and kept there until the needling sensation is induced to the patient and the needle shakes by itself. Then, the needle is inserted to the middle portion (the man portion). The fingers with the actions of alternate twirling and releasing in performing the manipulations of lifting and thrusting the needle in different directions and of twirling it are like spreading wings of a flying phenix (See Fig. 4—48).

This method is suitable for clearing the collateral (i. e. dredging the collateral), belonging to one of the four methods of flying the channel and circulating qi, and frequently applied in treatment of soreness, heaviness, and wandering pain of muscles and joints.

(5) Zi Wu Dao Jiu Needling

This is a needle manipulation in which the twirling method and lifting and thrusting methods are combined. "Zi Wu" refers to twirling the needle clockwise and anti—clockwise; "Dao Jiu" refers to lifting and thrusting the needle upwards and downwards. To the operation, following insertion of the needle and arrival of qi, the needle is thrust quickly and lifted slowly for 9 times, and then lifted quickly and thrust slowly 6 times. Meanwhile, the needle is twisted clockwise and anti—clockwise in cooperation. This procedure is repeated for several times (See Fig. 4—49). This method is suitable for reinforcing and reducing in combination and subducing swelling and inducing diuresis.

(6) Dragon-tiger Fighting

It is a manipulation of the needle in which "rotating method" plays the main role. "Dragon" refers to twirling the needle clockwise, "tiger" refers to twirling the needle anti—ciockwise, and "fighting" refers to the alternation of the anti—clockwise and clockwise twirling in manipulation. To its operation, the needle is twirled forcefully clockwise 9 times at first, then twirled forcefully anti—ciockwise 6 times. This course is repeated for several times (See Fig. 4 — 50). This method is suitable for inducing analgesic effect.

(7) Dragon—Tiger Ascending—Descending Method

It is a needle manipulation to promote circulation of qi. To its operation, firstly, insert the needle into the acupoint to its heaven portion (i. e. the shallow portion), rotate the needle clockwise a turn at this portion, and quickly insert it by pressure to the man portion (i. e. the middle portion). Then, lift the needle up to the heaven portion again, rotate it anticlockwise a turn at this portion, and quickly thrust the needle by pressure to the man portion. Finally, slowly lift the needle up to the heaven portion again. Repeat this course nine times. (See Fig. 4 — 51A). Secondly, thrust the needle to the earth portion (i. e. the deep portion) and , at that portion, rotate the needle anti—clockwise a turn, quickly lift and slowly thrust it . Then rotate the needle clockwise and quickly lift and slowly thrust it. Repeat this course 6 times (See Fig. 4 — 51B). Or, at first, insert the needle into the acupoint to its heaven portion, and rotate the needle clockwise a turn with the finger force somewhat focusing in the thumb and pressing the needle down to the man portion. Then, at that portion rotate the needle anticlockwise a turn with the finger force somewhat focusing in the middle finger, slowly lift the needle upward to the heaven portion again, and hold the middle portion of the needle shaft to press the needle downward to the man portion again. Repeating this course nine times is taken as the "dragon descending". At second, thrust the needle to the earth portion and, at that portion, rotate the needle clockwise a turn and anticlockwise a turn. Then, quickly lift the needle to the man portion and slowly push it by pressure downward to the earth portion again. Repeating this course six times is taken as "tiger ascending".

(8) Qi—Enterring Method

It is a comprehensive needling method formed by combination of lifting and thrusting methods with the method of manipulating the needle in cooperation with the patient's respiration. To the operation, insert the needle into the acupoint to its deep portion and perform reinforcing manipulations such as the manner by inserting the needle quickly and lifting it slowly nine times. Then, direct the needle tip obliquely toward the diseased area and apply deep puncture. Meanwhile, ask the patient to breathe in 5 — 7 times. This method is suitable for promoting circulation of qi to induce analgesic effect.

(9) Qi—Retaining Method

It is a needle manipulation by taking lifting and thrusting manners as the main method. To the operation, insert the needle into the acupoint to its middle portion (for about 0.7 cun deep) and perform reinforcing manipulations such as the manner by inserting the needle quickly and lifting it slowly nine times. Then, thrust the needle to the deep portion and withdraw it to the original place. The method is suitalbe for promoting circulation of qi to dispel accumulation.

(10) Chou Tian Method

"Chou" refers to lifting the needle, and "tian" to thrusting the needle. This is a needle manipulation taking "lifting and thrusting" as the main. To the operation, following inserting the needle into the acupoint and inducing needling sensation, lift and thrust the needle in various dirctions. Then, puncture perpendicularly with the pressure from the finger force. This method can serve to activate the meridian and its collateral and be applicable to treatment of paralysis, pyogenic infecton of skin and tinea capitis.

七、留针与出针

1. 留针：针刺入选定的腧穴施行各种手法后，为加强针刺作用，便于继续行针施术，或施行手法未能得气有待候气，均可将针留置穴内。留针时间一般为10～20分钟，特殊病症如急性腹痛、顽固性麻痹、痉挛症，可留针1～2小时或数个小时。

2. 出针：是针刺技法中最后一环，出针时一般以左手拇、食指按住针孔周围皮肤，右手持针将针轻微捻动并提至皮下，然后将针抽出（图4—52）。根据病情需要，揉按或摇大针孔，但在血管丰富处出针时，一般应将消毒棉球压按针孔，以防出血。确需出血者例外，

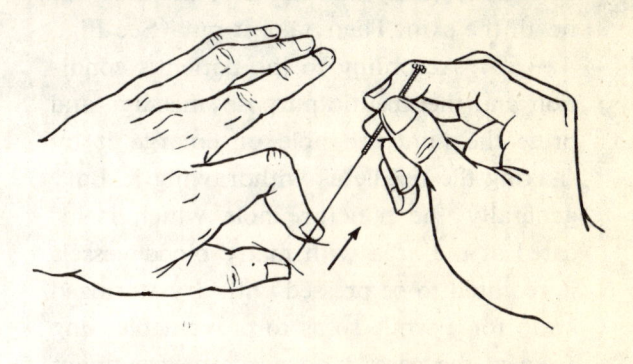

图 4—52 出针
Fig. 4—52 Withdrawing the Needle

Ⅶ. RETAINING AND WITHDRAWING THE NEEDLE

1. *Retaining the Needle*

After the needle is inserted into the selected acupoint and the required manipulation are performed, the needle may be kept in place in the acupoint in order to strengthen the needling sensation and to continue to manipulate the needle, or to wait for the needling sensation which should but has not been induced by some manipulations. Generally, the period of retention of the needle is 10—20 minutes at one session of treatment, but in treating some specific disorders such as acute abdominal pain, stubborn numbness or spasm, it may be 1—2 hours or more.

2. *Withdrawing the Needle*

It is the last step in acupuncture manipulation. In withdrawing a needle, generally, press the skin around the needle with the thumb and index finger of the left hand, hold the needle with the right hand to twirl it gently and lift it to the area beneath the skin. Then, take it out (See Fig. 4—52). According to the patient's condition and therapeutic purpose, massage and press the puncture hole or enlarge it by shaking the needle as withdrawing it. But, generally, the puncture hole which is located at the area with many blood vessels is required to be pressed with dry sterilized swab for a while so as to prevent bleeding (except the cases who need the treatment to cause bleeding by acupuncture).

八、异常情况处理与注意事项

（一）异常情况处理

1. 滞针：由于行针时用力过猛，或向一个方向捻转时，致使肌纤维缠绕针身而致滞针。可将针向相反方向退转，并左右轻捻使针松弛。若因患者精神紧张致肌肉痉挛而使针下涩滞，行针困难，可嘱病人放松肌肉延缓留针时间，并在其邻近部位配合按摩以消除痉挛。如因移动体位而致滞针，可将患者体位复原，即可顺利出针。

预防滞针，必须要对初诊及精神紧张的病人，先作解释工作，消除紧张情绪，以便配合医师接受治疗。行针时捻转角度不宜太大，更不要朝一个方向强行捻转，进针后不可随便移动体位。

2. 弯针：医师手法不熟练，用力过猛或患者移动体位，均能造成弯针，针弯角度小者可顺针弯曲度慢慢退出，如角度大则必须轻微摇动针身，边摇边顺其弯曲方向将针退出。如针身弯曲度不止一处，须视针柄扭转倾斜的方向逐渐分段退出（图4—53）。切勿猛拔，以防断针，若因体位而致弯针，应加复原来体位，使局部肌肉放松再行退针。

预防弯针要求先选好合格的针具，施术者手法要轻巧熟练，针刺部位与针柄不能受外物碰压，选择好舒适，便于患者能持续操作的体位。

3. 断针：临床上较为少见，多因针具质量差，针身或针根剥蚀，加之医师操作用力过猛，患者移动体位，或滞针，弯针处理不当，或电针时突然加大电流强度而致断针。一旦发现断针，当嘱患者保持体位，以防断针向肌肉深处陷入，若折针的断端尚留出体表，可立即用左手拇、食二指挤压指折针周围的皮肤，使断端暴露更多（图4—54），右手持镊子夹住断端取出。如断端完全陷入肌肉层或体腔内，应手术取出，必要时应在X线投照下定位，再施手术取出。

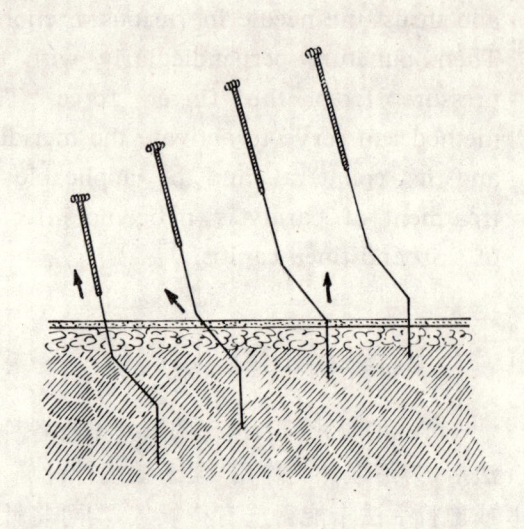

图4—53 弯针处理
Fig. 4—53 Withdrawing the Bent Needle

预防断针的可靠方法，是选择好光滑、质地紧韧、针根牢固的针具，进针时不能将针身全部刺入体内，当留出2～3分（6～9毫米）在体外，以防万一断针时便于取出。

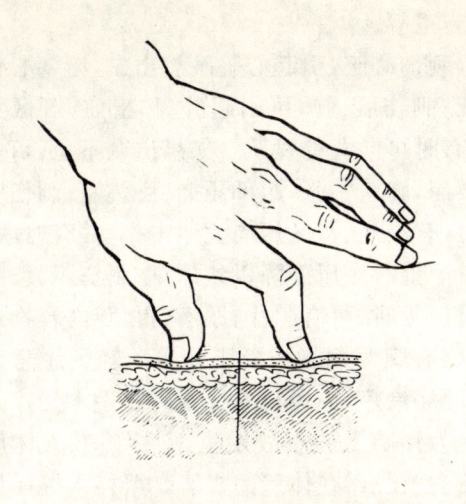

图 4—54 断针处理
Fig. 4—54 Withdrawing the Broken Needle

4.晕针：患者初诊或精神紧张，过度疲劳、饥饿、过饱、久病、大汗、体位不当，或施术者手法过重，致使病人突感胸闷、恶心、头晕、目眩、继而面色苍白，四肢厥冷，出汗，脉沉细，甚或血压下降，神志昏迷倒地，唇爪青紫，二便失禁等。

一旦发现上述现象，应立即将针抽出，让患者平卧，或头低足高位松开衣领、腰带，躺在空气流通处，轻者休息片刻，饮温开水或糖开水即可缓解；重者可掐人中穴，刺内关穴或灸足三里，膻中，气海，百会等穴，即可缓解。若出现呼吸微细、脉搏微小、晕厥不醒者，可嗅以氨水，并视情况施用人工呼吸，注射强心剂。低血压者，可口服麻黄素，静注50%葡萄糖等，亦可对症采取其他措施急救。

预防晕针，要先做好患者解释工作，消除精神紧张，尽可能采用卧位扎针，手法不宜过重，体位要求舒适，针刺前当令患者休息片刻，若饥饿者待稍加进食后，方可施术。行针期间，当时时注意病人表情，一旦出现晕针先兆，应立即采取处理措施。

5.血肿：针刺时，有时难免伤及小血管，尤其是针尖带钩时易引起出血，小的渗血或皮下出血，可不必处理，让其自行消退。若局部血肿较大，胀痛，影响活动，当先行冷敷或压迫止血，后作热敷、揉按，帮助消散瘀血。为减少针抽出后产生血肿，当严格选好针具，尽可能避开血管进针，在血管丰富处不宜大幅度捻转提插。

6.后遗感：多因手法过重刺激太强，致抽出针后，仍有酸痛、重胀、麻木不适感觉。轻者自行消失；重则可局部按摩，配合艾灸，1～3天后自然消失。为避免出现后遗感，应掌握好针刺时的强度，在神经干分布处要避免大幅度捣动提插。

（二）注意事项

1.体质虚弱、初诊病人、精神紧张者、施术手法不宜过强，并尽量选用卧位。

2.怀孕3个月的妇女，不宜刺小腹部腧穴，怀孕3个月以上，腹部、腰骶部腧穴也不宜刺。三阴交、合谷、至阴、昆仑等穴，孕妇及月经期经量正常的妇女，在行经期不宜刺。

3.不能合作的小儿，针后不留针，囟门未合时，头顶部不宜刺。

4.自发性出血疾患及凝血机制较差的患者一般不宜刺。

5.胸、肋、背、腰部为重要脏器所在，针刺过深，可刺伤内脏，发生意外，引起不良后果。故施术者一定要熟悉腧穴下的解剖结构，严格把握进针的角度与深度。

6.眼眶周围血管丰富的穴位，不可大幅度捻转提插，以防出血。

7.皮肤有感染、溃疡、瘢痕、肿瘤时，不宜针刺。

（三）针刺事故的预防

1.创伤性气胸：多因针刺前胸部、侧胸部和锁骨上窝及胸骨切迹上缘腧穴时，由于针刺深度,角度与方向不正确,致使毫针刺破脏层胸膜,使气体流入胸腔所致。

易刺伤肺脏的常用穴(本书所采用的穴位,下同),如天突、俞府、乳根、中府、大包、极泉、肩井、肩外俞、期门、大杼、风门、肺俞、厥阴俞、心俞、膈俞、肝俞、胆俞、脾俞、膏肓俞、定喘等。

发生气胸,多在针后突感胸闷,胸痛,甚则呼吸困难,心跳加快,紫绀、出汗、血压下降等休克症状。叩诊时患侧胸部有过度反响,肺泡呼吸音明显减弱或消失,严重者可发生气管向健侧移位。X线胸透可进一步确诊。少数病例当时无明显异常,几小时后才感胸闷或胸痛,以及呼吸困难。

一旦发现气胸,即应取半卧位休息,轻者由于少量气体进入胸膜腔,尚可自然吸收,注意休息,密切观察,给予抗菌药物防止感染,有咳嗽时给予镇咳药。一旦出现呼吸困难、发绀,甚至休克时,当立即抢救。迅速将消毒粗短注射针头插入锁骨中线第二、三肋间,自然排气。或用50~100毫升消毒注射器,以胶管连接胸腔穿刺进行抽气。或采取其他方法排气,并送急诊处理。

为防止气胸发生,必须严格掌握针刺角度、深度及操作规程。前胸壁一般直刺2~3分(同身寸)深,背部腧穴一般直刺以不超过中指同身寸3~5分深(约0.5~1厘米左右)为宜,最多不超过8分深。为安全起见,均采用斜刺。

2. 刺伤心、肝、脾、肾……等内脏:在心、肝、脾、肾……等内脏的体表相应部位腧穴进针过深时,也会引起严重后果,特别是肝、脾肿大,膀胱充盈的病人,尤须注意。

易刺伤心、肝、脾、肾、胆、胃、大肠小肠、膀胱的常用穴如鸠尾、巨阙、中脘、下脘、气海、石门、关元、中极、天枢、水道、归来、大横、日月、京门、带脉、章门、三焦俞、肾俞、大肠俞、志室等。

刺伤心脏,引起心脏破裂出血,堵塞心包致死;刺伤肝、脾,可引起肝、脾出血,肝区疼痛,有时可向背部发散。如果出血不止,可伴有腹痛,腹肌紧张,腹部压痛、反跳痛;刺伤肾脏时,有腰痛、肾区压痛及叩击痛,并有血尿。出血严重时血压下降以致休克;刺伤胆囊、膀胱、胃、肠时,可有胆汁、尿液、胃、肠内容物外溢,则有腹膜刺激或急腹症等。轻则注意休息,对症治疗,尚可自愈。重则需手术治疗。

为预防上述事故发生,必须熟知人体解剖结构及脏器在体壁的投影。严格掌握操作规程与进针深度,不可麻痹大意。剑突下心窝附近穴位以1寸针为宜,注意选择体位与取穴姿势。如刺鸠尾穴时,要两臂上举以利抬高胸腔内的脏器;脐周及下腹穴位,以1.5寸针为宜。对肝、胆、脾肿大的病人,严禁深刺期门、日月、章门、梁门等穴;对膀胱尿潴留的病人,严禁深刺曲骨、中极、关元等穴;对食后过饱的病人,严禁深刺上、中、下脘穴及其附近穴位;对肠粘连、肠梗阻病人的腹部穴位如天枢、大横、水道、归来等穴,严禁将针刺透腹壁进入腹腔。

3. 刺伤脑、脊髓:凡在颈项部正中线上的哑门、风府、和两旁的风池、天柱等穴进行针刺时,如角度、方向、深度不当,针由颅底枕骨大孔进入颅腔,可伤及延髓、桥脑、小脑及血管,危及生命。在背部正中线督脉,针刺第一腰椎以上棘突间穴位,和华佗夹脊穴向棘间方向深刺,皆可刺中脊髓,出现触电样感觉向肢体远端放散。重者可因刺激部位的不同,产生暂时的肢体瘫痪,若属轻症经安静休息,对症治疗,多能逐渐恢复。如有头痛、恶心、呕吐,应注意观察。若进而神志昏迷,就应及时抢救。

为避免针刺意外发生,应严格掌握针刺角度、方向与深度。一旦刺入深部,病人有触电感时,应立即退针,切勿捣刺。

VIII. PRECAUTIONS AND MANAGEMENT OF POSSIBLE ACCIDENTS IN ACUPUNCTURE AND MOXIBUSTION TREATMENT

1. *Management of Possible Accidents*

(1) Stuck Needle

Cause and Management: It may be due to too strong manipulation or rotating the needle in a single directon only, resulting in entangle of the needle with the muscle fibers. When it happens, withdraw the needle as rotating it in the opposite direction and twirling it left and right gently to make the needle released from being entangled. If it is caused by the patient's muscular spasm due to nervousness, advise the patient to relax his or her muscle, prolong the period of retention of the needle, and massage the area close to the acupoint to relieve the muscle spasm. If it is caused by changing of the posture of the patient, move the patient to the original position and then withdraw the needle.

Prevention: Say some wards to the first — visiting patient or the nervous patient to even him or her and make him or her be in cooperation prior to the operation. Avoid twirling the needle in a too large amplitude or in a single direction by force, and avoid changing the patient's posture after insertion of the needle if possible.

(2) Bent Needle

Cause and Management: It may be due to unskillfull manipulation, or over violent manipulation, or changing of the patient's posture. If the bend is slight, withdraw the needle by following the course of the bend slowly; if pronounced, shake the needle shaft slightly and withdraw the needle by following the course of the bend with the needle shaked; if the needle is bent in several places, withdraw it section by section, following the course of bends (See Fig. 4—53). Never withdraw the bent needle suddenly and forcefully; otherwise, the needle may be broken; if it is caused by changing of the patient's posture, move the patient to the original position to relax the local muscle and then withdraw the needle.

Prvention: Only the qualified needles are selected for treatment, the manipulation should be gentle and skillful, the area to be punctured and the needle shaft should not be impacted and pressed by some foreign material, and a comfortable posture which is suitable for the patient to accept the constant operation should be chosen.

(3) Broken Needle

Cause and Management: It occurs occasionally, which may be due to poor quality of needle, corrosion of the needle shaft, violent manipulation, changing of the patient's posture, improper management of sticking or bending of the needle, or sudden increase of the electric current in the electric needling. Once the needle is broken, ask patient not to chagne the posture so as to prevent the distal broken fragment of the needle from going deeper into the muscle. If the end of the broken fragment of the needle is above the skin, immediately press the skin around it with the thumb and index finger of the left hand to make the end exposed more, then pull it out with the forceps held with the right hand (See Fig. 4—54). If the broken fragment end is completely under the skin surface or in the organ in the body, perform the surgical operation to take it out or, if necessary, do the operation under X—ray examination.

Prevention: A dependable method of preventing the needle from being broken is to make inspection of the quality of the needle prior to treatment and to use only the smooth and flexible needle with its root fixed. The complete insertion of the whole shaft of the needle into the body is not allowed and the shaft should be left 0.2—0.3 cun (6—9mm) above the skin so as to take the fragment of the broken needle out easily if the needle is broken.

(4) Needling Fainting

Cause and Management: It may be due to the patient's receiving the treatment of acupuncture for the first time, or the patient's nervous tension, fatigue, hunger, overeating, prolonged illness, oversweating, improper posture, or the operator's too violent manipulation. It is manifestated by sunden attack of oppressed feeling in the chest, nausea, dizziness and vertigo, followed by pallor, cold extremities, sweating, deep and thready pulse, even lowering of blood pressure, unconsciousness and coma, falling down the ground, cyanosis of the lip and claws, incontinence of urine and stool, etc. Once the phenomena mentioned above happen, take the needle out immediately, keep the patient in recumbent position, or help the patient lie with the head lower and the feet higher, the collar and the waistband loosed or lie in a room with fresh air.

For the milder case, advise the patient to take a short rest and drink some warm water or sugar solution, resulting in disappearance of the patient'a symptoms. For severe cases, it is needed to press Renzhong (DU 26) with the finger-nail, puncture Neiguan (PC6) and apply moxibustion on Zusanli (ST36), Danzhong (RN 17), Qihai (RN 6), Baihui (DU 20), etc. Throuh this treatment the patients, generally, will respond. If the patient has faint respiration, faint pulse and loss of consciousness, help the patient smell ammonia water, apply artificial respiration, and inject cardiac stimulant to the patient. In case with lower blood pressure, administer peroral ephedrine and inject 50% glucose injection to him or her, or give some other emergency treatments according to symptoms.

Prevention: Say some words to the patient to relieve his or her nervous tension prior to the treatment, choose the recumbent position for the patient as far as possible, avoid too violent manipulation of the needle, and advise the patient to have a short rest prior to insertion of the needle. If the patient is hungry, apply puncture after the patient takes some food. During manipulation of the needle, pay close attention to the patient's expression from time to time, and apply the management immediately whenever the prodromal symptoms and signs of fainting appear.

(5) Hematoma

Cause and Management: It may be due to injury of some small blood vessels by needling, which is some times unavoidable, especially when the tip of the needle is hooked. If there is a little oozing of blood or subcutaneous bleeding, give no treatment to it but leave it to disappear of its own accord. If there is a local bigger hematoma with distention, which disturbes the body activity, apply cold compress or press the punctured area to stop bleeding at first. Then, apply hot compress and massage to promote absorption of the extravasculated blood.

Prevention: In order to reduce the possibility of inducing hematoma after withdrawing the needle, select the needle to be used strictly, avoid the blood vessels in insertion, and avoid twirling, lifting and thrusting the needle in a great amplitude at the area with rich distribution of blood vessels.

(6) Sequelae

Cause and Management: After withdrawal of the needle, there may still remain an uncomfortable feelings such a soreness, pain, heaviness, distension and numbness, which are known as sequela. The sequela in acupuncture treatment may be mainly due to too violent manipulation and too strong stimulation. In milder cases, apply no management to it because it may disappear of its own accord. For severe cases, massage the local area in coordination with moxibustion, resulting in its disappearence within 1—3 days.

Prevention: Choose the proper stimulation intensity in puncture, avoid shaking, lifting and thrusting the needle in a large amplitude at the area distributed with the nerve trunk.

2. Precautions

(1) For the patient who is weak, nervous, or at first — visiting, a recumbent posture should be chosen.

(2) It is contraindicated to puncture acupoints on the lower abdomen for women pregnant within the first three months. And for those beyond the first three months it is also contraindicated to puncture acupoints on the abdomen and lumbo—sacral region. Sanyinjiao(SP 6), Hegu(LI 4), Zhiyin(BL 67) and Kunlun (BL 60) should not be punctured for pregnant women and the women who have a normal menstruation and now are at the menstruation period.

(3) Retention of the needle should not be given to children who may not be in cooperation. Acupoints on the vertex of infants should not be punctured when the fontanel is not closed.

(4) It is contraindicated to apply puncture to patients with spontaneous bleeding or poor blood coagulation mechanism.

(5) Special attention must be paid in puncturing acupoints on the chest, hypochondrium, back and loin, where the important viscera are located. Over deep puncture to acupoints on these areas may injure the cooresponding internal viscera, leading to accident and bad result. So an operator must know well the anatomy of acupoints and control the angle and depth of puncture strictly.

(6) In acupoints at the area around

the orbital region, where the blood vessels are rich, the needle should not be rotated, lifted or thrust in a large amplitude, so as to prevent bleeding.

(7) The skin with infection, ulcer, scar, or tumor, should not be punctured.

3. Prevention of Acupuncture Accidents

(1) Traumatic Pneumothorax

Causes: It is usually due to incorrect depth, angle, and direction of puncture at points on the anterior or lateral chest, on the supraclavicular fossa, or on the upper border of the costal incisures of the sternum, resulting in that the visceral pleura is broken and air enters the thoracic cavity.

Possible common acupoints relating to injury of the lung by puncture: Tiantu (RN 22), Shufu(KI 27), Rugen(ST 18), Zhongfu(LU 1), Dabao(SP 21), Jiquan (HT 1), Jianjing(GB 21), Jianwaishu(SI 14), Qimen (LR 14), Dashu (BL 11), Fengmen (BL 12), Feishu (BL 13), Jueyinshu (BL 14), Xinshu (BL 15), Geshu(BL 17), Ganshu(BL 18), Danshu (BL 19), Pishu(BL 20), Gaohuanshu(BL 43), Dingchuan (EX—BI).

Manifestations: Sudden occurrence of depressed feeling in the chest, chest pain, or even such shock manifestations as dyspneic respiration, tachycardia, cyanosis, sweating, lower blood pressure. Percussion and auscultation will find that percussion note of the diseased side of the chest increases and vesicular breath sound of the diseased side largely decreases or even disappears as compared with the healthy side of the chest. In severe case, tracheal displacement to the healthy side of the chest may be found. X—ray examination on the chest helps the diagnosis. The manifestations usually occur just a little time after the puncture. But in a few cases, they may occur several hours after the puncture.

Management: As soon as finding some manifestions of traumatic pneumothorax, help the patient lie at semireclining position. To mild case with a little air entering the thoracic cavity, which can be absorbed in its own accord, just give close observation on the patient, administer some antiseptic to prevent infection, and prescribe some antitussive if the patient has cough. But to severe case with dyspnea, cyanosis or even shock, first aid measurement should be applied immediately. At first, insert a steriliged thick and short syringe needle into the thoracic cavity through the 2nd intercostal space at the midclavicular line of the diseased side of the chest to make the air go out of the cavity automatically, or insert a pnenmothorax puncture needle which, through a plastic pipe, is connected with a sterilzed 50—100 ml syringe to aspire the air, or apply some other exsufflation methods. Then, send the patient to the emergency room for further treatmant.

Prevention: The rule of correct depth, angle and direction of puncture should be obeyed strictly. Generally, the depth of perpendicular puncture at points at the anterior or lateral chest should not be more than 0.2—0.3 cun (referring to the proportional unit of the body). The depth of perpendicular puncture at points at the upper back should be less than 0.8

cun (referring to the proportional unit of the body with the middle finger), and it is proper to keep the depth of puncture at 0.3—0.5 cun (0.5—1cm). For safe, all of these points should be punctured obliquely.

(2) Injury of the Heart, Liver, Spleen, Kidney and Some Other Internal Organs.

Cause: It may be due to over deep puncture at the points on the body surface corresponding to the internal organs. Especially, when the patient has hepatomegoly, splenomegaly, or filling of the bladder, the liver, spleen, or bladder is more easily injured by improper puncture.

Possible common acupoints relating to injury of the heart, Liver, spleen, kidney, gallbladder, stomach, large and small intestines, and bladder: Jiuwei (RN 15), Juque (RN 14), Zhongwan (RN 12), Xiawan (RN 10), Qihai (RN 6), Shimen (RN 5), Guanyuan (RN 4), Tianshu (ST 25), Shuidao (ST 28), Guilai (ST 29), Daheng (SP 15), Riyue (GB 24), Jingmen (GB 25), Daimai (GB 26), Zhangmen (LR 13), Sanjiaoshu (BL 22), Shenshu (BL 23), Dachangshu (BL 25), Zhishi (Bl 52).

Manifestations:

Impairment of the heart by puncture: Symptoms and signs due to bleeding from the heart may be caused and, in severe case, the manifestations caused by filling of the pericardium with blood can be seen and even death caused.

Impairment of the liver or spleen by puncture: Hepatalgia due to bleeding of the liver or spleen, which, sometimes, can spread to the back. If the bleeding is not stopped, abdominal pain, tension of the abdominal muscles, abdominal tenderness and rebounding pain may be accompanied.

Impairment of the kidney by puncture: Lumbago. tenderness over the kidney region by percussion or pressing, hematuria, or lowering of blood pressure and shock due to large bleeding in severe case.

Impairment of the gallbladder, bladder, stomach, intestine due to puncture: Signs of peritoneal irritation or even manifestation of acute abdomen may be caused due to that some contents of these organs go out of them.

Management: To mild case, apply expectant treatment, and advise the patient to have rest, having the impairment cured in its own accord. To severe case, surgical operation is needed sometimes.

Prevention: Before giving puncture, you should have a sound knowledge about the human anatomy as wall as the projection locations of the internal organs on the corresponding regions of the body surface. And yor should obey the manipulation rules, control the puncture depth strictly, and have no carelessness. When puncturing points below the xiphoid process and near the epigastric region, it is proper to select needles about 1 cun long and pay attention to selection of the patient's position. On puncturing Jiuwei (RN 15), for example, ask the patient to raise the arms to lift the internal organs in his or her chest. When puncturing points around the umbilicus and points at the lower abdomen, select 1.5 cun long needles. To case with liver enlargement, gallbladder enlargement, or spleen enlargement, deep insertion is forbidden on puncture at Qimen (LR 14). Riyue (GB 24), Zhangmen (LR 13) and Liangman (ST 21). To case with retention of urine, deep insertion is forbidden when puncturing at Qugu (RN 2), Zhongji (RN 3) and Guanyuan (RN 4). To case with filling of the stomach due to over eating, it is forbidden to apply deep puncture at Shangwan (RN 13), Zhongwan (RN 12), and Xiawan (RN 10), as well as the points around them. And to case with intestinal adhension or intestinal obstruction, it is forbidden to insert the needle throughout the abdominal wall into the abdominal cavity when puncturing points at the abdomen such as Tianshu (SR 25). Daheng (SP 15), Shuidao (ST 28) and Guilai (ST 29).

(3) Injury of the Brain and Spinal Cord

Causes: The bulb, pons and cerebellum can be injured when a needle enters the cranial cavity through the great occipital foramen. This condition is usually due to incorrect angle, direction or depth of puncture at the points on the posterior median line of the neck such as Yamen (DU 15) and Fengfu (DU 16), or at the points lateral to the line such as Fengchi (GB 20) and Tianzhu (BL 10). The spinal cord may be injured by deep puncture at the points locating between the spinous processes above the first lumbar vertebra or by deep puncture at Jiaji (EX—B2) with the needle directing towards the interspinal area.

Manifesfations and treatment:

Injury of the brain: Headche, nausea and vomiting in mild case; and loss of consciousness or even death in severe case. Take out the needle immediately whenever finding any manifestation of it, and pay close attention to the patient's condition. If finding that the patient is at coma, apply emergency treatment immediately.

Injury of the spinal cord: Electrifying sensation radiating to the distal ends of the extremities in mild case, and temporary paralysis of the extremities in severe case. Remove the needle out as soon as finding any manifestation of it, advise the patient to have rest, and give some expectant treatment to the patient. Usually, the injury will be cured in its own accord.

Prevention: When puncturing the points at the areas mentioned above, control the angle, direction and depth of insertion of the needle strictly. In case of electrifying sensation is induced to the patient by puncturing points at these areas, never take it as good needling sensation and never apply thursting-lifting manipulation forcefully, but withdraw the needle immediately.

第二节 三棱针

古称"锋针"。临床上用于刺破患者一定穴位或浅表血管，放出少量血液以治疗疾病的方法。具有活血消肿、开窍泄热、通经活络的作用。

一、适应范围

主要用于各种热病、实证与痛证，如高热、中暑、急性扁桃体炎、咽喉肿痛、眼结膜炎、扭伤、以及疖肿、淋巴管炎、神经性皮炎等。

SECTION 2 ACUPUNCTURE WITH THE THREE — EDGED NEEDLE

The three — edged (triangular prismatic) needle is called the sharp needle in ancient times. Acupuncture with the three — edged needle is a needling method of treatment by prisking the acupoint or the superficial blood vessel with a three — edged needle to obtain a little bloodletting. This mehod functions to promote the blood circulation for disappearing swelling, causing resuscitation, reducing heat, cleaning and acitivating the meridian and collateral (i. e. , dredging the meridians and collaterals and ensuring the flow of qi and blood through them).

I. INDICATIONS

Acupuncture with the three — edged needle is applicable to various heat syndromes, excess syndromes and pain syndromes[①]. It is usually employed in treating high fever, heat — stroke, acute tonsilitis, sore and swelling throat, conjunctivitis, sprain, furuncle, lymphangitis, neurodermatitis, etc.

二、实用技法

针具及刺血部位常规消毒后，根据病情需要有如下几种刺法：

1. 点刺法：先在针刺穴位或患处上下推按，使之局部充血，医师左手挟持或扶持治疗部位，右手持针，拇、食指捏住针柄、中指指腹紧靠针身下端，露出针尖3毫米左右，对准已消毒的部位迅速刺入1～2毫米深(图4—55)，立即出针并轻轻挤压针孔周围，使之出血数滴，然后用消毒棉球按压针孔片刻。本法多用于治疗高热、惊厥、中风昏迷、中暑、急性扁桃腺炎、急性腰扭伤。尤其在医疗条件较差的地区或临时缺少医疗服务的情况下，常可收到意外的效果。

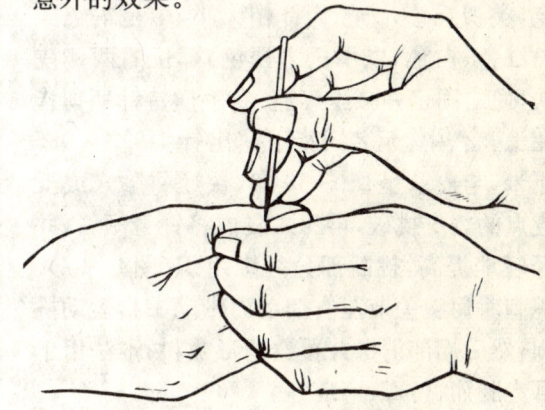

图4—55　点刺法
Fig. 4—55 Spot Pricking

2. 散刺法：又称"围刺"。医生左手用舒张法按压应刺部位皮肤，右手如上法持针，在病

---

① A heat syndrome refers to a morbid condition due to attack of pathogenic heat or hyperactvity of yang—qi, usually seen in infectious disease and those caused by abnormal hyperactivity of the body, with manifestations such as fever, fidgets, flushed face, congested eyes, dry mouth and throat, red and dry lips, thirst with preference for cold drink, constipation, scanty dark urine, reddened tongue with dry brownish or black coating, and rapid pulse.

　　A excess syndrome is characterized by presence of excessive pathogenic factors which lead to intense body reaction, or by the presence of pathological products due to dysfunction of the internal organs, such as stagnant qi and blood, excessive fluid, retained phlegm and undigested food.

　　A pain syndrome refers to a morbid condition taking pain as the main manifestation.

灶周围的上、下、左、右快速垂直点刺(图4—56)后,即轻轻挤压针孔使之出血。本法多用于外伤性瘀血疼痛、丹毒、疖疮等。

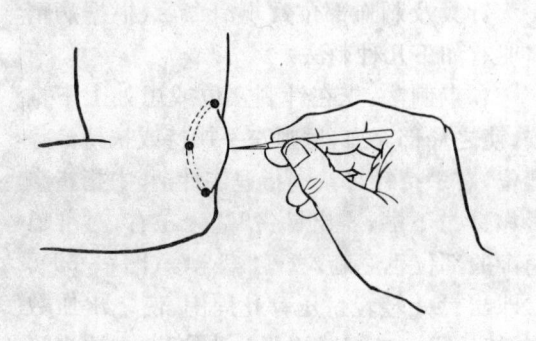

图4—56 散刺法
Fig. 4—56 Scattering Pricking

3.挑刺法:医师以左手按压腧穴或反应点(类似丘疹,一般为针帽大小,多呈褐色或粉红色、白色,以手压之褪色)部位的两侧皮肤,使之固定并减少疼痛。右手横持针柄拇指在上,食、中、无名三指下露出针尖0.3～0.5厘米,与皮肤呈15°～30°角,快速将腧穴或反应点的表皮挑破,再深入皮内将针身倾斜,并轻轻地提高,挑断部分纤维组织(图4—57)。挑刺时用腕关节左右摆动力带动手指运动挑刺,然后局部消毒并覆盖消毒敷料。本法用于目赤肿痛、丹毒、痔疮等。

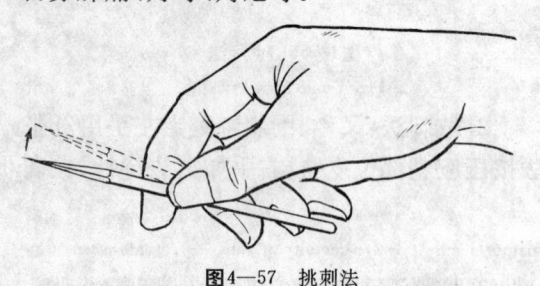

图4—57 挑刺法
Fig. 4—57 Fibrous—Tissue—Broken Pricking

II. MANIPULATIONS

There are following methods of puncture with the there-edged needle, all of them being carried out with the routine local sterillzation as the beginning.

1. Spot Pricking

This is a method knwon as collateral pricking in ancient times. To the operation, press and push the site to be pricked to cause local congestion, hold the needle with the right hand, the thumb and index finger griping its handle, and the belly of the middle finger supporting the lower portion of its shaft, exposing proximately 0.3cm from the tip of the needle, direct the tip precisely at the spot to be punctured and swiftly prick it 0.1 — 0.2 cm deep (See Fig. 4—55), and withdraw it immediately. Then, squeeze out a few drops of blood by pressing the skin around the punctured hole, and press over the hole with a sterilized swab for a moment. This method is mainly applicable to high fever, convulsion, apoplexy with coma, heat—stroke, acute tonsilitis, and acute lumbar sprain. Eespecially, at the area with poor medical service, this method is usually very important and causes miraculous effect in treatment of these diseases.

2. Scattering Pricking

This method is also termed surrounding needling. To the operation, stretch the skin to be punctured with the fingers of the left hand, hold the needle with the right hand in the same way as in "spot pricking method", and prick the skin around the affected focus perpendicularly and rapidly (see Fig. 4—56). Then, gently press the skin to obtain a little bloodletting. This method is mainly applicable to traumatic pain due to stagnant blood, erysipelas, carbuncle, sore, etc.

3. *Fibrous — Tissue — Broken Pricking*

This method is also termed "breaking". To the operation, press the skin at two sides of the acupoint or sensitive spot(like a rush, 2 — 4 mm in diameter, usually with dark — yellow, green — dark — yellow, reddish, or white colour, which is disappeared if pressing it) with the left hand to fix the skin, hold the needle with right hand, the thumb above the middle, index and ring fingers, exposing the tip of the needle for 0.3 — 0.5cm. Then, quickly prick and break the skin of the acupoint or responsible spot at an angle of 15 — 30° formd by the needle with the skin surface punctured, insert the needle deep to the subcutaneous tissue, make the shaft of the needle tilted and then gently moved upwards to break some of fibrous tissues (See Fig. 4 — 57). When pricking and breaking, it is advisable to use the force formed by left — right movement of the wrist joint, making the finger's movement for pricking and breaking. This method is applicable to redess, swelling and pain of eye, erysipelas, hemorrhoids, etc.

三、注意事项

1. 严格遵守无菌操作规程，避免感染。
2. 手法宜轻快，出血不宜过多，勿刺伤深部大血管。
3. 出血性疾病患者禁用，如血小板减少、血友病等均不宜使用。孕妇、产后、过饥、过饱、过劳患者慎用。
4. 一般1日1次，或隔日1次，或3～7日挑刺一次，3～5次为一个疗程。

III. PRECAUTIONS

(1) Strictly observe the aseptic operation rule to prevent infection.

(2) It is advisable to manipulate gently and swiftly. No more than a few drops of blood should be squeezed out. Never injure the deep big artery.

(3) This method should not be used in patients with hemorrhagic diseases, shch as thrombocytopenia, hemophilia. It should be used with a great care in patients who are preganant, postpartal, famished, over-eating, or over — fatigued.

(4) Generally, this method is carried out once every day or once every other day, or once per 3 — 7days. One therapeutic course needs 3 — 5 times.

第三节 皮内针

皮内针又称"埋针"。是将特制的小型针具刺入皮内，固定并留置一定时间，利用其持续的刺激作用，调整经络脏腑功能来治疗疾病的一种方法。

一、适应范围

本法宜应用于需要较长时间留针的慢性、疼痛性疾患，如头痛、三叉神经痛、牙痛、胃痛、哮喘、失眠、月经不调、痛经、遗尿，以及其他病症。

SECTION 3 ACUPUNCTURE WITH THE INTRADERMAL NEEDLE

Acupuncture with the intradermal needle, also termed the needle—embedding therapy, is a treatment method by inserting and leaving a small needle beneath the skin so as to give the body a long—lasting continuous stimulation for regulating the visceral functions.

a, irregular menstruation, dysmenorrhea, enuresis, and some other painful syndromes.

二、实用技法

首先将皮内针、镊子、及欲埋针的部位皮肤进行消毒。麦粒型或环型皮内针可用于躯干、四肢部腧穴,操作时医师左手拇、食指将所刺部位皮肤撑开,右手持镊子挟住针柄,对准穴位垂直刺进真皮后,与经脉循行呈交叉方向,沿皮横刺入皮内,针身埋入皮内约0.5～1厘米(图4—58),然后用胶布将露在皮外的针柄粘贴固定;图钉型皮内针(揿针)多用于耳穴埋针。操作时,用镊子挟住针柄,将针对准穴位刺入,使针之环状针柄平整地留在局部穴位皮肤上(图4—59①)用胶布固定,亦

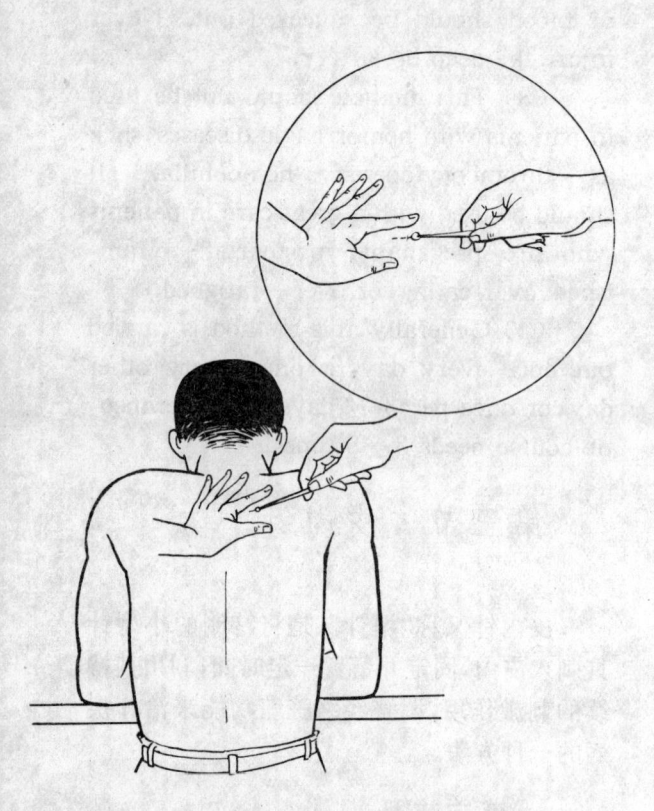

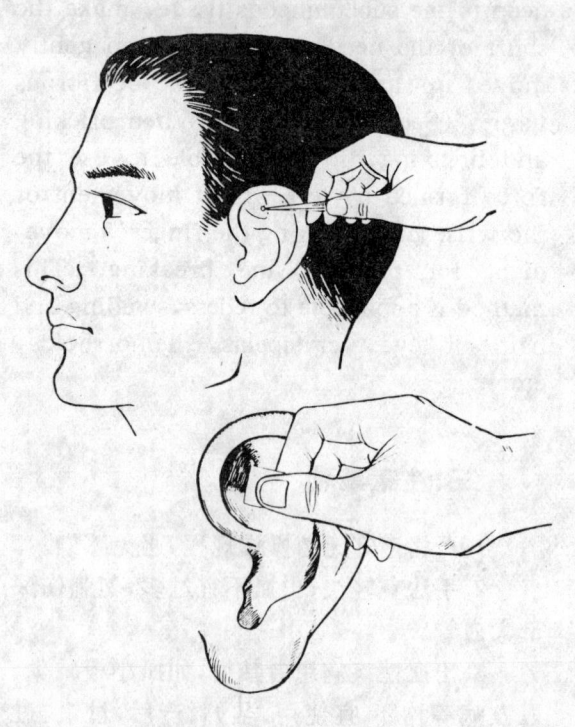

图4—58 皮内针埋针法
Fig. 4—58 The Needle—Embedding Method

I. INDICATIONS

It is applicable to chronic and painful disorders, in which prolonged retention of needle is needed for treatment purpose, including headache, trigeminal neuralgia, toothache, stomachache, asthma, insomni-

图4—59 揿针埋针法
Fig. 4—59 Embedment of the Thumb—Tack—Shaped Needle

可将针柄放在预先剪好的小方胶布上粘住，手持胶布拇指压住针柄，对准穴位将针贴刺在穴位的皮内（图5—59②），埋针的时间视季节而定，夏天一般留置1～2天，秋冬季节可留置3～5天。撤针埋针期间可每天用手按压数次，每次1～2分钟，以增强刺激提高疗效。

Ⅱ. MANIPULTIONS

Sterilize the intradermal needle, forceps and skin area to be punctured. If the acupoint is located at the trunk or limb, the intradermal needle with wheat-granule shape or circle shape is seleted. To the embedding method, push the skin at the acupont area in two opposite directions with the thumb and index fingter of the left hand, hold the needle handle with a pair of the forceps held with the right hand, and insert the needle perpendicularly directly into the acupoint to the dermis. Then, horizontally puncture in a direction crossing the meridian course along the skin, and embed the needle shaft 0.5—0.1 cm inside the skin (See Fig. 4—58). Finally, fix the handle of the needle left outside on the skin with a piece of adhesive plaster. If the acupoint is located at the auricle, hold then needle handle whice is usually with a thumb—tack shape (namely, thumb—pin shape) with a pair of the forceps, direct the needle tip at the acupoint and insert it into the acupoint, making the flat—expanded handle of the needle lie flat on the skin (See Fig—4—59A). Then, stick and fix the handle with a piece of adhesive tape. Or, paste the needle handle on a piece of adhesive plaster, hold the plaster and press the handle with the thumb to paste and insert the needle accurately at the acupoint, embeddimg the needle shaft into the skin (See Fig. 4—59B). The duration of embedment varies with the season, generally, 1—2 days in summer, and 3—5 days in autumn or winter. During embedding period, the patient should press the thumb—tack needle several times daily, each time lasting 1—2 minutes, so as to strengthen the stimulation and increase the therapeutic effect.

三、注意事项

（1）关节附近不可埋针，因活动时会导致疼痛。

（2）皮肤有化脓性炎症或破溃处不宜埋针。

（3）为防止感染，针具及施术处应严格消毒，埋针处不可着水，热天因出汗较多故埋针时间不宜过长。

（4）针埋入皮内如患者感觉疼痛，或防碍肢体活动时，应将针取出重埋。

Ⅲ. PRECAUTIONS

(1) No needle embedment is allowed over the joint, otherwise pain may be caused by movement.

(2) It is not suitable to embed the needle at the purulent infected skin or at the broken and ulcer skin.

(3) In order to prevent infection, the needle apparatus and the site to be punctured should be sterilized stictly, and the punctured site should be prevented from being wetted. It is inadvisable to have the needle imbedded too long in summer as

druing that times the patient may be liable to profuse sweating.

(4) If the patient feels pain or has disorders of body movement after imbedment, the embedded needle should be taken out and then embedded again.

第四节 皮肤针

皮肤针又称"梅花针"、"七星针",是一种多针浅刺皮肤相应部位治疗疾病的方法。

一、适应范围

高血压病、头痛、近视、神经衰弱、胃肠病、斑秃、痛经、关节痛、腰背痛、肌肤麻木、肋间神经痛、面瘫、神经性皮炎等。

SECTION 4 ACUPUNCTURE WITH THE SKIN NEEDLE

Acupuncture with the skin needle, also known as the plum—blossom needling, seven — star needling, or cutaneous needling, is a needling method of treatment by using several small needles to tap on the skin of the corresponding area shallowly.

Ⅰ. INDICATIONS

It is applicable to hypertension, headache, myopia, neurasthenia, gastrointestinal disorder, alopecia areata, dysmenorrhea, arthralgia, pain of back and loin, numbness of skin, intercostal neuralgia, facial paralysis, neurodermatitis, etc.

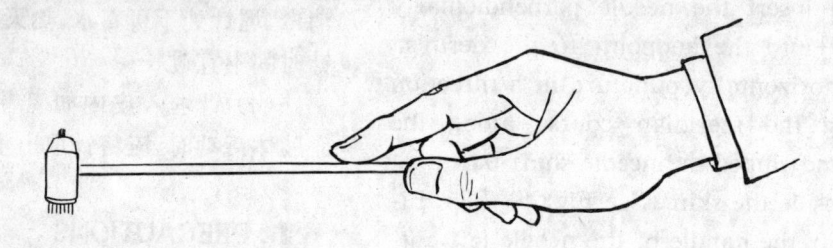

图4—60 皮肤针持针法
Fig. 4—60 Holding the Skin Needle

二、实用技法

将针具及施术部位常规消毒后,医生右手无名指与小指将针柄的后端固定于手掌小鱼际处,再以中指及拇指挟持针柄、食指压在针柄的中段(图4—60),悬肘,利用腕关节的弹力,似小鸡啄米状将针垂直叩打在皮肤上,并立即提起(图4—61),此时可发出短促的"哒"声,整个过程好似敲扬琴。要注意弹刺时一定要平刺,着力要均匀平稳、集中,不能斜刺或拖刺(图4—62)。轻叩以局部红晕充血为度;重叩以微微出血为度。叩打手法的轻重及次数,视病情及体质而定,一般叩打5~7次,叩打间距1~2厘米,叩打频率约每分钟80次左右。

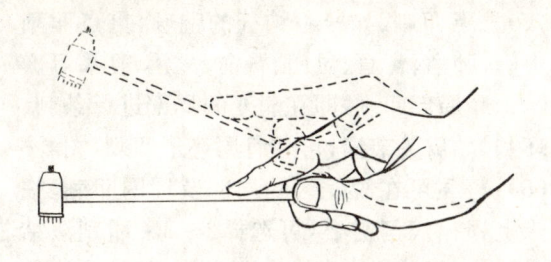

图4—61 皮肤针操作
Fig4—61 The Correct Way of Manipulating the Skin Needle

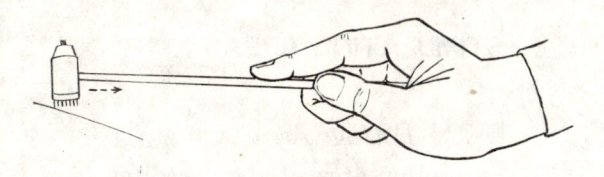

图4—62 不正确操作
Fig. 4-62 The Inccorect Way of Manipulating the Skin Needle

亦可将晶体管电针仪的一对输出导线,其中一根接在皮肤针针组上,另一根接在铜棒上,常用输出峰值电压100~120伏;输入锯齿波频率16~300次次/分;电源电压用9伏(直流)干电池;电流小于5毫安,以病人能耐受为宜(钟海泉:《中国梅花针》)。操作时,患者手握铜棒,医者持皮肤针如上法进行叩刺。

Ⅱ. MANLPULATIONS

After routine and local sterilization, fix the end of the needle handle with the ring and small fingers of the right hand at the small thenar eminence of the palm, hold the needle handle with the middle finger and the thumb of the right hand, the index finger pressing over the middle of the handle (See Fif. 4－60), tap quickly and perpendicularly on the skin with a flexible movemt of the wrist , like a chiken pecking at the rice (See Fif. 4—61), causing the short sound "da". The tapping force should focus, and no oblique or slipping puncture is allowed (See Fig. 4—62). If a gentle tapping is needed, tap until the local area appears redness and congestion; if a heavy tapping needed, tap until the local area appears bleeding . The tapping manipulation depends on the pathological condition and the patient's physical constitution. Generally , in one treatment session 5 — 7 times of tapping are done with frequency of proximately 80 times per minute and interval space being 1—2 cm.

Or, this method may be combined with electroacupuncture. To the operation, connect one of a pair of the output leads from a transistor electroacupuncture unit to the skin needle and the other to a copper stick. Usually, select 100—120 volt as the peak voltage of output, 16—300 times per minute as the frequency of output of irregular wave, and a dry batter with 9 volt and a current below 5mA (direct currect) as the power. Druing the operation, the patient is asked to hold the copper stick, and the operator holds the skin needle to tap in the same way mentioned above.

三、刺激部位

1. 常规刺激部位:背部脊正中线(督脉)及足太阳膀胱经第一侧线(脊正中线旁开1.5寸)、第二侧线(脊正中线旁开3寸)。由颈椎

（只叩督脉）、胸椎、腰骶椎，从上而下，左右共叩打五行（图4—63）。

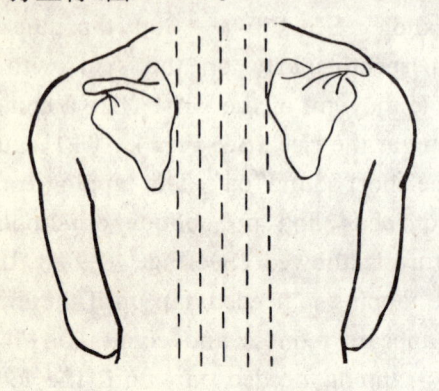

图4—63 常规刺激部位
Fig. 4—63 The Routine Stimulating Area in skin Needling

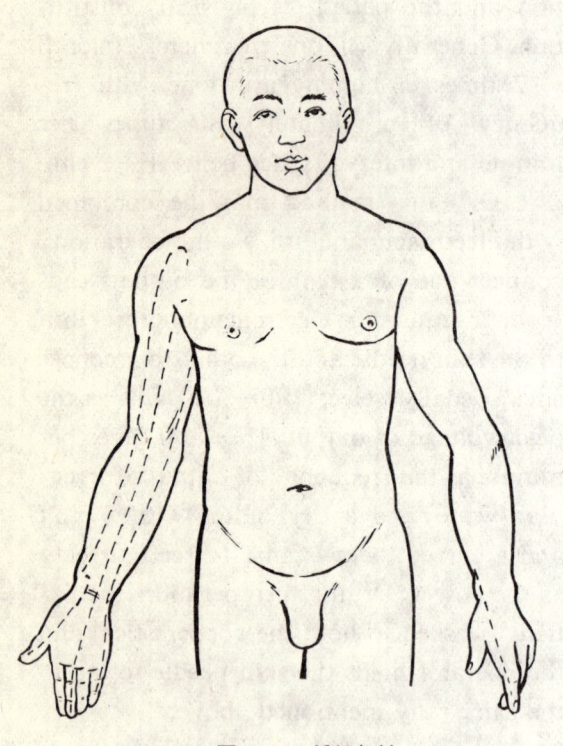

图4—64 循经条刺
Fig. 4—64 Tapping along the Meridian with Skin Needle

2. 循经条刺：即在辨证的基础上，确定病变属何脏何经后，取其相应经脉沿线叩刺。如喘咳叩刺手太阴肺经体表的循行线；偏头痛叩刺足少阳胆经及手少阳三焦经在头颈部的循行路线（图4—64）。

3. 穴位叩刺：在辨证的基础上，根据穴位的主治特点，选择一定的穴位（主要为特定穴）重点叩刺。如肾不纳气的喘咳，重点叩刺中府、肺俞、膏肓、风门、肾俞、太溪、复溜等。

4. 局部叩刺：即在病变的局部进行条刺、环刺，如肩关节痛，可在肩周环形叩刺（图4—65）；斑秃可在脱发区的局部及周围叩刺。临床上根据病情需要，可选择2～3种叩刺法结合治疗，如神经衰弱可先刺常规区，结合穴位重点叩刺心俞、肾俞、肝俞等。又如肋间神经痛，可选叩肝经循行处，结合痛处的肋间由内向外横行叩刺。

III. STIMULATING AREAS

1. The Routine Area

The routine area of skin needling includes the posterior median line on the spinal column (namely, the course of the Du Meridian on the spinal column), and the four lines respectively 1.5 cun and 3 cun lateral to the posterior median line on the back (i.e. the branches of the Bladder Meridian on the back), five lines in total (See Fig. 4—63).

2. The Corresponding Meridian Area

Take the corresponding meridian course as the stimulating area, namely, based on the differentiation of the syndromes (i.e., the patient's symptoms and signs are collected, analyzed and summarized, under the guidance of the theories of TCM, so as to identify the etiology, the location of the disease, the pathologic changes and the body conditions, etc), termime which viscus or meridian the disease is closely related to, tap on the skin along the corresponding meridian course. For example, tap on the skin along the course of the Lung Meridian of Hand—Taiyin for asthma and cough; tap on the skin at the head and nape along the courses of the Gallbladder Meridian of Foot—Shaoyang and the Triple Energezer Meridian of Hand—Shaoyang for migraine (See Fig. 4—64)

3. *The Corresponding Points*

Based on differentiation of syndromes and chief indications of the acupoint, choose some acupoints (mainly referring to the special acupoints) as tapping area. For example, asthma and cough due to failure of the kidney in receiving air may be treated by tapping on Zhongfu (LU1), Feishu (BL13), Gaohuang (BL43), Fengmen (BL12), Shenshu (BL23), Taixi (KI3), and Fuliu (KI7).

4. *The Affected Area*

Take the diseased area as the tapping area. Usually the line—puncture or circle—puncture is given to the area. For example, in treating pain of the shoulder joint, a circle—puncture over the shoulder joint is given (See Fig. 4—65); in alopecia areata, the local diseased area and the area around it may be selected in combination. In order to meet the needs of the treatment, 2—3 tapping methods may be used in coordination. In treating neurasthenia, for example, the routine stimulating area is tapped first, then some related acupoints

such as Xinshu (BL15), Shenmn (BL23), Ganshu (BL18) are tapped; and in treating intercostal neuralgia, some area along the course of the Liver Meridian is tapped in combination with tapping the painful intercostal area from middle side to the lateral side.

四、注意事项

1. 术前、术后均要注意清洁消毒,以防感染。

2. 操作前应检查针具,要求针尖平齐,无钩。

3. 局部皮肤外伤及溃疡者,不可叩刺。出血性疾病患者不可刺。

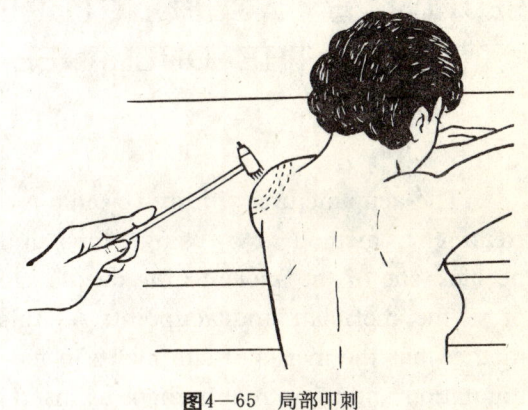

Fig. 4—65 Tapping at the Affected Area

IV. PRECAUTIONS

1. Pay attention to sterilization before and after operation so as to prevent infection.

2. Check the needle apparatus prior to operation. It is required that the tips of the needles be even and free of any hook.

3. Tapping is not allowed to the local trauma and ulcers. It is also contraindicat-

ed in the patients with hemorrhagic diseases.

第五节 鍉针

鍉针为古代九针之一,用于按压经络穴位的表面以治疗疾病。由于操作简便、无须刺入皮肤,故病人乐于接受,适宜于小儿、老人及体弱病人,亦可指导病人自行使用。

一、适应范围

宜用于经气虚弱的病症,如胃痛、腹痛、消化不良、神经性呕吐、妊娠呕吐以及神经症等。

SECTION 5 ACUPUNCTURE WITH THE DULL NEEDLE

The acupuncture with dull needle is a treatment method by using the dull needle, one of the ancient nine needles, to press the meridian and acupoint. As this method has the merits of simplicity in manipulation and of no requirement of inserting the needle into the skin, patients like to accept it, it is suitable to children, the aged or weak persons, and it can be applied to patients by the patients themselves after accepting the guidance from the doctor.

I. INDICATIONS

It is applicable to disorders caused by deficiency of qi of channel, such as stomachache, abdominal pain, indigestion, neurogenic vomiting, pregnant vomiting, and neuresis.

二、实用技法

以拇指、中指及无名指挟持针柄,食指抵压针尾(图4—66),或取用拇、食、中指捏合针柄,无名指抵住针身的四指持针法(图4—3),将针尖按压在经络穴位表面,推压时亦可以指甲上下刮动针柄增强感觉,压按轻重程度可根据病人体质与病情分为强弱两类。虚证用弱刺激,即将针轻轻压在经穴上,待局部皮肤周围发生红晕或症状缓解时,慢慢起针,起针后局部稍加揉按;实证用强刺激,即将针重压于经穴上,待病人感觉疼痛或酸胀向上下扩散时,迅速起针。

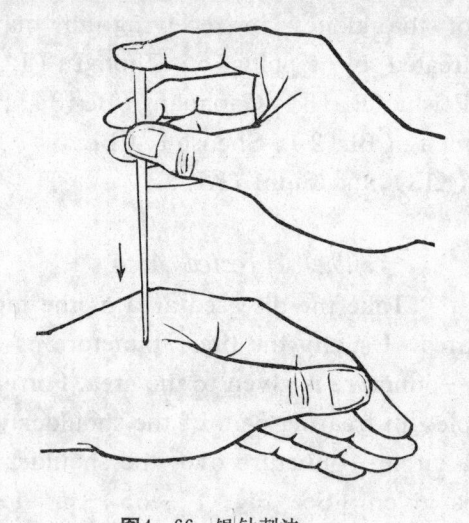

图4—66 鍉针刺法
Fig. 4—66 Pressing with the Dull Needle

10次为一疗程,轻症1~2次即可,10次后仍无效者,可结合或改用其他技法。

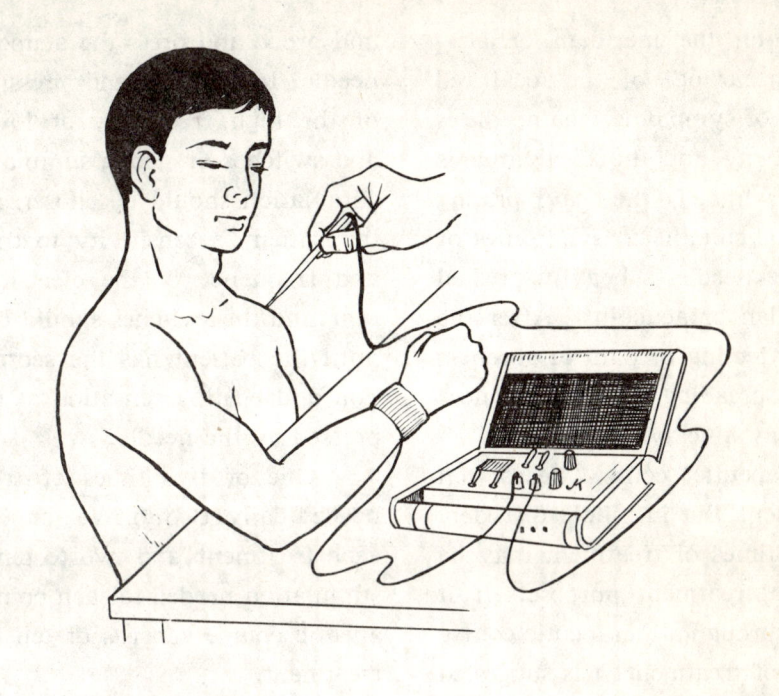

Fig 4—67 The Electrical Dull Needle

亦可利用低频脉冲电波经过锟针输入人体穴位，激发经气传导，治疗神经系统常见病和各种炎症。临床常用 ZKC—2 型电锟针治疗仪，使用前将手夹接头同负极端相接，固定在患者任一手腕上；将探针（锟针）同输出端相接用于探压穴位（图 4—67），并将电锟针频率、幅度调至最小，然后打开电源开头，探压穴位。根据病人对脉冲幅度和频率的敏感程度，选择高低频开关与强弱开关，并调节幅度和频率旋钮，待探针（锟针）头所压穴位有烧灼样感及跳动感为止。每日 1～2 次，每次选 2～5 穴，每穴刺激 2～10 分钟，10 次一个疗程。

II. MANIPULATIONS

Hold the needle with the thumb, middle and ring fingers, the index finger resisting the needle tail (See Fig. 4—66). Or hold the needle handle with the thumb, index and middle fingers, the ring finger resisting the needle shaft (See Fig. 4—3). Then, press the needle tip over the meridian or acupoint. When pressing, the needling sensation may be strengthened by scraping the needle handle with the nail of the finger. The manipulation of the dull needle may be classified, according to the intensity of the pressing force, into two: the gentle pressing and the heavy pressing. The gentle or heavy pressing method is chosen based on the patient's constitution and pathological condition. In the gentle pressing method which is suitable to syndromes of deficidncy type, the needle is gently pressed on the meridian or acupoint. After appearance of the local red areola or relief of symptoms, the needle is slowly taken away and the local area is massaged for a while. To the heavy prssing method which is suitable to syndromes of excess type, the needle is heavily pressed over the meridian or acupoint. After the patient has the feeling of pain or soreness and distension spreading upward, the needle is taken away quickly.

One therapeutic course needs ten times of treatment. But in milder disroders, one or two times of treatment may be enough for the treatment purpose. If it does not work through a therapeutic course with ten times of treatment, it is suggested that this needling method should be in combinaion with or replaced with some other therapeutic methods.

Additionally, the dull needle can be employed in treatment of disorders of the nerve system and various inflammations by conducting the pulse wave current at lower freqrency from an electric acupuncture unit through the dull needle to the acupoint of the body to induce the qi of channel to circulate and spread. Clinically, ZKC—2 type of electric dull—needling unit (made in Beijing Motomatiom Equipment Factory) is frequently employed. In the operation of this unit, connect the hand —holding junction with the negative and fix it on the wrist of one hand, connect the probing needle (i. e. a dull needle), which is used to probe and press the acupoint, with the output (See Fig. 4—67), and set the frequency and amplitude at the lowerest degree. Then, turn on the electric power and probe and press the acupoint with the needle. In probing and pressing, switches of the high frequency or low frequency and switches of strong stimulation or faint stimulation should be chosen according to the patient's sensitivity to the amplitude and frequence of the electric pulse current, and the switches should be readjusted until the patient has the scorching sensation and beating sensation at the acupoint pressed by the needle.

One or two times of treatment are needed daily, two to five acupoints selected each treatment, and two to ten minutes of stimulation needed to each point. One therapeutic course consists of ten times of the treatment.

第六节 火 针

火针是一种特制的粗针,烧热后刺入一定部位以治疗疾病的一种古老方法。

具有温经散寒、通经活络的作用。

一、适应范围

临床常用于治疗风寒湿痹,虚寒痈肿等症。除外尚有用于治疗瘰疬(淋巴结核)、顽癣、扁平疣、痣、血丝虫病象皮腿等。

SECTION 6 ACUPUNCTURE WITH THE HOT NEEDLE

The acupuncture with the hot needle is an ancient needling metod of treatment by inserting a thick needle having been warmed into a certain area. It can serve to warm the meridian, to clear and to activate the channel and collateral.

I. INDICATIONS

It is usually indicated in arthralgia due to wind—cold—dampness (wind, cold and dampness combined as a pathegen), swelling and pain due to cold of deficiency type. Additionally, it can be used in treatment of scrofula, neurodermatitis, flat wart, nevus, elephantiasis crus, filarial infection.

二、实用技法

在选定的穴位或部位上，用2％碘酊消毒后，再以75％酒精脱碘，根据患者适应情况，为减除恐惧心理及疼痛感，可选用1％普鲁卡因（也可加入0.1％盐酸肾上腺素以防出血）作浸润麻醉，2分钟后即行针。按不同病情与体质，操作可分深刺与浅刺两种。

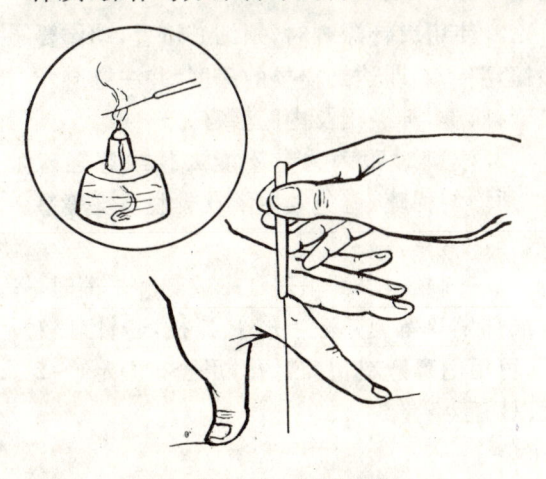

图4—68 火针深刺法
Fig. 4—68 Deep Puncture with the Hot Needle

1. 深刺：适宜于外科疾患，如痈疽、瘰疬、象皮腿等。用于排脓时选择粗些的针；用于阴症坚肿如瘰疬等，选择细些的针。一般左手用舒张法或挟持法或爪切法固定穴位，右手持针，将针身下端向针尖逐渐在酒精灯上烧红，对准穴位或一定部位迅速刺入（图4—68）立即退出，随即用消毒棉球按住针孔。

2. 浅刺：多用于治疗风湿痛及肌肤冷麻、顽癣等症。操作时右手持针，将针烧红轻轻地在皮肤表面叩刺。若治疗顽癣，可将木制皮肤针针束的针尖烧红在治疗部位叩刺，即为多针浅刺（图4—69）。

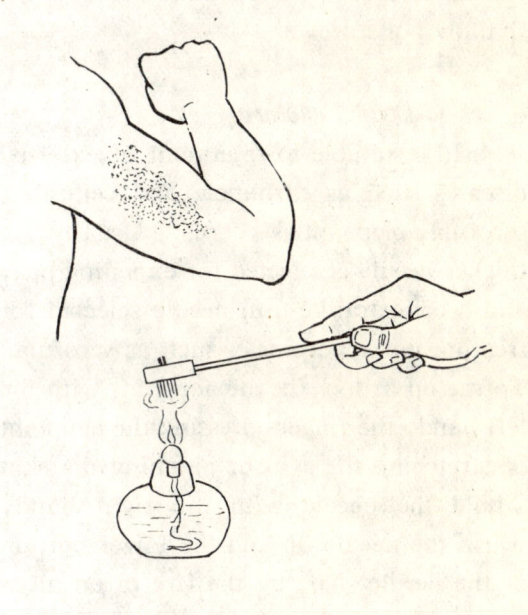

图4—69 火针浅刺法
Fig. 4—69 Shallow Puncture with the Hot Needle

一般间隔3～6天治疗1次，疗程根据病情需要确定。

II. MANIPULATIONS

Sterilize the skin of the selected acupoint or area with 2% of iodine and then swab away the iodine with 75% of alcohol. Then, according to the patient's adaptability, the infiltration anesthesia with 1% procaine (or added with 0.1% of adrenalin hydrochloride in order to prevent bleeding) may be given to minimize the patient's possible pain and terror. Two minutes later, the puncture can be carried out. The manipulation of the hot needle may be classified, according to th patient's constitution and pathological condition, into the deep puncture and the shallow puncture.

1. Deep Puncture

It is suitable to treatment of external diseases such as carbuncle and cellulitis, scrofula, elephantiasis crus. Usually, a thicker needle is selected for expelling pus, and a comparative thin needle selected for treating yin syndromes[①] such as scrofula. To the opeartion, fix the acupoint with the left hand, the fingers pressing the acupoint or stretching the skin or pinching the skin, hold the needle with the right hand, warm the needle tip and the lower portion of the needle shaft by the fire of an alcohol lamp unitl the colour of these parts of the needle becomes red, insert the needle accurately into the acupoint or a required area quickly (See Fig. 4—68) and draw it immediately. Then, press the needle hole with a sterilized cotton ball.

2. Shallow Puncture

It is mainly used in treatment of arthralgia due to wind — dampness, coldness and numbness of skin, and neurodermatitis. In the operation, hold the needle with the right hand and warm the lower portion of the needle on the fire until the colour of this portion becomes red. Then, gently tap on the skin surface with the needle. In treatment of neurodermatitis, the shallow puncture may be carried out with a skin needle (i.e. seven — star needle) which replaces the hot needle, termed as shallow puncture with multi — needles (See Fig. 4—69).

Generally, the treatment is given once per 3 — 6 days, and a therapeutic course may be long or short according to the pathological condition.

三、注意事项

1. 火针刺激强烈,体弱患者及孕妇与面部慎用或不用。

2. 使用火针深刺时,须细心慎重,动作要敏捷,要一刺即达到需要的深度,并注意避开血管,肌腱,神经干及内腔器官。

3. 浅刺时叩刺力量不能太猛或忽轻忽重,须均匀稀疏,避免发生随针剥脱表皮等事故。

4. 针刺后,局部呈现红晕或红肿未消时,或局部发痒等,应避免洗浴、抓搔,若针刺较深,可用消毒敷料覆盖针孔,用胶布固定1~2天以防感染。

III. PRECAUTIONS

---

① The symptoms and signs which are chronic, cold, inactive, weak, depressed, hypofunctional, hypometabolic, retrogressive, inward, or downward in nature are classified as the yin syndrome, which belongs to yin in nature.

1. The hot needling should be used with a great care or even should be contraindicated to patients with a week constitution or to pregnant women because the stimulation caused by hot needling is strong. It is contraindicated to the face.

2. In applying deep puncture, the operator should be carefull, manipulating the needle swiftly, inserting it to the required depth by one motion and avoiding the blood vessels, muscular tendons, and nerve trunks, as well as internal organs.

3. In applying shallow puncture, the operator should not tap too forcefully or with an uneven force. The tapping should be even and loose in space so as to prevent incidents such as epidermal desquamation with withdrawing the needle.

4. After puncture, the patient should not bathe or scratch the skin until the local redness and swelling are disppeared. If tapping too deep, the needle hole should be covered with the sterilized dress and the dress be fixed with the adhesive plaster for one to two days so as to prevent infection.

第七节 电 针

针刺穴位得气后,在针上通以接近人体生物电的微量电流,以加强对穴位的刺激,从而达到治疗疾病的一种方法。它具有调整人体功能,加强镇痛、镇静、促进血液循环,调整肌张力等作用。

电针的配穴处方与毫针取穴大致相同。一般以取两侧肢体1～3对穴位为宜(即1～3对导线)。过多会刺激太强,患者难以忍受。

一、实用技法

针刺穴位得气后(神志失常、知觉麻木、小儿患者例外),将输出电位器调至"0"度,负极接主穴,正极接配穴,也有不分正负极,将两根导线任接两只针柄上(图4—70),一般将同一对输出电极连接在身体的同侧,胸背部的穴位使用电针时,更不可将两个电极跨接在身体的两侧。拨开电源开关,选择所需波型与频率,逐渐调高输出电流至所需的电流量,使病人出现酸麻等感觉又能耐受为度。通电时间一般为10～20分钟。治疗完毕,把电位器回到"0"度,关闭电源拆去输出导线退出毫针。治疗中由于人体经过多次刺激后会产生适应性,感觉亦会由强变弱,此时可加大输出电流量或改变频率,以保持恒定的刺激作用。

如果病情只需用一个穴位,可把一根导线接在针柄上,另一根导线接在一块约2×3厘米大小的薄铅板上,外包几层湿纱布,平放在离针稍远的皮肤上(一般为大椎穴或一侧的三阴交或内关穴),用带子固定(图4—71),

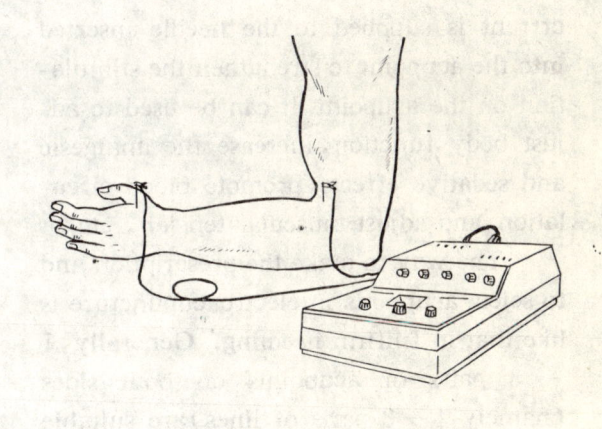

图4—70 两穴通电法

Fig. 4 — 70 The Way of Applying Electroacupuncture to Two Points

然后如同上法操作,即打开电源,调好应选的波型与频率,再慢慢调高至病人能耐受的电流量。

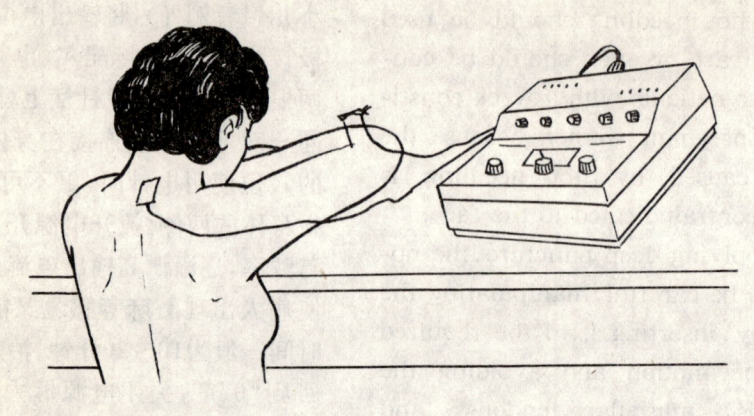

Fig. 4—71 The Way of Applying Electroacupuncture to One Point

SECTION 7 ELECTROACUPUNCTURE

Electroacupuncture is a kind of therapeutic technique in which an electric current which is almost as weak as bioelectric crrrent is supplied to the needle inserted into the acupoint to strengthen the stimulation on the acupoint. It can be used to adjust body function, increase the analgesic and sedative effects, promote blood circulation, and adjust muscular tension, etc.

The way to make the prescription and to select acupoints in electroacupuncture is like that in filifirm needling. Generally, 1 — 3 pairs of acupoints on both sides (namely 1 — 3 paris of lines) are suitable in number. Too many acupoints used once may induce too strong stimolation for the patient to stand it.

I. MANIPULATIONS

After needling sensation is induced, a required electroacupuncture unit is selected. The output potentiometer in the electroacupuncture unit is set to "0", the negative electrode is connected to the main acupoint and the positive one to the corresponding acupoint. But it is allowed to attach the lines to the needles without considering the negative or the positive, namely, a pair of output leads are connected to the handles of a pair of needles with no choice (See Fig. 4—70). Generally, two output electrodes of a pair should be connected to the same side of the body. Moreoer, when the electroacupuncture is applied to the acupoints on the back and chest, it is forbidden to connect a pair of output electrodes to two sides of the body, otherwise a serious accident may occur. Then, the power switch is turned on, the designed wave mode and frequency are selected, and the output crrrent is gardually increased until tolerable soreness and numbness are induced to the patient. The duration of electric stimulation is usually 10 — 20 minutes. At the end of the operation, the potentiometer is set back to "O", the power switch is turned off, the output lead to the needle is disconnected, and the filiform needles are withdrawn. The patient who has experienced electroacupuncture many times may become gradually tolerant to this stimulation and his or her needling sensation may decrease gradrally. For this kind patient, the increase of electric current and change of the frequency are necessary in maintaining constant stimulation.

If only one acupoint is needed in treatment, one of a pair of leads is connected to the handle of the needle, and the other connected to a thin piece of black about 2×3 cm in size, which is wrapped by several layers of wet cloth and laid on the skin somewhat remote to the needle (usually on Dazhui Du 14, or Sanyinjiao SP 6, or Neiguan PC 6 on the one side), and fixed there with the thread (See Fig. 4 — 71). Then, the rest operation procedure is done in the same way mentioned above.

二、波型的选择与适应范围

低频脉冲电流的波型、频率不同,其作用也不同,临床使用时应根据病情选择适当的波型,频率,以提高疗效。

密波(或叫高频):频率快,一般在每秒50～100次,能降低神经应激功能,先对感觉神经起抑制作用,接着对运动神经也产生抑制作用。常用于镇痛、镇静、缓解肌肉和血管痉挛,治疗各种痛症,并用于针刺麻醉等。

疏波(或叫低频):频率慢,一般在每秒2～5次,刺激作用较强,能引起肌肉收缩,提高肌肉韧带的张力,对感觉与运动神经的抑制发生较迟。常用于治疗痿证,各种关节、肌肉、韧带的损伤等。

疏密波:是疏波、密波自动交替出现的一种波型,能克服单一波型易产生适应性的缺点,治疗时兴奋效应占优势,能促进代谢、气血循环,改善组织营养,消除炎性水肿。常用于疼痛、扭挫伤、关节炎、气血运行障碍、坐骨神经痛、面瘫、肌无力、局部冻伤等。

断续波:为有节律地时断时续自动出现的一种疏波。能提高肌肉组织的兴奋性,对横纹肌有良好的刺激作用。常用于痿证、瘫痪。

锯齿波:为脉冲波幅按锯齿型自动改变的起伏波。其频率接近于人体的呼吸规律,故又称呼吸波。可用于刺激膈神经,作人工电动呼吸,抢救呼吸衰竭。还有提高神经肌肉兴奋性,调整经络功能,改善气血循环的作用。

II. SELECTION AND INDICATIONS OF THE WAVE FORMS

The function of a low — frequency pulse current varies with its wave and frequency. In clinical practice, the proper wave and frequency should be selected by considering the patient's condition so as to enhance the therapeutic effect.

High Frequency: also termed dense wave. Its frequency is high, usually at 50 — 100 pulses per second, it can serve to lower nerve irritability by inhibiting the sensory nerve at first and then motor nerve. This frequency is usually selected to induce analgesic and sedative effects and to relax spasm of muscle and blood vessels, for treatment of painful syndromes and for anaethesia, etc.

Low Frequency: Also termed sparse wave. Its frequency is low, generally at 2 — 5 pulses per second, and its stimulation is comparatively strong. It may induce contracture of muscle and increase tension of muscle and ligament. Its result to inhibite the sensory and motor nerves occurs comparatively late. This frequency is usually indicated in atrophy, impairment of joint, muscle, and ligament, etc.

Irregular Wave: Also termed alternately dense and sparse wave. This wave is formed by spontaneously alternate appearance of low and high waves, which has merit to avoid the patient's toleration which is easily caused by application of only one kind of wave. As having the excitation function in domination, it can serve to promote metabolism and circulation of qi and blood, to improve tissue nutriton, and to subdue inflammatary swelling. It is usually applied to painful syndromes, injuries due to sprain and contusion, arthritis, disorders of circulation of qi and blood, sciatic neuralgia, facial paralysis, amyostenia, local cold injury, etc.

Intermittent Wave: It is a special kind of low frequency, appearing regularly and intermittently. It can serve to enhance irritability of muscular tissue, and to effect a good stimulation to strained muscle. It is seleted for atrophy, and paralysis.

Sawtooth Wave: This wave appears in a way with its wave shape like the sawtooth. Its frequency is almost like that of person's respiration, so it is also termed resperatory wave. It may serve to stimulate the phrenic nerve and to be used as an electric spirophorus to salvage the patient with respiratory failure, and it may also serve to enhance the irritability of nerve

and muscle, to adjust the channel function and to improve circulation of qi and blood.

三、注意事项

1. 若电流输出时断时续，须注意导线接触是否良好，应检修后再用。

2. 有心脏病者，应避免电流回路通过心脏。靠近延髓、脊髓部位使用电针时，电流输出量宜小，以免发生意外。孕妇慎用。

3. 调节电流量应从小到大逐渐增加，以防突然增强引起肌肉强烈收缩，造成病人不能耐受，甚至折针、弯针或晕针的痛苦。

4. 电针器最大输出电压在40伏以上者，最大输出电流应控制在1毫安以内，以免发生触电危险。

5. 直流电或脉冲直流电有电解作用，容易引起断针和灼伤组织，不能作电针器的输出电流。

6. 毫针的针柄如因温针灸而表面氧化不导电，应将电针器输出的导线挟持在针身上。

III. PRECAUTIONS

1. If the output current is discontinuous, it may be due to poor connection of the lead. It is necessary to have a check and repair it.

2. In the patient with heart disease, the back flow of the current should be prevented from passing through the heart. In the area near the bulb and spinal cord, the output current should be low, otherwise an accident may occur. It should be given with a great care to the pregnant women in the operation.

3. The increase of the electroc current

should be gradrated, othertwise the patient may not stand it, or even the needle be broken or bent, or needling fainting be caused, as sudden increase of electric current will cause contructure of muscle.

4. The direct current or direct pulse current which has electrolysis and is liable to causing fracture of needle and the burn of the tissue should not be used as output current of the electroacupuncture unit.

5. If the electroacupuncture current has its output voltage above 40 volts, the output current should be limited to below 1 mA so as to avoid electric shock.

6. If the surface of the handle of the needle having been burnt in the warming needling method through moxibustion (a kind of moxibustion method, by burning the pulp of mugwort on the handle of the needle after inserting it into the body) is oxidizied and poor in electric conduction, the output lead of the unit should be connected to the shaft of the needle instead of the needle handle.

第八节 水 针

水针，是选用某些药物注入穴位及局部痛点内，以充分发挥针刺及药物的综合效能，达到防治疾病的一种治疗方法。

一、适应范围

各种类型腰腿、肩背、关节疼痛，软组织损伤、肌肉麻木、萎缩、胃肠、肝胆疾患，以及毫针的一般适应症等。

SECTION 8 HYDRO—ACUPUNCTURE (POINT INJECTION)

Hydro — acupuncture, also termed point injection, is a needling therapy by injection of some liquid medicine into the acupoint or local painful spot for the purpose of prevention and treatment of diseases. It has the merit to promote the synthetic effect of acupuncture and drug.

Ⅰ. INDICATIONS

Various pains of the loin and leg, shoulder and back, and joint, injuries, numbness of the muscle, atrophy, gastrointestinal disorders, liver and gallbladder disorders, as well as the disorders which the filiform needle is applicable to.

二、实用技法

1. 根据注射部位及所需注射药量，选用不同类型的注射器及针头。一般多用5号、6号、7号针头。深部穴位如环跳等，可用9号针头、耳穴可选用1～2毫升注射器，5号针头。

2. 根据病情选用有效穴位，一般每次以1～3对穴位为宜。常以特定穴多用，也可选择压痛点以及病损肌肉的起止点。

3. 注射的药量视病情及穴位而定，头面部穴位可注射0.3～0.5毫升；耳穴注射0.1～0.2毫升；四肢部1～2毫升；胸背部0.5～1毫升；腰臀部2～5毫升。治疗瘫痪及各类肌病时，可于肌肉的起止点进针，注射剂量可大，一般10～20毫升(可将药液用生理盐水或5%葡萄糖注射液稀释)。

4. 将药液注入穴位时，应先将注射器及针头严格消毒，选择相宜的注射器，用消毒镊子挟住大小合适的针头,紧套在注射器上(图4—72①),医者左手拿住药瓶,并固定注射套管,右手挟住注射器轴心尾端(图4—72—②),抽足应注药液量,再缓慢地推动轴心朝着气泡的方向排空注射器内空气(图4—72③)。然后在穴位局部皮肤常规消毒下,右手拇、食、中指持注射器、无名指扶住针头柄部,左手撑开应注射部位周围的皮肤(手不要碰到已消毒的针头及施术处),对准穴位快速刺入皮下,缓慢进针寻找针感,待出现酸、胀、重

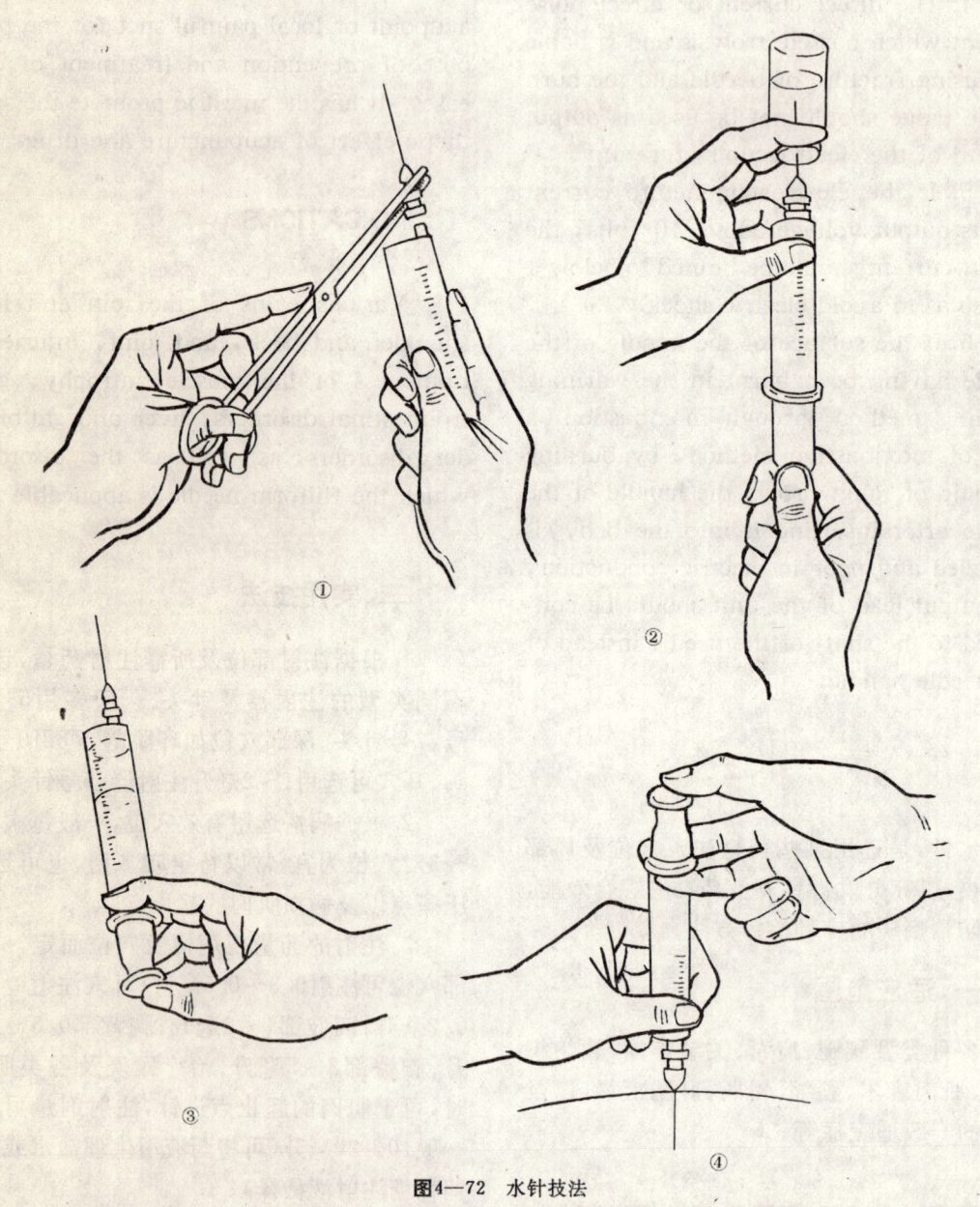

图4—72 水针技法

Fig. 4—72 Manipulating in the Hydro-Acupuncture

感后,略回抽注射器轴心,若无回血即可注入药液(图4—72④),肌肉萎缩、瘫痪的病人,选择病肌起止点进针后,即将针呈15～45°角深刺入到肌腹,边注边将针后退,使其药液浸入瘫痪或萎缩的肌肉内。

急症每日1～2次,慢性病一般每日或隔日1次,5～10次为一疗程。

Ⅱ. MANIPULATIONS

1. Selection of the syringe and syringe needle depends on the location to be injected and the amount of solution to be needed. Generally, No. 5, No. 6 and No. 7 needles are usually selected. But if the acupoint is at the area with rich muscle, such as Huantiao (GB 30), No. 9 needle may be used. For the acupoint on the auricle (i. e. otopoint) 1 — 2 ml syringe and No. 5 needle may be used.

2. The effective acupoints should be selected according to the patient's condition. Usually, it is suitable to use 1 — 3 pairs of acupoints once, in which the special acupoints are often chosen, and sometimes the tender spot and the beginning and ending spots of the diseased muscle may also be chosen.

3. The dosage to be injected depends upon the patient's conditions and the acupoint selected. Generally, 0. 3 — 0. 5ml drug fluid may be injected to one acupoint at the head and face; at the auricle, 0. 1 — 0. 2ml can be injected; in the limbs, 1 — 2ml injected; in the chest and back, 0. 5 — 1ml injected; and in the loin and buttock, 2 — 5 ml injected. For treatment of paralysis and various muscular disorders, the beginning and ending spots of the muscle are injected with large amount of dose, which generally is 10 — 20ml (the drug fluid may be diluted with normal physiological saline or 5% of glucose solution).

4. Strictly sterilize the syringes and syringe needles before they are used, select a proper syringe and hold a proper syringe needle with the sterilized forceps to fix it on the syringe (See Fig. 4—72A). Hold the drug bottle and fix the syringe tube with the left hand. Then, hold the end of the piston of the syringe with the right hand (See Fig. 4—72B). After aspiring enough durg fluid, slowly push the piston to expel the air in the cavity of the syringe (See Fig. 4—72C). Then, hold the syringe with the thumb, middle and index fingers of the right hand, the ring finger holding back the handle of the needle, stretch the skin around the puncture point where the routine local sterilization has been given with the fingers of the left hand moving in the opposite directions (but not touch the sterilized area to be injected and the needle), and swiftly insert the needle into the acupoint to the subcutaneous tissue. Then, slowly insert it to induce the needling sensation. After the patient complains of soreness, distension and heaviness, inject the drug fluid if no blood is aspired into the syringe by slightly withdrawing the piston (See Fig 4—72D). For treatment of muscular atrophy and paralysis, the initial point and the terminal point of the diseased muscle are selected for insertion of the needle. After the needle tip is pierced through the skin, the needle is further inserted deep obliquely to the belly of the muscle in an angle of 15—45° to the

skin. Then, the drug is injected into the muscle while the needle being withdrawn, making the drug fluid filtrate into the diseased muscle.

For acute cases, injection is given 1 — 2 times daily; for chronic cases, it given once every day or every other day. One therapeutic course needs 5 — 10 times of treatment.

三、注意事项

1. 所选穴位附近有疖肿、湿疹、炎症等情况时,可另选其他功效相同的穴位注射。

2. 进针后如回抽有血,可稍退针避开血管再行回抽,无血方可注药。

3. 药液一般不能注入关节腔、脊髓腔,否则会引起关节红肿热痛,及脊髓损伤;针尖也不可碰到骨膜,以免引起骨膜刺激症状。

4. 颈项、胸背部注射时切勿过深,以免伤及内脏。注射速度宜慢。

5. 在有神经干的部位注射时,应避开神经干,针进入一定深度如出现触电感时,应立即退针,改换角度再进,以免损伤神经。

6. 要注意所选用药物的性能、剂量、副作用等,凡能引起过敏反应的药物,如普鲁卡因等,必须先作皮内试验。副作用较强的药物不宜采用。

7. 孕妇下腹,腰骶部,三阴交,合谷等穴位不宜作水针;年老体弱者选穴宜少,药量酌减。

8. 注射器如有漏气,针头有钩者,均剔除不宜使用。

III. PRECAUTIONS

1. If there are carbuncle and swelling, eczema, or inflammation near the selected acupoint, another acupoint having the same function as the selected one may be used instead of the selected one.

2. If blood is aspired into the syringe by withdrawing the piston after insertion, the needle should be drawn a little to avoid the blood vessel, then the drug fluid is injected after no blood is aspired into the syringe by withdrawing the piston again.

3. The ordinary drug fluid is not allowed to be injected into the joint cavity and spinal canal, otherwise swelling, heat and pain of the joint and impairment of the spinal cord may be caused. The tip of the needle is not allowed to touch the periosteum, otherwise the irritable symptoms of the periosteum may occur.

4. In the nape, chest and back, no deep injection is allowed, otherwise the internal organ may be injured. Moreover the speed of injection at these places should be slow.

5. In the region with main nerve trunk passing through, pay attention to avoiding the nerve trunk in insertion and injection. When causing an electrifying sensation to the patient, the needle should be drawn immediately and try to insert the needle in a different angle so as to prevent injuring the nerve.

6. Pay attention to the property, dosage and side — effect of the drug fluid to be used. The drugs which can induce the allergic reaction, including penicillin, procaine, etc. should be used after the skin test is done. The drug with too strong side — effect is not suitale to be used in hydro

—acupuncture。

7. To the pregnant women, it is not allowed to apply hydro—acupuncture to the acupoints at the lower abdomen, lumbo—sacral region, and some acupoints on which acupuncture is not allowed during pregnancy, such as Sanyinjiao(SP 6)and Hegu(LI 4). To the aged and weak patients, it is suitable to use fewer acupoints and to reduce the dosage。

8. The syringe with air going out freely or the needle with its tip hooked is not allowed to be used.

第九节 耳 针

耳针是借助耳廓穴位诊治疾病的一种方法。早在《灵枢、邪气脏腑病形》篇就记载:"十二经脉,三百六十五络,其血气皆上于面而起空窍……其别气走于耳而为听"。说明耳不单纯是个听觉器官,并与全身经脉皆有联系。此外,耳还能通过经络与肾、心、脾、肺、脑等脏器密切联系。为此,观察耳部的变化,刺激相应的耳穴与反应点,又可达到诊治疾病的目的。

耳针操作简便,适应症广,功能性疾病、器质性疾病用之均有效果。对于某些病,如流行性腮腺炎,治疗时针腮腺、屏间(内分泌);晕车、晕船者在乘坐车船前针脑(皮质下)、神门、枕穴,可达预防目的。此外,耳穴还可对疾病的临床诊断起辅助作用,凡属毫针的适应症,均宜于耳针治疗。手术时,对耳穴进行针刺可作麻醉用。

一、实用技法

(一)耳穴探查

1. 肉眼观察法:清洁患者耳廓,医者用拇、食指牵拉耳轮后上方(图4—73),自上而下用肉眼或借用放大镜,直接观察病变相应区形态,色泽等的变化。如丘疹、脱屑、结节、充血、小水泡、凹陷等。这些现象即称为阳性反应点。

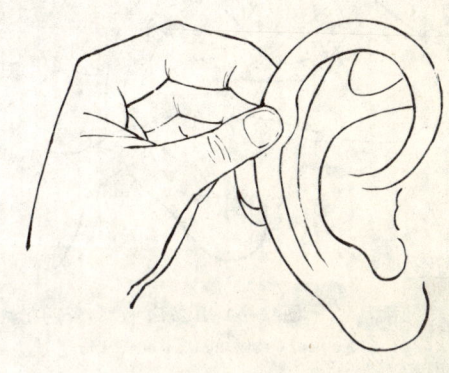

图4—73 肉眼观察法

Fig. 4—73 Detecting on the Auricle with the Naked Eye

(1)变色:临床上常见的有红晕、白色、暗红色、褐色、暗灰色。形状可有点状、片状或环状。常见于急慢性胃炎、胃、十二指肠溃疡、阑尾炎、气管炎以及各种关节炎、肝胆疾患、头痛、神经痛等。

(2)变形:医者肉眼观察或用手触摸耳部,发现耳穴形状有点状凹陷、条索状或结节状隆起等。多见于器质性病变,如肝脾肿大、肿瘤、骨质增生等。

(3)丘疹:呈红色或白色点状。红色为急性或炎症性疾病;白色为慢性或器质性疾病。

(4)脱屑:呈白色片状,似糠皮样物,一般不易剥落。多见于耳甲腔、三角窝、耳轮脚周围、耳舟等处。临床常见于各种皮肤病、便秘以及吸收、代谢功能不良,内分泌功能紊乱等病症。

2. 耳穴压按法:即用毫针针柄、探针、火柴梗等,以均匀的压力在病变相应区压按(图4—74),当压到敏感点时,病人会出现皱眉、呼痛、躲闪等反应，以最痛点作为针刺点。

3.电阻测定法：用耳穴探测仪或经络探测仪，在耳壳相应区探查低阻点，即导电性能良好的"良导点"，作为判定耳穴或刺激点的参考。

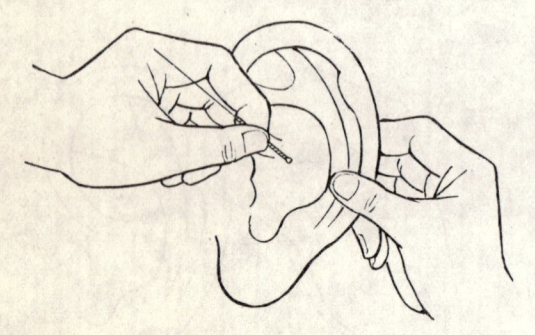

图4—74 压按法
Fig. 4—74 Pressing on the Auricle

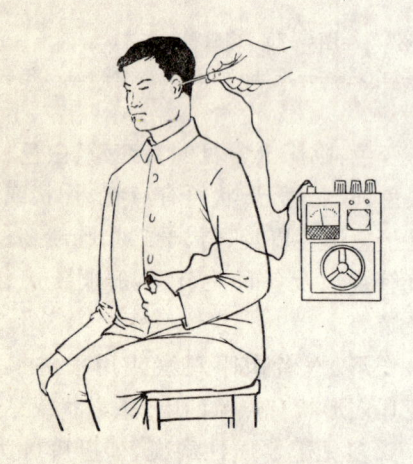

图4—75 耳穴电阻测定法
Fig. 4—75 Measuring the Electrical Resistance of the Otopoint

耳穴探测仪品种多样，测定时无关电极若为棒式，可由病人用手握住；若为片状，可固定在病人大椎穴上。医者手持探测电极，在病人耳廓上的相应区着力轻而均匀缓慢探测（图4—75），当喇叭声音增强，或表图指针摆动加大读数明显增高时，这点即为"低阻点"。若患者双耳均查找不出痛点或低阻点，亦可直接在选定的耳穴上施术。

（二）消毒

耳穴消毒要求严密，先用2%碘酒涂擦，后用75%酒精脱碘。针具也要求严密消毒。

（三）刺激方法

1.毫针刺法：找准穴位后用针柄按压标记，局部消毒，选用1寸左右的短毫针，术者左手拇、食指固定耳廓，中指抵托针刺部位的耳背（图4—76），使之便于掌握针刺深度和减轻针刺时的疼痛。然后右手拇、食、中三指持针，在所标记的敏感点或耳穴处捻转进针。一般以刺透软骨，不刺透对侧皮肤为度，刺激强度和针刺手法视病人的具体情况而定，多捻转而不提插。留针时间约15～30分钟，慢性病或疼痛性疾病亦可留针1～2小时，每间隔5～10分钟捻转一次，每次几秒钟至1分钟。起针时左手托住耳背，右手起针并立即用消毒干棉球或干棉扦压迫针眼，以防出血，再以酒精涂擦消毒。本法可用于一般常见病多发病，尤以胃肠、心血管病及神经系统病与各种痛症、炎症多用。

2.贴敷法：又称压丸法。是一种代替埋针（揿针）的简易方法，安全无痛苦易于接受。操作时先将耳区局部常规消毒，左手固定耳廓，右手用镊子夹取黏有中药王不留行籽或绿豆、小米、油菜籽、磁珠等物（以王不留行籽多用）的胶布，对准已选好的耳穴贴敷（图4—77），按压数秒钟或1～2分钟。儿童、老人轻压刺激，急性病或痛症重压强刺激。并嘱患者每日在贴敷处自行按压2～3次，每次每穴按压1～3分钟，每次贴敷3～5天，按病情予以增减或更换耳穴，10次一个疗程，必要时间隔3～5天后再作第二疗程。本法宜于老年慢性支气管炎、胆结石、高血压、近视、失眠等病症。

3.梅花针法：患者先行按摩双耳数分钟，待耳廓呈轻度充血状态后，消毒所选耳区，医师左手固定托住耳廓，右手持消毒的梅花针

（药液浸泡消毒），运用针的集束端，选定的耳穴或敏感点，利用腕力，轻巧、快速地如雀啄样点刺（图4—78）。以耳区充血、发热，局部少量渗血为度，先用消毒干棉球或棉扦将渗血按擦一下，然后再以75％酒精棉球消毒。每日1～2次，10次为一疗程。

4. 刺血法：刺血前以手按摩耳廓使之充血，严密消毒应刺部位，右手持消毒三棱针，对准耳穴快速点刺，并以手挤压出血。如刺耳

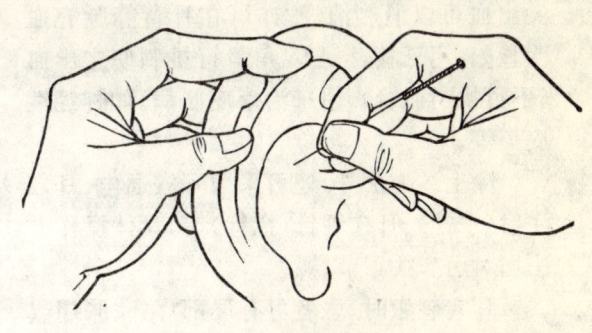

图4—76 耳穴刺法
Fig. 4—76 Puncturing at the Otopoint with the Filiform Needle

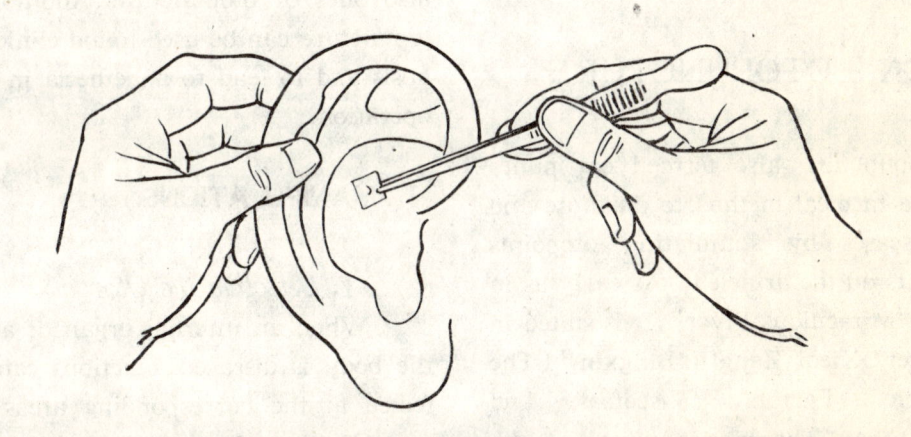

图4—77 耳穴贴敷法
Fig. 4—77 The Otopoint-Mounting Method

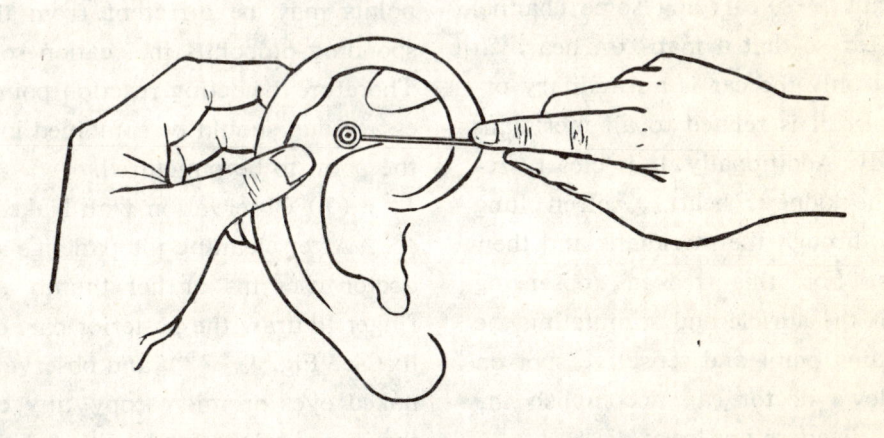

图4—78 耳穴皮肤针刺法
Fig. 4—78 Puncturing at the Otopoint with the Plum-Blossom Needle

尖出血可以退热消炎；亦可在耳背静脉充血明显处，用三棱针呈45°角斜行挑刺使之出血（不可挑断血管），用来治疗皮肤病。如神经性皮炎等。

除上述方法外，还可采用耳穴通电、耳穴注射（水针）、耳穴埋针（揿针）等，具体操作方法均对照有关章节。

耳穴刺激时，患者可有局部疼痛、胀痛或热感、酸麻感，个别患者尚有感觉沿经放散的特征。

SECTION 9 OTOPUNCTURE

Otopuncture, also termed ear puncture, is a medical method to diagnose and treat diseases by stimulating otopoints (acupoints on the aruicle). As early as in the book "Miraculous Pivot", It is stated in its chapter "Xieqi Zangfu Bingxin" (The Pathogenic Factors, Viscera, And Diseases) that "The blood and qi of the twelve regular meridians and their 365 collaterals ascend to the face and into the sense organs, ... carrying some channel qi to the ear so that a man can hear." It means not only the ear is an auditary organ, but also it is related to all meridians of the body. Additionally, it is closely related to the kidney, heart, spleen, lung and brain through the meridians and their collaterals. For this reason, observing changes of the auricle and stimulating the corresponding point and sensative spot on the auricle, a doctor can accomplish the prupose to diagnose and treat diseases.

Otopuncture has the advantages of simplicity and convenience in operation and a wide range of indications on its applying. It is effective to both functional and organic diseases. Moreover, It has preventive effect to some diseases. For example, otopoint (Ot.) Parotid Glands and Endocrine are punctured to prevent mumps during its epidemic season; Ot. Brain, Ot. Shenmen and Ot. Occiput are punctured before taking boat or bus to prevent sea disease. In a word, all indications of acupuncture with the filiform needle are also ones of otopuncture. Additionaly, otopuncture can be used to aid clinical diagnosis and to lead to anaethesia in surgical operation.

I . MANIPULATIONS

1. *Detecting the Otopoint*

When an internal organ or a part of the body is diseased, reactions can be detected at the corresponding areas on the auricle. Clinical practice has proved that stimulating these reaction points yields good therapeutic results. But the reaction points may be different from the corresponding otopoints in location sometimes. Therefore, detecting reaction points is necessary and should be combined in selecting the point to be punctured.

(1) Observation with Naked Eye

After cleaning the patient's auricle, a doctor uses his or her thumb and index finger to draw the posterior part of the helix (See Fig. 4—73), and observe, with the naked eyes or microscopy, any change in the form, colour, and lustre of the corresponding area on the auricle, such as rush, desquamation, tubercle, congestion, small blister, depression, and so on, from the upper to the lower of the auricle. The area with the change is termed positive reaction spot (i. e. reaction point, tender or sensitive point).

a. Change in colour: It is usually seen in clinic that the colour becomes white, dark—red, brown, or gloomy. The form with changed colour may be like spot, patchy or circle. These changes in colour are easily seen in chronic and acute gastritis, gastronal and duodenal ulcers, pendicitis, tracheitis, arthritis, disorders of liver and gallbladder, headache, neuralgia, etc.

b. Change in the form: The changes such as depression, streak or nodular prominence may be found by observing the aurick with the naked eyes or touching it with the finger. The changes are usually seen in organic diseases such as hepatosplenomegaly, tumor, hyperosteogeny.

c. Rush: It seems like red or white spot. The red one indicates acute or inflammatory diseases, and the white one, chronic or organic disease.

d. Desquamation: It is white and patchy, and like branny. It is usually difficult to be taken away. It mainly occurs at the cavum concha. triangular fossa, area around the helix crus, and scapha. In clinic it is usually found in skin disorders, constipation, dysfunction of absorption, metabolic disorder, dyshormonism, etc.

(2) Detecting the Tender Spot

The disease — related corresponding area on the auricle is evenly pressed with a probe, match, or the needle handle (See Fig. 4—74). When the sensitive spot is pressed, the patient will have reactions such as frowning, dodging or calling out with pain. The most tender spot should be taken as the puncture point.

(3) Detacting Electrical Changes

An otopoint—probing apparatus or a channel—probing apparatus is used to detect the corresponding areas on the auricle to look for the spot with lower electrical resistance (namely, good — conducted spot), which is good in conducting electricity. The spot is taken as the reference for determining the puncture point or stimulating point.

There are various otopoint — probing —apparatuses. If an apparatus is with a stick — like free electrode, the electrode may be held by the patient with his hand; if with a patchy — like one, it may be fixed on the patient at Dazhui (DU 14). The doctor holds the probing electrode with hand to probe the corresponding area on the auricle evenly and slowly (See Fig. 4—75). During probing, when the trumpet of the apparatus sounds alouder or the swing finger of the apparatus becomes large and its reading increases obviously at some spot, the spot is right the "lower resistance spot" or "good—conducting spot". If a painful spot or lower resistant spot is not found, the designed otopoint may be directly punctured.

2. *Sterilization*

A strict sterilization with 2% of iodine and then with 75% of alcohol to disappear the iodine is required at the area to be punctured on the auricle. The needles are also required to be sterilized with high temperature and pressure or in the drug fluid.

3. *Method of Stimulation*

(1) Puncture with the Filiform Needle

After locating the point accurately, press it with the needle handle to make a mark on it, and give a routine local sterilization. Then, fix the auricle with the thumb and index finger of the left hand, and hold back the posterior area of the puncture area with the middle finger of the left hand (See Fig. 4—76) in order to control the depth of insertion of the needle and to relieve pain due to insertion. Then, hold the needle with the thumb, index and middle fingers of the right hand, and insert it into the marked spot as twirling it. The depth of insertion is just to pierce through the cartillage but not through the skin of the oppsite srurface. The stimulation intensity and manipulation depends upon the patient's condition, and usually, the manipulation is twirling more without lifting or thrusting. The retention of the needle is usually for 15—30 minutes, but in treating chronic or painful diseases, it may be for 1—2 hours. During the retention, tweirl the needle for several seconds to one minute per 5—10 minutes. When withdrawing the needle, hold the back of the auricle with the left hand, withdraw the needle and immediately press over the punctured hole with a sterilized dry cotton ball to prevent bleeding. Finally, use alcohol to sterilize the area.

The puncture with the filiform needle may be applicable to common diseases, especially to gastrointestinal disorder, cardiovascular disorder, neuropathy, as well as painful syndromes and inflammation.

(2) Mounting

The mounting method is also termed "pill—pressing". It is a simple way instead of embedding the intradermal needle beneath the skin. It is safe and painless, as well as easily acceptable to the patients. To the operation, give a routine and local sterilization to the selected area on the auricle, fix the auricle with the left hand, grip a piece of adhesive plaster on which a vaccaria seed, magnet drop or muny been is stuck (usually, the vaccaria seed is employed). Then, paste it with the right hand on the auricle with the seed or some other material directly pressing at the otopoint selected (See Fig. 4—77). Finally, press it for several seconds or 1—2 minutes. In treating children or aged persons, slightly press the seed to lead to mild stimulation, while in acute or painful disease, press heavily to lead strong stimulation. Advise the patient to press the seed by himself 2—3 times daily, and every time for 1—3 minutes on each point. The plaster is kept for 3—5 days in one treatment session, The number of plaster or the otopoints may be changed according to the pathological condition. Ten times of treatment is needed in one therapeutic course, and the next course will begin after an interval of 3—5 days if it necessary.

(3) Puncture with the Plum—Blossom Needle

Sterilize the selected area on the auricle after asking the patient himself to massage the auricle for several minutes to lead to slight congestion in the aruicle. Hold the plum—blossom needle sterlized in the drug fluid with the right hand, and use it to prick the selected otopoint or sensitive spot swiftly and quickly with the wrist force like a bird pecking until the puncture area appears congestion, heat, and oozing of blood (See Fig. 4—78). Then, sterilize the area with 75% alcohol cotton ball after pressing and wiping out oozed blood with sterilized dry cotton ball. The treamtment is given once or twice daily and for ten times as a course.

(4) Pricking to Causing Bleeding

Massage the auricle to induce congestion, and sterilize the area to be punctured strictly. Then, hold sterilized three—edged needle with the right hand, prick at the otopoint with it quickly, and squeeze the local area to cause bleeding. It may be applicable to some diseases with fever and some skin disorders. For example, pricking at the auricle apex to cause bleeding can disappear fever and eliminate inflammation; and pricking at the area with obvious congestion at the retroauricular veins to cause bleeding is employed for treating neurodermatitis.

In addition to the methods mentioned above, the electroacupuncture, hydro—acupuncture, or needle embedding may be applied to the otopoints. The concrete operation methods are referred in the related chapters.

During stimulation on the otopoint, the patient may feel local pain, distension, or heat, soreness and numbness. A few pateints may feel the needling sensation spreading along the meridian.

二、注意事项

1. 严密消毒预防感染。出针后若见针孔发红耳廓胀痛，有轻度感染时，应即刻涂擦2.5%碘酒或用消炎药治疗。夏天埋针时间以1～3天为宜。炎症及冻伤部位禁针，以免引起软骨感染。

2. 正常人耳廓不同部位电阻大小也不一致，在分析时务必结合临床检查和症状。

3. 耳针治疗扭伤及肢体活动功能障碍的疾患，要求患者在接受治疗时配合活动患部，以增强疗效。

4. 耳针适应症广，凡毫针能治疗的疾患均可耳针治疗，但有的病证亦应与其他疗法综合使用提高疗效。

5. 耳针刺激时比较疼痛，注意防止晕针，一旦晕针可按毫针晕针方法处理。孕妇、年老体弱者慎用或暂时不用。

II. PRECAUTIONS

1. Strict sterilization should be given to prevent infection of the auricle. In case of redness of teh needle hole, or distension or pain in the auricle after puncturing, which may be due to mild infection, timely and appropriate measures should be taken for it, such as applying 2.5% iodine or oral administration of anti—inflammation drugs. Duration of no more than 1—3 days of keeping the skin needle embedded beneath the skin is allowed in summer. The area with inflammation or cold injury is forbidden to be punctured, otherwise chondric infection may occur.

2. A normal person has different electric resistances at the different places of the auricle, therefore, clinical signs

and symptoms should be considered in analysis.

3. In treating sprain or impairment of movement of the limb, the therapeutic effect may be enhanced by patient's movement of the diseased limb during the treatment procedure in cooperation.

4. Otopuncture has various indications, which can be applied to treat any disease which can be treated with the filiform needle. But it still has its limitation. Therefore, in treating some disorders it shoule be combined with other therapeutic methods in order to enhance the effect.

5. Pay attention to preventing needing fainting because the stimulation caused by otopuncture may lead to serious pain. If the fainting occurs, it may be treated with the same way as in filiform needling. It should be carefully applied or even forbidden temporally to the pregnant, the aged, or the weak patients.

第十节 头 针

头针又称头皮针。是在头部的特定区、线,进行针刺治病的一种方法。其流派多种,现介绍根据中国医学的针刺方法,结合现代医学关于大脑皮层功能定位的理论,在大脑皮层相应的头皮投射区针刺的技法。

一、特点与适应范围

1. 头针选用的是刺激区而不是穴位。
2. 快速持续捻转,手法固定。
3. 针刺部位大部分在体征的对侧。
4. 主要适宜于脑源性疾病,如中风、瘫痪、麻木、失语、眩晕、舞蹈病、震颤性麻痹(帕金森氏病),以及腰腿痛、夜尿,各种神经痛等。

SECTION 10 SCALP ACUPUNCTURE

Scalp acupuncture is a therapeutic method by needling the specific areas or lines of the scalp. There are many schools of the thought about it. Out of them, only one, the acupuncture method based on combination of the acupuncture method of TCM and the theory of location of corticocerebral function of modren medicine, is introduced here, which is performed by needling the corresponding projection areas of the cerebral cortex on the scalp.

I. THE CHARACTERISTICS AND INDICATIONS

1. In scalp acupuncture, the selected puncture area is not acupoints but the stimulation lines on the scalp.

2. The manipulation is only quick and constant twisting method without any change.

3. The area or line to be punctured is usually at the side opposite to that with clinical signs and symptoms.

4. It is mainly indicated in diseases originated at the brain, such as paralysis due to apoplex, numbness, aphonia, dizziness, chorea, Parkinson's disease, as well as lumbago, pain of the leg, nocturia, or various neuralgias.

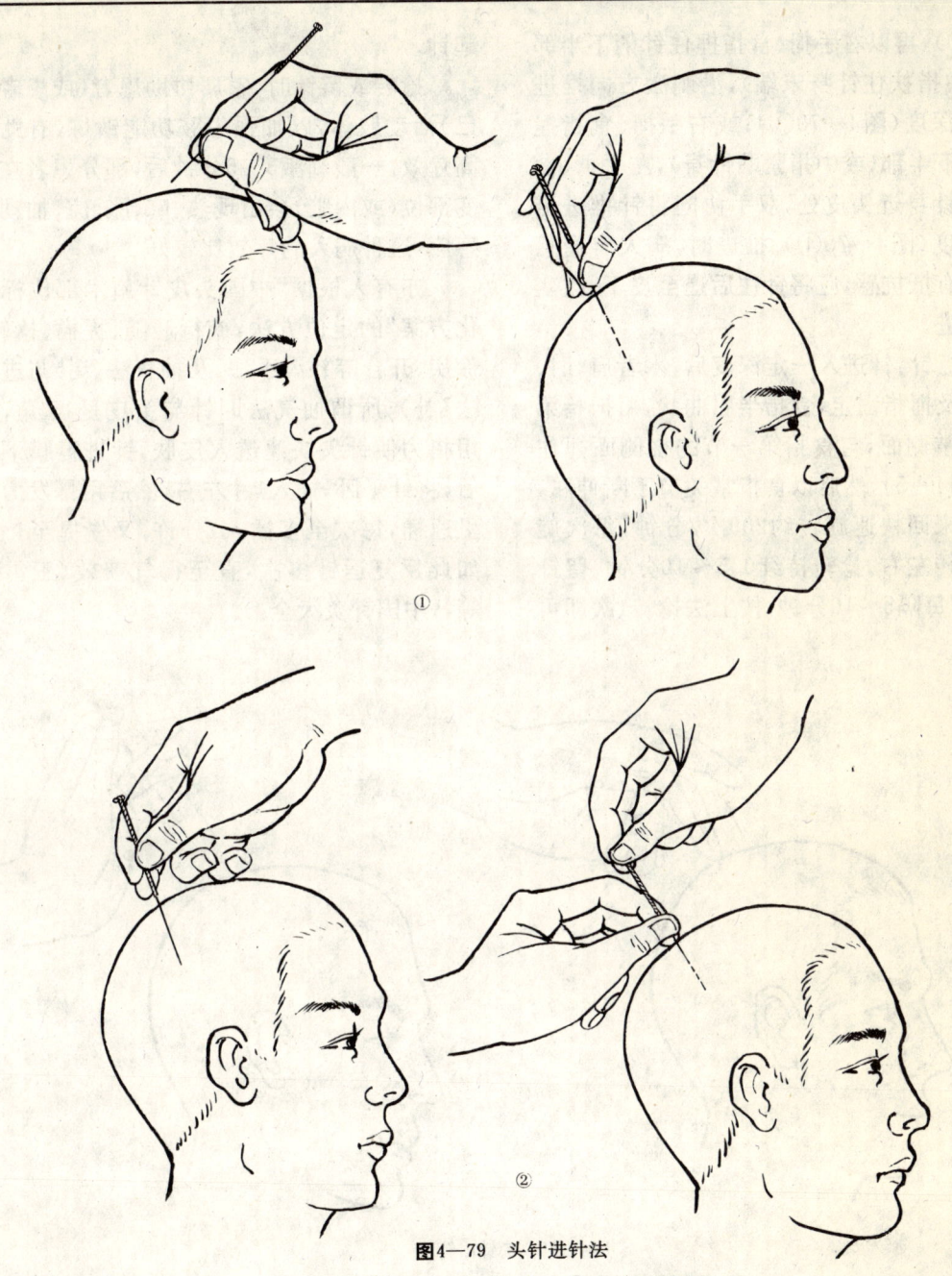

图4—79 头针进针法
Fig. 4-79 Inserting the Needle in Scalp Acupuncture

二、实用技法

1. 进针：取消毒过的26～28号1.5～2.5寸长的毫针，针尖与头皮呈30°左右夹角，医者右手拇、食指捏住针身露出针尖2毫米，沿刺激区的方向对准进针点，手指距头皮约5～10厘米（图4—79①），然后手腕突然用力往掌侧屈曲，使针尖快速冲刺进头皮下或肌层（图

4—79②），再以右手拇、食指捏住针柄下半部（或将中指扶住针身末端），沿刺激方向推进至所需深度（图4—79③）；或右手拇、食指捏住针柄下半部（或中指紧贴针身），左手拇、食指捏住针身近头皮处，双手协同将针推进至一定深度（图4—79④）。推进时，病人有痛感或针下有抵抗感，应将针往后退至皮下，改变角度推进。

2. 行针：针进入一定深度后，术者肩、肘、腕关节及拇指固定，食指半屈曲状，用拇指第一节的掌侧面，与食指第一节的桡侧面捏住针柄（图4—5），然后以食指掌关节不断伸屈，使针身来回快速旋转约200次/分钟，每次旋转各两转左右。捻转持续0.5～10分钟、留针30分钟，每隔5～10分钟，按上法捻转1次即可起针。

捻转或留针时，家属协助患者（或患者自己）活动肢体，以加强患肢功能锻炼，有助提高疗效。一般刺激3～5分钟后，部分患者在病变部位（或内脏）会出现热、麻、胀、凉、抽动等感应，这种病人的疗效比较好。

亦有人根据"中国头皮针施术部位标准化方案"的定位方法，施行迎随、提插、捻转、徐疾、开合等补泻手法，及抽气法（泻）与进气法（补）。所谓抽气法即针与头皮呈15°角，运用指力使针尖快速透入皮肤，针进腱膜下层后，将针平卧，插入1寸左右，然后用暴发力向里速插，每次至多插入1分许，又慢提至1寸。如此反复运针多次，直至得气获效（王雪苔等，《中国针灸大全》）。

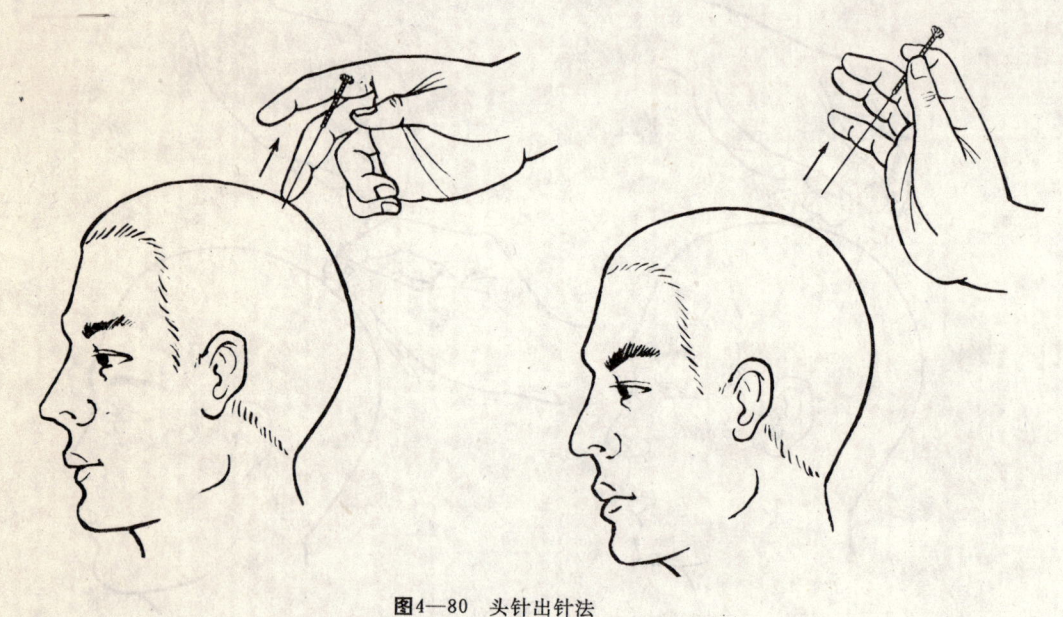

图4—80 头针出针法
Fig. 4—80 Withdrawing the Needle in Scalp Acupuncture

3. 出针：起针时，如针下无沉紧感，可快速拔出针。即左手持消毒棉球对准针孔附近，右手的中指或无名指沿着针柄快速往下滑（图4—80①），然后拇指和食指（或拇、食、中指）捏住针柄快速往外拔出（图4—80②）。也可右手边捻转边缓缓出针，起针后必须用消毒干棉球按压针孔片刻，以防出血。

一般每日或隔日针1次，10～15次为一个疗程,间隔5～7天后再继续下一疗程。

II. MANIPULATIONS

1. *Insertion of the Needle*

Select the sterilized filiform needle 1. 5—2.5 cun long and at the gauge No. 26—28. Hold the shaft of the needle with the thumb and index finger of the right hand, exposing the needle tip for 2mm, direct the needle tip at the area to be inserted accurately, and keep the finger tip 5—10cm far from the scalp and the needle tip 10—20cm far from the point (See Fig. 4—79A). Then, swiftly insert the needle at 30° angle to the scalp by sudden and forceful palmar flexion of the wirst through the scalp or into the muscular layer (See Fig. 4—79B). And then, hold the lower half of the needle handle with the thumb and index finger of the right hand (or support the needle shaft with the middle finger), push the needle along the direction of stimuation to the depth needed (See Fig. 4—79C). Or hold the lower half of the needle handle with the thumb and index finger of the right hand (or support the needle shaft with the middle finger) and grip the portion of the needle near the scalp with the thumb and index finger of the left hand, push the needle to a certain depthe with the two hands acting in coordination (See Fig 4—79D). In pushing, if the patient feels pain or there is resistance feeling aroucd the needle, the needle should be withdrawn to the subcutaneous layer for another try in a different direction.

2. *Manipulation of the Needle*

After the needle is inserted to a certain depth, make the joints of shoulder, elbow and wrist and the thumb at the fixed position, and keep the index finger at half flexion. Then, hold the needle handle with the palmar side of the tip portion of the thumb and radial side of the tip portion of the index finger (See Fig. 4—5), twirl the needle by continuous and alternate flexion and extension of the metacarpal phalangeal joint of the index finger in frequency of about 200 times per minute, every time having about two clockwise and anti—clockwise turns, for 0.5—1 minute. Then, retain the needle for 30 minutes. During retention, twirl the needle in the way mentioned above one time per 5—10 minutes. Finally, withdraw the needle.

During twirling or retaining the needle, ask the patient's relative to help the patient or ask the patient to move his affected limb so as to enhance the therapeutic effect by strengthening fucntional excercise of the affected limbs. Generally, through the stimulation for 3—5 minutes, if the patient has reaction at the affected area, including heat, numbness, distension, cold or trembling, the patient may get a good therapeutic effect.

Another method in manipulation of scalp acupuncture is mentioned by prof. Wang Xuetai, general secretary of World Association of Acupuncture and Moxibustion. Based on the Standard Nomenclature and Location of Scalp Acupuncture Lines recommended by the Regional Consulation Meeting on the standardization of acupuncture nomenclature, Tokyo, May, 1984, vatrious reinforcing and reducing manipulations, including those by lifting and thrusting the needle, twirling and rotating the needle, punctuing along and against the direction of the course of the meridian, rapid and slow insertion and withdrawal of the needle, and keeping the needle hole open or close, as well as the qi — entering reinforcing manner and the qi — withdrawing reducing mannner, are applied. All manipulations mentioned above except qi — withdrawing reducing manipulation and qi — entering manipulation are the same as in body puncture. Qi — withdrawing reducing manipulation refers to the following needling method. The needle is inserted to the selected line through the skin quickly at an angle of 15° to the scalp to the subfascial layer, and pushed horizontally for about 1 cun along this layer. Then the needle is lifted quickly for about 0.1 cun and thrust to the original depth again. This course is repeated for sevral times to induce the needling sensation.

Qi — entering reinforcing manipulation: The needle is inserted quickly through the skin at an angle of 15° to the scalp to the subfascial layer, and pushed horizontally for about 1 cun along this layer. Then, the needle is thrust quicly for about 0.1 cun and lifted slowly to the originnal place. This course is repeated for several times to induce needling sensation.

3. *Withdrawal of the Needle*

In withdrawal, if there is no heavy — tight sensation along the needle, put off needle swiftly. To the operation, hold the sterilized swab with the left hand and direct it at the puncture hole area, move the middle or ring finger of the right hand downwards along the needle handle smoothly and qucikly (See Fig. 4—80A), hold the needle handle and put out the needle qucikly with the thumb and index finger (or with the thumb, index and middle fingers) (See Fig. 4 — 80B). Or withdraw the needle slowly as twirling the needle. Then press over the needle hole with the sterilized cotton ball for a moment to prevent bleeding.

Genrally, the scalp acupuncture is done once daily or every other day, 10 — 15 times as a therapeutic course, and repeated after 5—7 day interval.

三、注意事项

1. 头部因长有头发尤需严密消毒，以防感染。

2. 由于头针刺激较强，术者须注意观察患者表情，以防晕针。一旦晕针，可按毫针晕针方法处理。

3. 对脑溢血患者，须待病情及血压稳定后方可做头针治疗。凡并发有高热、心力衰竭等症时，不宜立即采用头针。

Ⅲ. PRECAUTIONS

1. As the hair on the head makes difficulty in sterilization, a strict sterilization should be given so as to prevent infection.

2. The patient's expression should be closely observed in order to prevent needling fainting, because the stimulation

caused by scalp acupuncture is strong. In case of fainting, it should be treated in the same way as in the filiform needling.

3. In patients with cerebral vascular hemorrhage, scalp acupuncture should not be done until the patient's condition and blood pressure is improved. It is inadvisable to do scalp acupuncture to patients who have high fever or heart failuar.

第十一节 腕踝针

腕踝针,是在经络学说与神经学说的启发下,针刺腕踝关节以上的六个区点,治疗人体相应部位疾病的一种方法。具有取穴少、适应症较广、操作简单的特点。

操作时,选用已消毒的28～30号1.5～2寸长毫针,进针点常规消毒后,医生左手固定针刺部(腕或踝部)周围皮肤,右手用拇指在下、食、中指在上挟持针柄,针身与皮肤呈30度角,快速进针(图4—81)。针进入皮肤后,针身贴近皮肤表面,将针身推进在皮下浅表层,针下有松软无痛感为宜。若病人有酸、麻、胀、沉、痛等感觉,说明针身深入筋膜下层,进针过深,宜将针退至皮下浅表部位,或检查针尖是否沿纵行线方向插入,然后作适当偏斜或表浅刺入。进针深度一般为3.5厘米左右,针尖方向一般朝上刺,若病症在手、足部位,针刺方向则可朝下。

进针后不作捻转、提插。留针30分钟,慢性病留针时间可适当延长,一般每日或隔日针刺1次,10次为一疗程。

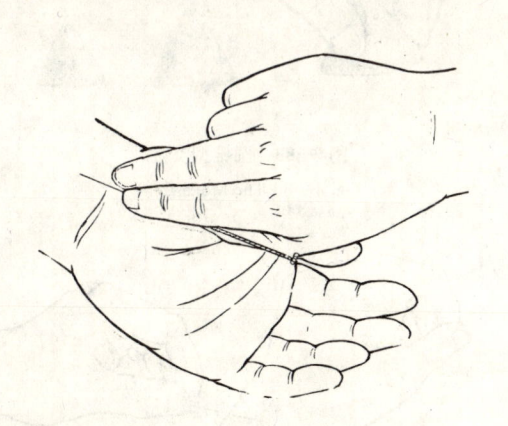

图4—81 腕踝针刺法
Fig. 4—81 Wrist-Ankle Needling

SECTION 11 WRIST — ANKLE ACUPUNCTURE

Wrist — ankle acupucture is a therapeutic method, based on the channel theory and neurology, by puncturing six pairs of spots proximal to the wrist and ankle to treat disease of the corresponding areas. It is characterized by fewer points to be punctured, wider range of indications, and simplicity in operation.

To the operation, select 1.5 — 2 cun long No. 28 — 30 filiform needles for usage. Sterilize the point to be punctured in routine way, fix the skin around the area to be punctured (i. e. wrist or ankle) with the left hand, and hold the needle handle with the thumb, index and middle fingers of the right hand, the thumb being below the others. Then, swiftly insert the needle at 30° angle formed by the skin surface and the needle shaft (See Fig. 4 — 81) through the skin. And then, horizontaly push the needle along the superficial layer of subcutaneous tissue. If feeling soft under the needle and causing no pain to the patient, this manipulation is better. If the patient complains of soreness, numbness, distension or pain, it indicates the needle has been over deep inserted to the subfascial layer or the direction of the needle has been along a vertical straight line, the needle should be withdrawn to the superficial layer of the subcutaneous tissue and pushed shallowly for another try, or the direction of insertion should be changed slightly for another try. Generally, the needle is pushed for about 1.2 cun and the direction of the needle tip is upwards in puncture. But if the disease is located at hand and foot, the direction of needling may be downwards.

Never twirl, rotate, lift, or thrust the needle after insertion of the needle. Retain the needle for 30 minutes, but in chronic diseases, the duration of needle retention may prolong properly. This acupuncrture is done once daily or every other day, one therapeutic course needs 10 times of the treatment.

第十二节 灸 法

灸法是利用某种易燃材料和药物,在穴位或患病部位上燃灼、薰熨和贴敷,借温热的物理效能刺激穴位,通过经络传导作用,达到调整机体生理功能而却病消疾的一种治疗方法。

灸法的应用范围颇为广泛,无论急症、热症、经络体表的病症,还是慢性病、虚寒证,或脏腑的病证均可治疗。归纳起来有温经散寒、活血镇痛、消瘀散结、疏风解表、回阳固脱、补中益气、防病保健等作用。临床治疗风寒湿痹、痛经、腹痛泄泻、内脏下垂、遗尿、阳萎、寒疝、虚脱、休克,以及疮疡初起,久溃不愈等病症。

一、常用灸法

(一)艾炷灸

艾炷是用艾绒加工特制而成的圆柱形小体(图4—82),或将纯净艾绒放在平版上,人工用手搓捏而成的圆锥形小体。分大、中、小三种(图4—83),大者高1厘米,炷底0.8厘米;中者为大炷一半如枣核;小者如麦粒,每燃完一炷称为一壮。

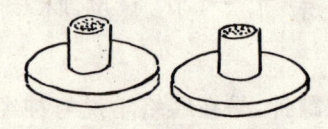

图4—82 圆柱型艾炷
Fig. 4—82 The Moxa Cylider

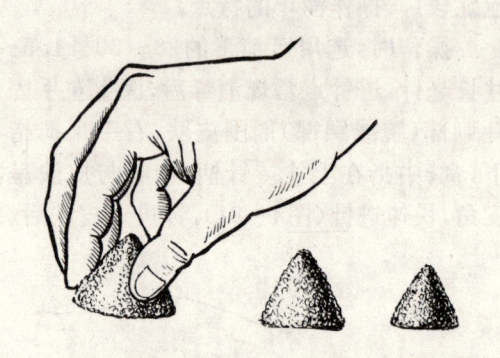

图4—83 圆锥型艾炷
Fig. 4—83 The Moxa Cone

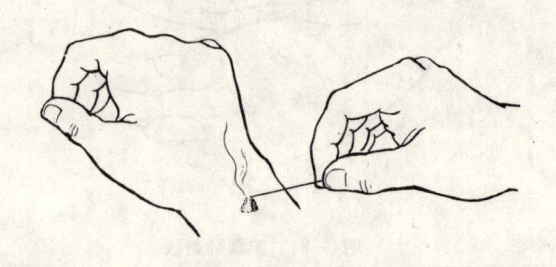

图4—84 直接灸
Fig. 4—84 Direct Moxibustion

艾可分为直接灸与间接灸两种。

1. 直接灸：是将大小适宜的艾炷，直接放在皮肤上施灸（图4—84）。由于对皮肤刺激程度的不同，临床上又分为瘢痕灸与无瘢痕灸两类。

(1) 无瘢痕灸：又称非化脓灸。灸后皮肤不起泡，不化脓，不留瘢痕。临床上多用中、小艾炷置于腧穴上点燃，当燃至3/5左右病者感到微有灼痛时，立即更换艾炷再灸，将规定艾炷数灸完为止，此时局部皮肤可见红晕。本法用于虚寒性疾病，如慢性腹泻、哮喘等。

此法有时也可出现水泡，不要挑破，任其自行吸收。

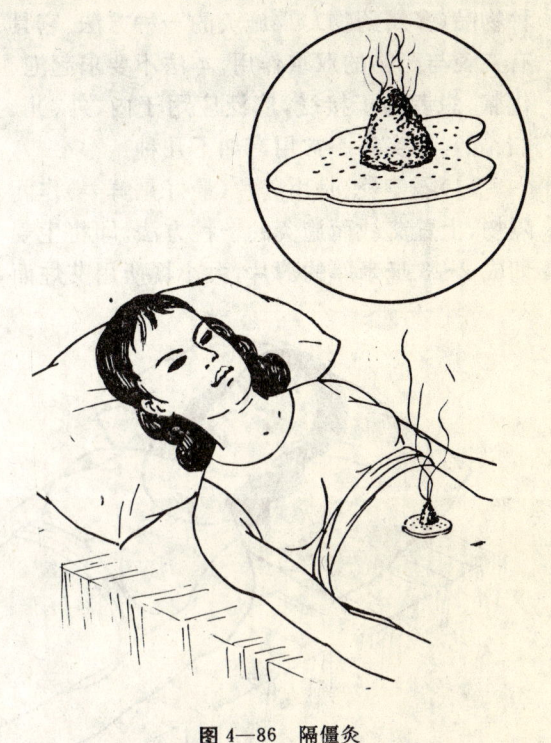

图4—86 隔姜灸
Fig. 4—86 Ginger Moxibustion

(2) 瘢痕灸：又称化脓灸。是指用艾炷直接置于穴位上施灸，灸至皮肤起泡，局部化脓，疮口结痂，痂脱后遗留瘢痕。一般每穴每次灸3～6壮，宜用小艾炷。小儿及体弱者可酌情减少炷数。施灸前在准备施灸的穴位上涂上蒜汁，将艾炷立即黏上并点燃艾炷，待艾炷燃尽再挟除艾灰（图4—85①），更换新艾炷继续施灸，直至规定艾炷数燃完为止。每灸完一炷需再涂蒜汁1次，施灸完毕后局部皮肤起泡，一般一周左右化脓，45天左右愈合结痂、痂脱留下瘢痕，因而必须先征得病者的同意，为了减轻或解决施灸时的烧灼痛，医生可在艾炷周围用手轻轻拍打（图4—85②），亦可将0.2%盐酸普鲁卡因1～2毫升，注入施灸穴位皮内或皮下。本法临床上常用于治疗哮喘、肺结核、癫痫等慢性、顽固性疾病。

2. 间接灸：是将艾炷与皮肤之间垫上某

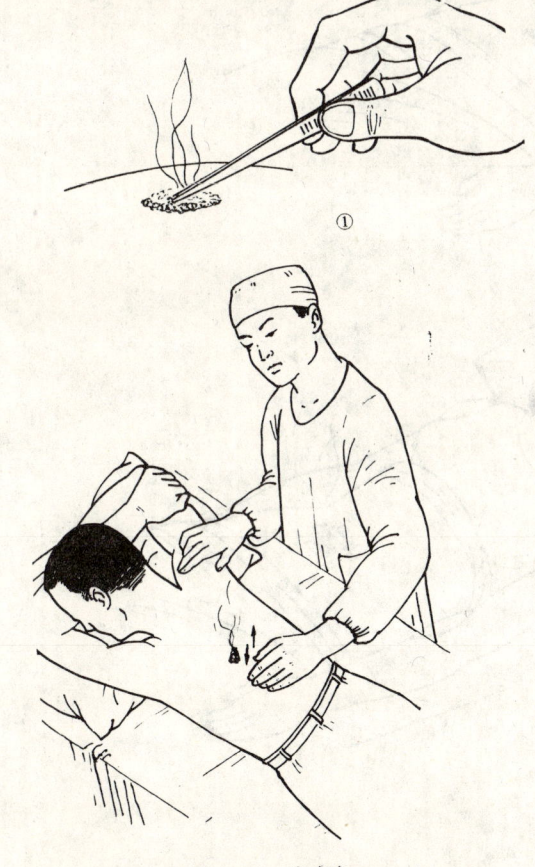

图4—85 瘢痕灸
Fig. 4-85 Scarring Moxibustion

种物品（多属药物），再施灸的一种方法。它具有艾灸与药物的双重作用。本法不要求起泡、化脓，患者易于接受，广泛应用于内、外、儿、妇、五官等疾病。常用有如下几种：

（1）隔姜灸：是用姜片（最好是鲜姜）作间隔物，上置艾绒而施灸的一种方法。即将生姜切成2～3毫米厚的薄片，大小视所用艾炷而定，中间刺数个小孔放于穴位上，再在姜片上置艾炷并点燃施灸（图4—86）。如病人在施灸过程中感觉局部有灼痛感，可将姜片连同艾炷向上略微提起，稍顷放下再灸。亦可随即更换艾炷再灸，一般施灸5～10壮，以局部皮肤出现红晕为度。

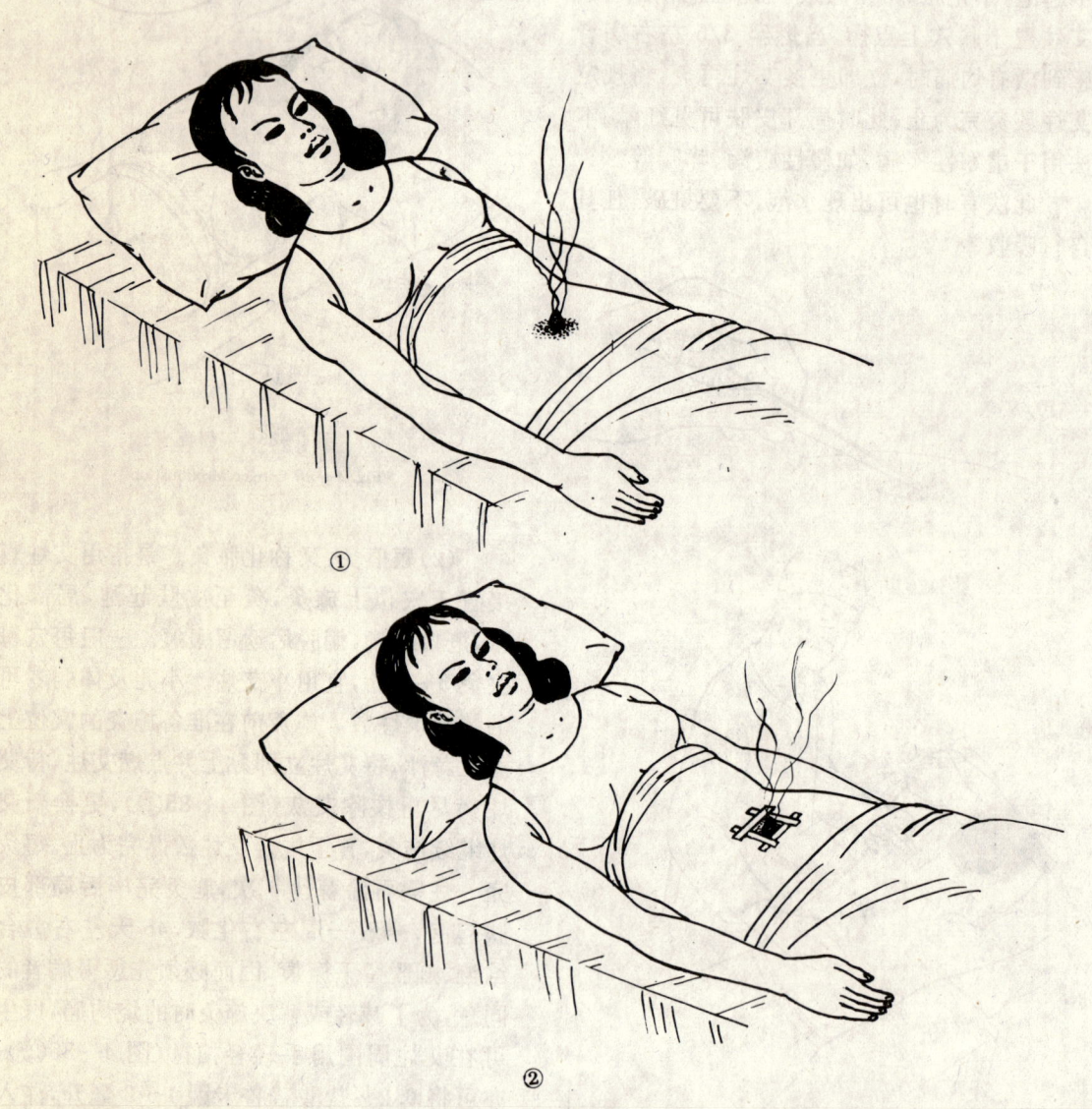

图 4—87 隔盐灸
Fig. 4—87 Salt Moxibustion

由于生姜功能调和营养、散寒发表、调中宽胃、驱积下气、开宣肺气、消水化食,所以本法对于一切虚寒病症,如呕吐、泄泻、胃痛、腹痛、风寒湿痹等,有较好疗效。

(2)隔蒜灸:是用蒜作为间隔物,上置艾炷而施灸的一种方法。即将新独头大蒜切成2～3毫米的薄片,以针刺数个小孔放于穴位上,再在蒜片上置艾炷点燃施灸。每灸2～3壮后,可换去蒜片继续灸治,一般5～10壮,局部皮肤红晕为度。

由于大蒜能祛寒湿、辟邪恶、开胃健脾、消肿化结,所以本法可用于治疗痈疽、疮、疖、蛇咬伤等疾患,亦可治肺结核、腹中积块等症。

(3)隔盐灸:是用食盐作间隔物,上置艾炷点燃施灸的一种方法。由于本法只适用于脐部,它处禁用,故又称神阙灸。其方法是以纯白干燥食盐(或炒热)填平脐孔,上置艾炷点燃施灸(图 4—87①)。亦有的于盐上放置姜片,再置艾炷点燃施灸的。其目的是避免食盐受火爆起而致烫伤。如病人脐部凸出,可在周围用物将脐周如"#"状圈定,再填盐于其内施灸(图 4—87②)。本法可用于急性胃肠炎、绕脐痛、疝痛、大汗、肢冷之脱症等。

(4)隔附子灸:临床上常用的有隔中药附子片灸,与隔附子饼灸两种。操作时,将附片或附子饼针刺数孔放于穴位或患处,上置艾炷点燃灸之。一般5～10壮,以局部温热皮肤红晕为度。

由于附子可逐风驱寒、补肾壮阳,故本法适用于各种阳虚病症,如阳萎、早泄、晨泄、肢厥等。

(二)艾条灸

将艾条或药条一端点燃在穴位上或患处施灸的一种方法。常分为温和灸、回旋灸、雀啄灸三种:

1.温和灸:将艾条的一端点燃,悬于施灸穴位上固定不移(图 4—88),当病人感到皮肤灼痛时,可适当拉开距离,至皮肤出现红晕为度。本法能温通经脉,祛除风寒湿邪。

2.回旋灸:将燃着的艾条悬于施灸穴位上,再将艾条回旋移动(图 4—89),使穴位皮肤有温热感。

3.雀啄灸:将燃着的艾条对准穴位皮肤处,一上一下如雀啄食一样地移动(图 4—90)。

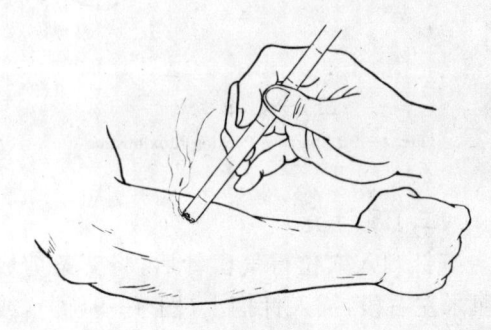

图 4—88 温和灸
Fig. 4—88 Mild Warming Moxibustion

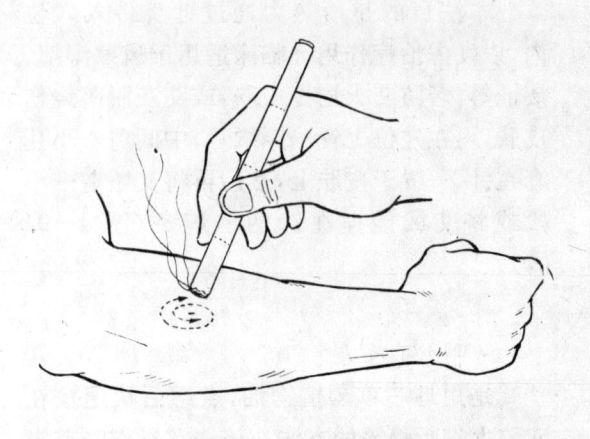

图 4—89 回旋灸
Fig. 4—89 Rounding Moxibustion

上述三法,一般能灸的病症均可采用,其中温和灸、回旋灸多用于治疗慢性病,如风寒湿痹;雀啄灸多用于灸治急性病,如昏厥及儿

· 287 ·

童疾患。

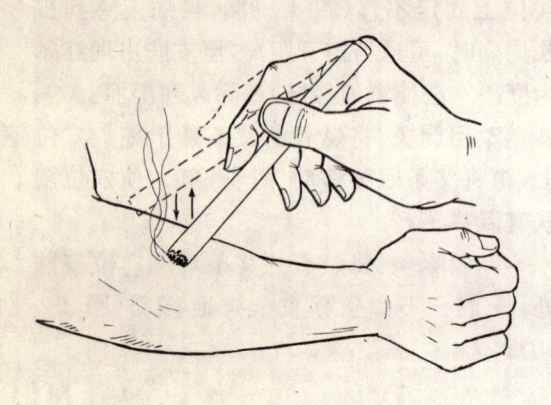

图 4—90 雀啄灸
Fig. 4—90 Sparrow-Pecking Moxibustion

(三) 温针灸

毫针刺入穴位得气留针后,将艾条剪成2厘米左右段,插入针柄上(图 4—91①),或将艾绒捏黏在针柄上点燃施灸(图 4—91②)的一种方法。

本法目的是使热力通过针身传入穴位内,以发挥治疗作用。临床适用于风寒湿痹、痿证等。若防艾火灼疼皮肤,或艾灰脱落烧伤皮肤,可在穴位上置一厚纸片,中间剪一小孔套在针下,置于皮肤上,然后再将艾条剪一小段或将艾绒插捏在针柄上施灸(图 4—91③)。

(四) 灯火灸

是用灯芯草蘸植物油,点燃后快速按在穴位上进行焠烫的方法。该法在操作时首先选定穴位作好标记,取灯芯草 4～5 厘米长,将一端浸入油中约 1～2 厘米,点火前用卫生纸吸去灯草上浮油,术者右手拇、食指捏住灯草露出草端 1 厘米左右点燃,对准穴位快速点按,一触即离(图 4——92),此时即出现"叭"的爆碎声,表明施述成功,如未闻爆碎声

可再重复一次,灸后注意局部清洁,防止感染。

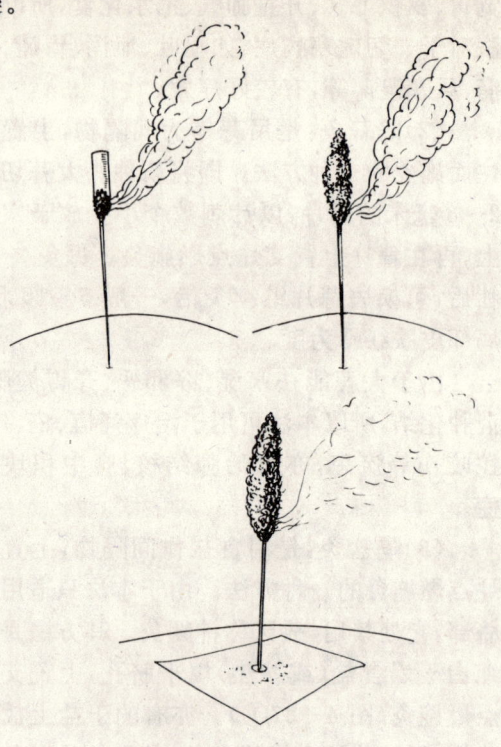

图 4—91 温针灸
Fig. 4—91 Moxibustion with Warming Needle

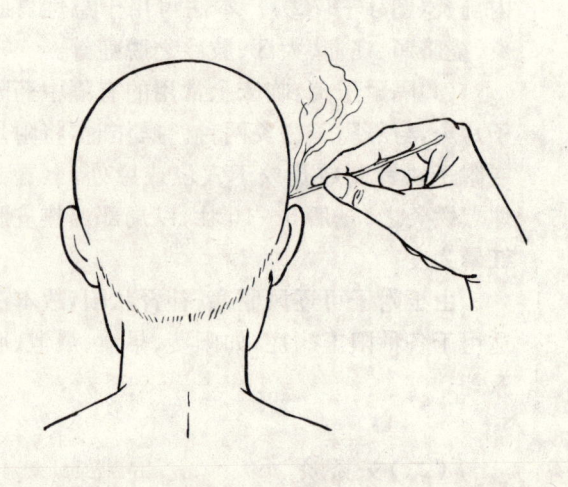

图 4—92 灯火灸
Fig. 4—92 Rush-Buring Moxibustion

本法有疏风解表、行气利痰、解郁开胸、开窍熄风的作用。主治流行性腮腺炎、小儿抽搐、昏迷、胃痛、腹痛等症。

（五）天灸

是用对皮肤有刺激性的药物，敷贴于穴位或患处，使之局部充血，起泡的一种方法。常用有如下几种：

1. 蒜泥灸：将食用大蒜捣成泥状，取3～5克置于穴位或一定部位上，覆盖塑料膜，再以大于塑料膜范围的胶布敷贴固定（图4——93）。敷灸时间为1～3小时，以局部皮肤发痒、发红或起泡为度。如敷涌泉穴治疗咯血、衄血；敷合谷穴治疗扁桃腺炎；敷鱼际穴治疗咽喉肿痛等。

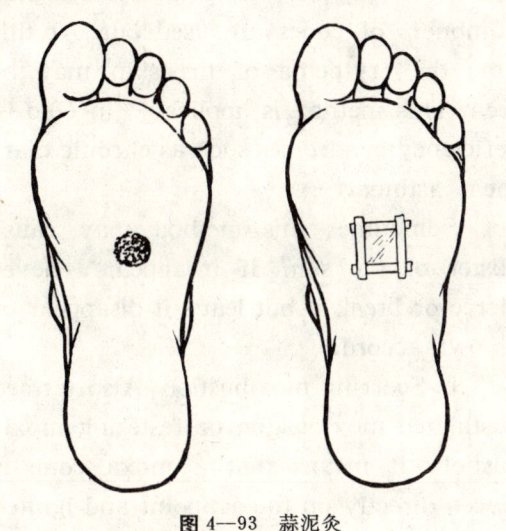

图4—93 蒜泥灸
Fig. 4—93 Mashed Garlic Moxibustion

2. 蓖麻子灸：蓖麻子去壳取仁适量捣成泥状，按蒜泥灸法敷贴于穴位上。如敷涌泉穴治疗滞产；敷百会穴治疗子宫脱垂、胃下垂、脱肛等。

3. 吴茱萸灸：取中药吴茱萸适量，研为细末，用醋调成糊膏状，按蒜泥灸法贴敷于穴位上，每日敷1次。如敷涌泉穴治疗高血压、口腔溃疡、小儿水肿等。

此外，中药毛茛叶敷贴内关穴、大椎穴可治疟疾；寒湿性疼痛可敷贴患处局部。白芥子灸贴肺俞、膏肓等穴可治哮喘、肺结核等病。操作方法均同蒜泥灸。

SECTION 12 MOXIBUSTION

Moxibustion is a therapeutic method by burning some combustible materials or applying some drug—compress or drug—plaster over the acupoint or affected area to produce warm—hot stimulation to the patient, which acts on the acupoint or the affected area and is conducted through the channel so that the equilibrium of bodily physical function would be adjusted.

The moxibustion is applied widely, which may be employed for either acute diseases, heat syndromes, diseases of the channel, and exterior syndromes[①], or chronic syndromes[②], and diseases of viscera. It may serve to warm the meridian to expel cold, to promote blood circulation to cause analgetic effect, to relieve depression of qi to remove obstruction, to dispel

---

① Exterior syndrome refers to superficial and mild illness, chiefly manifested by chilly sensation, fever, headanche, general and limb aching, stuffy running nose, cough, floating pulse, thin coating of the tongue. It is usually seen in common cold, influenza, and the prodromal or early stage of various acute infections diseases.

② Cold—deficiency syndrome, also termed cold syndrome of deficiency type, refers to a morbid condition resulting from insufficiency of genuine qi with endogenous cold, marked by pale complexion, loss of appetite, chilliness and aversion to cold, abdominal distension and pain, lumbogo, loose stools, pale tongue with whitish coating, deep and slow and weak pulse.

wind to relieve the exterior syndrome, to recuperate yang and rescure the patient from collapse(resurrect), to reinforce middle—jiao and replenish qi, to prevent diseases and keep healthy, and so on. In clinical practice, moxibustion is applied in treatment of arthralgia due to wind—cold—dampness, dysmenorrhea, abdominal pain and diarrhea, prolapse, visceroptosis, enuresis, cold hernia, collapse, and shock, as well as carbuncle at the first stage or with untractable ulcer, and some other disorders.

I. COMMONLY USED MOXIBUSTION TECHNIQUES

1. *Moxibustion with Moxa Cone*

Moxa cone is made of moxa wool into the small cylinder shape(See Fig. 4—82), or into the small cone shape by artificial rbbing of the pure moxa woll with the hand. The moxa cone may be small, medium, or large in size(See Fig. 4—83). The large one is 1 cm high, with a bottom 0.8cm in diameter; the medium one is just as big as a half of a large one in size, like a jubepit; and the small one is as big as big as a grain or a wheat. One moxa cone is called a cone(壮 zhuang, the number of moxa cones used in moxibustion, taken as unit for measurement).

The moxibustion with the moxa cone includes two kinds: the direct moxibustion and the indirect moxibustion.

(1) Direct Moxibustion

It means that a moxa cone in proper size is put directly on the skin and ignited for moxibustion (See Fig. 4—84). This type of moxibustion is subdivided into the scarring moxibustion and the non—scarring moxibustion according to whether the local scar is formed or not after moxibution.

a. Non—scarring moxibustion: Also termed non—pustulated moxibustion. It is so named because this moxibustion will not cause blister, pus and scar of the skin after moxibustion. In clinical practice, usually put a medium or small moxa cone on an acupoint and ignite it. When about 2/5 of it is burnt out or the patient feels burning discomfort, remove the cone and place another one. Replace the moxa cone one by one in this way until the designed numbners of cones are used out. At this time the erythema of the skin may be seen. This method is applicable in cold—deficiency syndromes such as chronic diarrhea, asthma.

Sometimes this method may cause blister of the skin. If it appears, never pierce or break it but leave it disappear of its own accord.

b. Scarring moxibustion: Also termed pustulated moxibustion or festering moxibustion. It means that a moxa cone is placed directly on the acupoint and ignited for moxibustion, the moxibustion continues until a blister appears, by which local purulence and crusta will be formed after moxibustion, and after decrustation there will be a scar left. Generally, 3—6 moxa cones are employed on each acupoint for one treatment session, and if the moxa cone is at small size, it is better. The number of cones may be reduced for children and for the weak persons according to the patient's condition. To its operation, smear some garlic juice on the skin of the selected point, place a moca cone on the point and ignite it for moxibustion. After it is completely burnt out, take away the ashes, swab some garlic jucie again and apply another moxa cone for moxibustion (See Fig. 4—85A). Repeat this course until the designed cones are all burnt out. After moxibustion, there is local blister on the skin, which will become purulent about one week later and heal with decrustation in about 45 days, and a scar will be left. This method can done only with patient's consent because it causes severe pain and scar. The scroching pain caused in operation can be relieved by gently tapping on the skin around the moxa cone (See. Fig. 4—85B), or giving intradermic or subcutaneous injection of 2—3 ml of 0.2% of procaine hydrochloride into the acupoint area. In clinic, this method is usually applied to chronic and intractable diseases, such as asthma, pulmonary tuberculosis, epilepsy, etc.

(2) Indirect Moxibution

Indirect moxibution refers to the moxibustion performed with some material (usually with drug) placed between the smoldering moxa cone and the skin, which can serve as both of treatment with moxibustion and treatment with drug in the same time. As this moxibustion does not require plister and purulence to be caused for therpapeutic purpose, patients are usually willing to accept it, It has a very wide arange of indications in the spheres of internal medicine, surgery, pediatrics, gynecology, otolaryngology, ophthalmology and stomatology. Its commonly used methods are as follows:

a. Ginger moxibustion: It is a moxibustion method with a slice of ginger (the raw one is better) placed between the moxa cone and the acupoint. To its operation, cut a slice of raw ginger about 2—3 mm thick, with its size as large as that of the moxa cone used, punch several holes at its center, and place it on the acupoint selected. Then, place a moxa cone on the ginger and ignite it for moxiubustion (See Fig. 4—86). When the patient complains of burning pain, slightly lift the ginger and the moxa cone for a short time and put them down again, or replace the moxa cone with another one and ignite it. Repeat at this way until there is a local erythema of the skin. Generally, 5—10 cones are used to each point selected at one treatment session.

As ginger has the property to regulate ying and wei (ying refers to nutrients or the materialistic founndation for body function, and wei, to the defensive mechanism or the yang principle for defense at the body surface), to dispel cold to relieve the exterior syndrome, to regulate middle —jiao to comfort stomach, to dispel the acumulation and regulate qi, to ventilate the lung, and to dispel water and promote digestion, this method can produce good therapeutic effect in treating cold syndromes of deficiency type such as vomiting, diarrhea, stomachache, abdominal pain, and arthritis due to wind—cold—dampness.

b. Garlic moxibustion: It is a moxibustion method with a slice of garlic placed between the moxa cone and an acupoint. To its operation, cut a slice of raw one-head garlic 2—3 mm thick, punch several holes in its center, and place it on the acupoint selected. Then, place the moxa cone on the garlic and ignite it for moxibustion. After 2—3 cones are burnt out in moixibustion, replace the garlic with another one and continue to perform moxibustion until there is an erythema of the skin. Generally, 5—10 cones are used to each point at one treatment session.

As the garlic can serve to dispel cold —damp factor and expel the pathogen, to strengthen spleen and stomach, and to relieve swelling and resolve masses, this method may be employed in treating diseases in the spheres of surgery and traumatology, suchy as carbuncle, deep rooted carbuncle, sore, furuncle (boil), and snake bite, as well as some internal diseases such as pulmonary tuberculosis, abdominal masses.

c. Salt moxibustion: It is a moxibustion method with salt placed between a moxa cone and an acupoint. It is also termed moxibustion at Shenque point because it is applied only on the umbilicus. To the operation, fill the umbilicus with dry salt (or fried hot salt) to the level of the skin, place moxa cone on the salt and ignite it for moxibustion (See Fig. 4—87A). Or place a slice of ginger between the salt and the moxa cone. The ginger can serve to prevent the patient from scald, which may be caused by explosion of the salt when it directly touches the fire. If the patient's umbilicus is not concave in shape, a piece of wet noodle or other material can be put around the umbilicus, and then, the salt is filled in the umbilicus area for moxibustion (See Fig. 4—87B). This method is applicable to acute gastroenteritis, pain around umbilicus, dysentery, hernia, prostration syndrome[①] with profuse sweating and cold limbs, etc.

d. Monkshood moxibustion: It has two types commonly used in clinic; one is to place a slice of aconite root between a moxa cone and an acupoint; and the other is to place a cake of monkshood between a moxa cone and an acupoint. To the operation, cut a slice of mokshood or select a monkshoodcake (the materials seen Chapter 3, Part one). Then, punch numerous holes on it and place it on the acupoint selected. And then, place a moxa cone on it and ignite the cone for moxibustion. The moxibustion continues until there are heat and erythema of the local skin. Generally, 5—10 cones are burnt out on each point selected at one treatment session.

As the aconite root has the property to dispel wind and cold, and to reinforce kidney—yang, this method is applicable to various syndromes of insufficiency of yang, including impotance, diarrhea at down, cold limb, etc.

2. Moxibustion with Moxa Stick

Moxibustion with the moxa stick is a moxibustion method by igniting one end of

---

[①] A prostration syndrome refers to a morbid condition with severe exhaustion of yin, yang, qi and blood, manifested as profuse sweating, cold limbs, openig of mouth and closing of eyes with hands relaxed, incontinence of urine, small and imdistinct pulse.

a moxa stick or a drug stick. It is classified into the mild — warm moxibustion, the rounding moxibustion and the sparrow — pecking moxibustion.

(1) Mild—Warming Moxibustion

Ignite one of the ends of the moxa stick, hold the stick and keep the ignited end above the selected acupoint from a distance without moving (See Fig. 4—88). when the patient complains of burning pain of the skin, properly lift the ignited end of the moxa stick. Apply the moxibustion until there is erythema of the skin, this method has the property to promote flow of qi by warming the channel, and to dispel wind, cold and damp pathogens.

(2) Rounding Moxibustion

Also termed circling moxibustion. To the operation, keep the ignited moxa stick above the selected acupoint in a distance from it. Then, round move the moxa stick horizontally (See Fig. 4—89)so as to cause warm sensation of the skin of the acupoint area to the patient.

(3) Sparrow—Pecking Moxibusgtion

Hold an ingnited moxa stick with its ignited end directed at the acupoint, and move it up and down. like a sparrow pecking foods (See Fig. 4—90).

The three moxibustion method above may be used in diseases which can be treated with moxibustion. But the mild — warming and rounding moxibustion methods are mainly applied in chronic diseases such as arthritis due to wind — cold — dampness; and the sparrow — pecking moxibustion mainly in acute diseases such as coma and syncope, as well as in child diseases.

3. Moxibustion with Warming Needle

Moxibution with the warming needle, also termed warm needling, is a method of acpuncture combined wtih moxaibustion. after arrival of qi and with the needle retained at the point, a segment of a moxa stick about 2 cm long is pierced through the needle handle (See Fig. 4—91A), or the needle handle is pinched with some moxa wool, and then the moxa wool or stick is ignited for moxibustion (See Fig. 4—91B).

The purpose of this moxibustion is to conduct heat power through the needle shaft into the acupoint, so as to produce the therapeutic effect. It is clinically applicable to arthritis due to wind — cold — dampness, flaccidity syndrome[①], etc. In this moxibustion, the skin may be injured by fire of ignited moxa or fall of ashes from the burnt moxa to it. The method of prevention of this condition is to place a piece of thick paper with a small hole in its center, through which the needle pierces, on the skin before putting the moxa strick or moxa swool on the needle for moxibustion (See Fig. 4—91C).

4. Rush—Burning Moxibustion

Rush — burning moxibustion, also termed lampwick moxibustion, or moxibustion with medulla junci, is a moxibus-

---

① A flaccidity syndrome refers to a morbid condition marked by weakness, limited morement and muscular atrophy of the limbs, especially, the lower limbs.

tion methos performed by pressing a burning oiled rush directly over an acupoint and immediately moving it away. In the operation, make a mark in the selected acupoint, select a segment of rush pith 4—5 cm long and put its one end into the vegetable oil to 1—2 cm depth. Then, take it out of the oil and dry it slightly with some piece of soft paper. And then, hold the rush with the thumb and index finger of the right hand, exposing the oiled end of the rush about 1 cm, ignite the end, quickly press it directly over the acupoint, and immediately take the rush away (See Fig. 4—92). If a sound "pa" is heard when the ignited end of the rush touches the skin, it indicates the operation is successful; if not, repeat the operation course in the same way once。 Be cautious to keep the local area clean after moxibustion so as to prevent infection. This method may serve to dispel wind for relieving exterior syndrome, to promote flow of qi for dispelling phlegm, to relieve stagnant qi for soothing the chest oppression, and to induce resuscitation for calming the endogenous wind[①]. It is mainly indicated in mumps, infantile clonic convulsion, coma, stomachache, abdominal pain, etc.

5. Crude Herb Moxibustion

Crude herb moxibustion is a therapy by pasting some irritant medicines on skin at certain acupoints or affected areas to cause local congestion and blister. The commonly used methods are as follows.

(1) Mashed Garlic Moxibustion

Mash some garlic well, place 3—5 g of mashed garlic on the skin with a piece of plastic film. Then, cover and fix the plastic film on the skin with a piece of adhesive plaster (See Fig. 4—93). Keep the mashed garlic on the acupoint or area until there are itching, redness or plisters of the local skin. Usually, the duration of keeping garlic on the skin is 1—3 hours. This method can be used in treating some diseases. For example, hemoptysis and epistaxis are treated by performing mashed garlic moxibustion at Yongquan (KI 1); and tonsilitis treated by perfoming it at Yuji (LU 10).

(2) Castor Seed Moxibustion

Take away the shell of a caster seed, mash the seed, plaster the mashed seed on the selected point in the same way as above, using mashed seed of castor instead of mashed garlic. This method can be used in treating some diseases. For example, prolonged labour may be treated by applying castor seed moxibustion at Yongquan (KI 1); and prolapse of uterus, gastroptosis and prolapse of anus treated by applying it at Baihui (DU 20).

(3) Fructus Euodiae Moxibustion

Grind a proper amount of fructus euodiae into powder, make it into paste with vinegar, plaster the paste on the acupoint in the same way as above, using the paste instead of the mashed garlic. This method is performed once daily, and can be used in treating some diseases. For example,

---

[①] Endogenous wind refers to a morbid condition manifested as tremor, dizziness caused by hight fever, deficiency of yin and blood, hyperactivity of the liver-yang or adverse flow of qi and blood.

hypertension, canker sore, and infantile edema are treated by performing fructus euodiae moxibustion on Yongquan(KI 1).

Additionally, moxibustion with folium ranunculus japonucus covering over Neiguan(PC 6)and Dazhui(DU 14)can be indicated in malaria, and over the affected area for pain due to cold—dampness; and moxibustion with semen cleomis covering on Feishu(BL 13)and Gaohuang(BL 43) can be used in treating asthma, pulmonary tuberculosis. These procedures of operation are the same as in mashed garlic moxibustion.

二、艾灸补泻

艾灸补泻主要指艾炷灸的补泻。临床上在应用灸法时,对于邪气偏盛的用泻法,正气虚弱的用补法。施灸时,点燃艾炷后不吹其火,等待它慢慢徐燃自灭,火力微而温和,且时间宜长,壮数较多,灸治完毕后再用手按其施灸穴位,使真气聚而不散者为补法;反之,点燃艾炷后以口速吹其火,促使其快燃,火力较猛,且快燃快灭,当患者感觉局部热烫时,即迅速更换艾炷再灸,灸治时间较短,壮数较少,施灸完毕后不按其穴,使邪气外散者为泻法。

II. REINFORCING AND REDUCINE IN MOXIBUSTION THERAPY

Reinforcing and reducing in moxibustion are mainly seen in those with moxa stick. In clinic application of moxibustion, reducing is used when pathogen is dominant; and reinforcing used when the vital—qi is weak. On performing moxibustion, it is taken as reinforceing that, after the moxa stick is ignited, the fire directing at the point selected is not blowed but burns slowly and goes to extinction of its own accord, with milder fire produced and lasting for a comparatively long time, and with more cones used once, and the area to which moxibustion is applied pressed with the hand as soon as the moxibustion is over so as to keep the genuine qi (i. e., vitality qi, dynamic force of all vital functions, origiating from the combination of the originated qi inherited and the acquired energy derived from food and air.) inside and prevent it from escaping; otherwise, it is taken as reducing, namely, the fire of igneted moxa stick is blowed by the mouth to quicken its burning speed and to produce a big fire power, with quick burning and quick extinction, when the patient feeling local heat and burning, the moxa stick is qucikly replaced with another one, the duration of moxibustion is comparatively short and rather fewer moxa sticks are used once, and after moxibustion the applied acupoint is not pressed so as to make the pathogen go out.

三、施灸禁忌及注意事项

1. 头面部,重要脏器及大血管附近、肌腱处避免施灸,禁用瘢痕灸。妇女孕期、腰骶部和少腹部、乳头、阴部均不宜施灸。

2. 外感温病、阴虚内热及其他实热证,一般不宜施灸。

3. 过劳、过饥、过饱、醉酒、大惊、大恐、大怒、大渴者不宜施灸。

4. 体弱者,施灸艾炷不可过大,刺激量不可过强。

5. 胸部、四肢施灸,艾炷数可少,头项部更少。腰、背、腹部施灸,艾炷数可多。老年人、小儿施灸,艾炷数宜更少,时间要短。青年人施灸,艾炷数应多,时间较长。

6. 施用瘢痕灸法,在化脓期间不宜做重体力劳动,若局部因感染发炎时,可进行消炎处理。为防止污染可在局部用消毒敷料覆盖保护。

7. 施灸后,皮肤微红灼热为正常现象,当不予处理,待其自行消失。如因施灸过量或时间过长而出现水泡,小者不必挑破,任其自然吸收,水泡较大可用消毒毫针挑破放出液体,敷以消毒纱布固定。

8. 对昏迷,肢体麻木不仁及感觉迟钝患者,不可施灸过量,并时时观察,避免灼伤局部皮肤。

III. CONTRAINDICATIONS AND PRECAUTIONS

1. It is inadvisable to apply moxibustion and forbidden to apply scarring moxibustion to the face, and to the area near the important viscera, large blood vessels and tendons. In the pregnant women, it is inadvisable to apply moxibustion to lumbar—scaral region, lower abdomen, nipple and lower orifice region.

2. Generlly, it is inadvisable to apply moxibustion to febrile disease due to exogenous pathogen, interior heat — shyndrome due to yin deficiency[①], and excess heat syndrome[②]

3. It is inadvisable to apply moxibustion to the patients who are over fatigue, famished, over-eating, tipsy, over fear, over angry, over—thirsty, or in terror.

4. In weak patients, it is inadvisable to apply moxibustion with too large moxa cone and too strong fire stimulation.

5. Generally, a faw moxa cones should be used to the chest and limbs; fewer moxa cones used in the head and neck; but more moxa cones may by used to loin, back and abdomen. Only a few moxa cones are used and the duration of moxibustion should be shorter for the aged or children, but for the young, more moxa cones may be used and duration of moxibustion may be comparatively longer.

6. To scarring moxibustion, advise the patient not to do heavy physical labour during the purulence period. If the local area occurs inflammation due to infection, give anti — inflammatory treatment and cover the area with sterilized dress to prevent it from being polluted further.

7. Do not deel with the reddish colour and burning heat of the local skin area appearing after moxibustion, but wait them to disappear of their own accord. when plisters appear due to excessive or prolonged moxibustion, to the small one, not break it but leave it disap-

---

① An interior heat—syndrome due to yin deficiency refers to a morbid condition showing heat syndrome due to impairment of yin and blood, usually at the advanced stage of febrile disase, marked by malar flush, low fever, hot sensation in palms and soles, restlessness, insomnia, night sweat, dry mouth and throat, reddened tongue with little or no coating, thready, rapid and weak pulse.

② An excess heat syndrome refers to a morbid condition due to affection by excessive exogenous pathogens which enter the interior of the body, transform into heat and lead to fierce struggle with the undiminished body resistance, manifested as high fever, fidgets, thirst, constipation, abdominal pain and tenderness, deep—coloured urine, yellowish dry coating of the tongue, full and rapid pulse.

pear of its own accord; to the large one, break it with a sterilized needle to drain the fluid out and then cover it with sterilized dress and fix the dress on the skin.

8. To the patient with coma, or numbness of limbs, or dysesthesia, and excessive moxibustion is contraindicated and close attention should be paid to preventing the local skin from being burnt.

〔附〕拔罐法

拔罐法是以罐为工具，借助热力排除其中的空气，造成负压使罐吸附于皮肤上，形成局部瘀血的一种方法。本法有行气活血、止痛消肿、散风驱寒、祛湿的作用。

常用的罐多为竹筒制成的竹罐，也有用玻璃制成的光滑透明的玻璃罐及陶土烧制而成的陶罐等。

APPENDIX: CUPPING METHOD

Cupping is a therapeutic method in which a jar or a cup is attached to the skin surface to cause local congestion through the negative pressure created by introducing heat in the form of an ignited material. This method serves to promote circulation of qi and blood, to induce manlgesic effect, to subdue swelling, and to expel wind and cold and damp pathogens.

The commonly used cupping apparauses are made of bamboo, glass, or pottery. (the apparatuses seen Part One in detail)

一、适应范围

风湿痹痛、急性扭伤、面瘫、半身不遂、感冒、咳嗽、胃痛、腹痛及痈、疽、疮疡初起等。

I. INDICATIONS

The indications of cupping method include arthritis due to wind — cold — dampness, acute sprain, facial paralysis, hemeplegia, common cold, cough, stomachache, abdominal pain, furuncle, carbuncle, deep — rooted carbuncle and ulcer which are at the early stage, etc.

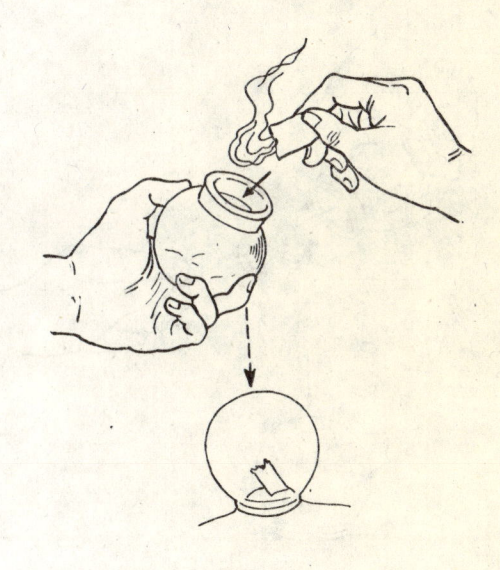

图4—94 投火法

Fig. 4—94 Fire—Throwing Method

二、实用技法

（一）扣罐的方法

1. 投火法：用酒精棉球或纸片，点燃后投入罐内，立即将罐罩在所取穴位或患病部位的皮肤上。此法宜于火罐横扣(图4——94),以免纸片掉落皮肤上造成灼伤。

2. 闪火法:用摄子挟住已经点燃的酒精棉球,在罐内壁回旋一下并迅速抽出、立即将罐罩在应拔穴位或患处皮肤上(图4—95)。此法安全多用。

3. 贴棉法:将酒精棉球贴在罐内壁底处,点燃棉球后立即罩在穴位皮肤上(图4—96)。此法酒精不宜太多,以免滴在皮肤上引起灼伤。

4. 架火法:用一圆形硬质橡皮或胶木瓶塞,置于应拔部位皮肤上,其上放95%酒精棉球一个,点燃后将火罐(最好是玻璃火罐)立即扣上,火罐自然吸附于皮肤上(图4—97),该法安全牢固。

一般疾病均可采用此法。

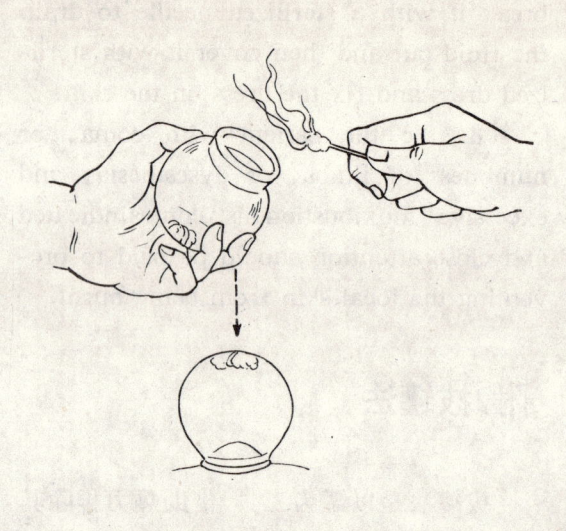

图4—96 贴棉法
Fig. 4—96 Cotton—Attaching Method

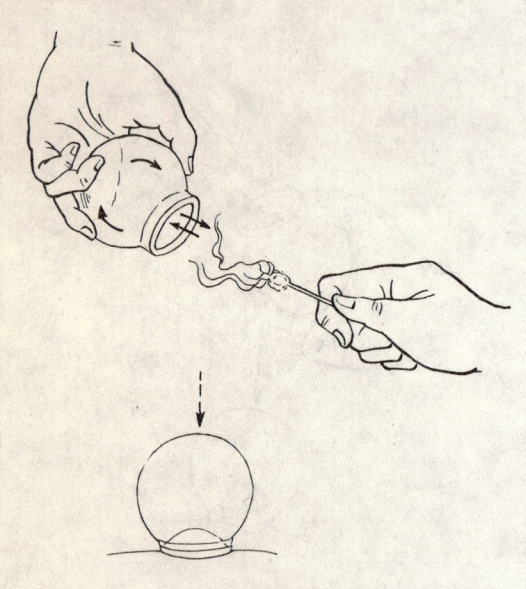

图4—95 闪火法
Fig. 4—95 Fire—Twinkling Method

(二)罐的用法

1. 坐罐:也叫留罐。当罐扣在一定的部位后,留置10~20分钟再起掉。此法可一次拔一罐,或在其肌肉丰厚处的局部拔2~5罐不等,

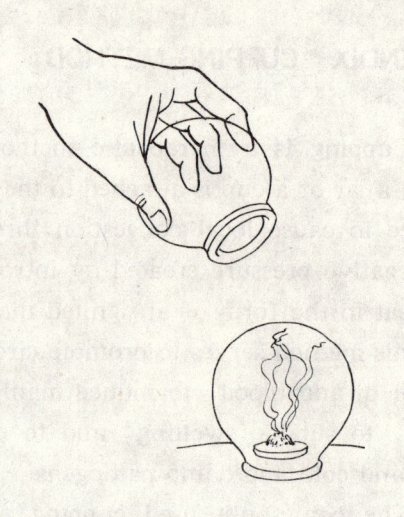

图4—97 架火法
Fig. 4—97 Material—Placing Method

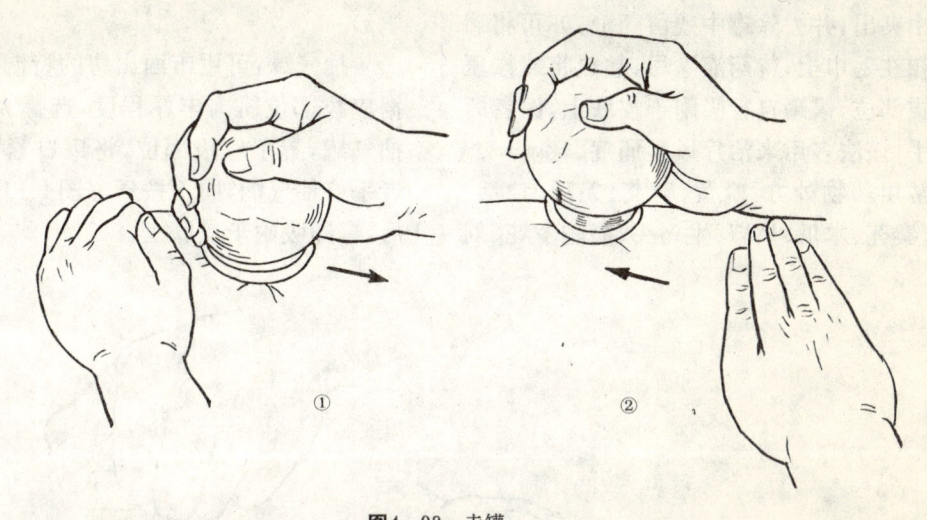

图 4—98 走罐
Fig. 4—98 Moving Cupping

2. 闪罐：即运用闪火法将罐扣上后立即起下，然后再次闪火扣上又起下，如此反复多次。适宜于局部皮肤麻木，或功能减退的虚证。

3. 走罐：又称推罐。此法宜于在肌肉丰厚，面积大的部位如背腰、臀、大腿等处进行。即将拔罐部位涂上凡士林，再将罐扣拔在一定部位的皮肤上，右手握好罐子，左手拉罐向下滑移（图4—98①），达到一定距离再将左手紧按下端皮肤、右手推罐向上滑移（图4—98②）。如此反复数次，见所过处皮肤红晕即止，起罐擦去油脂。此法多用于脉络阻滞或有窜痛的疾病。

4. 针上套罐：此法可起到针、罐双重作用，即在选定穴位或部位，针刺得气留针，将火罐用闪火法迅速套扣在留针的皮肤上（图4—99），多用来治疗深部顽疾。

5. 刺络拔罐：用消毒的三棱针点刺或散刺，或梅花针叩刺一定穴位后，立即将罐扣拔在其处，使之出血。一般留罐10～15分钟，取罐擦去血迹。适用于治疗各种气血瘀滞的疾病，如扭伤，毒蛇咬伤等。

近些年来，除普遍使用火罐外，尚采用药罐，抽气罐。其具体方法如下：

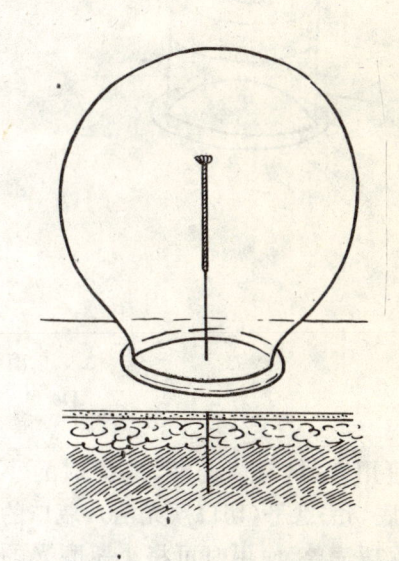

图4—99 针上套罐
Fig. 4—99 Cupping with the Needle inside the Jar

药罐：将配制成的中药装入布袋内，扎紧袋口，放入清水煮至适当浓度，再把竹罐投入药汁内,煮15分钟左右。使用时用镊子将罐从药液中夹出,并去除罐中残留药液,亦可将罐口倒扣在毛巾上,待药液除尽,趁热将罐按压在应拔部位,候罐自行吸附于皮肤上,医者即可松手。该法多用来治疗风湿痛症。

常用药物处方:麻黄、蕲艾、羌活、独活、防风、秦艽、木瓜、川椒、生乌头、蔓陀罗花、刘寄奴,乳香,没药各6克(奚永红等:《针法灸法学》)。

抽气罐:可用市面出售的特制抽气罐、根据应拔部位肌肉丰厚程度,选择大小适宜的抽气罐,置于应拔部位,将罐口紧贴皮肤,医者手持抽气柄,向下按压,(图4—100①)松手后,罐即吸附于皮肤上。

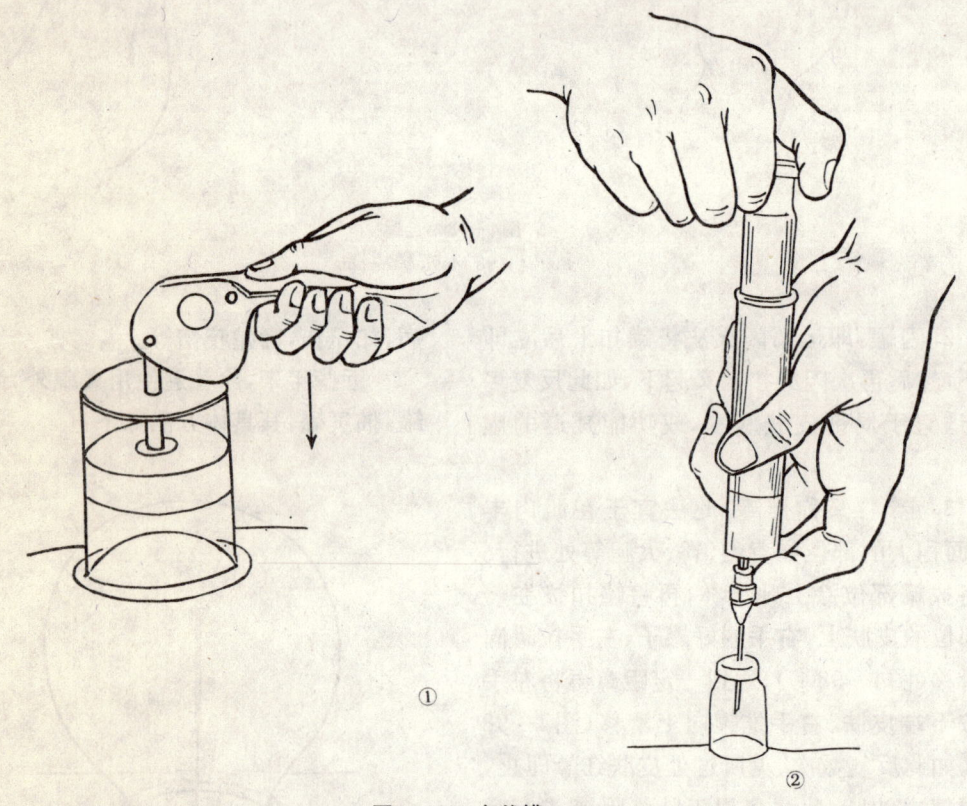

图4—100 气拔罐
Fig. 4—100 Aspirating Cupping

亦可用青、链霉素药瓶,或类似的小药瓶,将瓶底切去磨平(切口须光洁),瓶口的橡皮塞须保留完整。使用时可将小瓶磨光的瓶底面紧置于应拔部位,将5~10毫升注射器套上6~7号针头,穿刺进瓶口的橡皮塞内,以手抽气拔注射器针轴(图4—100②),小瓶即可吸附于应拔部位上。

II. MANIPULATIONS

1. *Cup—Placing Method*
(1) Fire—Throwing Method
Throw an ignited alcohol ball or a piece of ignited paper into a jar, and immdiately place the mouth of the jar firmly a-

gainst the skin on the desired location, making the jar attached on the skin. This method is applied only when the jar is required to be attached horizontally, otherwise the burning material may fall to and hurt the skin(See Fig. 4—94).

(2) Fire Twinkling Method

Clamp an alcohol cotton ball with the forceps, ignite it and put it into the jar, Then, immediately take it out and place the jar on the selected point or area (See Fig. 4—95). This method is frequently applied because it is safe to the patient during the opertion.

(3) Cotton—Attaching Method

Attach an alcohol — wetted cotton ball to the bottom of the internal wall of the jar, ignite it, and immmediately place the jar to the selected point (See Fig. 4—96). In this method, It should be cautious to avoid too much alcohol wetting the cotton in this operation, otherwise fall of the alcohol to the skin may hurt the skin due to burning.

(4) Meterial—Placing Method

Place a circle—shaped hard rubber or a bakelite stopper over the skin of the selected area, and place a cotton ball wetted with 95% of alcohol on the hard rubber or bakelite stopper. Then, ignite the ball, and immediately place a jar(select a glass jar as far as possible)to the skin where the rubber or stopper is on (See Fig. 4—97). This method is safe to the patient and mades the jar sucked firmly.

2. *Cup—Manipulating Method*

(1) Retaining Cupping

After a jar is sucked on the skin of the selected area, retain it there for 10—20 miuntes before removing it. With this method, one jar may be employed at one treatment or 2—5 jars employed to the local area with abundant muscle. This method may be applicable to most of diseases which can be treated with cupping.

(2) Successive Flash Cupping(Quick Cupping)

Make a jar sucked on the skin with fire — twinkling method and immediately remove it. Repeat this course for several times. Theis method is suitable for treating numbness of local skin, or deficiency syndrome due to hypofunction.

(3) Moving Cupping

Also termed pushing cupping. This method is suitable for cupping to the area with abundant muscle, such as back and loin, buttock and thigh. In its operation, smear vaseline over the selected area skin, make a jar sucked on the area. Then, hold the jar with the right hand, and draw it with the left hand to slide downwards (See Fig. 4—98A)for certain distance. Then, forcefully press the skin below the jar with the left hand and push it with the right hand, to slide upwards(See Fig. 4—98B) for certain distance. Repeat this course several times. After the skin of the local area a ppears erythma, take the jar away and wipe the vaseline out. This method is mainly used in treatimg disorder of obstruction of the channel or wandering pain.

(4) Cupping with the Needle inside the Jar

This method serves as therapy of both of puncture and cupping. In its operation, insert a filiform needle into a selcected acupoint to induce needling sensation, retain the needle there. Then quickly place a jar with the fire—twinkling method over the skin where the needle is retained, the needle being inside the jar (See Fig. 4—99). This method is mainly used in treating intractable diease of deep area.

(5) Blood—Letting Puncture and Cupping

After pricking the selected acpoint or area with a sterilized three—edged needle or plum—blossom needle, apply cupping there immediately to cause bleeding. Generally, retain the jar for 10—15 minutes. Then take away the jar and wipe out blood print. This method is used in treating various diseases due to stagnation of qi and blood, such, as sprain, and snake—bite.

Besides the cupping methods metioned above, drug—cupping and aspirating cupping are applied recent years.

Drug Cupping : Make a prescription with some chinese herbal drugs, boil the drugs with water to proper consistency, and add bamboo jar needed into the drug fluid to boil for about 15 minutes. Take the jar out with the forceps, eliminate the fluid in the jar, and press the hot jar over the selected area to make the jar sucked to the skin spontaneously. This method is usually used to treat painful syndromes due to wind-dampness.

The commonly seen drug prescription: Herba Ephedrae, Folium Artemisiae Argyi, Notopterygium, Radix Angelicae Pubescentis, Radix Ledebouriellae, Radix Gantianae Macrophyllae, Fructus Chaenomelis, Pericrpium Zanthoxyli, Fresh Radix Aconiti, Flos stramonii, Herba Serissae, Resina Boswelliae Carterii, Myrrha, each of them being 6 g.

Aspirating cupping: Select proper specially—made aspirating jars (See chapter three, part one) in different sizes according to the cupping area, attach the mouth of the jar to the skin of the selected area, hold the pistal handle with hand and withdraw it upwards a littlle, the jar being sucked to the skin. (See Fig. 4—100A) Or use a special drug bottle to replace the aspirating jar and aspirate the air in the bottle with a syringe (See Fig. 4—100B).

三、注意事项

1. 罐口需圆滑而无缺口，否则会损伤皮肤。

2. 所选部位应肌肉丰厚，且体位要适当，毛发，关节凸凹处不宜拔罐，否则易于脱落。

3. 火罐留置时间一般为15分钟，过久易于引起水泡。

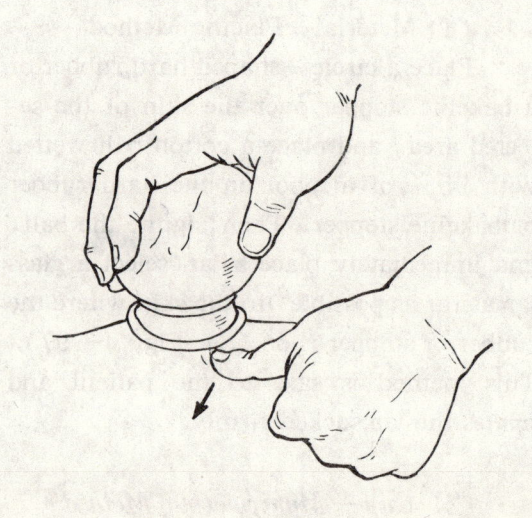

图4-101 起罐
Fig. 4—101 Removing the Jar

4. 起罐时手法要轻缓,用手按压罐口肌肉,使空气进入,则火罐自行脱落(图4—101),切不可强行旋拉,以防损伤皮肤。

5. 采用闪火法时,火焰一定要旋燃在罐内,不可烧热罐口,以免引起烫伤。

6. 根据不同部位,选择口径大小相宜的火罐。

7. 施用本法后,局部会出现瘀血现象,此属正常,可自行消退,不需处理。如瘀血严重者,暂时不要再在原位拔罐,若拔罐后皮肤起泡,小的可自行吸收,大的可用消毒针从底部刺破,放出水液,盖上消毒敷料即可。

8. 高热、抽搐、痉挛;孕妇腰骶部及腹部;皮肤过敏或溃疡破裂处不宜拔罐。

Ⅲ. PRECAUTIONS

1. The mouth of the jar should be round and smooth, without break, otherwise the skin may be injured.

2. The site with abundant muscular mass should be selected , and the patient should be put in a comfortable position. The site with hair, prominence or depression of the joint is not suitable for cupping, otherwise the jar may easily fall off.

3. The duration of the retention of a jar is usually 15 minutes, prolonged duration may be liable to causing blister.

4. The hand maneuver to take away the jar should be gentle and slow. When removing a jar it is needed to press the skin around the mouth of the jar to make the air enter the jar so as that the jar would fall spontaeously (See Fig. 4—101). It is forbidden to use strong force draw and turn the jar, otherwise the skin may be injured.

5. When the fire—twinkling method is used, the fire flame should be moved around inside the jar but not near or at the mouth of the jar so as to prevent burn injury.

6. Jars in different sizes are used according to the area to be applied with cupping.

7. There may be local blood stasis after cupping , this is considered normal, and it may disappear of its own accord, without need of treatment. But when the blood stasis is severe, the cupping should not be applied there temporally. If there are blisters after cupping, the small one can be absorbed of its own accord , however, the large one should be treated by piercing through it from its bottom with a sterilzed needle and covering it with the sterilized dress after the fluid flowing out.

8. It is inadvisable to apply cupping to the patient with fever , clonic convulsion, or spasm, or to the lumbo—sacral region and abdommen of the women during pregnancy, or to the area with leptochroa or broken ulcer.

第五章
针灸技法的临床运用

CHAPTER FIVE
CLINICAL APPLICATION OF SKILL OF ACUPUNCTURE AND MOXIBUSTION

　　针灸治病如同中药治病一样，以望、闻、问、切四诊所取得的资料为基础，运用表里、阴阳、寒热、虚实八纲进行辨证，从复杂的病情变化中，找出疾病的规律予以针灸施治。

　　针灸治病的准则，不外乎补虚、泻实、平补平泻三大类。虚寒证多用补的手法，其中寒证又多久留针，阳气虚陷配合艾灸；实热证多用泻的手法，其中热证或脉络瘀滞，又可用速刺疾出法或刺血法；虚实难辨的经脉病，取相关经穴用平补平泻法，掌握了针灸治病的准则，还必须结合腧穴的主治功能选穴配穴，常用有近部选穴、远道选穴、对症选穴三种。

　　1. 近部选穴：是指在病痛的局部和邻近部位选穴。多用于局部症状比较显著的器官、经脉、经筋以及四肢关节等病痛。如眼病选睛明、太阳；鼻疾选迎香、印堂；肩痛选肩髃、天宗等。

　　2. 远道选穴：是指在距离病痛较远的部位选穴，它包括在病变部位所属经脉的循经选穴，或相关经脉的远道选穴。如胃脘痛取所属胃经远端的足三里穴，也可取与胃相表里的脾经远端的公孙穴。

　　3. 对症选穴：是针对全身性的某些疾病，结合腧穴特殊作用的一种取穴方法，多以特定穴及经验穴为主。如感冒发热选督脉大椎穴，恶心呕吐选心包经内关穴等。除外，尚可根据中医理论辨证选穴，如年高头晕耳鸣，选肾经复溜穴；呕吐呃逆反酸，选肝经太冲穴。上述三种选穴原则，可根据患者具体情况单独运用，也可配合运用。

　　除此以外，耳针治病也有其一定的选穴原则，即：

　　1. 按疾病的相应部位选穴：当某组织或器官发生病变时，可取耳廓上相应的耳穴或敏感点（包括压痛点、低阻点）治疗。如胃病选胃穴；心悸选心穴；肩痛选肩穴或肩关节穴。

　　2. 按中医理论选穴：根据中医经络脏腑学说辨证选用相应耳穴。如"肺主皮毛"，皮肤病可选用肺穴；肝气犯胃致呕吐呃逆，选肝穴与胃穴。

　　3. 按现代医学生理、病理知识选穴：如恶心呕吐，选下脚端（交感）；月经不调选屏间

（内分泌）等。

4.经验选穴：如目赤肿痛选耳尖；高血压选降压沟等。

As the same as in the other branches of TCM, the treatment with acupuncture and moxibustion is carried out based on the four diagnostic methods (i.e. inspection, ausculation and olfaction, interrogation, pulse feeling and palpation) and on application of analysing and differentiating pathological conditions in accordance with the eight principle syndromes (i.e. yin and yang, exterior and interior, cold and heat, and deficiency and excess syndromes serving as guidelines in diagnosis), through which the disease nature, no matter how complicated it is, is determined and known.

The principles of treatment with acupuncture and moxibustion include reinforcing insufficiency, reducing excess, and uniformly reinforcing—reducing some other conditions in which insufficiency is ususlly acompaning with excess and vice versa. In the concrete, reinforcing method is frequently employed in treatment of deficiency — cold syndromes, in which a long retaining of the needle is usually seen in treatment of syndrome of cold[①], and moxibustion is combined in treatment of syndrome of deficiency and sinking of yang—qi[②]. Reducing method is frequently employed in treatment of excessive and heat syndromes, in which heat syndrome or stagnant blood in collaterals may be treated with the method of quick insertion and swift withdrawal of the needle, or by pricking to cause bleeding. The uniform reinforcing — reducing method is usually employed in treatment of channel disorders to which the nature is difficultly determined.

Additionally, the principles of treatment should be considered in combination with selection of acupoint according to the indications and functions of the acupoint. There are three commonly used methods of selection of point in acupuncture and moxibustion: the selection of nearby points, the selection of distant points, and the selection of symptomatic acupoints

1. *Selection of Nearby Points*

Selection of nearby acupoints refers to selection of the acupoints on the local area of the disease or the adjacent area of the disease. It is usually employed in treatment of diseases of the oragan, channel, tendon and joint of limb, which are manifested by marked local symptoms. For example, Jingming (BL1) and Taiyang (EX—HN5) are selected for eye disease; Yingxiang (LI 20) and Yintang

---

① A syndrome of cold or cold syndrome refers to a morbid condition caused by invasion of pathogenic cold, or insufficiency of yang and excess of yin which leads to hypofunction and reduced metabolism, and lowered resistance of the body, marked by aversion to cold, cold limbs, pale complexion, lassitude, huddling up with cold, preference for warmth, epigastric and abdominal pain which may be relieved by heat, absence of thirst, or predilection for hot drinks, loose stools, copious clear urine, pale tongue with whitish slippery coating, deep and slow pulse, frequently seen in chronic and hypofunctional diseases。

② A syndrome of deficiency of sinking of yang—qi: refers to a morbid condidtion due to yang deficiency and sinking of qi of middle—jiao, marked by the flaccidity of tissues and prolapse of visceral organs, fatigue, shortness of breath, intolerance of cold, cold limbs, pallor, polyuria with watery urine, diarrhea, pale and tender tongue, deep and small pulse.

(EX — HN3) for nose problem; and Jianyu (LI 15) and Tianzong (SI 11) for pain in the shoulder.

2. Selection of Distant Points

Selection of distant acupoints refers to selection of acupoints on the area far from the diseased area, which includes selection of acupoints along the affected meridian or along the corresponding meridian. For example, epigastric pain, a disorder of stomach or the Stomach Meridian, is treated by selection of Zusanli (ST36) at the leg, which belongs to the Stomach Merician and is distant to the epigastric region, or by selection of Gongsun (SP4) at the foot, which belongs to the Spleen Meridian which is exteriorly—interiorly related with the Stomach Meridian and is distant to the diseased area.

3. Selection of Symptomatic Acupoints

Selection of symptomatic acupoints refers to selection of the corresponding acupoints in treatment of some general diseases according to the specific functions of the acupoints and some prominent symptoms. The corresponding acupoints mainly refer to the specific acupoints and the empirical points. For example, Dazhui (DU 14) is selected to treat common cold with fever; and Neiguan (PC 6) selected to treat nausea and vomiting. Additionally, it may include selection of acupoints based on differentiation of syndromes according to the theory of TCM. For example, Fuliu (KI 1) is selected for dizziness and tinnitus; and Taichong (LR 3) for vomiting, hiccup and acid regurgitation.

The three methods for acupoint selection metioned above can be applied singly or in combination.

Additionally, there are three commonly used methods of selection of points in otopuncture as follows.

1. Selection of Otopoint According to Disease Location

It refers to selection of the otopoints or sensitive points (including tender points or lower resistance points) on the auricle corresponding to the diseased organs. For example, Ot. Stomach is selected for stomach disease; Ot. Heart for palpitation; and Ot. Shoulder or Shoulder Joint for pain in the shoulder.

2. Selection of Otopoints According to Theories of TCM

According to theories of the channel, zang—fu organ and differentiation of syndromes, the corresponding otopoints are selected. For example, Ot. Lung can be employed for skin promblems because the lung dominates the skin and hair; and Ot. Liver and Stomach for vomiting and hiccup caused by attack of stomach by liver — qi. (i. e., a disorder involving the stomach by transverse invasion of the hyperactive liver — qi, manifested as dizziness, chest distress, hypochondriac pain, irritability, epigastric distension and pain, anorexia, nausea, vomiting, acid regurgitation, hiccup, and taut pulse.)

3. Selection of Otopoints According to Modern Medical Theories

Selection of otopoints depends upon the knowledge of physiology and pathologg of modern medical science. For example, Ot. Endocrine is selected for irregular menstruation; and Ot. Sympathetic for nausea and vomiting.

4. Selection of Otopoints According to Clinical Experience

For example, Ot. Ear Apex is selected for pain, redness and swelling of the eyes; and Ot. Groove of Inferior Helix Crus, also termed Groove for Lowering Blood Pressure for hypertension.

第一节 内科病症

一、流行性腮腺炎

流行性腮腺炎,中医称为"痄腮"。临床以发热、耳下腮腺部漫肿疼痛,咀嚼困难,张口不利为主要表现。初起时可有恶寒发热并见,头痛等症,严重时可伴有睾丸肿痛。

技法运用

1. 毫针:外关、颊车、曲池、下关、合谷、翳风、痄腮穴(耳垂下3分处。图5—1)。

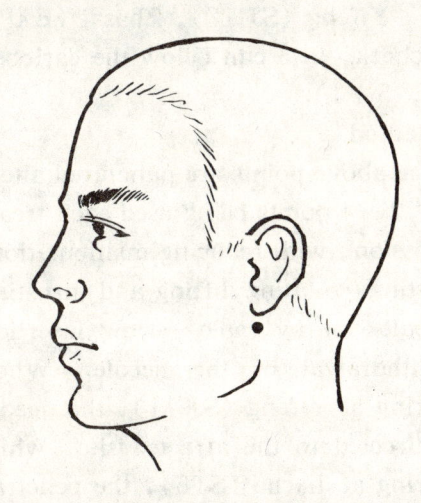

图5—1 痄腮穴

Fig. 5—1 Zhasai (Extra point)

上穴交替针刺。针翳风时,针尖斜向患处;针颊车向大迎方向透刺。均用捻转、提插、徐疾泻法。留针20～30分钟,隔10分钟捻针1次,日针1次。(小儿不留针)

若睾丸肿痛,可加刺太冲、曲泉、三阴交用平补平泻法;高热时可用三棱针点刺少商或商阳放血。

有人取阿是穴,用圆形刺法,即先在肿块顶端向其中心刺1针,再根据肿块大小在肿块周围基底部向对侧刺3～5针,针尖刺至对侧皮下,均用提插捻转手法,留针30～60分钟,10分钟行针1次,每日1次。若出现高热配大椎、(徐徐提插手法,短促行针)合谷、曲池、(提插捻转手法);并发睾丸配大敦,用捻转手法,短促行针后再用艾炷隔姜灸3～5壮,也可针太冲3～5分,捻转手法短促行针,或留针15～30分钟,5～10分钟行针1次。(孙学全.《针灸临证集验》)

2. 灯火灸:取角孙穴。

用2寸长灯草1根,蘸清油点燃后,对准患侧角孙穴(剪去头发)快速点灸,亦可配合点灸患侧颊车,翳风等穴,每日点灸1次,1～3次即应见效,若不效则改用他法。

有报道用火柴棒灸角孙穴治疗痄腮。方法:医者以右手拇、食指持火柴,棒头对准角孙穴(局部头发要剃光),擦燃火柴棒,随即用闪电式动作,点烧在穴位皮肤上,一点即起(图5—2),以发出清脆"喳"声为准。(王松荣.《第一届世界针灸学术大会针灸论文摘要选编》)

3. 电针:双侧合谷、少商及患侧腮腺炎刺激点(肿大腮腺上缘处)。

针呈45°角,由肿大腮腺上缘刺入,深约1～1.5寸,通电10～15分钟,起针后再刺双侧少商出血。(靳志英.上海针灸杂志2:5;1984)

4. 耳针:腮腺穴(平喘穴的内侧,即对耳屏的尖角内侧,若此角不明显,则取对耳屏边缘中点的内侧。图5—3)、面颊区、神门、屏间、脑、耳轮4、5、6。强刺激,每次选2～3穴,留针30～60分钟,每日针1～2次。

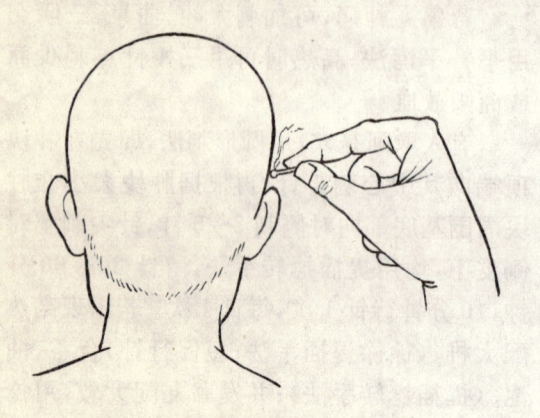

图5-2 火柴棒灸
Fig. 5-2 Moxibustion with the Lighited Match

腮腺穴
Ot. Parotid Glands

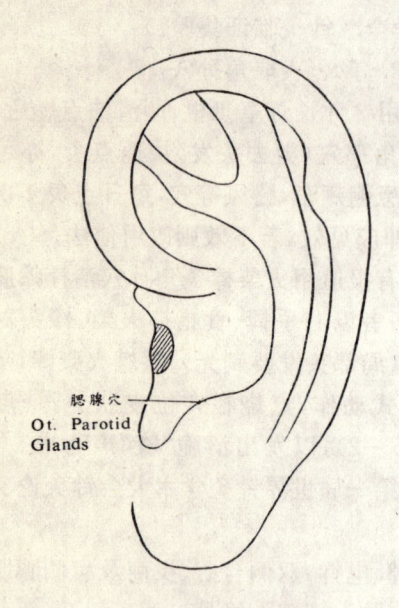

图5-3 腮腺穴
Fig. 5-3 Ot. Parotid Glands

SECTION 1 DISEASES OR SYNDROMES IN INTERNAL MEDICINE

1. MUMPS

Manifestations

Mumps, infectious parotitis, termed Zha Sai (痄腮) in TCM, is manifested clinically by swelling and pain in the parotid region, fever, difficulty in chewing and opening the mouth. Intolerance to cold and headache may be accompanied at the first stage, and swelling and pain in the testicle in the severe stage.

Treatment by Applying Acubustion (i. e. acupuncture and moxibustion) Techniques

(1) *Filiform Needling*

Selection of Points

Waiguan (SJ 5), Jiache (ST 6), Quchi (LI 11), Xiaguan (ST 7), Hegu (LI 4), Yifeng (SJ 17), Zhasai (EX[①], at the cheek, 0.3 cun below the earlobe, see Fig. 5-1).

Method

The above points are punctured alternately, 2-4 points being used each treatment session, with reducing manipulations by twisting, rotating, lifting and thrusting the needle, or by rapid — slow insertion and withdrawal of the needle. When puncturing at Yifeng (SJ 11), the needle tip is directed to the affected site, while puncturing at Jiache (ST6), the penetration needling (透针 or 透刺, Touzhen or Touci, a needling method performed by

---

[①] Ex. is from extra point or extraordinary point, including the points determind after determination of those of the fourteen Meridians.

piercing two or more points or channels simultaneously in one insertion) towards Daying (ST5). The needles are retained in each point selected for 20—30 minutes and twisted per ten minutes during the retention. The puncture is given once daily. Note: retention of the needle is forbidden to children.

Supplementary Points and Method

Taichong (LR 3), Ququan (LR 8) and Sanyinjiao (SP 6) are added for swelling in the testicle with uniform reinforcing — reducing manipulation applied, and Shaoshang (LU 11) or Shangyang (LI 1) is pricked with the three—edged needle to cause bleeding in addition for high fever.

Introducing Some Experiential Techniques

It is recorded in Collection of Clinical Experiences of Acupuncture & Moxibustion that Ashi points (i.e. painful points) are punctured with the manipulation by circling needling. To the operation, first, the center of the swollen parotid region is punctured perpendicularly deep to the diseased center at the bottom, then three to five points around the swollen parotid region are punctured with the needle tips respectively arriving at the area beneath the skin opposite to its own puncturing point. The puncture is given with the manipulations by lifting, thrusting and twisting the needle, the needles retained at each point for 30—60 minutes and manipulated per ten minutes during the retention. Dazhui (DU 14), Hegu (LI 4) and Quchi (LI 11) are added for high fever, Dazhui (Du 14) being punctured with the needling method of slow lifting and thrusting for a moment, and the other points punctured with lifting, thrusting and twisting manipulations. For orchitis, Dadun (LR 1) and Taichong (LR 3) are added, the former being puntured with twirling manner and a short and quick manipulation of the needle, followed by ginger moxibustion with three to five moxa cones applied to it, and the latter punctured 0.3—0.5 cun deep with twirling method as well as short and quick manner, or the needle retained for 15—30 minutes and manipulated per five to ten minutes during the retention.

(2) *Moxibustion with Medulla Junci (Rush—Burning Moxibustion)*

Selection of Point

Jiaosun (SJ 20)

Method

A 2 cun long segment of rush pith soaked with vegetable oil is lighted and aimed at Jiaosun (SJ 20) where the hair is cut out, It is removed quickly as soon as there is a sound of burning of the skin. Or, the moxibustion mentioned above may be applied on Jiache (DT6) and Yifeng (SJ 17) of the diseased side in addition. The moxibustion is given once daily. Generally, one to three times of the treatment will lead to cure of the disease. If not, other method of treatment should be given to replace it.

Introducing An Experiential Technique

It is reported by Dr. Wang Shongyong, a famous acupuncturist, that the moxibustion with an ignited match on Jiaosun (SJ 20) is also effective in treating mumps. To the operation, hold the match with the thumb and index finger of the right hand, with its head aimed at Jiaosun (SJ 20) where the local hair has been cut away. Then, ignite match and presse it over the point and remove it quickly as soon as there is a sound of burning of the skin (See Fig. 5-2).

(3) *Electroacupuncture*

Selection of Points

Hegu (LI 4) and Shaoshang (LU 11) of both sides, the stimulation point of mumps (at the upper border of the swollen parotid region).

Method

Insert a needle obliquely 1-1.5 cun deep at an angle of 45° into the upper border of the swollen parotid region, and connect the needle with an electric current from an electric therapeutic unit for 10-15 minutes. After withdrawal of the needele the bilateral Shaoshang (LU 11) are pricked to cause bleeding and bilateral Hegu (LI 4)puncdtured.

(4) *Otopuncture*

Selection of Otopoints

Parotid Glands (medial to Ot. Soothing Asthma, i.e., medial to the antitragus apex. If the the apex is not obvious, the point medial to the midpoint of the lower border of the antitragus is taken, (see Fig. 5-3). Cheek, Shenmen, Endocrine, Brain, Helex 4,5, and 6.

Method

Two to three otopoints are punctured with strong stimulation and the needles are retained at each point for 30-60 minutes in each treatment session. Give the puncture treatment one to two times daily.

二、急性传染性肝炎

急性传染性肝炎，属于中医"黄疸"、"胁痛"范畴。临床以肝区痛、食欲不振、恶心、乏力为主要表现，部分病人可有黄疸（色黄如桔为阳黄，色黄晦暗或如烟薰为阴黄）和发热、肝脏肿大，肝功能有不同程度的损害。

技法运用

1. 毫针：阳黄主穴：胆俞、阳陵泉、内庭、太冲。每次2～3穴，用捻转、提插、疾徐泻法。每日针1次，留针20分钟。脘闷食少加中脘、足三里；胸闷呕恶加内关、公孙；腹胀便秘加天枢、大肠俞。

阴黄主穴：至阴、脾俞、胆俞、中脘、足三里、三阴交。每次2～3穴，用平补平泻法，每日针1次，留针20分钟，可配合艾灸。神疲恶寒加命门、气海；大便溏泻加天枢、关元。胁痛加支沟、丘墟透照海、肝俞，用捻转、提插、疾徐泻法；复溜、肾俞用疾徐、捻转、提插补法。

有人针刺治疗急性传染性黄疸型肝炎，取穴分三组，第一组以中封为主穴，后溪、合谷、足三里为配穴；第二组为中封、后溪；第三组为中封。均用泻法，特别运用了复式泻法，即针尖取逆经方向，一进三退，起针时不闭其孔。针刺后溪穴时深达劳宫；针合谷穴时，可以合谷透劳宫。每日取单侧穴位治疗，左右交替使用，两周为一疗程（钟英，等．上海中医药杂志2：23；1962）。

2. 电针：取穴同毫针。选用疏波或疏密波，输出电量为中等度刺激，频率40～60次/分钟。每日1次，每次15～30分钟，10次为一疗程。

3. 耳针：胆、肝、脾、胃、神门、下脚端、三焦、耳迷根。每次取2～3穴。中等刺激，留针20分钟，每日1次。

2. ACUTE INFECTIOUS HEPATITIS

Manifestations

Acute infectious hepatitis, belonging to the disease or syndrome categories of Huang Dang (黄疸 jaundice) and Xie Tong (胁痛 hypochondriac pain) in TCM, is manifested clinically mainly by hepatalgia, poor appetite, nausea and lassitude. Jaundice (yang jaundice is termed according to lustrous yellow skin and sclera, and yin jaundice, according to dusky yellow skin), fever, hepatomegaly and manifestations of impairment of the liver function are accompanied in some cases.

Treatment by Applying Acubustion Techniques

(1) *Puncture with the Filiform Needle*

a. For yang jaundice:

Selection of Points

Main points: Danshu (BL 19), Yanglingquan (GB 34), Neiting (ST 44), Taichong (LR 3).

Suppelementary points according to symptoms: Zhongwan (RN 12) and Zusanli (ST36) are added for oppressed feeling in the chest with loss of appetite; Neiguan (PC6) and Gongsun (SP 4) added for oppressed feeling in the chest with nausea; and Tianshu (ST25) and Dachangshu (BL25) added for abdominal distension and constipation.

Method

Two or three points are selected each treatment session and punctured daily, and reducing manipulations by twirling, rotating, lifting and thrusting the needle, and by slow — rapid insertion and withdrawal of the needle are applied. The needles are retained in the acupoints for twenty minutes.

b. For Yin jaundice:

Selection of Points

Main points: Zhiyin (BL67), Pishu (BL20), Danshu (BL19), Zhongwan (RN 12), Zusanli (ST36), Sanyinjiao (SP6).

Method

Two or three points are selected each treatment session and punctured daily, with uniform reinforcing — reducing method applied and the needles retained at each point for twenty minutes. Moxibustion may be applied in cooperation.

Supplementary points according to symptoms and method: Mingmen (DU 4) and Qihai (RN 6) are added for general lassitude and aversion to cold; Tianshu (ST25) and Guanyuan (RN4) added for loose stools; Zhigou (SJ6), Qiuxu (GB40) and Ganshu (BL18) added for hypochondriac pain, with reducing manipulations by twisting, lifting and thrusting the needle and by rapid — slow insertion and withdrawal of the needle, and with the penetration needling at Qiuxu (GB40) to Zhaohai (KI6); Xingjian (LR2) added with reducing manipulations by twisting, lifting and thrusting the needle and by rapid — slow insertion and withdrawal of the needle; and Fuliu (kI7) and Shenshu (BL23) added with reinforcing manipulations by twisting, lifting and thrusintg the needle and by rapid — slow insertion and withdrawal of the needle for dryness of the mouth and heat sensation in the palms and soles.

Introducing Some Experiential Techniques

It is reported in Shanghai Journal of Acupuncture & Moxibustion that the following three groups of points are selected in treatment of acute infectious icterohepatitis. The first group consists of Zhongfeng (LR4) which is the main point, Houxi (SI3), Hegu (LI4) and Zusanli (ST36) which are the secondary; the second group, ZhongFeng (LR4) and Houxi (SI3); and the third group, Zhongfeng (LR4). The points are punctured with reducing manipulations, especially with compound reducing manipulations. That is, make the needle tip direct against the running course of the punctured meridian in needling, thrust the needle once followed by lifting it three times, and leave the needle hole opened after withdrawal of the needle. Houxi (SI3) and Hegu (LI4) are punctured with penetration needling to Laogong (PC8). The points at the same side are selected in one treatment session, and the left points and the right points are selected alternately. Fourteen treatment sessions constitute a therapeutic course.

(2) *Electroacupuncture*

Selection of Points

The same as in puncture with the filform needle.

Method

Two to four points are selected each treatment session. An electric stimulation with a low or irregular wave, a frequency at 40 — 60 turns/min., and a medium strength intensity is given for fifteen to thirty minutes daily. Ten treatment sessions constitute a therapeutic course.

(3) *Otopuncture*

Selection of Otopoints

Gallbadder, Liver, Spleen, Stomach, Shenmen, Sympathetic, Sanjiao, Ergenmi.

Method

Two or three otopoints are punctured daily, with a medium strength stimulation applied and the needles retained at each point for twenty minutes.

三、细菌性痢疾

细菌性痢疾，中医称"痢疾"、"滞下"。临床以腹痛、里急后重、痢下赤白粘液脓血为主要表现，可同时伴发热、畏冷等症状。

技法运用

1．毫针：刺天枢、足三里、上巨墟。

发热加刺曲池、大椎；恶心加内关、中脘；里急后重加大肠俞、白环俞、长强。急性患者用提插捻转泻法，留针30分钟，每日1～3次。慢性者用提插、捻转补法。

有报道针刺"三合穴"治痢疾。"三合穴"即胃经合穴足三里、大肠下合穴上巨墟、小肠下合穴下巨墟。先针双腿足三里，深1.5～2寸，次针上巨墟1.5寸左右，后针下巨墟1.2寸左右（光明日报．1980年5月8日）。

发热加刺曲池或合谷；腹痛厉害或久病不愈加针气海或关元。留针30分钟，每隔10分钟行针1次。

有人取脾经过敏点（三阴交穴上约一横指处）、地机（或在地机穴上下5分左右）、阴陵泉（或在阴陵泉穴上下5分～1寸左右）。一般用泻法，采取逆经络捻针，双手同时进针，用食指向前，拇指向后的迎随捻转法。一般每日针1次，重者每日针2次，留针30分钟至1小时

或2小时,留针期间每隔20分钟用泻法1次。(焦国瑞,等.《针灸临床经验辑要》)

2. 灸疗:取神阙、天枢、关元、足三里、上巨墟、小肠俞等穴。

用艾卷回旋灸及温和灸,亦可用艾炷隔姜或隔蒜灸,以及神阙隔盐灸。每穴每次用艾卷点10～15分钟,或艾炷灸3～5壮,每日1～2次。本法对急性菌痢无高热者效果较好,对慢性菌痢坚持长期灸治优于其他方法。

3. 刺络拔罐:取穴大椎、脾俞、大肠俞。用三棱针点刺穴位出血,然后再加拔火罐。(陈佑邦,等.《当代中国针灸临证精要》)

4. 耳针:大肠、小肠、下脚端、脾、胃、肾、直肠下端。每日1～2次,每次3～5穴,急性用强刺激;慢性用轻刺激,亦可隔日1次,每次留针15～30分钟。

3. BACILLARY DYSENTERY

Manifestations

Bacillary dysentery, belonging to the disease or syndrome categories of Li Ji（痢疾）, Zhi Xia（滞下）in TCM, is manifested clinically cheifly by abdominal pain, tenesmus and evacuation of purulent or bloody stool. Fever and aversion to cold may be accompanied.

Treatment by Applying Acubustion Techniques

(1) *Puncture with the Filiform Needle*

Selection of Points

Main points: Tianshu (ST25), Zusanli (ST36), Shangjuxu (ST31).

Supplementary points according to symptoms: Quchi (LI 11) and Dazhui (DU 14) for fever; Neiguan and Zhongwan (RN 12) for nausea; and Dachangshu (BL25), Baihuanshu (BL30) and Changqiang (DU 1) for tenesmus.

Method

Two to four points are punctured each treatment session. For acute cases, the treatment is given one to three times daily, reducing manipulations by twisting, lifting and thrusting the needle are applied, and the needles retained at each point for thirty minutes. But for chronic cases, the points are punctured with reinforcing manipulations by lifting, thrusting and twisting the needle, and the treatment is given once daily.

Introducing Some Experiential Techniques

It is reported in Guangming Daily that "three He—Sea acupoints" are punctured for treatment of dysentery. The three He—Sea points refer to Zusanli (ST36), the He—Sea point of the Stomach Meridian, Shangjuxu (ST37), the Lower He—Sea point of the Large Intestine Meridian, and Xiajuxu (ST39), the Lower He—Sea point of the Small Intestine Meridian. To the operation, first, left and right Zusanli (ST36) are punctured to a depth of 1.5—2 cun. Then, left and right Shangjuxu (ST37) punctured to a depth of about 1.5 cun. Finally, left and right Xiajuxu (ST39) punctured to a depth of about 1.2 cun. Quchi (LI 11) or Hegu (LI 4) is punctured additionally for fever, Qihai (RN 6) or Guanyuan (RN 4) added for severe abdominal pain or protracted cases. In the treatment, the needles are retained at each point for thirty minutes and twisted per ten minutes during the retention.

In the Collection of Outstandings of Clinical Experiences of Acupuncture & Moxibustion another method is recorded. The sensitive spot of the Spleen Meridian, which is one finger—breadth above Sanyinjiao (SP 6), Diji (SP 8) or the points at the line stretching from Diji (SP 8) upward and downward 0.5 cun respectively, and Yinlingquan (SP 9) or points at the line stretching from Yinlingquan (SP 9) upward and downward 0.5—1 cun respectively are taken as the puncture points, and reducing manipulations are applied. In the operation, insert the needle with the two hands acting in coordination into the point, and twirl the needle against the running course of the punctured meridian with the thumb of the right hand moving backwards. Usually, puncture once daily, but for severe cases, give the puncture treatment two times daily. The needles are retained at each point for thirty minutes to one hour or two hours, and manipulated with reducing manner per twenty minutes during the retention.

（2）*Moxibustion*

Selection of Points

Shenjue (RN 8), Tianshu (ST25), Guanyuan (RN 4), Zusanli (ST36), Shangjuxu (ST37), Xiaochangshu (BL27).

Method

Apply the circling moxibustion or mild — warming moxibustion with the moxa roll, or the ginger moxibustion or the garlic moxibustion, or the moxibstuion with some salt on Shenjue (RN 8) one to two times daily. Give the moxibustion to the each point with the moxa roll for ten to fifteen minutes or with the moxa cone until three to five cones have been burnt out. The moxibustion is effective in treating acute bacillary dysentery without high fever, and provides a better effect in treating chronic bacillary dysentery as compared with other treatment methods.

（3）*Blood—Letting Puncture and Cupping*

Selection of Points

Dazhui (DU 14), Pishu (BL20), Dachangshu (BL25)

Method

Prick the points with the three—edged needle to cause bleeding and apply cupping on the pricked points.

（4）*Otopuncture*

Selection of Otopoints

Large Inestine, Small Intestine, Sympathetic, Spleen, Stomach, Lower Portion of Rectum

Method

Three to five otopoints are punctured one or two times daily or once every other day, with the needles retained at each point selected for fifteen to thirty minutes, and with a strong stimulation applied for acute cases and a mild stimulation applied for chronic cases.

四、疟 疾

疟疾，临床表现为先寒颤后高热，而后全身大汗，体温降至正常。本病多为周期性发作，有1日一次的"一日疟"；隔日一次的"间日疟"；2日一次的"三日疟"，也有发作不规则的发作者。

技法运用

1．毫针：取大椎、间使、后溪、陶道、至阳等穴。

于发作前1～2小时施针，或三棱针点刺大椎出血，再酌取其他穴位。新病用提插捻转泻法，久病用提插捻转补法，留针30分钟，并可配合艾灸，每隔5～10分钟行针1次。

有报道取疟门穴（即四、五掌指关节前凹陷中）治疗有良效，嘱患者两手四指并拢作轻握拳式，术者左手食指作押手固定穴位，右手以15°角（针尖向掌心），徐徐将针刺入0.8～1寸深（图5－4）。捻转得气后留针20～30分钟，每隔5～15分钟捻转1次（朱复林，等．江苏中医，11：～32；1961）。亦有人取大椎、间使、陶道、合谷、后溪、内关、疟门穴，在发作前2～3小时针刺，以泻法为主，留针30分钟，每隔3～5分钟行针1次。（田丛豁，等．《针灸医学验集》）。

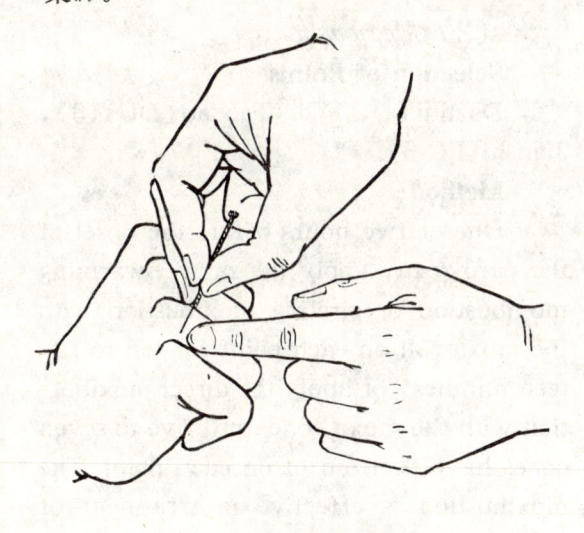

图5－4 疟门穴刺法

Fig. 5—4 Puncturing at Nuemenxue (Extra point)

2．灸法：取大椎、陶道、间使等穴。

于发病前1～2小时用艾条温和灸或回旋灸，每穴灸10～15分钟，亦可艾炷着肤灸5～7壮。本法对间日疟效果满意，但对恶性疟疾疗效较差。

有人用朝天辣椒、野薄荷、鲜毛茛、白芥子四药，任选一种捣烂如泥状，制成杏仁大小的丸，贴于大椎、内关穴上，固定了3～6小时。取下后可见皮肤上起泡即可，有的也不一定起泡。（陈积祥．《针术临床实践》）

3．耳针：下屏尖、脑、屏间、肝、脾。

取双侧，在发作前1～2小时针刺，用较强刺激，留针1小时，连续针刺3次。

4．三棱针刺血：选腘窝（委中）小静脉，于发作前1～2小时，将患者腘窝部常规消毒后，用三棱针刺入小静脉上，出针时血随针出，放血1毫升左右，然后用干棉球压迫止血。每次取一侧，左右交替。（田丛豁，等．《针灸医学验集》）

4. MALARIA

Manifestations

Malaria is manifested clinically by regular paroxysms of sever chills and high fever followed by sweating and lowering of the body temperature. The daily malaria, the malaria tertiana and the quartan malaria are termed according to the frequency of the paroxysm. But some cases with malaria do not present a regular paroxysm.

Treatment by Applying Acubustion Techniques

(1) *Filiform Needling*

Selection of Points

Dazhui (DU 14), Jianshi (PC 5), Houxi (SI 3), Taodao (DU 13), Zhiyang (DU 9)

Method

Apply acupuncture treatment one to two hours prior to the onset of the paroxysm. Puncture at two to four points each treatment session with reducing manipulations by lifting, thrusting, twirling and rotating the needle for acute malaria, and reinforcing manipulations by lifting, thrusting, twirling and rotating the needle for chronic malaria, and with the needles retained for thirty minutes and manipulated per five to ten minutes during the retention.

Note, pricking at Dazhui (DU 14) with the three — edged needle to cause bleeding may be applied before the puncture, and moxibustion may be given in cooperation.

Introducing Some Experiential Techniques

In Jiangsu Journal of TCM it is reported that Nuemenxue (Ex., located at the depression between the fourth metacarpophalangeal joints of the middle and ring fingers) is punctured for treatment of malaria. To the operation, ask the patient to make a loose fist, fix the point with the index finger of the left hand, insert the needle slowly to a depth of 0.5 — 1 cun and at an angle of 15°, with the needle tip directed to the center of the palm (See Fig. 5 — 4). Then, twirl and rotate the needle to induce the needling seasation to the patient. Finally, retain the needle for twenty to thirty minutes during the retention.

Another method is recorded in Collection of Experiences of Acupuncture & Moxibstion. Dazhui (DU 14), Jianshi (PC5), Taodao (DU 13), Hegu (LI 4), Houxi (SI 3), Neiguan (PC6) and Nuemenxue (Ex., located at the depression between the fourth and fifth metacarpophangeal joins) are punctured two to three hours prior to the onset of the paroxysm for treatment of malaria. The puncture is given with the reducing manipulations applied and with needles retained at each point for thirty minutes during which the needles are manipulated per five to ten minutes. Or the puncture is given with the needles lifted, thrust, tiwisted and rotated for twenty minutes, and then retained for thirty minutes. But for the weak patients or the patients sensitive to needling, the uniform reinforcing — reducing manipulation is applied and, after arrival of qi, the needles are retained for one to two hours and manipulated per three to five minutes.

(2) *Moxibustion*

Selection of Points

Dazhui (DU 4), Taodao (DU 13), Jianshi (PC 5)

Method

One or two hours before the onset of the paroxysm, apply the mild — warming moxibustion or circling moxibustion with the moxa roll on each point for ten to fifteen minutes, or apply the direct moxibustion with the moxa cone until five to seven cones have been burnt on each point. The moxibustion is effective in treatment of malaria tertiana, but poor in treatment of pernicious malaria.

Introducing An Experiential Technique

It is recorded in Clinical Practice of Acupuncture & Moxibustion that a drug — moxibustion is applied for treatment of malaria. To the method, select any one from the very hot pepper, wild pepermint, fresh buttercup and white mustard seed and pound it into paste with which pills like a bitter apricot kernel in size are made up. The pills are stuck and fixed on Dazhui (DU 14) and Neiguan (PC 6) for three to six hours. A blister may or may not occur on the local skin after moving away the pill.

(3) *Otopuncture*

Selection of Otopoints

Infratragic Apex, Brain, Endocrine, Liver, Spleen

. Method

Two to four of bilateral otopoints are punctured one to two hours prior to the onset of the paroxysm, with strong stimulation administered and the needles retained at each otopoint for one hour. The otopuncture is repeated consecutively for three times.

(4) *Pricking with the Three — Edged Needle*

Selection of Point and Method

The treatment is given one to two hours prior to the onset of the paroxysm. A routine and local sterilization is given to the popliteal fossa, the small vein at the popliteal fossa is selected and pricked with the three — edged needle to cause letting out of the blood about 1 ml, and the needle hole is pressed to stop bleeding with the dry sterilized cotton ball. Only one side is pricked in each session and the two sides are pricked alternately.

五、感 冒

感冒，属中医"伤风"范畴。临床分为两型。风寒型症见恶寒发热、无汗、头痛、鼻塞、流涕、喷嚏、咳嗽、痰液清稀、四肢酸痛、苔薄白、脉浮紧；风热型症见发热重恶寒轻，头痛、目赤、咳嗽、痰黄稠、有汗不解、苔薄黄、脉浮数。若暑热夹湿，则兼见头重如裹、胸闷、呕恶，甚至腹胀、便溏、口淡不渴、苔厚腻或黄腻、脉缓或浮数。

技法运用

1. 毫针：取合谷、列缺、风池等穴。

用平补平泻手法。风寒型无汗，合谷穴用捻转、提插、疾徐补法，或烧山火手法，使其发汗；风热型加大椎、曲池，用捻转、提插疾徐泻法，或透天凉手法，以清其热；暑热加阴陵泉、曲池、内关等穴，用捻转、提插泻法，或透天凉手法。

有报道，治疗感冒用毫针顺四、五掌骨间隙（液门穴）刺0.5～1寸，捻转数次。一般取单侧，10分钟效果不好者，加刺对侧，留针15～30分钟（申健．河南中医，4：19；1988）

另有报道，感冒早期用长3.5厘米，直径0.3毫米的毫针，针刺大椎穴。针刺时患者侧卧，两腿屈曲，用力以手抱头后枕部，使颈部最大限度向前弯曲，医者一手持针柄自大椎穴徐徐刺入，针尖刺透皮肤后，继续与脊柱成15°角，向尾侧探进约1.5～2厘米，另一手从大椎穴下方沿脊柱至尾部施以巡按法，然后捻转施用透天凉手法，捻针时腰部或尾部产生发凉的感觉，可作为正确的刺激标志，每人只针1次，捻针5～15分钟。

恢复期根据临床尚存的不同症状，分别选取足三里，内关、合谷。一般都针一侧足三里，气短配一侧内关；咳嗽配一侧合谷，与皮肤表面呈垂直方向进针，采用平补平泻法，捻针5分钟，留针10分钟，每人只针1次。

预防流感针一侧足三里，采用补法，酸麻感觉达足背时，立即起针。每人只针1次（延安县医院内科．中医杂志，2；1960）

还有人在外感初起,如恶寒重发热轻、口中和、舌苔白、头身痛、无汗、脉浮紧时,取天柱、大椎、身柱、风门、合谷等穴,用"烧山火"手法。令患者鼻孔吸气1次,口呼5次,以左手拇指或食指紧按其穴,随其呼气进针于天部(皮内浅层),找到酸胀感觉,向一个方向用手指轻捻3次或9次(如无感觉,少停,轻弹3次,再捻3次,若针下特别沉紧,则轻提动针头),即将针急插于人部(中层),操作方法与天部(浅层)相同。捻毕轻提豆许,再急插于地部(筋骨间,亦即该穴的深层),操作方法与天部(浅层)相同,捻毕轻提少许,再急插慢提各3次,手法操作完毕,随其吸气,慢慢将针提出,急按其穴。

外感末期,发热重恶寒轻、口渴、舌红、苔黄、脉浮数时,取大椎、陶道、风门、肺俞或后溪、申脉等穴,用"阳中隐阴"手法,以左手拇指或食指紧按其穴,进针于天部(浅层),找到酸或胀的感觉,即将针急插于人部(中层),向一个方向轻捻9次,或急插慢提各3次,如觉微热或微汗,稍停针便慢慢插于地部(深层),向一个方向捻6次,或慢插急提各3次,找到凉的感觉,即将针提于天部(浅层),少停,即提出,慢慢揉按其穴或不按其穴,不留针。有时先用"烧山火"手法,针1、2个穴法,见到汗出适宜,再用"透天凉"手法,令患者口中吸气1次,鼻孔出气5次(自然呼吸),随其气慢慢进于地部(深层),找到麻或触电样感觉,向一个方向捻6次,急提至人部(中层),慢插急提各3次(如无感觉,少停,再搓6次,如针下特别紧涩,则摇针),急提至天部(浅层),少停,手法用毕,随鼻孔出气急速将针提出,慢慢揉按其穴,或不扣闭其穴,有时不利用呼吸也可以。(刘冠军,等.《中医针法集锦》)。

2.拔火罐:选用风门、肺俞、大椎拔火罐,也可针上套罐、留罐10~15分钟。本法宜于风寒型感冒。

5. COMMON COLD

Manifestations

Common cold, belonging to the disease or syndrome category of Shang Feng (伤风, a disease due to attack by wind—evil) in TCM, is classified into two types, the wind cold and the wind heat. The type of wind cold is manifested by aversion to cold, fever, anhidrosis, headache, nasal obstruction, running nose, sneezing, cough with thin sputum, soreness and pain of the limbs, thin and white tongue coating, superficial and tense pulse; while the type of wind heat manifested by fever, slight aversion to wind, headache, congestion of eye, cough with yellow and thick sputum, sweating, thin and yellowish tongue coating, superficial and rapid pulse. If the type of wind heat is due to summer heat evil complicated with damp evil, heaviness of head, oppressed feeling in the chest, vomiting and nausea, even abdominal distension, loose stool, thick and sticky tongue coating, slow or superficial and rapid pulse are seen.

Treatment by Applying Acubustion Techniques

(1) *Puncture with the Filiform needle*

Selection of Points

Hegu(LI 4), Lieque(LU 7), Fengchi (GB 20)

Method

The uniform reinforcing — reducing needling is applied. For wind cold type with anhidrosis, Hegu (LI 4) is punctured with reinforcing manipulations by twirling, lifting, and thrusting the needle and by insertting and withdrawing the needle slowly and rapidly, or with heat—producing needling to induce diaphoresis; for wind heat type, Dazhui (DU 14) and Quchi (LI 11) are additionally punctured with reducing manipulations by twisting, rotating, lifting and thrusting the needle and by inserting and withdrawing the needle rapidly and slowly, or with the cold—producing needling to eliminate heat; for summer heat—damp evil, Yinlingquan (SP 9), Quchi (LI 11) and Neiguan (PC 6) punctrued additionnally with reducing manipulations by twirling, rotatng, lifting and thrusting the needle, or with the cold—producinhg needling.

Introducing Some Experiential Technigues

It is reported in Henan Journal of TCM that Yenmen (SJ 2) is punctured for treatment of the disease. To the operation, left or right Yemen (SJ 2) is punctured to a depth of 0.5—1 cun, with the needle twisted for several times and then retained for fifteen to thirty minutes. If the effect is not present ten minutes later, the opposite Yemen (SJ 2) is added.

Another acupuncture method for treating common cold is introduced by Journal of TCM. To the operation, a filiform needle 3.5 cun in length and 0.3 mm in diameter is used and Dazhui (DU 14) is selected. The patient is asked to lie on one side, with the lower extremities at flexion and hands crossing at the occiputal area, so as to make the neck at the maxium flexion. The needle is inserted slowly into the point. Through the skin ., the needle is pushed slowly at an angle of 15° formed with the spinal column, with the needle tip directing to the lower portion of the spinal column to a depth of about 1.5—2 cun with great care. Then, the portion of the spinal column below Dazhui (DU 14) is pressed from the above downwards with the other hand, and the cold—producing needling by twirling and rotating the needle is applied to induce the cold sensation in the lower back and buttock. The puncture treatment is given once only to each patient and the needlde is twisted for five to fifteen minutes in the treatment.

For the cases at at convalescence, puncture at Zusanli (ST 36), Neiguan (PC 6), or Hegu (LI 4) is given according to different symptoms left. Generally, Zusanli (ST 6) of one side is selected, perpendicular puncture with the uniform reinforcing—reducing manipulation is applied, and the needle is retained for ten minutes. For shortness of breath, Neiguan (PC 6) of one side is added, and Hegu (LI 4) added for cough. The puncture is given only once to each patient.

For the purpose of preventing common cold, Zusanli (ST 36) of one side is punctured with reinforcing manipulation. When the needling sensations of soreness, numbness and heaviness are propagated to the dorsum of the foot, the needle is withdrawn immediately. The puncture is given once only to each paitent.

Besides, some other methods for treating common cold are recorded in Collection of Outstandings of the Needling Methods of TCM. At early stage with aversion to cold, slight fever, white tongue coating, pain of the head and the trunk, anhidrosis, and superficial and tense pulse, Tianzhu (BL 10), Dazhui (DU 14), Fengmen (BL 12) and Hegu (LI 4) are punctured with the heat—producing needling applied. To the operation, ask the patient to inspire with the nose once and expire with the mouth five times. As the patient expiring, insert the needle into the acupoint to its heaven portion (beneath the skin) to induce soerness and distension to the patient, then, twirl he needle gently in a single direction three or nine times. If the needling sensation is not induced to the patient, retain the needle for a short time, then, tap and twirl it three times respectively. If feeling very tense under the needle, lift the needle gently and, immediately, insert it swiftly to the man portion (inside the muscle) and manipulate it with the same way as at the heaven portion. After lifting the needle about 2 cm, thrust it quickly to the earth portion (between the tendon and bone, i. e. the deepest area of the acupoint) and manipulate it with the same way as at the heaven portion. After lifting the needle about 1 cm further, thrust it swiftly and lift it slowly three times respectively. Finally, withdraw the needle slowly as the patient inspires and press the needle hole immediately.

For the cases at the final stage of the common cold with fever, slight aversion to cold, thirst, red tongue with yellow coating, superficial and rapid pulse, Dazhui (DU 14), Taodao (DU 13), Fengmen (BL 12) Feishu (BL 13) or Houxi (SI 3) and Shenmai (BL 62) are punctured with the manipulation of yin occluding in yang. To the operation, press the acupoint heavily with the thumb or the index finger of the left hand, and insert the needle into the acupoint to the heaven portion. After inducing soreness or distension to the patient, thrust the needle to the man portion quickly, and twirl it in a single direction gently for nine times, or thrust it quickly and lift it slowly three times respectively. When the patient complains of slight fever or sweating, stop manipulating the needle for a short time. Then, thrust the needle to the earth portion slowly and twirl it in a single direction six times, or thrust it slowly and lift it quikly three times respectively. After the cold sensation is induced to the patient, lift the needle to the heaven portion and retain it there for a short time. Then, withdraw it, massage and press the acupoint punctured, or do not so. Sometimes, puncture at one or two acupoints first with the heat — producing needling applied to induce a little sweating, then with the cold — producing needling applied. To the operation, ask the patient to inspire with the mouth once and expire with the nose five times, insert the needle into the acupoint to the earth portion as the patient expires. After inducing the soreness or electrifying sensation to the patient, twirl the needle in a single direction six times. Then, lift the needle to the man portion quickly. At this portion, thrust the needle slowly and lift it quickly three times respectively. If the needling sensation is not induced to the patient, stop manipulating the needle for a little while, then twist it six times. If feeling strong tense under the needle, shake the needle. After these, lift the needle to the heaven portion quickly, stop manipulating it there for a short time, withdraw it quickly as the patient expires with the nose, massage and press the acupoint after withdrawal. But the withdrawal of the needle can be done without cooperation with the patient's respiration, and the needle hole can not be pressed.

(2) *Cupping*

Selection of Points

Fengmen(BL 12), Duzhui(DU 14), Feishu(BL 13)

Method

Apply cupping on the acupoint which is being punctured with the needle or not for ten to fifteen minutes. The cupping treatment is suitable for wind cold type of common cold.

六、急、慢性支气管炎

急、慢性支气管炎，属中医学"咳嗽"范畴。临床表现急性初起除咳嗽、咯痰外，还伴有发热恶寒、头痛等症，慢性多为长期反复发作，早晚加重，或气喘、咯泡沫白痰或白色粘液痰，还可兼见盗汗、纳呆、腰腿酸软等表现。

技法运用

1. 毫针

急性取太渊、列缺、肺俞、合谷、风门穴。用捻转、提插、呼吸泻法或平补平泻法。如喉肿痛加刺少商穴放血；发热加大椎（针感向下传至十二胸椎部，上传至颈椎）、曲池。每日针刺1～2次，每次留针15～20分钟。中间捻转行针1次。

慢性取丰隆、肺俞、脾俞、太渊、足三里、肾俞。用捻转、提插、呼吸补法配合艾灸，每日或隔日针治1次，留针15～20分钟，中间捻转行针1次。若慢性急性发作，仍可用泻法。

有报道针刺定喘、合谷、太渊为主治疗外感咳嗽。采用平补平泻法，缓慢进针。针定喘穴要求针感酸、麻、胀上行至颈，下行至背及两肩，捻针2～3分钟，不留针。继针合谷、太渊。一般针3～5次能取得显效。（田丛豁，等．《针灸医学验集》）

也有人采用大椎穴扎针拔火罐，治疗小儿慢性支气管炎。方法是令小儿侧伏于助手大腿部，固定其头足两手，穴位常规消毒后，用三棱针扎大椎穴，并在其四周约6厘米处各刺2针（上下左右共8针），以微出血为佳，然后用中型玻璃火罐，燃酒精棉球或纸片投入罐内，罩于应拔部位上，约20～30分钟去掉即可。（楚金荣．浙江中医杂志，12；1965）

2. 耳针：气管、神门、枕、下脚端、下屏穴。用中等刺激，针双侧，每次3～4穴，留针20分钟。慢性可加刺脾、肾。急性每日针1次，慢性可隔日针1次。亦可用王不留行籽贴压耳穴，每日按压3次。

3. 水针：定喘、曲池、尺泽、丰隆、足三里、风门、肺俞、脾俞、肾俞。

用维生素 B_1 100毫克，或鱼腥草注射液2毫升，或黄连素注射液4毫升，亦可用胎盘组织液，每次取2～3穴，每穴注射0.5毫升，每日1次。

4. 灸疗：天突、风门、肺俞、大椎、膏肓。采用艾炷灸，3～5天治疗1次，5次为1疗程，或艾条灸，每日1次，每次5～10分钟，以皮肤潮红为度，本法宜于慢性支气管炎。

有报道用线香点燃后，快速按在上述穴位上（膏肓除外）进行焠烫，点灸时听到皮肤表面发出一声微响声即可，每穴1次。对急性支气管炎、咽痒咳嗽有良效。（陈佑邦，等．《当代中国针灸临证精要》）

6. BRONCHITIS

Manifestations

Bronchitis, belonging to the disease or syndrome category of Kesou (咳嗽 cough) in TCM, is manifested clinically by cough with sputum, fever, aversion to cold, and headache in early stage of the actue type. In chronic type, it is manifested by prolonged course with repeated attacks of paroxysmal cough with white and sticky mucoid sputum, which is aggravated in early morning and night, asthma, accompanied by night sweating, poor appetite, soreness and weakness of lower back and lower extremities.

Tteatment by Applying Acubustion Techniques

(1) *Filiform Needling*

a. *For Acute Bronchitis*

Selection of Points

Taiyuan (LU 9) Lieque (LU 7), Feishu (BL 13), Hegu (LI 4), Fengmen (BL 12)

Method

Select reducing manipulations by twirling, rotating, lifting and thrusting the needle and by manipulating the needle in cooperation with the patient's respiration, or apply the uniform reinforcing—reducing needling. The puncture treatment is given once or twice daily, with the needles retained at each point for fifteen to twenty minutes and twisted and rotated once during the retention.

Supplementary points and method: For sore throat, Shaoshang (LU 1) is pricked additionally to cause bleeding; and Dazhui (DU 14) and Quchi (LI 11) added for fever (in puncturing at the former, make the needling sensation propagated downwards to the 12th thoracic vertebra and upwards to the cervical vertebrae).

b. For chronic Bronchitis:

Selection of Points

Fenglong (ST 40), Feishu (BL 13), Pishu (BL 20), Taiyuan (LU9), Zusanli (ST 36), Shenshu (BL 23)

Method

Three to five points are punctured each treatment session, and the punture is given once dialy or every other day, with the reinforcing manipulations by twirling, lifting and thrusting the needle and by manipulating the needle in cooperation with the patient's respiration. The needles are retained in each point for fifteen to twenty minutes and twisted once during the retention. Moxibustion may be given in cooperation. But, it should be known that reducing manipulation may be used for acute onset of the chronic bronchitis.

Introducing Some Experiential Techniques

A method by puncturing at Dingchuan (EX—B1), Hegu (LI 4) and Taiyuan (LU 9) for treatment of cough due to invasion by exogenous pathogenic factors is recorded in Collection of Experiences of Acupuncture &. Moxibustion. To the operation, insert the needle slowly and apply the uniform reinforcing — reducing manipulation. On puncturing at Dingchuan (EX—B1), twirl the needle for two to three minutes to induce soreness, numbness and distension to the patient and to make these needling sensation propagated upward to the neck and downwards to the back and shoulder, and withdraw the needle without retention. After Puncturing at Dingchuan (EX—B1), give puncture at Hegu (LI4) and Taiyuan (LU9). Generally, an obvious effect will be caused by the puncture treatment three to five times.

Anther acupuncture mehthod for treatment of childish chronic bronchitis is reported in Zhejiang Journal of TCM. To the method, make the child lie prone on one side on the assistant's thigh, ask the assistant to fix the child's head and extremities, select Dazhui(DU 14) and give a routine and local sterilization. Then, prick the point and other eight points respectively 6 cm above, below, left and right to it with the three edged needle to course bleeding slightly. After pricking, select a medium size glass jar and apply cupping with it on the pricked site for twenty to thirty minutes. Then, remove the jar.

(2) *Otopuncture*
Selection of Otopoints
Trachae, Shenmen, Occiput, Sympathetic, Infratragic Apex
Method
Three or four otopoints are punctured each treatment session, with a medium strength of stimulation administered and the needle retained for twenty minutes in each point. For chronic type, Ot. Spleen and Kidney are punctured additionally. The otopuncture treatment is given once daily for the acute type and once every other day for the chronic type. Or the vaccaria seeds are stuck on the otopoints and pressed three times daily for the treatment purpose.

(3) *Hydro—Acupuncture*
Selection of Points
Dingchuan (EX — B1), Quchi (LI 11), Chize (LU 5), Fenglong (ST 40), Zusanli (ST 36), Fengmen (BL 12), Feishu (BL13), Pishu (BL20), Shenmen (BL 23)
Seletion of Drugs
Vitamin B_1 100 mg, Houttuynia Injection Solution 2ml, Berberian Injection Solution 4 ml, Injection Solution Made of Placental Tissues.
Method
Two or three acupoints are injected with 0.5 ml of drug solution from anyone of the drugs metioned above once daily, and for ten times as a course.

(4) *Moxibustion*
Selection of Points
Tiantu (TN 12), Fengmen(BL 12), Feishu(BL 13), Dazhui(DU 14), Gaohuang(BL 43)
Method
Three to five points are employed each session, moxibustion with the moxa cone is given once per three to five days and five times constitute one therapeutic course. Or moxibustion with the moxa roll is given until the local skin becomes reddish (for about five to ten minutes)once daily. The moxibustion is suitable for chronic bronchitis

Introcucing An Experiential Technique
In Outstandings of Clinical Experiences of Modern Chinese Acupuncture & Moxibustion, the moxibustion with the thread incense burner for treatment of bronchitis is recorded. To the method, the

burner is ignited and directely pressed over the acupoints mentioned above (but except Dazhui, DU 14) quickly, and removed quickly as soon as there is a sound of burning of the skin. The moxibustion treatment is given to each point once only, leading to an effective result for acute bronchitis, itching of the throat, and cough.

七、支气管哮喘

支气管哮喘，监床表现以喉中痰鸣、喘息、呼吸急促、张口抬肩，不能平卧为特征。初起多咳嗽痰粘稠，以后咳出泡沫样痰液而感到松快，发作可在数分钟内缓解，也有持续几天而不停止的，严重时动则汗出，肢冷神疲、脉沉细。

技法运用

1. 毫针：取定喘、天突、肺俞、膻中、列缺、足三里、丰隆等穴。

急性发作期以捻转提插泻法为主，每次取3～5穴，留针20～30分钟，每日1次。风寒重者配合拔火罐；脾气虚见食少、脘痞、便溏、加脾俞、三阴交穴；肾俞见气促自汗，加复溜、太溪用捻转提插补法。缓解期可用捻转提插补法加艾灸。

有报道针刺双侧孔最穴，针深1～2公分（厘米），得气后要求针感呈双向传导，向下传至拇、食指端，向上传至胸部，刺激频率120～180次/分，捻转90°～180°之间，留针30～60分钟，每隔10分钟行针1次，每次3分钟左右。（田丛豁，等.《针灸医学验集》）

2. 灸疗：取大椎、肺俞、定喘、天突、膻中、足三里、孔最穴。

用艾条温和灸或回旋灸，每次2～4穴，每穴灸5～10分钟，每日1次。亦可艾炷隔姜灸，每次2～4穴，每穴灸5～7壮，每日1次。若用化脓灸，疗效亦佳，即在穴位处涂上大蒜汁，将黄豆般或碗豆般大小艾炷置于其上，为减少病人疼痛，医者可用手轻轻拍打施灸处周围，以分散注意力，或穴位常规消毒后，注射1%普鲁卡因0.5～1毫升后，再涂上大蒜汁置黄豆般大小艾炷灸之。每次施5～9壮，灸毕后贴上消毒敷料，待局部化脓。一般于夏季伏天（7～9月）灸治，隔日1次，每次1～3穴，3次一疗程，每年灸一疗程。

3. 耳针：取平喘（图5—5）、下屏尖、气管、脑、肺、下脚端穴。脾虚加脾；肾虚加肾。每次3～5穴，留针30分钟，每日1次。缓解期可用耳穴贴敷王不留行籽，以巩固疗效。

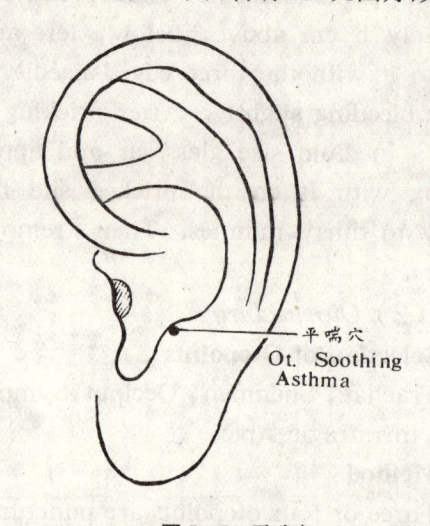

图5—5 平喘穴
Fig. 5-5 Ot. Soothing Asthma

4. 电针：取孔最、鱼际、定喘、肺俞，配合合谷、天突、膻中、内关穴。

每次取2～4穴，上穴交替使用，多采用密波（也可用连续波），5分钟后改用疏密波，刺激量可由中等度逐渐增加到强刺激。根据病情需要每日1～2次，也或隔日1次，每次15～60分钟，10次为一疗程。

据报道电针双侧孔最穴，对控制支气管

哮喘发作疗效满意。患者取坐位，孔最穴常规消毒后，以28号1寸长不锈钢毫针，快速刺入腧穴，进针3～5分深，待得气后施以泻法，要求针感出现双向传导后通电，采用连续波，频率160次/分，通电时间30～60分钟。（田丛豁，等.《针灸医学验集》）

5.挑治：取崇翼穴（第六颈椎棘突下的崇骨穴旁开5分）、喘息穴（大椎穴旁开1寸）。患者俯坐，上穴常规消毒，用三棱针挑破0.1～0.5厘米，每穴连挑3针，病人自觉如弹弦感，皮肤略有出血。挑后用碘酒消毒，外盖消毒纱布，每隔3～5天挑治1次，连续10次为一疗程。（刘冠军，等.《中医针法集锦》）

7. BRONCHIAL ASTHMA

Manifestations

Brochial asthma is characterized clinically by burgling with sputum in the throat, dyspnea, rapid and short breathing, indrawing of the soft tissues of the neck, and orthopnea. The attack of the paroxysm usually begins with cough with sticky and thick sputum, is relieved somewhat by coughing frothy sputum, and ends several minutes later or lasts for several days in some cases. Sweating on exertion, cold extremities, lassitude, and deep and thready pulse may be seen in severe cases.

Treatment by Applying Acubustion Techniques

(1) *Puncture with the Filiform Needle*

Selection of Points

Dingchuan (EX—B1), Tiantu (RN 22), Feishu (BL 13), Danzhong (RN 17), Lieque (LU 7), Zusanli (ST 36), Fenglong (ST 40)

Method

During the attack period, three to five acupoints are punctured with reducing manipulations by twisting, lifting and thrusting the needle applied, and with the needles retained at each point selected for twenty to thirty minutes. The treatment is given once daily. For severe wind cold type, cupping is given in coordination. If the spleen—qi is deficient, manifested by decreased digestive and aborsptive functions, Pishu (BL20) and Sanyinjiao (SP 6) are punctured additionally; and if kidney-qi is insufficient, manifested by short breathing and spontaneous sweating, Fuliu (KI 7) and Taixi (KI 3) are additionally punctured with reinforcing manipulations by twirling, lifting and thrustintg the needle.

At remission state, puncture with reinforcing manipulations by twirling, lifting and thrusting the needle is given in coordination with moxibustion with the moxa roll.

Introducing An Experiential Technique

An acupuncture method for treamtent of bronchial asthma is recorded in Collection of Experiences of Acupuncture & Moxibustion. To the method, Kongzui (LU6) of both sides are selected, the needle is inserted into the acupoint 1—2 cm deep, twisted at the range between a quarter turn and a half turn, and manipulated with the stimulation at frequency of 120—180 times/min, inducing and making the needling sensation propagated downwards to the distal ends of the thumb and index finger and upwards to the chest. Then, the needle is retained for thirty to sixty minutes, and manipulated per ten minutes during the retention.

(2) *Moxibustion*
Selection of Points

Dazhui(DU 14), Feishu(BL 13), Dingchuan(EX—B1), Tiantu(RN 22), Danzhong(RN 17), Zusanli(ST 36), Kongzui(LU 6).

Method

Two or three acupoints are selected each treatment session, and the mild — warming or circling moxibustion with the moxa roll is given to each point for five to ten minutes and once daily, or the ginger moxibustion is given to each point with five to seven cones once daily. Additionally, the scarring moxibustion is also effective. To the operation, smear some garlic juice over the point, place a moxa cone like a yellow bean in size on the acupoint and ignite it. In order to relieve the possible pain caused by burning to the patient, gently tap the area around the acupoint during the moxibustion, or inject 0.5—1 ml of 1% procanie into the acupoint area before the moxibustion. Five to nine cones are used for each acupoint in each session. After the moxubustion, the acupoint is covered over by the sterilized dress, and the local area will be purulent. Generally, the scarring moxibustion is given during the period from July to September and once every other day. The moxibustion is given to one to three acupoints in each session, and ten sessions constitute one therapeutic course. The next course is given in next year.

(3) *Otopuncture*
Selection of Otopoints

Main points: Soothing Asthma (See Fig. 5—5), Infratragic Apex, Trachea, Brain, Lung, Sympathetic.

Supplementary points according to symptoms: Spleen for hypofunction of spleen (manifested by decreased digestive and absorptive functions); and Kidney for hypofunction of kindney (manifested by dizziness, tinnitus, lumbago, nocturnal emission, impotence, sterility, lassitude, and forgetfulness).

Method

Three to five otopoints are punctured once daily, with the needles retained at each point for thirty minutes. During the remission stage, stick the vaccaria seeds over the otopoints in replace of the needling on them to consolidate the therateutic effect.

(4) *Electroacupuncture*
Selection of Acupoints

Kongzui(LU 6), Yuji(LU 10), Dingchuan(EX—B1), Feishu(BL 13), Hegu(LI 4), Tiantu(RN 22), Danzhong(RN 17), Neiguan(PC 6)

Method

The electroacupuncture is given to two to four acupoints each session, with the dense wave administered in the first five minutes and irregular wave in the rest time, and with the stimulation being graduately increased, from the medium to the large intensity. The electroacupuncture is applied for fifteen to sixty minutes and one or two times daily or once every other day. Ten treatment sessions constitute a therapeutic course.

Introducing An Experiential Technique

Another electroacrpuncture method is recorded in Collection of Experience of Acupuncture & Moxibustion. To this method, left and right Kongzui (LU 6) are selected when the patient is at the sitting position, and a routine and local sterilization is given. Then, the point is punctured with No. 28 stainless filiform needle 1 cun long to the depth of 0.3—0.5 cun. After arrival of qi, a reducing manipulation is applied to make the needling sensation propagated in bidirectional ways. Then, the needles are attached with the electric leads with the continuous wave and the frequency of 160 times/min. for thirty to sixty minutes.

(5) *Breaking Therapy*
Selection of Points

Chongyi (EX., 0.5 cun lateral to Chonggu, which is located below the spinous process of the sixth cervical vertebra) Chuanxi (EX., 1 cun lateral to Dazhui DU 14).

Method

The patient is at the prone—sitting position. After the local and routine sterilization, break the skin of the acupoint 0.1—0.5 cm with the three—edged needle, and consecutively break the fibrous tissues of each point for three times. During pricking, the patient may feel like flicking a string and the skin may bleed slightly. After breaking, sterilize the pricked area with iodine and cover it with the sterilized dress. The pricking therapy is given once per three to five days and ten times contitute a therapeutic course.

八、急、慢性胃炎

急慢性胃炎，属中医学"胃脘痛"、"呕吐"、"伤食"范畴。临床以上腹不适、疼痛、呕吐、恶心为主症。实证兼见胃痛拒按，呕吐频繁，嗳气吞酸，可伴发腹泻；虚证兼见胃痛隐隐，喜温喜按。急性发病迅速；慢性多由急性转变而来，起病隐匿，发展缓慢。

技法运用

1. 毫针：取中脘、内关、足三里穴。

实证用捻转、提插泻法，留针15～20分钟，每日针1～2次。腹胀痛而泻者加天枢、大肠俞；吐泻急重兼口干、烦热者可于曲泽、委中点刺出血；发热重者加曲池、大椎用捻转、提插、呼吸泻法；嗳气吞酸，攻痛连胁加太冲、内庭。虚证加脾俞、胃俞、气海用捻转、提插迎随、疾徐补法。

有人针刺一侧内关透外关，反复行雀啄提插手法，并轻揉腹部1～2分钟，同时嘱患者行深呼吸5～7次，患者即感腹部舒适。以后每隔5分钟重复上法1次，待腹痛消失后，留针15分钟即可出针。（熊新安．中医杂志，2：48；1981）

有报道治食停胃脘不能消化，胸腹胀满疼痛，取内关穴，以左手紧切其穴，右手持针刺入2～3分，找到麻或触电似的感觉，用"关闭法"，左手托起患者手腕放平拇指，压在针的下方。右手持针的针尖和左手拇指压按的指力，向肩头努力推进少许（约0.5～1厘米，图5—6），使感觉传导到胸部或腋窝；如感觉传导达不到要求时，则在3分至5分间反复提插几次，或者左手将患者之中指捏住，再将第一、第二指骨关节2/3倒向前，以右手轻弹其中指关节，感觉就能传导到胸部或腋窝，即将针拔出。两侧的内关穴针毕，再取中脘穴，针刺时以左手紧按其穴，右手持针刺入8分之中，找到感觉，用"关闭法"。以中指压在针的下方,其他四指压按在两侧,右手持针的针尖和左手压按的指力,随其出气向胸部努力推进少许(约 0.5~1 厘米),随其入气左手减轻压按将针尖提出少许,反复操作几次,使感觉向上传导,上涌作呕,急速将针拔出。即可以将胃脘停留难以消化食物呕吐而出。(刘冠军,等.《中医针法集锦》)

2. 灸疗:取中脘、天枢、内关、足三里穴。

本法适宜于脾胃感受寒湿患者,用艾炷隔姜灸,每日 1 次,每次 2~3 穴,每穴 3~5 壮。或艾条温和灸及回旋灸,每次 15~20 分钟,每次 1 次。

3. 耳针:取下脚端、脑、胃、神门、肝、脾穴。中等刺激,每次 2~3 穴,每穴留针 30 分钟,每日 1 次。宜于慢性浅表性胃炎。

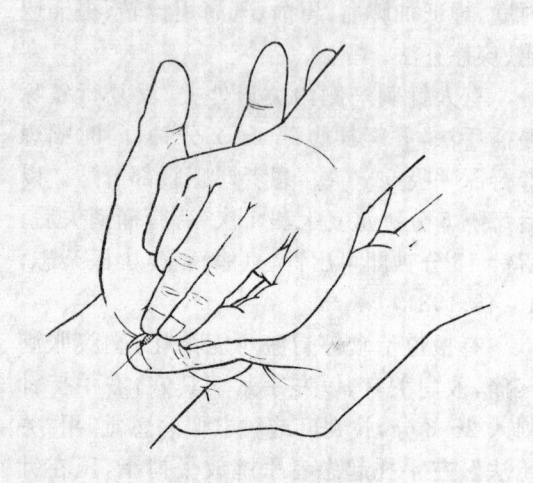

图 5-6 关闭法刺内关
Fig. 5-6 Puncturing at Neiguan(PC 6)for Gastritis

4. 挑治:适宜于感冒或暴食冷饮诱发。初起头痛,全身发胀,胃脘痛如刀绞,可见心窝、腰背两旁有疹,顶稍带黄白透明点,出现于皮毛,或稍陷于皮内。取三棱针行针挑,皮肤常规消毒,针对疹子以 30~40°角刺入 2 分许,旋将针尖向上挑起,拔出白色蚕丝样的纤维,反复 4~5 次,以拔出更多纤维为度,挑完一个疹子,再挑第二个,直到胀痛消失或大减为止。(肖家琅:《江西中医药》,6;1957)

8. GASTRITIS

Manifestations

Acute or chronic gastritis, usually seen in the diseases or syndromes of Wei Wan Tong(胃脘痛, epigastric pain), Ou Tu,(呕吐 Vomiting), Shang shi(伤食, dyspepsea due to improper diet)in TCM, is manifested clinically mainly by discomfortable feeling and pain in the epigastric region, vomiting and nausea. The gastritis may be divded into two types, the excess type and the deficiency type, according to the differentiation with TCM theories. The excess type is characterized by stomachache aggravated by pressure, frequent vomiting and belching and regurgitation. The deficiency type is characterized by dull stomachache, relieved by warming and pressure. The acute gastritis onsets quickly, and the chronic gastritis onsets slowly, which is usually formed from the acute one.

Treatment by Applying Acubustion Techniques

(1) *Filiform Needling*
Selection of Points
Zhongwan (RN 12), Neiguan (PC 26), Zusanli(ST 36)
Method
a. For the excess type, the acupoints are punctured with the reducing manipulations by twirling, rotating, lifting and thrusting the needle, the needles at each point are retained for fifteen to twenty minutes, and the treatment is given one to

two times daily.

Supplementary points according to symptoms: Tianshu (ST 25) and Dachangshu (BL 25) are added for abdominal distension and pain with diarrhea; Quzei (PC 3) and Weizhong (BL 40) are pricked additionally to cause bleeding for acute and severe vomiting and diarrhea, accompanied with thirst and dysphoria with feverish sensation; Quchi (LI 11) and Dazhui (DU 14) are punctured additionally with the reducing manipulations by twisting, lifting and thrusting the needle and by manipualting the needle in cooperation with the patient's respiration for high fever; and Taichong (LR 3) and Neiting (ST44) added for belching with fetid odour, distension and pain in the epigastric region radiating to the hypochondriac region.

b. For the deficiency type, Pishu (BL 20), Weishu (BL 21), and Qihai (RN 6) are punctured additionally, and the reinforcing manipulations by twirling, lifting and thrusting the needle, by puncturing along the running direction of the meridian, and by slow — rapid insertion and withdrawal of the needle applied.

Introducing Some Experiential Techniques

Another acupuncture method for treatment of gastritis is reported in Journal of TCM. To the operation, select left or right Neiguan (PC 6), insert a needle into the point and apply penetration needling toward Waiguan (SJ 5). Then, apply bird — pecking needling repeatedly, and massage the patient's abdomen gently for one to two minutes as the patient is asked to breathe deep five to seven times. After this procedure, the patient will feel comfortable in his abdomen. Then, repeat this coruse once per five minutes until the abdominal pain disappears, and retain the needle for fifty minutes before withdrawal of it.

In Collection of Outstandings of the Needling Mothods of TCM the following acupuncture method for treating gastritits in which dyspepsea and distending pain in the chest and abdomen due to retention of food are the main symptoms is recorded. In the operation, press the acupoint area with the left hand and insert a needle into Neiguan (P 6) to the depth of 0.2 — 0.3 cun with the right hand. After inducing electrifying sensation or numbness to the patient, lift the patinet's wrist at the horizontal position with the left hand, and press the area distal to the acupoint with thumb of the left hand. Then, insert the needle deeper with the needle tip directing towards the shoulder and move the pressing finger and push the needle towards the shoulder 0.5 — 1cm (See Fig 5 — 6) in order to make the needling sensation propagated to the chest and axilla. If the needling sensation is not propagated to the designed area, lift and thrust the needle at the range between 0.3 — 0.5 cun of the acupoint depth repeatedly for several times, or grip the patient's middle finger of the punctured hand with the left hand to make the first and the second finger joints at flexion position, and flick the points gently with right hand. Through the manipulation, the needling sensation can be propagated to the chest or the axilla. After puncturing at Neiguan (PC 6) of the both sides, Zhongwan (RN 12) is punctured. With the left hand pressing the acupoint area tightly, the needle is inserted by the right hand to the depth of 0.8 cun. After inducing needling sensation, press the area distal to the acupoint with the middle finger of the left hand and the areas lateral to the acupoint with the rest fingers of that hand, insert the needle towards the chest 0.5—1 cm, with the needle tip directing to and the pressing fingers of the left hand pressing towards the chest, as the patient breathes in. Repeat this course for several times to make the needling sensation propagated upwards. When the patient has the sensation of vomiting, withdraw the needle immidiately. Through these manipulations, the accumulated food which is difficult to be digested in the stomach can be expelled through vomiting.

(2) *Moxibustion*

Selection of Points

Zhongwan (RN 12), Tianshu (ST 25), Neiguan (PC 6), Zusanli (ST 36).

Method

Select two or three points each treatment session, and apply the ginger moxibustion until three to five moxa cones have burnt on each point, or apply the mild-warming or circling moxibustion with the moxa roll to each point for fifteen to twenty minutes. The moxibustion treatment is given once daily, which is suitable for the type of the disease due to attack by cold and damp evil.

(3) *Otopuncture*

Selection of Otopoints

Sympathetic, Brain, Stomach, Shenmen, Liver, Spleen.

Method

Two or three otopoints are punctured with the medium strength stimulation, and the needles are retained in each point for thirty minutes. The otopuncture is given once daily, which is suitable for chronic superficial gastritis.

(4) *Pricking Therapy*

The pricking therapy is suitable for the gastritis induced by common cold or by over — drinking of cold fluid, which is manifested by colic epigastric pain with headache and general distension at the beginning, followed by rushes with yellow, white and transparant spot on the heads of the rushes which are distributed over the skin of the areas of the xiphoid process and the upper and lower back. To the operation, following a routine and local sterilization, insert a three—edged needle into the rush about 0.2 cun deep at an angle of 30—40° formed by the needle with the local skin surface, and make the needle shaft tilted and moving upward to break the white and silk fiber until many fibers are broken. After one rash is pricked, the next one is pricked in same way. The pricking is given until the epigastric distending pain is relieved.

九、胃、十二指肠溃疡

胃、十二指肠溃疡,归属于中医"胃脘痛"、"肝胃气痛"范畴。临床主要症状是上腹疼痛、时发时止,有周期性与规律性。胃溃疡多在饭后半小时至2小时发作;十二指肠溃疡疼痛多在饭后2～4小时,进食后可缓解,夜间发作加重。随着病情变化可出现恶心、呕吐、吞酸、嗳气等症状,严重者可伴发出血及穿孔等。

技法运用

1.毫针：取内关、中脘、足三里、公孙、梁丘、肝俞、脾俞、胃俞。

每次3～5穴，用平补平泻法，留针30分钟，每隔10分钟行针1次，每日1次。失眠加神门、通里、三阴交；嗳气加太冲、行间；腹胀加天枢。胃神经症亦可参照上穴治疗。

有人取脊柱痛点针刺。方法：取俯卧位，胸腹部稍垫高，使脊柱略成弓形，医者用拇指腹面，从第1胸椎用力大小一致地按压至第12胸椎，压痛点处即为针刺点，压痛点多少不一，每次针2～3个，若压痛点多时，可分2组，交替选用。间日针1次，若无压痛时，在此部选择2～3个椎间隙针刺亦有良效。操作时针尖顺棘突间隙方向缓慢进针0.8～1.2寸，徐徐提插和刮针手法，持续行针至疼痛减轻或消失后，留针30～60分钟。留针期间，若痛有反复时，仍用上法行针，直至疼痛不再发作时，方可起针。针刺时，当注意穿透黄韧带时，阻力突然消失，说明针尖已进入椎管内之硬膜外腔，严禁刺伤脊髓，深度一般不应超过同身寸之2寸。（孙学全.《针灸临证集验》）

2.灸疗：可单用，亦可在针刺起针后再灸，取穴同毫针。适宜于胃痛隐隐，喜暖喜按、纳少神疲、大便溏薄等虚寒性胃脘痛。用隔姜灸、隔附子饼灸，或艾条悬灸，温针灸。每次灸1～2小时，每日1次，一般灸后都能迅速止痛，若坚持长时间的施灸，可获良好效果。

3.耳针：取胃、脾、十二指肠、神门、肝、下脚端、脑穴。双耳交替治疗，每次留针1～2小时，每日1次。亦可配合耳穴贴压王不留行籽，每日按压2～3次。

若见胃穿孔、胃出血，当采取中西医综合治疗。

9. GASTRIC AND DUODENAL ULCER

Manifestations

Gastric ulcer and duodenal ulcer, belonging to desease or syndrome categories of Wei Wan Tong (胃脘痛 epigastric pain), and Gan Wei Qi Tong (肝胃气痛 stomachache due to attack by the liver gi) in TCM, is manifested clinically by timed and regular onset and relief of the paroxysmal pain in the epigastric region. The onset of the paroxysmal pain usually occurs 0.5—2 hours after eating in the gastric ulcer, and 2—4 hours after eating in the duodenal ulcer which is relieved by eating again and aggravated in the night. Nausea, vomiting, belching, acid regurgitation may be accompanied with the change of the disease condition, and bleeding from the stomach and duodenum or even gastric perforation may be accompanied in severe cases.

Teratment by Applying Acubustion Techniqes

(1) *Filiform Needling*

Selection of Points

Neiguan (PC6), Zhongwan (RN 12), Zusanli (ST 36), Gongsun (SP 4), Liangqiu (ST 34), Ganshu (BL 18), Weishu (BL 21).

Method

Three to five acupoints are punctured once daily, with the uniform reinforcing—reducing manipulation applieed and with the needles retained at each point for thirty minutes and manipulated per ten minutes during the retention.

Supplementary points according to symptoms: Shenmen (HT 7), Tongli (HT

5) and Sanyinjiao(SP 6) are added for insomnea; Taichong (LR 3) and Xingjian (LR 2) added for belching; and Tianshu (ST25) added for abdominal distension.

Note: gastroneurosis may be treated by referring to the method metioned above.

Introducing An Experiential Technique

In Collection of Clinical Experiences of Acupuncture and Moxibustion the following acupuncture method for treating gastric and duodenal ulcer is recorded. To the method, select the prone position to the patient, with something placed under the patient's abdomen to make the spinal column slightly bow — shaped, press the spinal column with the palmar surface of the trumb from the 1st thoracic vertebra to the 12th thoracic vertebra evenly and forcefully to find the tender spots, and puncture at two to three tender spots in each treatment session. If there are many tender spots found, divide them into two groups and puncture at them alternately. Give the puncture once every other day. If no tender spot is found, select two or three points located at the interspaces of the thoracic vertebrae and insert the needle slowly along the interspace of the vertebrae to the depth of 0.8—1.2 cun. Then, lift, thrust and scrape the needle, and manipulate it until the pain is relieved or eliminated. And then, retain the needle for thirty to sixty minutes. If the pain relapses during the retention of the needle, manipulate the needle in the same way as above until the pain does not relapse. Finally, withdraw the needle. Sudden disappearence of the resistance to the needle during puncturing indicates the needle tip has been inserted into the epidual space inside the vertebral canal and deeper insertion is forbidden so as to avoid injuring the spinal cord. Generally, the depth of insertion of the needle should be less than 2 cun (here, cun meaning the proportional unit of the patinet's own body).

(2) *Moxibustion*

Selection of Point

The same as in the puncture with the filiform needle.

Method

Three to five points are employed each treatment session, and moxibustion may be applied singly or after puncturing. The moxibustion treatment is suitable for epigastric pain of deficiency — cold type, manifested by dull pain in the epigastrium which may be relieved by pressure and warmth, poor appetite, general lassitude and loose stool. The ginger or monkshood — cake moxibustion, the suspended moxibustion (a moxibustion technique in which the lighted end of moxa roll is maintained a certain distance above the skin), or mild-warming moxibustion is given for one to two hours once daily. Generally, the pain is relieved immidiately after the moxibustion, and a better effect will be achieved if a long period of treatment with the moxibustion is given.

(3) *Otopuncture*

Selection of Otopoints

Stomach, Spleen, Duodenum, Shenmen, Liver, Sympathetic, Brain.

Method

Two to four otopoints are employed

each treatment session, the left and right otopoints are punctured alternately with the needles retained at each point for one to two hours, and the puncture is given once daily. Or the vaccaria seeds are stuck over the otopoints and pressed two or three times daily in cooperation.

If gastric perforation or stomach-bleeding occurs, the treatment with the western and traditional Chinese medicines in combination should be applied.

十、胃下垂

胃下垂,属于中医"胃脘痛"、"嗳气"、"嘈杂"范畴。临床主要症候为胃纳减少,胃脘胀满不舒,进食加重,有坠胀感,时有脘腹隐隐作痛、嗳气、吞酸、呕吐、大便溏或便秘,常伴有消瘦、乏力、心悸、头昏等。

技法运用

1. 毫针:取中脘、足三里、气海、关元、天枢、脾俞、胃俞、大横、下脘穴。

用捻转补法,其中气海穴沿皮透刺关元;中脘沿皮透刺下脘;大横沿皮透刺关元,每次除透穴外,再取2～3穴,得气后留针30分钟,隔日针1次。

有报道,长针治胃下垂,用28号8寸长毫针,由剑突下1寸刺入,约与皮肤呈30°角,沿皮捻转进针透至脐左侧0.5寸处(图5-7),此时患者有腰胀及下腹上抽感,术者提针有重力感时(如术者感到重力感消失或脱落时,可再捻转,重力恢复后重新提针),改为15°角,不捻转提针40分钟,出针前行抖动手法10～15次,然后出针,针刺结束后,平卧休息2小时,每周1次,亦可隔日针1次,10次1疗程。(高云.中国针灸 1982;5:9。)

2. 电针:中脘、气海、关元、足三里、提胃(中脘旁开4寸)、胃上(下脘旁开4寸)。

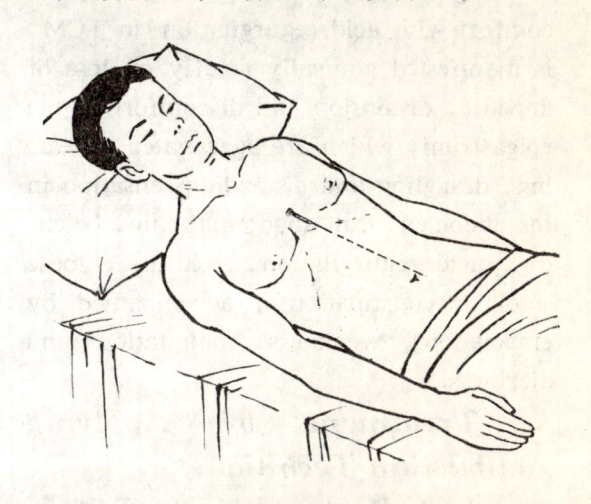

图 5-7 长针透刺
Fig. 5-7 Penetration Needling with the Long Needle

每次取2～4穴,断续波或疏密波,腹部穴位先通电,下肢穴位后通电,电流输出量为中等度,每天1次,每次15～30分钟。呕吐恶心加内关;腹胀加天枢;久病加三阴交、脾俞。

据报道,用4寸毫针取胃上穴沿皮下刺向天枢穴,隔日1次,电针断续波,每次行20分钟;中脘、足三里用补法,留针20分钟。无论毫针、电针,在治疗完毕时,应再次运针,待有针感后,引道经气上行,助升提之力。(陈佑邦,等.当代中国针灸临证精要)

3. 灸疗:取百会、足三里、关元、气海、中脘、胃俞、脾俞、天枢、三阴交穴。

艾条温和灸或回旋灸,亦可针上加灸。每次2～4穴,从下而上顺次施灸,每穴灸15～20分钟,每日1次。

10. GASTROPTOSIS

Manifestations

Gastroptosis, belonging to disease or syndrome categories of Wei Wan Tong, (胃脘痛 epigastric pain), Ai Qi, (嗳气

belching) and Cao Za, (嘈杂, gastric discomfort with acid regurgitation) in TCM, is manifested clinically chiefly by loss of appetite, distension and discomfort in the epigastrum, which are aggravated by eating, draggling and distending sensation in the abdomen, dull abdominal pain, belching, acid regurgitation, vomiting, loose stool or constipation, accompanied by emaciation, weakness, palpitation and dizziness.

Treatment by Applying Acubustion Techniques

(1) *Puncture with the Filiform Needle*

Selection of Points

Zhongwan (RN 12), Zusanli (ST 36), Qihai (RN 6), Guanyuan (RN 4), Tianshu (ST 25), Pishu (BL 20), Weishu (BL 21), Daheng (SP 15), Xiawan (RN 10).

Method

Qihai (RN 6), Zhongwan (RN 20) and Daheng (SP 15) are punctured with the penetration needling along the subcutaneous tissues respectively to Guanyuan (RN 4), Xiawan (RN 10) and Guanyuan (RN4), and two or three acupoints are punctured in addition in each treatment session. The needles are retained at each point for thirty minutes after arrival of qi. The puncture treatment is given once every other day.

Introducing An Experientiasl Technique

Another acupuncture method for treating gastroptosis is reported in Chinese Acupuncture & Moxibustion. To the operation, select a No. 28 needle (8 cun long), insert it into the point one cun directly below the xiphoid process at the angle of 30° formed by the needle with the local skin surface, and push it beneath the skin to the area 0.5 cun left to the ambilicus as twirling it (See Fig. 5—7). When the patient complains of distension in the lower back and feels like the lower abdomen is drawn upwards, and the operator feels force of gravity as the needle is lifted (if the operator feels the sensation of force of gravity disappears, twist the needle again to induce it), change the angle of insertion and puncture at an angle of 15° without twirling the needle but with lifting manipulation applied for forty minutes. After shaking the needle ten to fifteen times, withdraw it and advise the patient to rest on the bed for two hours. The puncture treatment is given once a week or once every other day, and ten treatmant sessions constitute a therapeutic course.

(2) *Electroacupuncture*

Selection of Points

Zhongwan (RN 12), Qihai (RN 6), Guanyuan (RN 4), Zusanli (ST 36), Tiwei (EX, 4 cun lateral to Zhongwan RN 12), Weishang (EX, 4 cun lateral to Xiawan RN 10).

Method

The electroacupuncdture is given to two to four acupoints once daily, with the intermittent or irregular stimulation and the medium strentth output current applied for fifteen to thirty minutes on each point. The current is connected with the acupoints first on the abdomen and second on the lower extremities. For vomiting and nausea, Neiguan (PC 6) is added; Tianshu

(ST 25) added for abddominal distension; and Sanyinjiao (SP 6) and Pishu (BL 20) added for the prolonged cases.

Introducing An Experiential Technique

In Outstandings of Clinical Experiences of Modern Chinese Acupuncture & Moxibustion, the following electroacupuncture method is recorded. Weishang (EX.) is selected and punctured with a 4 cun long needle with the needle tip moving along the subcutaneous tissues to Tianshu (ST 25). Then, the electric stimulation is applied to it for twenty minutes. In coordination, Zhongwan (RN12) and Zusanli (ST 36) are punctured additionally with the reinforcing manipulations applied and the needles retained for twenty minutes. The treatment is given once daily. In order to improve the lifting force on the stomach, before finishing the operation, the needles, no matter used for acupuncture or for electroacupuncture, should be manipulated again to induce the needling sensation and to make the channel—qi ascend.

(3) *Moxibustion*

Selection of Points

Baihui (DU 20), Zusanli (ST 36), Guanyuan (RN 4), Qihai (RN 6), Zhongwan (RN 12), Weishu (BL 20), Pishu (BL 21), Tianshu (ST 25), Sanyinjiao (SP 6).

Method

The mild—warming or circling moxibustion or the moxibustion with warming needle is given to two to four acupoints once daily, with the order of applying moxibustion from the lower to the upper. The moxibustion is applied to each point for twenty minutes.

十一、膈肌痉挛

膈肌痉挛，中医称为"呃逆"。临床上表现为呃逆连声，短促频繁，持续不断可达数分钟至数小时，严重者由于长时间发作而不停歇，可引致脘腹胀满而疼痛。

技法运用

1. 毫针：取内关、中脘、阴都（中脘穴旁开0.5寸）、膻中、脾俞、胃俞、足三里、天突、内庭穴。

每次3～5穴，用平补平泻手法，留针30～60分钟，每5分钟行针1次。此外，膻中、膈俞、中脘、尚可针后加拔火罐。亦可经渠穴透太渊，大陵透内关、公孙透太白、足三里透上巨墟，沿皮透刺用平补平泻法，留针20分钟。

有人采用针刺法通气于天治疗呃逆。令患者张口深长呼吸；取膻中穴，针尖向上沿皮刺3分～2寸，直至取效；取双列缺穴，向肘部斜刺2分～5分，强刺激，直到取效；针刺制止呃逆后，可按发作规律，适当针刺内关穴、足三里穴，以巩固疗效，一日一次，3～5日即可（陈高材．江西中医药，2：36；1986）

2. 耳针：神门、耳中（膈）、胃、肝、下屏尖、脾。强刺激，每次3～4穴，留针1～数小时。亦可贴压王不留行籽，每日按压3次。

3. 灸疗：灯火灸天突穴。方法：局部消毒后，按灯火灸法灼灸天突穴，灸后涂以消炎软膏预防感染，轻症灸1次，重症隔7天后再在原部位灼灸1次。（田丛豁，等.《中国灸法集粹》）

另外，有人将两手拇指压按在患者双侧攒竹穴，其余四指并拢紧贴在耳尖上的率谷

穴(图 5—8),指压由轻至重,持续约 3~5 分钟,呃逆即止。(龚瑞章. 中国针灸 1∶48,1981)

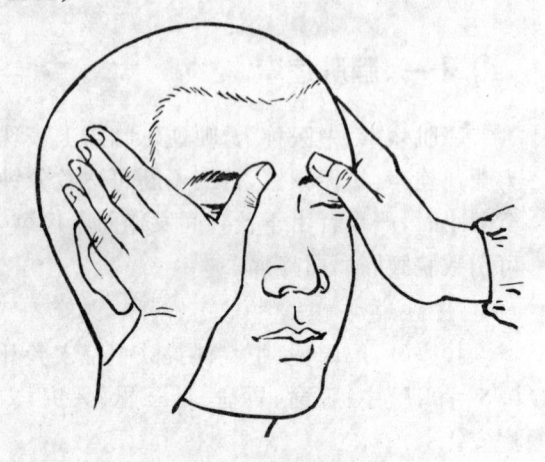

Fig. 5—8 Pressing Cuanzhu(BL 2)

11. PHRENOSPASM

Manifestaons

Phrenospasm, referring to E Ni (呃逆, hiccup) in TCM, is manifested clinically by frequent and quick hiccup which lasts for several minutes to hours. In severe cases epigastric distending pain due to long—term onset of the spasm of the diaphragm may be accompanied.

Treatment by Applying Acubustion Techniques

(1) *Puncture with the Filiform Needle*

Selection of Points

Neiguan (PC 6), Zhongwan (RN 12), Yindu (EX., 0.5 cun lateral to Zhonwan RN 12), Danzhong (RN 17), Pishu (BL 20), Weishu (Bl 21), Geshu (BL 17), Zusanli (ST 36), Tiantu (RN 22), Neiting (ST 44).

Method

Three to five acupoints are punctured with the uniform reninforcing — reducing manipulation applied, and with the needles retained at each point for thirty to sixty minutes and manipulated per five minutes. Additionally, the cupping may be given to Danzhong (RN 17), Geshu (BL 17) and Zhongwan (RN 12) after them being punctured. Or Jingqu (LU 8), Daling (PC 7), Gongsun (SP 4) and Zusanli (ST 36) are additionally punctured with the uniform renforcing — reducing manipulation, with the penetration needling respectively to Taiyuan (LU 9), Neiguan (PC 6), Taibai (SP 3) and Shangjuxu (ST 37), and with the needles retained at each point for twenty minutes.

Introducing An Experiential Technique

It is reported in Jiangxi Jorunal of TCM that hiccup is treated by puncturing to make the channel — qi ascend. To the operation, the patient is asked to breathe deep wtih the mouth, and Danzhong (RN 17) is punctured with the needle tip moving along the subcutaneous tissue upwards 0.3—2 cun until the effect is achieved. Then, the left and right Lieque (LU 7) are punctured obliquely 0.2—0.5 cun, with the needle inserted toward the elbow and with a strong stimulation applied until the effect is achieved. After the hiccup is stopped by needling, the following puncture is given in order to consolidate the effect. Neiguan (PC 6) and Zusanli (ST 36) are punctured properly according to the regularity of the paroxysm of hiccup, and once daily for three to five days.

(2) *Otopuncture*
Selection of Otopoints
Shenmen, Esophagus, Stomach, Liver, Infratragic Apex.
Method
Three or four otopoints are punctured with the strong stimulation applied and with the needles retained at each point for one to several hours. Or the otopoints are stuck with the vaccaria seeds and pressed three times daily. The puncture is given once daily and for seven days as a course.

(3) *Moxibustion*
Selection of Point
Tiantu(RN 22)
Method
Following the rourtine and local sterilization, the moxibstion with medulla junci is given to the acupoint. Then, the area burnt is smeared with anti—in flammatory ointment to prevent infection. The moxibustion is repeated to the same point seven days later for severe cases.

(4) *Massage*
A simple way to stop onset of hiccup is reported in Chinese Acupunture Moxibustion. The left and right Cuanzhu(BL 12) are pressded by the left and right thumbs respectivrly, with the rest fingers of two hands being close reaspectively to attach on bilateral Shuaigu (GB 8) closely (See Fig. 5—8). The pressure given to Cuanzhu(BL 2)is gradually increased and lasts about three to five minutes. Then, the hiccup is stopped.

十二、肠 炎

肠炎,属中医学"泄泻"范畴。临床主要表现为大便次数增多、粪便稀薄或水样、腹痛、肠鸣。若偏于寒湿则便清稀、水谷相杂、口不渴、身寒喜热、脉迟、苔白;偏于湿热则泻物热臭、肛门灼热、小便短赤、兼身热口渴、苔黄、脉濡数;慢性者,病程数月至数年不等,可见神疲、不思饮食、食谷不化、腰酸腿软、腹部寒冷等症。

技法运用

1. 毫针:取天枢、大肠俞、中脘、足三里、上巨墟穴。

急性湿热腹泻用捻转提插泻法,加刺关元穴;寒湿泄泻用平补平泻或烧山火手法;慢性腹泻用捻转提插补法。每日1次,重病者每日可2~3次,每次留针20~30分钟。发热加刺合谷、曲池用泻法;不思饮食、四肢无力加刺脾俞、公孙用补法;腰酸腿软、食谷不化、腹部畏寒加刺肾俞、命门、太溪用补法配合艾灸。

有人用28~30号毫针刺脐中四边穴(脐中上下左右各1寸),以上下左右为序进针,成人一般针3~5分深,小儿针2~3分深,不留针。对虚寒型患者,采用缓刺捻转半分钟,对湿热型患者取急刺捻转10秒钟左右。(田丛豁,等.《针灸医学验集》)

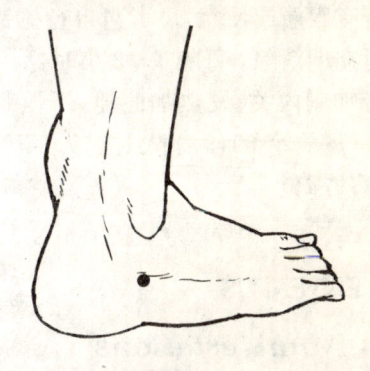

图 5—9 腹泻特效穴
Fig. 5—9 Fuxietexiaoxue (Extra point)

另有人取肓俞(神阙穴旁0.5寸)配足三

里。方法:先针肓俞(双),常规消毒后用1.5寸,30~31号毫针刺入穴位,针尖稍偏向脐中方向,进针1.2寸左右,每穴提插捻转约半分钟出针。对80余例小儿腹泻经1~3次针灸治疗均获痊愈。其1岁以内小儿只捻转不提插,较大者可于捻转过程中提插2~3次。出针后再刺双侧足三里穴,进针约1寸左右,每次提插捻转约半分钟左右出针。(田丛豁,等.《针灸医学验集》)

2. 灸疗:神阙、腹泻特效穴(足外踝最高点直下,赤白肉际交界处。图5—9)。

神阙可用艾炷隔盐灸。方法:取食盐适量研细末放脐中,凸出脐上0.5~1厘米,盐末上置姜片或蒜片,再置艾炷于其上点燃灸之,每次5~7壮;腹泻特效穴用艾条温和灸或回旋灸,每次15~20分钟,每日2~3次。(田丛豁,等.《针灸医学验集》)

3. 耳针:大肠、小肠、下脚端、神门、肝、脾、肾、三焦。急性用强刺激,慢性用中等刺激,每次选3~5穴,留针10分钟,每日1次。

有单位取左侧耳舟"肩关节穴",方法:沿耳舟皮下向上平行刺入1寸左右,捻转约5分钟,病人渐感耳廓似热水烫一样,肉眼亦可见耳廓发红。一般留针12~24小时。留针期间若有腹痛或便意,患者可自行捻针5分钟,多可立即消除。每隔1~2小时捻针1次。呕吐者加刺内关;发热加曲池,用强刺激,不留针。(解放军6919部队卫生队.新医学,10:532;1974。)

12. ENTERITIS

Manifestations

Enteritis, referring to Xie Xie (泄泻, diarrhea) in TCM, is manifeated clinically chiefly by abnormal and frequent fecal discharge with liquicity, abdominal pain and borborygma. In cases with cold and damp evil being predominant, watery diarrhea with undigested food, absence of thirst, chilliness which responds to warmth, slow pulse and white tongue coating are present, and diagnosis of "diarrhea of cold—damp type or syndrome is given; in cases with damp and heat evils being predominant, hot and fetid stools, burning sensation in the anus, yellow and scanty urine, or accompanied by general feverish feeling, thirst, yellow tongue coating, soft and rapid pulse are present, and dignosis of "diarrhea of heat —damp type or syndrome is given; and in chronic cases with the disease course lasting several months or years, general lassitude, anorexia, undigestion, soreness of the lower back and weakness of the lower extremities, and cold sensation in the abdomen may be present, and dignosis of "diarrhea of cold syndrome of dificiency type" is given.

Treatment by Applying Acubustion Techniques

(1) *Puncture with the Filiform Needle*

Selection of Points

Main points : Tianshu (ST 25), Dachangshu (BL 25), Zhongwan (RN 12), Zusanli(ST 36), Shangjuxu(ST 37)

Method and Supplementary Points

Three or four points are employed each treatment session. For acute diarrhea of heat-damp type, puncture is given with the reducing manipulations by twirling, rotating, lifting and thrusting the needle, and Guanyuan(RN 4) is added. For diarrhea of cold damp type, prncture is given with the uniform reinforcing — reducing manipulation or with the heat — producing needling. For chronic diarrhea, puncture is given with the reinforcing manipulations by twirling, lifting and thursting the needle. The puncture treatment is applied once daily but two or three times daily for severe cases, and the needles are rertained at each point for twenty to thirty minutes. For fever, Hegu(LI 4)and Quchi(LI1)are added with reducing manipulation; Pishu (BL 20) and Gongsun (SP 4) added with reinforcing manipuiation for anorexia and weakness of the extremities; and Shenshu (BL 23), Mingmen (DU 4) and Taixi (KI 3) added with reinforcing manpulation and in coordination with moxibustion for soreness of the lower back, weakness of the legs, undigestion, and aversion to cold in the abdomen.

Introducing Some Experiential Techniques

In Collection for Experiences of Acupuncture & Moxibustion the following method is recorded. No. 28 — 30 needles are employed and Sibian(EX., 4 points in total, 1 cun respectively left and right to, above and below the center of the umbilicus) are selected. The points are punctured in the order from above, below, left to right. The needles are inserted to a depth of 0.3 — 0.5 cun in adults and 0.2 — 0.3 cun in children and not retained. For the cold syndrome of deficiency type, the needles are inserted slowly and twisted for thirty seconds, But for the heat — damp syndrome, the needles are inserted quickly and twisted for ten seconds.

Another method is recorded in the same book mentioned above. Left and right Huangshu(Extra, 0.5 cun lateral to Shenque, RN 8) are selected and punctured wtih No. 30 — 31 needles 1.5 cun long, the needle tip moving slightly towards the center of the umbilicus and to a depth of about 1.2 cun. Then, the needle is twisted for thirty seconds, during which the needle may be lifted and thrust two or three times in child case whose age is above one year, but can not be lifted or thrust in child case whose age is below one year. After being twisted, the needles are withdrawn, and left and right Zusanli(ST 36) are punctured about one cun deep, with the needles lifted, thrust and twisted for about thirty seconds before withdrawal of them.

(2) *Moxibustion*

Selection of Points

Shenque (RN 8), Fuxietexiaoxue (Extra point, located at the dorso — ventral boundary of the foot, directly below the peak of the external malleolus) (See Fig. 5—9).

Method

To Shenque(RN 8), the salt moxibustion is applied. To the operation, a proper amount of salt powder is placed on the umbilicus, with the powder being 0.5 — 1 cun above the local skin surface around the umbilicus, a slice of ginger or garlic is placed on the salt, and a moxa cone is placed on the ginger or garlic and ignited for moxibustion. Five to seven cones are burnt in each session. To Fuxietexiaoxue (Extra point), the mild — warming or circling moxibustion with the moxa roll is given two or three times daily and for fifteen to twenty minutes each treatment session.

(3) Otopuncture
Selection of Otopoints

Large Intestine, Small Intestine, Sympathetic, Shenmen, Liver, Spleen, Kidney, Sanjiao.

Method

Three to five otopoints are punctured once daily, with the needles retained at each point for ten minutes, and with strong stimulation applied for acute cases and medium strength stimultion applied for chronic cases.

Introducing An Experiential Technique

The following method for treating diarrhea is reported in New Medicine. Ot. Shoulder Joint of the left side is punctured horizontally along the subcutaneous tissue upwards to a length of about 1 cun, with the needle twisted for about five minutes. On puncturing, the patient gradually feels the sensation like hot water scalding the auricle, and redness of the auricle may be seen in naked eye. Generally, the needle is retained for 12 to 14 hours, and the patient is asked to twirl the needle by himself per one to two hours during the retention, or for five minutes when he has abdominal pain or has the sensation of the bowel movements. For vomiting, Neiguan (PC 6) is added; and for fever Quchi (LI 11) added with strong stimulation administered and no retention of the needle given.

十三、阑尾炎

阑尾炎,归属于中医"肠痈"范畴。临床上主要症候为上腹正中或绕脐周围持续疼痛,阵发性加重,数小时后腹痛下移到右下腹,从右髂前上棘与脐作连线,当此线外1/3与内2/3交界处有明显压痛,右下腹不能伸直,局部有反跳痛,同时伴有发热、恶心、呕吐、腹泻或便秘等症状。血液中的白细胞计数可升高,若全腹压痛,反跳痛,腹肌紧张,体温明显升高,腹胀,脉数,当考虑阑尾炎穿孔而致腹膜炎。

针刺对急性单纯性阑尾炎效果满意,对慢性阑尾炎亦有一定效果。

技法运用

1. 毫针:取阑尾穴、天枢、上巨墟穴或阿是穴。发热加合谷、曲池;呕吐加内庭、中脘;腹胀加气海、大横。首先取阑尾穴、天枢、上巨墟、阿是穴,用捻转、提插、呼吸泻法或强刺激,持续捻转,行针至疼痛减轻或消失后,再留针1~2小时,每隔10分钟左右行针1次,每日2~3次。慢性阑尾炎亦可参考上穴治疗。

有人取①天井穴,当明显得气后用平补平泻手法,提插1~2次后,先向左再向右各捻转1~2次,最后轻轻提插1~2次,针后再艾灸天井穴上1.5寸处,共10壮(双);②大肠俞得气后,左侧穴朝反时针方向捻转30次,重提插40次,右侧穴朝顺时针方向捻转30次,重提插40次,出针后均不封口;尾骨尖穴,针沿尾骨尖刺入,针尖朝患者脐孔,得气后反时针方向捻转30次,重提插40次,出针后不封口。50例急性阑尾炎患者全部治愈。(张伟,《中国针灸》2:22,1986)

2. 耳针:取阑尾、下脚端、大肠、小肠、肺、神门穴。每次2~4穴。每穴持续捻转1分钟左右,强刺激,留针1~2小时,间隔20分钟行针1次,每日1~4次。两耳交替针刺。

有人取耳轮脚上缘及耳舟中段之痛点处(图5-10),用强刺激手法,留针30~60分

钟，以治疗早期急性阑尾炎为主。（上海耳针协作组．上海中医药杂志，2：20；1962）

3. 穴位注射：右侧足三里或阑尾穴。

患者取仰卧屈膝或屈膝端坐位，穴位常规消毒后，用5毫升注射器吸入注射用蒸馏水2～4毫升，以较快速度将针刺入3～4厘米，探索穴位刺激点，待有酸重麻胀感时，即将蒸馏水缓慢注入，患者立即感到沉重的麻酸胀感，沿经前外侧传至足背以至足趾。视病情每日注射1～2次，直至痊愈为止。（宋端麟，等．中华外科杂志，1：62；1960）

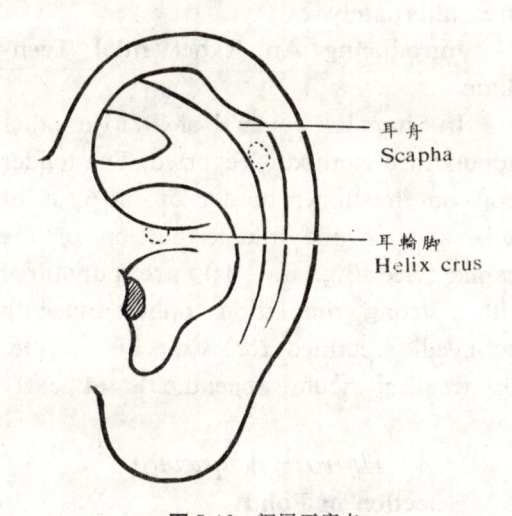

图 5-10 阑尾压痛点
Fig. 5-10 Tender Spots Relating to Appendix

13. APPENDICITIS

Manifestations

Appendicitis, chiefly referring to Chang Yong (肠痈, intestinal abscess) in TCM, is manifested clinicaly chiefly by pain felt first in the center of the umbilicus or around the umbilicus which is aggravated paroxysmally, and several hours later, felt and localed in the right lower abdomen, accompanied by obvious tenderness at the junction of external 1/3 portion and internal 2/3 portion of the line connecting the right anterior superior iliac spine with the umbilicus, difficulty in abduction of the right leg, local rebounding pain, fever, nausea, vomiting, diarrhea, or constipation. If there are general abdominal tenderness or rebounding pain, contructure of the abdominal wall, high fever, abdominal distension and rapid pulse, the condition indicates peritonitis due to appendicular perforation may occur.

Acupuncture is effective in treating simple appendicitis and helpful in treating chronic appendicitis.

Treatment by Applying Acubustion Techniques

(1) *Puncture with the Filiform Needle*

Selection of Points

Main points: Lanweixue (EX-LE7), Tianshu (ST25), Shangjuxu (ST37), Ashi Point.

Supplementary points according to symptoms: Hegu (LI 14) and Quchi (LI 11) for fever; Neiting (ST44) and Zhongwan (RN 12) for vomiting; and Qihai (RN 6) and Daheng (SP 15) for abdominal distension.

Method

For acute appendicitis, Lanweixue (EX-IE 7), Tianshu (ST 25), shangjuxu (ST 37) and Ashi Point are punctured two or three times daily, with the reducing manipulations by twisting, rotating, lifting and thrusting the needle and by manipulating the needle in cooperation with the patient's respiration, or with strong stimulation by continuous twisting and rotating movemont until the symptoms are relieved. Then, the needles are retained at each point for one to two hours and manipulated per ten minutes during the retension. Chronic appendicitis may be treated by selecting the same acupoints as in acute appendicitis.

Introducing An Experiential Technique

Another method is introduced by Chinese Acupuncture & Moxibustion. Tianjing (SJ 10), Dachangshu (BL 27) and Weigujianxue (Extra point) are selected. Firstly, the left and right Tianjing (SJ 10) are punctured with the uniform reinforcing — reducing manipulation applied after arrival of qi, the needles being lifted and thrust one or two times and twisted left and right one or two times respectively. Then, the needles are lifted and thrust one or two times gently. Following withdrawal of the needles, the moxibustion with the moxa cones is given to the left and right points 1.5 cun above Tianjing (SJ 10) until ten cones are burnt in total. Secondly, the left and right Dachangshu (BL 27) are punctured. After arrival of qi, the needle in the left point is twisted anticlockwise thirty times, and lifted and thrust forcefully forty times; while the needle in the right point twisted clockwise thirty times, and lifted and thrust forcefully forty times. The needle holes are not pressed after withdrawal of the needles. Finally, Weigujianxue (Extra point) is punctured with the needle inserted along the coccygeal apex towards the umbilicus. After arrival of qi, the needle is twisted anti—clockwise thirty times and lifted and thrust forcefully forty times. The needle hole is not pressed after withdrawal of the needle. 50 cases with acute appendicitis were cured by this treatment in that report.

(2) *Otopuncture*

Selection of Otopoints

Appendix, Sympathetic, Large Intestine, Small Intestine, Lung, Shenmen.

Method

Two to four otopoints are punctured one to four times daily, with the needles in each point twisted to cause strong stimulation for one minute. The needles are retained for one to two hours and manipulated per twenty minutes during the retention. The left and right auricles are punctured alternately.

Introducing An Experiential Technique

In Shanghai Journal of TCM another otopuncture method is reported. The tender spots on the upper border of the crus of helix and on the middle portion of the scapha (See Fig. 5 — 10) are punctured with a strong stimulation applied and with the needle retained for 30 — 60 minutes for treating acute appendicitis at early stage.

(3) *Hydro — Acupuncture*

Selection of Point

Right Zusanli (ST 36) or right Lanweixue (EX—LE 7).

Method

The patient is on the supine position with genuflex or on sitting position with genuflex, the local and routine sterilization is given. A needle in a 5 ml syrange with 2 — 4 ml of water for injection is inserted quickly into the acupoint to a depth of 3 — 4 cm. When needling sensations such as soreness, heaviness, numbness and distension are induced, the water is injected slowly into the point and the patient's needling sensation will be increased and propagated to the dorsum of the foot or even to the toes. The injection is given one or two times daily, according to the patient's condition, until the disease is cured.

十四、急性胆道疾患

急性胆道疾患，属中医学"胁痛"、"黄疸"、"厥"等范畴。临床主要表现为右上腹剧痛，或痛感放射至右肩及背部，可为阵发性绞痛，伴有恶心、呕吐、发热、黄疸等。

技法运用

1. 毫针：取胆囊穴、阳陵泉、支沟、足三里、内关、丘墟、肝俞、胆俞穴。

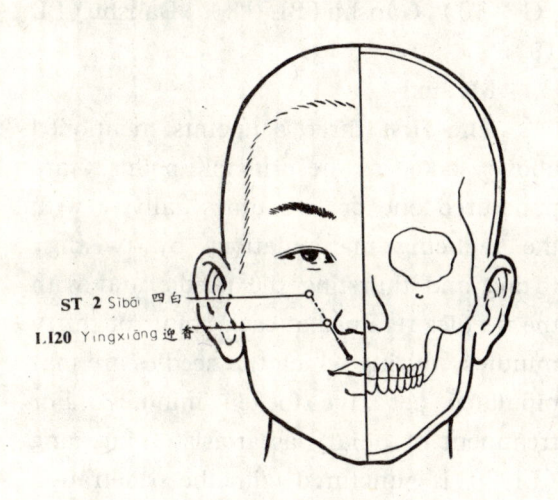

图 5-11 迎香透四白穴
Fig. 5-11 Penetration Needling from Yingxiang(LI 20) to Sibai(ST 2)

以前三穴为主穴，用捻转提插泻法。留针30分钟，每隔5～10分钟行针1次，每日1～2次。胆道蛔虫症可取迎香透四白穴，即由迎香穴垂直进针约0.5厘米，得气后将针斜向外上方，刺向四白穴（图5-11），用捻转提插泻法，留针1～2小时以上。

有报道针刺治胆石症，取穴①章门、期门、日月。②肺俞、胆俞。③足三里、合谷、太冲、阳陵泉、行间、足临泣。方法：患者先仰卧位，后俯卧位，或侧卧位，对主穴章门、期门、肝俞、胆俞均采用皮内推针法，在穴位表层上施按摇重震刮针术，每穴施用手法5分钟。四肢穴每天取2穴，深刺久留针（约半小时左右），每日1次，疼痛剧烈者可1日施针2次。（张子文，等.中医杂志，7：27；1959）

有人治胆道蛔虫症取鸠尾、阳陵泉，右上腹压痛点（一般在剑突上偏右方）。方法：鸠尾和压痛点呈15°角，向小腹方向斜刺0.5～1寸，针尖进入腹直肌即止；阳陵泉呈45°角针尖向内踝方向刺入1～3寸。均用提插捻转手法，持续行针至腹痛症状减轻或消失后留针，至疼痛再次发作时，仍用上法行针，如止反复操作至腹痛不再发作为止。留针期间并用艾条灸烤剑突下腹痛部位，灸至症状消失，起针时为止。

治急性胆囊炎，可取肩胛区压痛点，发烧配大椎、曲池；胁痛配阳陵泉；呕吐饱胀配中脘、足三里。操作取坐位，患者两前臂胸前交叉，双抱肩，使肩胛骨尽量外展。医生左手掌扶住患者左肩背部，右手拇指腹面由上而下按压脊椎右侧与肩胛之间，寻找压痛点。压痛点多在右肩胛区的中下部位。用1.5～2寸长毫针，呈30°角向下斜刺1～1.5寸，提插捻转手法，持续行针5～10分钟。起针后拔罐10～15分钟；大椎针0.5～1寸，提插刮针手法，短促行针；中脘针1.5～2寸，刮针手法，留针15～30分钟，每5分钟行针1次。（孙学全.《针灸临证集验》）

2. 耳针：取胆、肝、下脚端、神门、脑、屏间。用强刺激，每次取3～5穴，留针30分钟～1小时，每间隔10分钟捻转1次，或配合耳穴用王不留行籽贴压，每日按压2～3次，每次每穴1～2分钟。

有报道预先剪胶布2cm×0.4cm，将三粒留行籽均匀等距离沾上（简称长条），剪胶布

0.4cm×0.4cm,将1粒留行籽沾上(简称短条)。将长条胶布贴于耳穴肝、胆、胰、胃、十二指肠及腹外穴(肩穴的上方,对耳轮与耳舟交接处。图5-12),共三条。短条胶布贴于神门、交感(下脚端)、皮质下(脑),耳廓背面穴位相对处亦贴上王不留行籽,餐后按压药籽20~30分钟。疼痛明显时可增加按压次数,胶布隔日更换1次,左右耳交替,9次为1疗程,一般贴2~3疗程。(毛如宝,等.上海针灸杂志,3:27;1987)

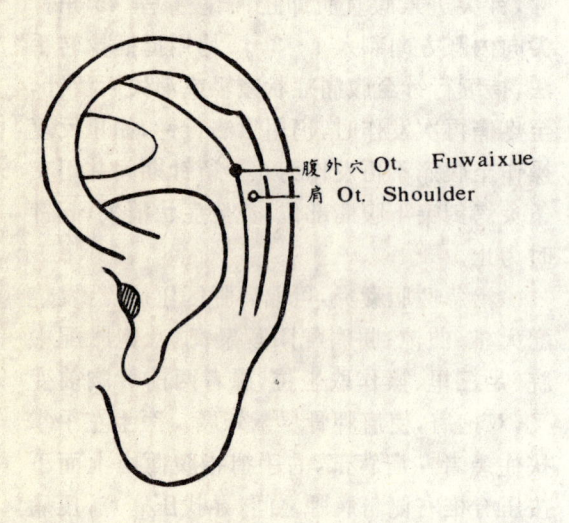

图 5-12 腹外穴
Fig. 5-12 Ot. Fuwaixue

3. 电针:取穴同毫针。用疏密波或密波,电流强度以病人能耐受为度,每日1~2次,每次30~60分钟。留针通电期间,可更换频率与加大电流量。

14. ACUTE BILIARY DISORDERS

Manifestations

Acute biliary disorder, belonging to Xie Tong, (肋痛 hypochondriac pain), Huang Dang (黄疸, jaundice), and You Jue (厥, colic caused by ascaris) in TCM, is manifested clinically chiefly by colic pain in the right upper abdomen which may radiate to the right shoulder or to the upper back, or be paroxysmal, accompanied by nausea, vomiting, fever and jaundice.

Treatment by Applying Acubustion Techniques

(1) *Puncture with the Filiform Needle*

Selection of Points

Dannanxue (EX — LE6), Yanglingquan (GB 34), Zhigou (SJ 6), Zusanli (ST 36), Neiguan (PC 6), Qiuxu (GB 40), Ganshu (BL 18), Danshu (BL 19).

Method

The first three acupoints mentioned above, taken as the principle points, are punctured one or two times daily, with the reducing manipulations by twistng, lifting and thursting the needle and with the needles retained at each point for thirty minutes, during which the needles are manipulated per five to ten minutes. For treatment of biliary ascariasis, Yingxiang (LI 20) is punctured with the penetration needling to Sibai(ST 2). Namely, Yingxaing (LI 20) is punctured firstly perpendicularly 0.5 cun deep, then, horizontally after arrival of qi, with the needle tip moving to Sibai(ST 2) but not piercing through the skin at Sibai(ST 2)(See Fig. 5—11). After the needle is pushed to the designed depth, the reducing manipulations by twisting, lifting and thrusting the needle are applied and the needle is retained for one to two hours.

Introducing Some Experiential Tech-

niques

A method for treatment of cholelithiasis is reporped in Journal of TCM. Zhangman(LR 13), Qimen(LR 14), Riyue(GB 24), Ganshu(BL 18), Danshu(BL 19), Zusanli(ST 36), Hegu(LI 4), Taichong (LR 3), Yanglingquan (GB 34) and Zulinqi(GB 41) are selected. On the operation, the patient is asked to be in the recumbent position, Zhangmen(LR 13), Qimen (LR 14), Ganshu (BL 18) and Danshu (BL 19), taked as the principle points, are punctured with the needles pushed forward beneath the skin and scraped, pressed, shaken and vibrated. This manner is applied to each point for five minutes. Moreover, other two of the acupoints on the extremities are punctured once daily or two times daily for severe cases, with the needles inserted deep and retained at each point for thirty minutes.

In Collection of Clinical Experiences of Acupuncture & Moxibustion the following methods are recorded. For treatment of biliary ascarialis, Jiuwei(RN 15) Yanglingquan (GB 34) and the tender spot on the right upper abdomen (usually near the xiphoid process) are selected. On the operation, Jiuwei (RN 15) and the tender spot are punctured at an angle of 15°, with the needles inserted obliquely towards the lower abdomen to a depth of 0.5—1 cun where the straight muscle of abdomen is located, Yanglingquan (GB 34)is punctured at an angle of 45°, with the needle pushed toward the internal malleolus to a depth of 2—3 cun. The puncture is given to the acupoints selected with the lifting, thursting and twisting manners applied until relief of abdominal pain. Then, the needles are retained. During retention of the needles, if the pain occurs again, the manipulations mentioned abvoe are repeated until the pain fails in attacking again. The moxibustion with the moxa roll is given to the painful spot on the abdomen in coordination until the symptoms are eliminated and the needles withdrawn.

For treatment of acute cholecystitis, the tender spots on the shoulder are selected as the main points. Dazhui(DU 14)and Quchi(LI 11) are added for fever; Yanglingquan (GB 34) added for vomiting and abdominal distension. To the operation, the patient is in the sitting position with the left hand holding the right slouder and the right holding the left shoulder, making the scapulae at the maximum abduction. The doctor holds the patient's left shoulder with the left palm, and press the area between the right border of the vertebrae and the right scapula from above down with the belly of the right thumb to find the tender spots which are usually located at the middle area of the lower portion of the right scapula area. Then, a 1.5—1 cun long needle is inserted into the tender spot at an angle of 30° and obliquely downwards to a depth of 1—1.5 cun. And then, the needle is lifted, thrust, twisted and rotated for five to ten minutes. Following withdrawal of the needle, cupping is given for ten to fifteen minutes on the spot in coordination. Besides, Dazhui(DU 14) is punctured 0.5 cun deep with manipulations by lifting, thrusting and scraping the needle quickly, and Zhongwan

(RN 12) punctured 1.5—2 cun deep with the manipulation by scraping the needle and with the needle retained for 15—30 minutes and manipulated per five minutes during the retention.

(2) *Otopuncture*

Selection of Otopoints

Gallbladder, Liver, Sympathetic, Shenmen, Brain, Endocrine.

Method

Three to five otopoints are punctured with strong stimulation applied, and with the needles retained at each point for thirty minutes to one hour and twisted per ten minutes during the retention. Or the vaccaira seeds are stuck on the otopoints and pressed two or three times daily and for one to two minutes on each point.

Introducing An Experiential Technique

In Shanghai Journal of Acupuncture & Moxibustion it is reported that some plasters with the vaccaria seeds on them are pasted on the otopoint for treatment of biliary diseases. To the operation, a piece of adhesive plaster 2×0.4 cm in size with three vaccaria seeds evenly placed on it, named long piece, is stuck on the area of Ot. Liver, Gallbladder, Pancrea, Stomach, Duodenum and Fuwaixue (above Ot. Shoulder, at the junction of antihelix and scalph, See Fig. 5—12). Another piece of adhesive plaster 0.4cm $\times$ 0.4cm in size and with one vaccaria seed on it, named short piece, is made up and stuck on the area of Ot. Shenmen, Sympathetic and Brain. The corresponding points on the back of the auricle are stuck with the plasters in the same way.

The seeds are pressed for twenty to thirty minutes after eating, and pressed more frequently when the pain is severe. The plasters are replaced once every other day and given to the left and right auricles alternately. Nine treatment sessions constitute one therapeutic course and two or three courses are usually needed.

(3) *Electroacupuncture*

Selection of Points

The same as in puncture with the filiform needle.

Method

Two to four acupoints are selected at each treatment session, and the electroacupuncture is given one or two times daily. The irregular or dense wave and a proper strength stimulation tolarable to the patient are administered for thirty to sixty minutes. During retention of the needles connecting with the current, the frequency may be changed and the current intensity can be increased properly.

十五、脱 肛

脱肛，临床主要表现为大便时肛门脱出，便后可自行回纳，严重时则咳嗽、起立、下蹲也会自行脱出，且不能自行回纳，须用手推回。时间日久局部可发生充血、水肿、出血、溃疡等。

技法运用

1. 毫针：取百会、长强、足三里、气海、承山、大肠俞、提肛（肛门两侧，各旁开肛门0.5厘米）穴。

以长强、百会为主穴，百会向上星方向沿皮刺0.5～1寸，用平补平泻法。留针30～60分钟，提肛穴针深1.5～2寸，针尖向同侧腹股沟方向直刺,并通电20～30分钟,使酸、麻、胀感向周围扩散。用断续波或疏密波,频率20次/分钟。通电强度以病人能耐受为度。

有人取百会、气海二穴治脱肛。操作即以上下为序,百会穴斜刺3分,留针5分钟;气海直刺8分～1寸深,将针进入到一定深度后,拇指向前捻,使穴下产生酸、麻、胀感,放散到阴部时将针退出,隔日针治1次。(光明中医函授大学.《针灸学》)

2.灸疗:取穴同毫针,以百会、气海为主穴。以小儿轻度脱肛效果为佳,医者灸百会穴时,分开患者头发以暴露穴位,右手持艾卷在其穴位上行温和旋灸5分钟,后改用雀啄灸15分钟。每日1次。

15. PROLAPSE OF RECTUM

Manifestations

Prolapse of rectum is manifested clinically chiefly by prolapse of rectum out of the anus during defecation, which returns itself to normal after the bowel movements. In severe cases, prolapse of rectum occurs with cough, or slight physical exertion, and the proalpsed rectum fails in retaining spontaneously without the aid of the hand. In prolonged cases, it may be accompanied by local congestion, swelling, bleeding and ulcer.

Treatment by Applying Acubustion Techniques

(1) *Puncture with the Filiform Needle*

Selection of Points

Baihui (DU 20), Changqiang (DU 1), Zusanli (ST 36), Qihai (RN 6), Chengshan (BL 57), Dachangshu (BL 25), Tigang (Extra point, 0.5 cm lateral to the anus).

Method

Three or four acupoints are selected each treatment session. Changqiang (DU 1) and Baihui (DU 20), taken as principle points, are puntured horizontally along the subcutaneous tissues to a depth of 0.5—1 cun, with the uniform reinforcing—reducing manipulation applied and the needles retained at each point for thirty to sixty minutes. Tigang (Extra point) is punctured to a depth of 1.5—2 cun, with the needle tip moving towards the groin of the same side and with electric stimualtion at intermittent or irregular wave and at frequency of 20 times/min., which is tolerable to the patient, administered to induce soreness, numbness and distension and to make them propagated all around.

Introducing An Experiential Technique

It is said in Acupuncture & Moxibustion, a textbook for acupuncture and moxibustion students, that Baihui (DU 20) and Qihai (RN 6) are punctured once every other day for treatment of prolapse of rectum. To the operation, first, Baihui (DU 20) is punctured obliquely to a depth of 0.3 cun, with the needle retained for five minutes. Then, Qihai (RN 6) is punctured perpendicularly to a depth of 0.8—1 cun, with the needle twisted clockwise to induce soreness, numbness and distension to the patient and to make them propagated to the anus.

(2) *Moxibustion*

Selection of Points

The same as in puncture with the filiform needle.

Method

Moxibustion is given to two to four acupoints once daily, first with the mild—warming moxibustion applied for five minutes, and then with bird—pecking moxibustion applied for fifteen minutes to each point. The moxibustion is effective in treating children with slight prolapse of rectum.

十六、痔 疮

临床上将痔疮分为外痔、内痔、混合痔三种。内痔是长于肛门内的小红疙瘩，质软，可逐渐增大，甚至脱出肛门，便秘时或便后可出血；外痔是长于肛门周围的状如樱桃的疙瘩，紫褐色，质硬，一般无疼痛；混合痔生于肛门内外，常为内外痔的合并症状。

技法运用

1. 毫针：取长强、承山、大肠俞、白环俞穴。

先针长强，用捻转泻法，使针感扩散至肛门周围，再针承山、大肠俞、白环俞，留针20～30分钟，每隔10分钟捻转行针1次，每日或隔日1次。痔疮出血可加刺孔最或二白穴（腕横纹直上4寸。桡侧腕屈肌腱左右两侧缘。（图5—13））

有人取长强穴治痔核，令患者腹卧位，两腿分成35°，经严密消毒后取2.5寸或3.5寸毫针，对准长强穴（图5—14），即以捻转的手法徐徐地将针刺入，使患者感到热、麻、胀。留针20分钟，每5分钟捻转1次，最初2天每日1次，以后隔日1次，5日为1疗程。（中医研究院医史文献研究室编.《中西医结合论文选编》，第一分册，1980年）

亦有人取承山穴（双）对痔疮疼痛100例的止痛效果进行了观察。方法：患者取俯卧位，术者一手托患者足跟，嘱其用力着术者掌心，术者另一手拇指标记穴位，然后用26号2寸毫针，于穴位皮肤常规消毒后，快速进针约1.5寸作强刺激捻转，每分钟约350次。以患者

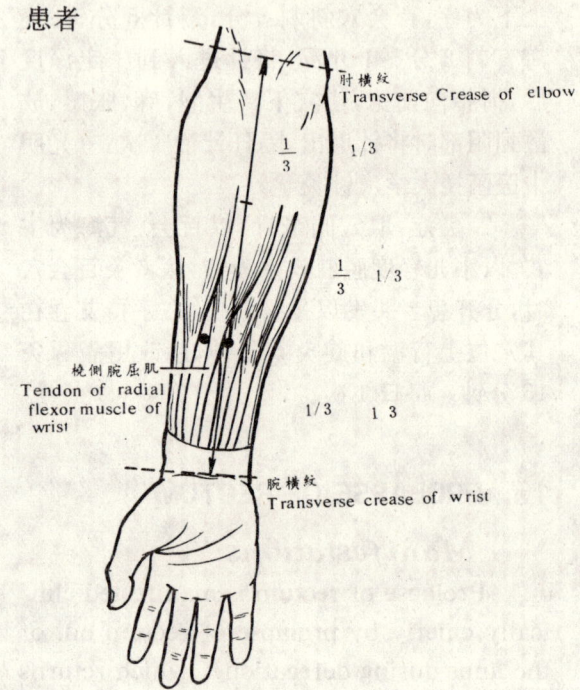

图5—13 二白穴
Fig. 5—13 Erbai(EX—UE 2)

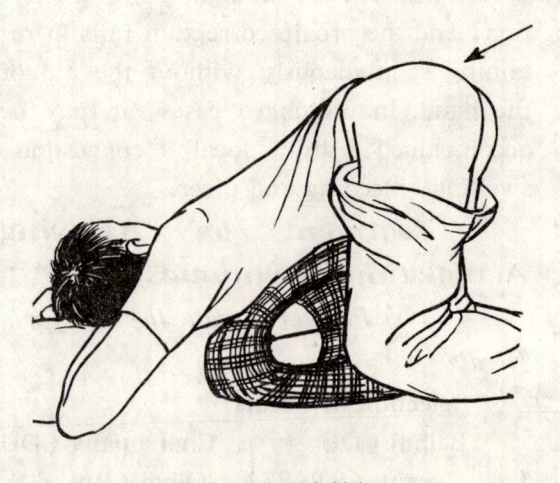

图5-14 长强穴刺法
Fig. 5—14 Puncturing at Changqiang(DU 1)

感到酸、麻、胀样的针感向腘窝、小腿、足底部放散(多数向小腿、足底放散),或局部胀痛为度,留针 30 分钟,5 分钟行针 1 次。(赵宝文.中国针灸,2:23;1986)

2.挑治:大肠俞、肾俞、次髎等穴,或腰骶部脊柱两侧,突出于皮面,状如大头针帽大小的红褐色小点。挑治部位及针具消毒,先以三棱针挑破表皮 2~3 毫米,再以圆利针挑断其纤维样物数根,碘酊消毒,盖上消毒敷料用胶布固定即可。每次挑治一对穴位,间隔 5~7 天挑治 1 次,挑治穴位或痔点轮换。

有报道,先找背部及腰骶部,圆形,有大头针顶大,稍高出于皮肤,呈灰白、棕褐色或暗红色,加压不褪色的痔点,然后消毒皮肤,用三棱针由下而上快速挑破表皮 0.5 厘米长,然后用弯缝针一层一层地向里挑,将白色纤维钩在针上,左右摇摆数次,以增强刺激,最后用力挑断,一般挑 10 针左右即可涂红汞,盖纱布,用胶布固定。若找不到痔点可挑大肠俞穴,一般 1 次挑 2 处,一周后再挑,3 次为一疗程。(刘冠军,等.《中医针法集锦》)

16. HEMORRHOID

Manifestations

Hemorrhoid may be classified into the internal, the external and the mixed types clinically. That situated above the anorectal line, being red, soft and small or gradually becoming larger, even prolapsed out of the anus, accompanied by bleeding on or after defecation belongs to the internal type; that below the anorectal line, like a cheer in size, being purplish brown and hard, the external, which generally does not cause pain to the patient; and that located both above and below the anorectal line, the mixed.

Treatment by Applying Acubustion Techniques

(1) *Puncture with the Filiform Needle*

Selection of Points

Changqiang (DU 1), Chengshen (BL 57), Dachangshu (BL 25), Baihuanshu (BL 30).

Method

First, Changqiang (DU 1) is punctured with reducing manipulations by twisting and rotating the needle, making the needling sensation propagated to the area around the anus. Then, Chengshan (BL 57), Dachangshu (BL 25) and Baihuanshu (BL 30) punctured with the needles retained for twenty to thirty minutes and twisted per ten minutes during the retention. The puncture is given once daily or once every other day. Kongzui (LU 6) or Erbai (EX—UE 2, 4 cun directly above the transverse crease of the wrist, lateral to the tendon of the radial flexor muscle of wrist, see Fig. 5—13) may be added for bleeding.

Introcucing Some Experiential Techniques

It is said that puncturing at Changqiang (DU 1) is effective in treatment of hemorrhoids. To the operation, the patient is on the prone position, with the legs at an angle of 35° formed by each other, strict local sterilization is given, and a 2.5 cun long or 3.5 cun long filiform needle is selected. The needle is inserted into the point to induce heat, numbness and distension to the patient. The puncture is given once daily in the first four days and once every other day in the following six days, with the needle retained for twenty minutes and twisted per five minutes during the retention. Five treatment sessions constitute a course (See Fig. 5—14)

Another method is reported by Chaniese Acupuncture & Moxibustion, which was effective in treating 100 cases with hemorrhoids. To the operation, the patient is on the prone position, and the doctor holds the patient's heel with the palm of the one hand and asks the patient to exert his leg forcefully. At the same time, the doctor makes a mark on Chengshan (BL57) with the thumb of the other hand. After a routine and local sterilization is given, a No. 26 filiform needle 2 cun long is inserted quickly into the marked point to a depth about 1.5 cun, and a strong twisting manner at a frequency of 350 turns/min is applied to induce soreness, numbness and distension to the patient and to make them radiated to the popliteal fossa, leg, and sole. Then, the needle is retained for thirty minutes and manipulated per five minutes during the retention. The Shengshan (BL57) at the other side is punctured with the same way and one treatment session needs selection of bilateral Shengshan (B 57).

(2) *Pricking Therapy*

Selection of Points

Dachangshu (BL25), Shenshu (BL23), Ciliao (BL32) or the red brown spots about 0.2 cm in diameter beside the lumbosacral vertebrae.

Method

A routine sterilization is given to the areas to be pricked and then to the needle. At first, at skin area of 2—3 mm in diameter of the point is pricked with the three—edged needle, then, some fiber—like tissues are broken with the round—sharp needle. Finaliy, the area is sterilized by iodine, covered with the sterilized dress and pasted with the adhesive plaster. The pricking therapy is given once per five to seven days and to a pair of acupoints in each treatment session. The points or spots are selected alternately.

Introducing An Experiential Technique

In Collection of Outstandings of the Needling Methods of TCM another method is recorded. Hemorrhoidal spots on the back and lumbosacral region which are round — shaped, 0.2 cm in diameter, above the skin surface, and of greyish white or brown or dark red colour which does not fade under pressure are selected as the pricking areas. Following sterilization, the spot is cut 0.5 cun long with the three—edged needle quickly pricking from the lower to the upper. Then, With the needle, the white fibral tissues are lifted, shaked several times to improve the stimulation, and then broken. The pricking course is repeated ten times in each spot. Finally, the area is smeared with mercurochrome, and covered with the sterilized dress and the adhesive plaster. If the hemorrhoidal spots are not found, left and right Dachangshu (BL25) may be selected. Generally, two spots are pricked in each treatment session, the pricking therapy is given once every week, and three treatment sessions constitute a course.

十七、高血压病

高血压病，属于中医"眩晕"、"头痛"、"中风"等病范畴。临床主要表现为头晕、头痛、心悸、失眠、耳鸣、心烦、肢体麻木，安静休息时收缩压≥21.3千帕，或/和舒张压≥12.7千帕。晚期可并发心、脑、肾病变。

技法运用

1. 毫针：取曲池、足三里、三阴交、内关、太冲穴。

用捻转提插泻法或平补平泻法。留针30分钟，每日1次，每次2～3穴。头痛加太阳、风池；耳鸣加翳风、中渚；失眠心悸加通里、神门；头重肢困加丰隆。

有人治高血压病取主穴内关。颈后痛配天柱、或风池；头顶痛而晕配上星、百会或头维；失眠配安眠₂，头两侧痛配太阳或头维。方法：刺天柱或风池，针尖向下颌方向刺0.5～0.8寸，单捻手法，捻针3～5次，此时患者局部可有强烈酸胀感，留针30～60分钟，10～15分钟用上法行针1次；头顶部刺百会或上星沿皮刺入0.5～1寸，留针1～2小时；头两侧胀痛时刺太阳或头维，刮针手法，5～10分钟行针1次，留针至胀痛减轻或消失后起针。配穴根据情况辨证选用。重者日针1次，轻者间日1次，一般7～10次为1疗程。（孙学全.《针灸临证集验》）

还有人对于不同类型的高血压，根据补虚泻实的原则，取绝骨、三阴交两穴施用补法或泻法。补法，即进针缓慢、针感轻微，并向四周扩散约1寸左右，留针15分钟，每隔5分钟用同样手法捻针1次；泻法，即进针较快、针感强烈，并向下扩散，留针15分钟，每隔5分钟用同样手法捻转1次。（李栋森.浙江医学，4：173；1961）

2. 耳针：降压沟、脑、神门、肝、下脚端、下屏尖。每日1次，每次3～5穴，留针1～2小时。亦可针刺后配合耳穴贴敷王不留行籽、或400高斯左右磁珠，或揿针，3～5天更换1次，每日按压2～3次。

3. 皮肤针：取颈后至尾骶脊柱两侧常规刺激区，气管两侧。按自上而下顺序进行轻度或中度叩刺，亦可根据症状重点叩刺肝俞、心俞、厥阴俞等穴。

4. 刺血：大椎穴附近常规消毒后，用三棱针刺入皮下，挑拨1～3次出针，随后将火罐扣于穴上，拔罐15分钟左右。或取曲泽、委中、太阳刺血，每次1穴（双侧），3～5天治疗1次，每次出血量5～10毫升。（田丛豁，等.《针灸医学验集》）

17. HYPERTENSION

Manifestations

Hypertension, belonging to disease or syndrome categories of Xun Yun（眩晕，dizziness）, Tou Tong（头痛, headache）, and Zhong Feng（中风, wind—stroke）in TCM, is manifested clinically chiefly by dizziness, restlessness, headache, palpitation, insomnea, tinnitus, numbness of the extremities, and systolic and diastolic pressure equal to or more than 21.3 kilopascal (160 mm/Hg) and 12.7 kilopascal (95 mm/Hg) respectively on rest. In severe cases, disorders in the heart, brain, and kidney may be accompanied.

Treatment by Applying Acubustion Techniques

(1) *Puncture with the Filiform Needle*

Selection of Points

Main points: Quchi (LI 11), Zusanli (ST36), Sanyinjiao (SP 6), Neiguan (PC 6), Taichong (LR 3).

Suppelmentary points according to symptoms: Taiyang (EX—HN5) and Fengchi (GB 20) are added for tinnitus; Tongli (HT 5) and Shenmen (HT 7) added for insomnea and palpitation; and Fenglong (ST 40) added for heaviness in the head and weakness of the limbs.

Method

Two or three points are punctured once daily, with the reducing manipulations by twisting, lifting and thrusting the needle, or with the uniform reinforcing reducing manipulation. The needles are retained at each point for thirty minutes.

Introducing Some Experiential Techniques

The following method for treatment of hypertension is introduced by Collection of Clinical Experiences of Acupuncture and Moxibustion. Neiguan (PC 6) is taken as the main point, Tianzhu (BL 10) or Fengchi (GB 20) selected for pain in the back of the head, Shangxing (DU 23) and Baihui (DU 20) or Touwei (ST 8) selected for pain in the vertex and dizziness, Anmian (Ex point) selected for insomnea, and Taiyang (EX—HN 5) or Touwei (ST 8) selected for pain in the temporal region. To the operation, Tianzhu (BL 8) or Fengchi (GB 20) is punctured towards the mandibular region to a depth of 0.5—0.8 cun with the needle twisted three to five times. When the patient complains of strong soreness and distension in the local area, the needle is retained for thirty to sixty minutes and twisted per ten to fifteen minutes during the retention; Baihui (DU 20) or Shangxing (DU 23) punctured with the needle inserted along the skin to a depth of 0.5—1 cun and retained for one to two hours; and Taiyang (EX—HN 5) or Touwei (ST 8) punctured with the needle retained and scraped per five to ten minutes until relief of the distending pain. The puncture treatment is given once daily for severe cases and once every other day for mild cases. Ten treatment sessions constitute a course.

Another method for treating hypertension is reported in Zhejiang Medicine. Xuanzhong (GB 39) and Sanyinjiao (SP 6) are punctured, and reinforcing or reducing manipulation is applied according to the patient's condition, namely, reinforcing needling is selected for deficiency type and reducing needling selected for excess type. To the reinforcing needling, the needle is inserted slowly to induce mild needling sensation to the patient and manipulated to make the needling sensation propagated about 1 cun around. Then, the needle is retained for fifteen minutes and twisted per five minutes during the retention. To the reducing needling, the needle is inserted quickly to induce strong needling sensation to the patient and make it propagated downwards. Then, the needle is retained for fifteen minutes and twisted per five minutes during the retention.

(2) *Otopuncture*

Selection of Otopoints

Groove for Lowering Blood Pressure, Brain, Shenmen, Liver, Sympathetic, Infratragic Apex.

Method

Puncture is given to three to five otopoints once daily, with the needles retained at each point for one to two hours. Or following puncturing at the otopoints, stick the vaccaria seeds or magnetic balls or embed thumb—tack needles over the otopoints punctured and press them two or three times daily. Three to five days later, remove them and give the therapy to some other otopoints.

(3) *Tapping*
Selection of Areas
The regular stimulation area beside the spinal column, the area beside the trachea.
Method
Tap on the areas gently or moderately from above down, or tap on them with emphasis on Ganshu (BL 18), Xinshu (BL 15) and Jueyinshu (BL 14) according to the patient's condition.

(4) *Pricking to Cause Bleeding*
Selection of Areas
Points around Dazhui (DU 14), Quze (PC 3), Weizhong (BL 40), Taiyang (EX—HN 5).
Method
After routine and local sterilization, prick the areas around Dazhui (DU 14) with the three—edged needle and shake the needle one to three times at each point. Following withdrawal of the needle, apply cupping to the Dazhui (DU 14) area for about fifteen minutes. Or select Quze (PC 3), Weizhong (BL 40) and Taiyang (EX—HN 5) alternately, pricking one pair of points to cause bleeding five to ten ml in each treatment session, and give the treatment once per three to five days.

十八、心绞痛

心绞痛,为"冠状动脉粥样硬化"的主症。归属于中医学"真心痛"、"厥心痛"范畴。临床特点为胸骨后或左前胸出现发作性绞痛,或压迫样紧闷、历时短暂(几秒到十几分钟),常放射到左肩、左臂、左手尺侧甚至颈部、喉部。多因体力活动、情绪激动、饱餐、受寒而突然发作,休息和治疗后可以迅速缓解。

技法运用

1. 毫针:取内关、膻中、郄门、足三里、神堂(第五胸椎棘突下旁开3寸)、通里。

先针左侧神堂穴,浅刺用捻转泻法,使针感向前胸及左臂放射,然后再取其他穴位用平补平泻法,留针20~30分钟,每日1次。

有报道取主穴膻中(沿皮下透向鸠尾,进针2.5~2.8寸),内关、足三里,配合通里、神门、间使、曲池、乳根、郄门,以补法为主,留针20分钟治疗冠心病心绞痛621例,总有效率89.2%。(北京市冠心病协作组.《全国针灸针麻学术讨论会论文摘要》(一),1979)

还有人取主穴心俞、厥阴俞,配穴内关、间使、通里、足三里。操作时每次取主穴1对,配穴1对。针刺背部穴位时,针左侧穴以左手持针,右手食指在椎间定向,针右侧穴位时反之。针尖斜向脊柱方向,与皮肤呈45°角迅速刺入皮肤后缓慢进针,直抵脊柱横突根部,可提插寻找敏感点,深度为1.5~2寸,施以轻、中刺激或轻刮针柄1~3分钟,不留针。针刺时勿垂直刺入,以防气胸。每日1次,12~15天1疗程。(解放军163医院.新医药学杂志,8:11;1973)

2. 耳针:取心、神门、脑、下脚端等穴。

中等刺激,留针30~60分钟,每日1次,留针期间每隔5~10分钟行针1次。

3. 灸疗:取膻中、膈俞穴。用艾灸每穴施15分钟,每日1次,6天为1疗程。(王富春.

江苏中医杂志,8：15;1987)

18. ANGINA PECTORIS

Manifestations

Angina pectoris, the main syndrome of coronary atherosclerotic cardiopathy, belonging to the disease or syndrome categories of Zhen Xin Tong (真心痛, real cardiac pain), or Jue Xin Tong (厥心痛, precordial pain with cold limbs) in TCM, is characterized chinically by paroxysmal pain or oppressed feeling in the precordial area, radiating to the left shoulder, left arm, or even to the neck and throat, induced by physical exertion, emotional disturbance, over—eating or attack by cold, and relieved quickly by rest and treatment.

Treatment by Applying Acubustion Techniques

(1) *Puncture with the Filiform Needle*

Selection of Points

Neiguan (PC 6), Danzhong (RN 17), Ximen (PC 4), Zusanli (ST 36), Shentang (BL 44, lateral to the lower border of the spinal process of the 5th thoracic vertebra, 3 cun lateral to the posterior median line), Tongli (HT 5).

Method

Three to five acupoints are selected each treatment session. Left Shentang (BL 44) is shallowly punctured first, with reducing manipulation applied to induce and make the needling sensation propagated to the precordial area and left arm. Then, the other acupoints selected are punctured with unifrom reinforcing — reducing needling applied and with the needles retained at each point for twenty to thirty minutes. The treatment is given once daily and for ten times as a course.

Introducing Some Experiential Techniques

Another method is reported, by which a total effective rate of 89.2% in treatment of 621 cases with angina pectoris of coronary atherosclerotic cardiopathy was achieved. To the operation, Danzhong (RN 17), Neiguan (PC 6) and Zusanli (ST 36) are punctured with reinforcing manipulations applied and with the needles retained at each point for twenty minutes. On punctruing at Danzhong (RN 17), the needle is pushed horizontally along the skin towards Jiuwei (RN 15) to a depth of 2.5 — 2.8 cun. Additionally, Tongli (HT 5), Shenmen (HT 7), Tianshu (PC 5), Quchi (LI 11), Rugen (ST 18), or Ximen (PC 4) is punctured according to the patient's condition.

In New Medicine the following method is reported for treatment of angina pectoris. Xinshu (BL 15) and Jueyinshu (BL 14) are taken as the main points, and Neiguan (PC 6), Jianshu (PC 5), Tongli (HT 5) and Zusanli (ST 36) taken as the supplementary. A pair of the main point and a pair of the supplementary point are punctured once daily for twelve to fifteen days as a course. On the back, the left point is punctured with the needle held by the left hand and the point fixed by the right index finger, and vice versa. The needle is inserted at an angle of 45° towards the spinal column quickly through the skin and then slowly pushed to the root area of the transverse process of the vertebra. Then, the needle is lifted and thrust between the depth of 1.5 cun and 2 cun, with mild or moderate stimulation applied or with the needle scraped one to three minutes. Finally, the needle is withdrawn. During the operation, the needles are not retained. It is forbidden to puncture at the point on the back perpendicularly, otherwise pneumothorax may be caused.

(2) *Otopuncture*

Selection of Otopoints

Heart, Shenmen, Brain, Sympathetic

Method

Moderate stimulation is applied, the needles are retained at each point for thirty to sixty minutes, and manipulated per five to ten minutes during the retention. The otopuncture treatment is given once daily and for ten sessions as a course.

(3) *Moxibustion*

Selection of Points

Danzhong (RN 17), Geshu (BC 17).

Method

Moxibustion with the moxa roll is given to each acupoint for fifteen minutes once daily and for six sessions as a course.

十九、高脂血症

血浆脂质浓度超过正常高限时，即为高脂血症。多见于未控制的糖尿病、动脉粥样硬化、肾病综合征，以及某些原发性、遗传性脂代谢紊乱等疾病。

技法运用

1. 毫针：取曲池、内关、三阴交、足三里、丰隆、太白、阳陵泉穴。

用捻转提插泻法或平补平泻法，或用轻捻转加震颤手法。每次3~5穴，每日1次，10次1疗程。本病因见于临床某些疾病中，故可根据具体病情随症加减，如伴高血压头胀痛、眩晕、耳鸣、面红目赤，加刺太冲；口渴多饮、消谷善饥者加刺内庭；畏寒肢冷、尿少身肿加太溪、阴陵泉、肾俞等穴。

有报道针刺内关穴可以降血脂。方法：每次仅取一侧内关穴，快速进针行捻转提插2分钟，引出酸、胀、麻或放射针感，留针20分钟，其间以同样手法刺激两次以保持针感。左右两穴交替针刺。（赵和熙，等.中西医结合杂志，11：666；1984）

2. 艾灸：用直接米粒灸法，灸双侧足三里、绝骨（交替使用），每周1次，每次3壮，致使三度烧伤起泡化脓，若破皮者，隔日换药1次，直至结痂形成瘢痕，以10次为1疗程，均只作1疗程。（蒋桂素.上海针灸杂志，3：11；1987）

19. HYPERLIPEMIA

Manifestations

Hyperlipemia is usually seen in uncontrolled diabetes mellitus, atherosclerosis, nephrotic syndrome, and some primary — hereditary disturbance of lipometabolism.

Treatment by Applying Acubustion Techniques

(1) *Puncture with the Filiform Needle*

Selection of Points

Quchi (LI 11), Neiguan (PC 6), Sanyinjiao (SP 6), Zusanli (ST 36),

Fenglong (ST 40), Taibai (SP 3), Ynaglingquan (GB 34).

Method

Three to five acupoints are punctured once daily and for ten times as a course, and reducing manipulations by twisting, lifting and thrusting the needle or the uniform reinforcing — reducing needling are applied. Or, gentle twisting and viberating manners are applied in coordination.

Supplementary points according to symptoms: As hyperlipoidemia may be seen in different diseases, the acupuncture prescription should be modefied according to the patient's condition. For example, Taichong (LR 3) is added for hypertension with distending pain in the head, dizziness, tinnitus, flushed face and congested eye; Neiting (ST 44) added for thirst, polydipsia, ravenous appetite and excessive hunger; and Taixi (KI 3), Yinlingquan (SP 9) and Shenshu (BL 23) added for aversion to cold, cold extremities, oliguria and edema.

Introducing An Experiential Technique

It is said that puncturing at Neiguan (PC 6) is effective in treating hyperlipemia. To the operation, Neiguan (PC 6) of one side is punctured with the needle inserted quickly and twisted and rotated for two minutes to induce needling sensation such as soreness, distension and numbness to the patient, or to make the needling sensation propagated. Then, the needle is retained for twenty minutes and manipulated with the same way two times to maintain the needling sensation during the retention. Left and right Neiguan (PC 6) are punctured alternately.

(2) *Moxibustion*

Selection of Points

Left and right Zusanli (ST 36) and Xuanzhong (GB 39).

Method

Left and right points are employed alternately. Direct moxibustion with the rice — size cone is given until three cones are burnt in each point, causing local third — degree burn, blister and purulence. If the local area is broken, it is covered with drug — dress and the drug — dress is replaced with a new one every other day until scar is formed. The moxibustion is given once per week and for ten sessions as a course.

二十、心律失常

心律失常,是指心率过快、过慢或心律不齐的一类病症,归属于中医学"心悸"、"怔忡"范畴。临床常见胸闷、心悸、怔忡、头晕、乏力、气短、失眠、易惊善恐等症候。

技法运用

1. 毫针:取内关、神门、心俞、厥阴俞、身柱(第3胸椎棘突下)、至阳、足三里穴。

胸闷气短加膻中;心动过缓加通里;早搏加阴郄透内关;心动过速加太冲或太溪。针四肢穴用平补平泻法,留针10~20分钟,中间间歇运针1~2次,每日针治1次;针背部穴时,针尖向前内与皮肤呈45°角,或将刺入点移至脊柱旁开一横指与皮肤呈75°角刺入。针刺深度1.5~1.7寸,有酸、麻、胀感即刮针柄1~3分钟后起针,每天1次,15~20天为1疗程。(解放军163医院.《全国针灸针麻学术讨论会论文摘要》(一)。1979)

2. 耳针:取屏间、心、下脚端、脑、肾穴。

每次取3~4穴,轻刺激,留针30~60分钟,每日1次。亦可针刺与王不留行籽贴敷穴位相配合,每日压按3~4次。

3. 电针:取内关、郄门、心俞、足三里、三阴交。每次2穴,选用疏密波,中等刺激以病人能耐受为度。每日1次,每次15~30分钟。

20. ARRHYTHMIA

Manifestations

Arrhythmia, including tachycardia, bradycardia and irregular heart beating rate, belonging to Xin Ji, Zhen Cong (心悸,怔忡, palpitation) in TCM, is manifested by oppressed feeling in the chest, palpitation, dizziness, lassitude, shortness of breath, insomnea, and fear and fright in clinic.

Treatment by Applying Acubustion Techniques

(1) *Filifrom Needling*

Selection of Points

Main points: Neiguan (PC 6), Shenmen (HT 7), Xinshu (BL 15), Jueyinshu (BL 14), Shenzhu (DU 12, below the process of the third thoracic vertebra), Zhiyang (DU 9), Zusanli (ST 36).

Supplementary points: Danzhong (RN 17) for oppressed feeling in chest and shortness of breath; Tongli (HT 5) for bradycardia; Yinxi (HT 6), punctured with penetration needling to Neiguan (PC 6), for premature beating; and Taichong (LR 3) or Taixi (KI 3) for tachycardia.

Method

Two to four points are employed each treatment session. The points on the extremities are punctured with the uniform reinforcing—reducing needling, and with the needles retained at each point for ten to twenty minutes and manipulated one or two times during the retention. To the points on the back, the needles are inserted obliquely at an angle of 45° to the skin or at 75° angle if the point is one cun lateral to the spinal column, and to a depth of 1.5—1.7 cun. When the patient complains of soreness, numbness, and distension, the needle handle is scraped for one to three minutes and the needle is withdrawn. The prncture treatment is given once daily and for fifteen to twenty days as a course.

(2) *Otopuncture*

Selection of Otopoints

Endocrine, Heart, Sympathetic, Brain, Kidney.

Method

Three or four points are selected each session, mild stimulation is applied, and the needle is retained in each point for thirty to sixty minutes. The puncture treatment is given once daily and for ten sessions as a course. Or, following the puncture, the vaccaria seeds are stuck on the otopoints and pressed three or four times daily in coordination.

(3) *Electroacupuncture*

Selection of Points

Neiguan (PC 6), Ximen (PC 4), Xinshu (BL 15), Zusanli (ST 36), Sanyinjiao (SP 6).

Method

Employ two points each session, and apply electric stimulation at medium strength and with sparse—dense wave, which is tolerable to the pateint, for fifteen to thirty minutes and once daily.

二十一、脑血管意外

脑血管意外，属于中医学"中风"、"卒中"、"类中"、"大厥"等范畴。包括近代所述的脑出血、蛛网膜下腔出血、脑栓塞、脑血栓形成、脑血管痉挛等。

临床归纳为闭证、脱证、后遗证三方面。

闭证，见突然昏倒不省人事、牙关紧闭、面赤气粗、鼾声如雷、脉弦滑；脱证，见骤然昏扑不语、目合口开、手撒遗尿、鼾睡肢冷、汗出如珠、脉微细欲绝；后遗证，见口眼歪斜、半身不遂、手足麻木、震颤、言语蹇涩等。

技法运用

1. 针灸

闭证取人中、十宣、风池、风府、内关、合谷、涌泉、太冲穴。用捻转提插泻法只针不灸，先刺人中、涌泉、内关、或十宣放血，后配合针刺其他穴位；脱证取人中、百会、涌泉、关元、气海、神阙、足三里。先刺人中、百会、涌泉用捻转提插补法，继之神阙用大灸炷隔盐灸，其他穴位均可针灸配合。留针30分钟，每日1次；后遗证，以局部与循经取穴相结合，用平补平泻法。如上肢瘫取肩髃、曲池、合谷、外关。下肢瘫取环跳、阳陵泉、绝骨、风市。语蹇取廉泉、风池、通里。面瘫取颊车、地仓、阳白、合谷等。每次取3～5穴，留针15～20分钟，每日或隔日1次。

有报道治中风取主穴内关、人中、三阴交、配穴取极泉、尺泽、委中。吞咽困难加风池、翳风；手指不能屈伸加合谷；失语配金津、玉液（舌系带两侧静脉上，左为金津、右为玉液）。（图5-15）。依次取双侧内关直刺0.8～1寸，施提插法使针感直达指端，行针1分钟；刺人中穴向鼻中隔斜刺0.3～0.5寸，用雀啄泻法以流泪或眼球湿润为度；三阴交，针尖沿胫骨后缘与皮肤呈45°角向后斜刺，进针1.5寸施提插补法，使下肢抽动3次；取极泉直刺1～1.5寸施提插泻法，以上肢抽动3次为宜；委中进针0.5～1寸，施提插泻法使下肢抽动3次。风池、翳风均向喉结方向深刺，进针2～2.5寸，采用小幅度、高频率捻转（补法）。每穴施手法1分钟。1日针2次，10天为1疗程。（翟义德.中国针灸，5：10；1988）

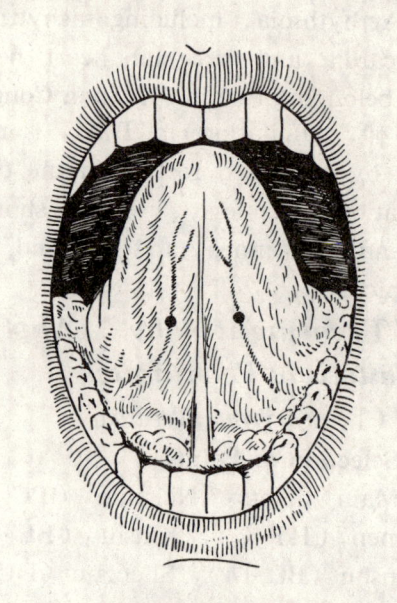

图5-15 金津、玉液
Fig.5-15 Jinjin and Yuye (L—X—HN 12,13)

有人治中风昏迷，先点刺十宣出血，再针百会、安眠、风府、涌泉、人中。风府向下颌方向针0.5～0.8寸，刮针手法；安眠针0.5～1.2寸，提插刮针手法；百会针0.5～1寸，捻转手法；刺人中时，医者左手先将鼻唇沟捏起，从鼻唇沟上1/3与下2/3交界处进针，针尖向鼻间隔方向斜刺0.3～0.5寸；涌泉直刺0.3～0.5寸。人中和涌泉均用提插捻转手法，持续行针至患者知觉恢复或苏醒后，再间歇行针1～2小时，10～15分钟捻针1次，余

穴均同。人中和涌泉约持续行针15～30分钟。患者昏迷仍不见好转时,应采取其他抢救措施。(孙学全.《针灸临证集验》)

另有报道针刺治脑血栓形成262例。方法:取穴分组,第一组上肢瘫取肩髃、曲池、合谷。下肢瘫取环跳、阳陵泉、昆仑。第二组上肢瘫取扶突或配臂中(位于腕横纹与肘横纹中央联系之中点,两骨之间)。失语或舌强语涩均配廉泉。

两组均采用泻法、重刺激,不留针。针扶突穴选用26号1.5寸毫针快速刺入皮下、进针后向颈椎后下方斜刺0.5～1寸深(刺时要谨慎,要熟悉局部组织解剖,以免发生医疗事故),使触电样针感传至手指,如针感不明显,可配用臂中穴。针臂中穴,选用26号1.5毫针直刺,待触电感传至手指时,不捻转,单纯提插5～6次,然后出针;针环跳穴,选用2.5～3寸毫针向前下方直刺2寸左右,待触电样针感传至足时,不捻转,单纯提插4～5次以加强针感。若针感不明显可配足三里,针足三里选用26号2寸毫针,直刺1.5寸左右,待触电样针感传至足时,反复提插5～6次,然后出针。针刺时均需取得要求的针感,以达到"气至病所",再施以提插手法,一般不留针。(徐笨人,等.中国针灸,6:13;1983)

2. 头针:选用瘫痪对侧的运动区、感觉区、足运感区、语言区。沿皮下刺入0.5～1寸,频频捻针,捻转角度在180°以内,频率为200次/分钟以上。

3. 电针:取穴同毫针,选四肢2～3对穴位,进针捻转得气或出现针感向远端扩散后再通电,用疏波或断续波,电流强度以患者能耐受为度,每次通电20分钟,每日或隔日1次。

有人用电头针治疗脑血管意外后遗症。运动障碍取对侧运动区上1/5～2/5处及足运感区;言语障碍取言语1区和言语2区;感觉障碍取对侧感觉区。进针后接通电针机,频率300～500/秒,先用连续波10分钟后,改为断续波或疏密波,电流强度以患者能耐受为度。每日或隔日1次,10次为1疗程。(田丛豁,等.《针灸医学验集》)

21. CEREBROVASCULAR ACCIDENT

Manifestations

Cerebrovascular accident, including cerebral hemorrhage, subarachnoid hemorrhage, cerebral embolism, cerebral thrombosis, cerebrovascular spasm, etc., belongs to Zhong Feng (中风), Zu Zhong (卒中), Lei Zhong (类中), Da Jue (大厥) in TCM. Its clinical manifestations can be classified into tense syndrome, the flaccid syndrome and the sequela syndrome.

The manifestations of the tense syndrome: Falling down in a fit with loss of consciousness, clenched jaws, flushed face, coarse breathing, string—taut and rolling pulse.

The manifestations of the flaccid syndrome: Falling down in a fit and sudden loss of consciousness with mouth agape and eyes closed, flaccid paralysis of limbs, incontinence of urine, snoring, cold extremities, profuse sweating, fading pulse.

The manifestations of the sequela syndrome: Deviation of mouth and eye, hemiplegia, numbness of the limbs, tremor, slurring of speech.

Treatment by Applying Acubustion Techniques

(1) *Filiform Needling*
a. For Tense Syndrome:

Selection of Points

Renzhong (DU 26), Shixuan (EX—UE 11), Fengchi (GB 20), Fengfu (DU 16), Neiguan (PC 6), Hegu (LI 4), Yongquan (KI 1), Taichong (LR 3).

Method

Three to six points are employed each treatment session. At fisrt, Renzhong (DU 26), Yongquan (KI 1), and Neiguan (PC 6) are punctured with reducing manipulations by twisting, lifting and thrusting the needle, or Shixuan (EX—UE 11) is pricked to cause bleeding. Then, the rest points selected are punctured. Moxibustion is forbidden.

b. For Flaccid Syndrome:

Selection of Points

Renzhong (DU 26), Baihui (DU 20), Yongquan (KI 1), Guanyuan (RN 4), Qihai (RN 6), Shenque (RN 8), Zusanli (ST 36).

Method

Firstly, Renzhong (DU 26), Baihui (DU 20) and Yongquan (KI 1) are punctured with reinforcing manipulations by twirling, lifting and thrusting the needle. Then, moxibustion with salt is given to Shenque (RN 8). Finally, Puncture and moxibustion are applied to the other points selected. Four or five points are employed each time, and the needles are retained at each point for thirty minutes. The puncture treatment is given once daily.

c. For Sequela Syndrome:

Selection of Points

Local points and the points along the corresponding meridian are selected. For example, Jianyu (LI 15), Quchi (LI 11), Hegu (LI 4) and Waiguan (SJ 5) are selected for paralysis of upper limb; Huantiao (GB 30) Yanglingquan (GB 34), Xuanzhong (GB 39) and Fengshi (GB 31) selected for paralysis of lower limb; Lianquan (RN 23), Fengchi (GB 20), and Tongli (HT 5) for slurring of speech; and Jiache (ST 6), Dicang (ST 4), Yangbai (GB 14) and Hegu (LI 4) for facial paralysis.

Method

Three to five acupoints are punctured once daily or every other day, with the needles retained in each point for fifteen to twenty minutes.

Introducing Some Experiential Techniques

Another method for treatment of wind stroke (Cerebrovascular accident) is reported in Chinese Acupuncture & Moxibustion. Neiguan (PC 6), Renzhong (DU 26) and Sanyinjiao (SP 6) are taken as the main points, and Jiquan (HT 1), Chize (LU 5) and Weizhong (BL 40) as the adjuvant. The supplementary points according to symptoms include Fengchi (GB 20) and Yifeng (SJ 17) for difficulty in swallowing, Hegu (LI 4) for disturbance in extension and flexion of fingers, and Yuye (EX—HN 13, on the veins at the lateral sides of the frenulum of tongue, left one being Jinjin and right one, Yuye, See Fig. 5—15) for aphasia. To the operation, left and right Neiguan (PC 6) are punctured perpendicularly 0.8—1 cun, with lifting and thrusting manner applied for one minute, inducing and making the needling sensation radiate to the finger tips; Renzhong (DU 26) punctured obliquely 0.3—0.5 cun, with the needle tip moving towards the nasal septum, and with the bird—pecking needling applied until the pateint is in lacrimation or his eyeballs are moist; Sanyinjiao (SP 6) punctured obliquely 1.5 cun deep, with the needle tip moving along the posterior border of the shin—bone, and with reinforcing manipulation by lifting and thrusting the needle applied, making the lower limbs trembled 3 times; Jiquan (HT 1) punctured 1—1.5 cun deep, with reducing manipulation by lifting and thrusting the needle applied, making the upper limbs trembled 3 times; Weizhong (BL 40) punctured 0.5—1 cun deep, with reducing manipulation by lifting and thrusting the needle applied, making the lower limbs trembled 3 times; and Fengchi (GB 20) and Yifeng (SJ 17) punctured towards the Adam's apple to a depth of 2—2.5 cun, with the needles twisted in a small amplitude and a high frequency (i. e., a kind of reinforcing manner). The manipulation is applied to each point for one minute, and four or five acupoints are employed each treatment session. The treatment is given twice daily and for ten days as a course, and it is mainly applicated to the sequela syndrome of cerebrovascular accident.

In Collection of Clinical Experiences of Acupuncture & Moxibustion the following method for treatment of coma due to cerebrovascular accident is reported. Shixuan (EX—UE 11) is pricked to cause bleeding firstly. Then, Baihui (DU 20), Anmian (EX—HN 17), Fengfu (DU 16), Yongquan (KI 1) and Renzhong (DU 26) are punctured. On puncturing at Fengfu (DU 16), the needle is inserted 0.5—0.8 cun deep towards the mandible and scraped; at Anmian (EX—HN 17), the needle inserted 0.5—1.2 cun deep, and lifted, thrust and scraped; at Baihui (DU 20), the needle inserted 0.5—1 cun deep, and twisted; at Renzhong (DU 26), the needle inserted obliquely 0.3—0.5 cun deep towards the nasal septum; and at Yongquan (KI 1), the needle inserted perpendicularly 0.3—0.5 cun. Manipulations by lifting, thrusting and twirling the needle are applied to Renzhong (DU 26) and Yongquan (KI 1) until the patient's consciousness is recovered. If the effect is induced within fifteen to thirty minutes, the needles are retained there for one to two hours and twisted every ten to fifteen minutes during the retention. If it is not induced, some other emergency methods should be given. The other points are punctured with the same way as above.

A method for treatment of cerebral thrombosis is reported in Chinese Acupuncture & Moxibustion, which was effective to 262 cases with cerebral thrombosis. Two groups of acupoints are selected. The first one includes Jianyu (LI 15), Quchi (LI 11) and Hegu (LI 4) for paralysis of upper limbs, and Huantiao (GB 30), Yanglingquan (GB 34) and Kunlun (BL 60) for paralysis of lower limbs; the second one includes Futu (LI 18) or Bizhong (at the midpoint of the line connecting the midpoints of transverse crease of the wrist and elbow, between the two bones, an extra point) for paralysis of upper limbs. The adjuvant point is Lianquan (RN 23) for aphasia or slurring of speech and stiff tongue. Reducing manipulations, strong stimulation and no retention of the needles are chosen. At Futu (LI 18), a 1.5 cun needle is inserted quickly through the skin, and obliquely towards the area posterior and inferior to the cervical vertebra to a depth of 0.5—1 cun, inducing electrifying sensation to the patient and making it propagated to his fingers (note: this puncture is given only when the operator has a good knowledge about the local anatomy otherwise a medical accident might be caused). If the patient complains of weak needling sensation, Bizhong (extra point) is punctured additionally, with a 1.5 cun long needle inserted into the point perpendicularly. After the patient complains of the electrifying sensation radiating to the fingers, the needle is lifted and thrust five to six times, and then withdrawn. On puncturing at Huantiao (GB 30), a 2.5—3 cun long needle is inserted perpendicularly 2 cun deep, inducing electrifying sensation radiating to the patient's foot, and lifted and thrust four or five times to consolidate the needling sensation. If the patient complains of a weak needling sensation, Zusanli (ST 36) is punctured additionally, and a No. 26 needle 2 cun long is inserted perpendicularly 1.5 cun deep to cause electrifying sensation radiating to the patient's foot and lifted and thrust five to six times before withdrawal of it. On puncturing, the required needling sensation should be induced by manipulation, so as to make "qi arrive the diseased site". After the needling sensation is propagated to the designed area, the needles are lifted, thrust and withdrawn.

(2) *Scalp Puncture*
Selection of Points
Motor Area, Sensory Area, Foot—Kinesthetic Sensory Area, Speech Area, which are at the diseased side of the cerebrum, namely, at the side without manifestations of paralysis.
Method
The needles are inserted into the areas selected, pushed beneath the scalp for 0.5—1 cun, and twisted at a frequency above 200 times/min. and within an amplitude of a half round.

(3) *Electroacupuncture*
Selection of Points
The same as in the filiform needling.
Method
Two or three pair of points are punctured at first. Following the needling sensation is induced to the patient and propagated to the distal end of the extremites, a tolerable electric current with sparse wave or intermittent wave is given to the needles in the points for twenty minutes.
Introducing An Experiential Technique
Electroacupuncture on the scalp for treatment of sequela of cerebrovascular accident is recorded in Collection of Experiences of Acupuncture & Moxibustion. Upper 2/5 of the Motor Area on the side without manifestation of paralysis and Foot—Kinesthetic Sensory Area are selected for dyskinesia, Speech Area 1 and 2 selected for disturbance of speech, and Sensory Area on the side without manifesta-

tions of paralysis selected for sensory disturbance. After being inserted into the scalp, the needles are connected with the electric current. The electric stimulation is adjusted at a frequency of 300 — 500 turns/second and tolerable to the patient. During the first ten minutes, continuous wave is administered. Then, intermittent wave or sparse — dense wave is applied. The treatment is given once daily or every other day and for ten times as a course.

二十二、癫 痫

癫痫,归属于中医痫症范畴。临床常见突然发作,短暂的感觉精神障碍、意识丧失、发出尖叫、跌扑在地、口吐白沫、肢体抽搐。每次发作约 5～10 分钟,醒后如常人。

技法运用

1. 毫针:取鸠尾、长强、腰奇穴(一说在尾骨尖端直上 2 寸;一说在两侧中髎穴之中点处)、丰隆。用泻法或平补平泻法,刺鸠尾时,针尖向下斜刺或沿皮刺 1 寸左右;刺腰奇时,针尖向上沿皮刺或斜刺 1～1.5 寸。

发作期加人中、内关、合谷、太冲用泻法,不留针。发作前加刺后溪、大椎、用平补平泻法,留针 20～30 分钟,每日 1 次。间歇期加风府,用平补平泻法,留针 30 分钟,每日 1 次。上穴亦可配合电针,用密波,每次 15～20 分钟,每日 1 次。

有报道用 26 号 2 寸毫针,由大椎穴进针向上约 30°角斜刺,针深 1.5 寸左右,若病人有触电感传至肢体时立即出针,勿反复提插。(徐笨人. 中国针灸,2:4;1982)

2. 挑治:取长强穴。方法:常规消毒后,以左手将穴位局部组织捏起,右手持三棱针重刺长强穴及其前后左右各 1 针,深达 6～9 毫米呈梅花状,四点距长强穴各 15 毫米,然后挤压使局部出血,如此每周针刺 1 次,10 次为 1 疗程,前后疗程间休一月,最多者为 3 个疗程。(光明中医函授大学.《针灸学》函授教材)

有人取风府至长强的每一脊椎棘突间,如大椎、筋缩(第 9 胸椎棘突下)、癫痫(十二胸椎与第 1 腰椎棘突间)、腰奇、长强,以及百会、神庭、鸠尾、中脘等穴,用消毒过的三棱针挑刺出血 2～3 滴,起初每周 1 次,随发作间距的延长,可半月或 1 月 1 次。(陈笑山. 浙江中医杂志,2:69;1983)

3. 灸疗:取身柱(第 3 胸椎棘突下)、神堂(第 5 胸椎棘突下旁开 3 寸)、膈俞。可单独使用,也可配合使用,用黄豆大小艾炷着肤灸,每次每穴各灸 3 壮,以灸疮化脓为好。(田丛豁,等.《针灸医学验集》)

22. EPILEPSY

Manifestations

Epilepsy, belonging to Xian Zheng (痫症)in TCM, is clinically manifested by sudden seizure, sensory and mental disturbance, loss of consciousness, screams, falling down in a fit, foam on the lips and convulsions. After five to ten minutes the patient's condition becomes normal.

Treatment by Applying Acubustion Techniques

(1) *Filiform Needling*

Selection of Points

Jiuwei (RN 15), Changqiang (DU 1), Yaoqi(EX—B6, 2 cun above the caudal end of the coccyx or between two Zhongliao, BL33), Fenglong(ST40).

Method

Reducing method or uniform reinforcing — reducing method is applied. On puncturng at Jiuwei (RN 15), the needle is inserted obliquely downwards or pushed downwards along the skin to a depth of about 1 cun; on puncturing at Yaoqi (EX —B6), the needle inserted upwards horizontally along the skin to a depth of 1—1.5 cun. On the seizure, Renzhong (DU 26), Neiguan (PC 6), Hegu (LI 4) and Taichong (LR 3) are added, reducing manipulation and no retention of the needle being applied. Before the seizure, Houxi (SI 3) and Dazhui (DU 14) are added, uniform reinforcing-reducing manipulation being applied and the needles retained for twenty to thirty minutes; and on the intermission, Fengfu (DU 16) punctured additionally, the uniform reinforcing — reducing manipulation being applied and the needle retained for thirty minutes, and the treatment being given once daily. Additionlly, electroacupuncture, in coordination with the puncture, may be given to the cases at the intermission with dense wave adminstered to the points mentioned above for fifteen to twenty minutes once daily.

Introducing An Experintial Technique

The following method is reported in Chinese Acupuncture & Moxibustion. A 2 cun long needle is inserted into Dazhui (DU14) and pushed upwards at an angle of 30° to a depth of 1.5 cun. When the patient complains of electrifying sensation radiating to his extremites, the needle is withdrawn immediately. The lifting or thrusting manner is forbidden.

(2) *Breaking with the Three —*

Edged Needle

Selection of Point

Changqiang (DU 1)

Method

After a local routine sterilization, hold the local tissue with the left hand, heavily prick Changqiang (DU 1) and 4 points 15 mm respectively anterior, posterior, left and right to Changqiang (DU 1) with the three — edged needle held by the right hand, and press the local area to cause bleeding. The treatment is given once every week, for ten times as a course, and for three courses as the maximum. The intermittent period between two courses is one month.

Introducing An Experiential Technique

Another method is reported by Chen Xiaoshan, a famous acupuncturist. The points located at every interspace of the spinal processes of the spinal column from Fengfu (DU 16) to Changqiang (DU 1), as well as Baihui (DU 20), Shenting (DU 24), Jiuwei (RN 15) and Zhongwan (RN 12) are selected as the pricking points. Each point is pricked with the three — edged needle to cause two or three drops of blood out. The pricking treatment is given every week at beginning, and then once every half or one month.

(3) *Moxibustion*

Selection of Points

Shenzhu (DU 12, below the spinal process of the third thoracic vertebra), Shentang (BL 44, 3 cun lateral to the spinal column, below the spinal process of the 5th thoracic vertebra), Geshu (BL 17).

Method

Direct moxibutstion is given to each point with soy bean—sized moxa cone until three cones are burnt out, causing plister and purulence left in several days.

二十三、神经衰弱

神经衰弱归属于中医学"心悸"、"虚损"、"郁证"等范畴。临床常见头晕、头胀、耳鸣、记忆力减退、失眠、情绪易于激动、白天精神萎靡、心悸、纳呆、腹胀等症。

技法运用

1. 毫针：取神门、内关、足三里、三阴交穴。

烦躁多怒加行间，太冲；心悸不宁，头晕目眩加通里，心俞，风池；喉中如梗加天突，膻中；脘腹胀满加中脘，公孙；遗精、阳萎、肢冷加肾俞、命门、关元、太溪、复溜等。用平补平泻法，留针10～15分钟，每日或隔日一次。

2. 耳针：取下屏尖、心、肾、神门、屏间、下脚端、枕、脾。

每次3～5穴，中等刺激，留针1～2小时，每日一次。亦可用王不留行籽贴敷，每日按压2～3次。有报道取双侧耳穴心，神门，将胶布剪成0.5×0.5厘米方形片，取王不留行籽一粒、粘于方形胶布片中央，备用。取火柴棒一根、将火柴头在上述穴位及其周围按压，测得敏感点（疼痛明显处）后，在原处轻轻加压，使该处留下压痕，然后将备用的胶布贴在穴位上（王不留行籽对准火柴头压痕）、医者以拇、食指分别置于耳廓前后，指腹相对，按压神门穴王不留行籽；再以食指或小指指端按压心穴王不留行籽，力度以患者有轻度刺痛为宜（不可过重、防止皮肤破损）。每穴按压1分钟，最后双手搓捻双耳，使之充血发热为度。患者如法每天自行按压耳穴3～5次，每次每穴1分钟，睡前必按压一次。胶布每天更换一次、7天为一疗程，需继续治疗者，休息一周再行第二疗程（王晓鸣.上海针灸杂志，1：31；1987）。

3. 皮肤针：背部督脉与膀胱经左右第一、二侧线，从大椎至腰骶、每线反复叩刺5～7回。至皮肤红润或稍见渗血为度。

头晕加叩百会、风池、头维；脘腹胀满加叩肝俞、胃俞、中脘、梁门；心悸失眠，健忘食减，便溏加叩内关、公孙、心俞、脾俞；面红耳鸣、头胀且痛，心悸失眠加叩肝俞、胆俞、太冲、三阴交；遗精阳萎加叩肾俞、命门。中度叩刺、每日一次。有报道用梅花针治疗神经衰弱，刺激部位除常规刺激部位外，重点刺激第8～12胸椎，腰椎及荐椎。另外，配合刺激两侧手掌的大、小鱼际、头部和颈部，用轻刺激手法（候沂，等.中华神经精神病杂志，2：91；1959）。

4. 灸疗：有报道每晚睡前用艾卷悬灸百会穴10～15分钟，一般患者在灸后5～15分钟即可入睡（焦国瑞.《针灸临床经验辑要》）。

23. NEURASTHENIA

Manifestations

Neurasthnia, belonging to disease or syndrome categories of Xin Ji (心悸, palpitation), Xu Sun (虚损, asthenic disease), and Yu Zhehg, (郁证 melancholia) in TCM, is manifested clinically by dizziness, distension in head, tinnitus, poor memory, insomnea, irritability, listlessness, palpitation, anorexia and abdominal distension.

Treatment by Appying Acubustion Techniques

(1) *Filiform Needling*

Selection of Points

Main points: Shenmen (HT 7), Neiguan (PC 6), Zusanli (ST 36), Sanyinjiao (SP 6).

Supplementary points accordingt to symptoms: Taichong (LR 3) for irritability; Tongli (HT 5), Xinshu (BL 15) and Fengchi (GB 20) for palpitation and dizziness; Tiantu (RN 22) and Danzhong (RN 17) for sensation of a plum pit stuck in the throat; Shenshu (BL 23), Mingmen (DU 4), Taixi (KI 3) and Fului (KI 7) for nocturnal emission, impotence and cold extremities; and Gongsun (SP 4), and Zhongwan (RN 12) for abdominal distension

Method

Three to five points are employed each treatment session, the uniform reinforcing — reducing manipulation is applied, and the needles are retained at each point for ten to fifteen minutes. The treatment is given once daily or every other day and for ten sessions as a course.

(2) *Otopuncture*

Selection of Otopoints

Adrenal Gland, Heart, Kidney, Shen-men, Endocrine, Sympathetic, Occiput, Spleen.

Method

Three to five points are punctured once daily, the medium strength stimulation is applied, and the needles are retained at each otopoint for one to two hours. Or the otopoints are stuck with vaccaria seeds and the seeds are pressed two or three times daily.

Introducing An Experiential Technique

Another otopuncture method is reported in Shanghai Journal of Acupuncture & Moxibustion. Left and right Ot. Heart and Shenmen are stuck with vaccaria seeds. To the operation, pieces of plaster 5×5 cm in size with vaccaria seeds on the centers are made for use, the otopoints and the area surrounding them are pressed with a match stick to find the sensitive spots and marks are made by pressure with the stick. Then, the sensitive spots are stuck with the plasters, the seed directing the mark. The seed on Ot. Shenmen is pressed with the thumb and the index finger placing on the two sides of the auricle and pressing towards each other for one minute, and the seed on Ot. Heart is pressed with the thumb and the index finger or the small finger placing on the two sides of the auricle and pressing towards each other for one minute, causing a tolerable stabbing pain to the patient. During pressure, heavy force is avoided so as not to break the skin. Finaly, the auricles are twisted to cause local congestion and fever. The patient is asked to press the otopoints by himself three to five times daily, especially before going to bed, each point for one minute. The plasters are replaced by new ones every day. A course needs seven days of treatment and next course begins after a week of interval.

(3) *Tapping*

Selection of Points

The Governor Vessel (the Du Meredian) and the branches of the Urinary Bladder Meridian on the back.

Method

Tap the channels from above downwards five to seven times to cause erythema and a little oozing of blood.

Supplementary points according to symptoms: Baihui (DU 20), Fengchi (GB 20) and Touwei (ST 8) for dizziness; Ganshu (BL 18), Weishu (BL 21), Zhongwan (RN 12) and Liangmen (ST 21) for abdominal distension and fullness; Neiguan (PC 6), Gongsun (SP 4), Xinshu (BL 15) and Pishu (BL 20) for palpitation, insomnea, poor memory, anorexia and diarrhea; Ganshu (BL 18), Danshu (BL 19), Taichong (LR 3) and Sanyinjiao (SP 6) for flushed face, tinnitus, distending headache, palpitation and insomnea; and Shenshu (BL 23) and Mingmen (DU 4) for nocturnal emission or impotence. The supplementary points needed are tapped once daily and with a medium strength force.

Introducing An Experiential Technique

The following tapping method for treatment of neurasthenia is reported. The regular areas and the areas of the spinal column region below the 7th thoracic vertebra as well as left and right large and small thenars, head and neck are selected. These areas are tapped alternately with the plum—blossom needle, causing mild stimulation to the points.

（4）*Moxibustion*

The following moxibustion method is recorded in Collection of Outstandings of Experiences of Acupuncture & Moxibustion. The moxibustion with moxa stick is given to Baihui (DU 20) for ten to fifteen minutes before the patient's going to bed. It is said the patients fall asleep five to fifteen minutes after the moxibustion.

二十四、癔 病

癔病归属于中医学"脏躁"、"郁证"、"厥证"、"百合病"等范畴。临床症状复杂，主要为精神、运动及感觉障碍，植物神经，内脏功能紊乱，如自觉喉中有物梗阻、吞之不下，吐之不出，哭笑无常或似痴呆，或失语，失明，失听，肢体僵硬，瘫痪或抽搐。

技法运用

1. 毫针：取人中、内关、神门、后溪穴。

失明加刺睛明，肝俞；失语加刺通里、廉泉；失听加刺翳风、听宫；咽喉梗塞加天突、膻中、足三里；上肢瘫痪或抽搐、震颤加肩髃、曲池、外关；下肢瘫痪或抽搐、震颤加环跳、阳陵泉、悬钟、昆仑；神志障碍加大陵、少冲等。发作时用捻转提插泻法，未发作时用平补平泻法，留针20分钟。每隔5分钟捻转一次，每日针一次。

有人在做好心理治疗的基础上，采用针刺疗法，上肢瘫痪取寸平穴（相当于内关穴），下肢瘫痪取泉中穴（相当于涌泉穴下1寸）。用22～26号2寸长的针刺入穴位，采用提插与捻转手法，不断加强刺激，刺入后一旦出现针感，可让其活动患肢，或针刺无恢复或不能自主运动时，可加用电针（赵吉明，等. 中国康复杂志1：19；1987）。

2. 耳针：下脚端、脑、心、神门、肾、枕。

强刺激，每次针3～5穴，留针20～30分钟，每日1次；亦可配合耳穴埋针或贴敷王不留行籽。

3. 电针：内关、神门、通里、足三里、人中、太冲。适宜于运动，感觉障碍。上肢或下肢运动障碍可参照毫针治疗取穴。用疏密波、中度刺激，每次5～10分钟，每日1次。

24. HYSTERIA

Manifestations

Hysteria, belonging to the disease or syndrome categores of Zang Zao(脏臊), Yu Zheng(郁证 melancholia), Jue Zheng (厥证), and Bei He Bin(百合病)in TCM, is complicated in clinical manifestations, which usually include psychonosema, dyskinesia, sensory disturbance, vegetative nervous function disturbance and vesceral function disturbance, such as subjective sensation as if something is stuck in the the throat which is difficult to be spitted out or swallowed downwards, capricious cry or laugh, or like dementia, or aphonia, blindness, loss of hearing, stiff trunk and extremities, paralysis or convulsion.

Treatment by Applying Acubustion Techniques

(1) Filiform Needling

Selection of Points

Main points: Renzhong (DU 26), Neiguan (PC 6), Shenmen (HT 7), Houxi(SI 3).

Supplementary points: Jingming (BL 1) and Ganshu (BL 18) for blindness; Tongli(HT 5) and Lianquan(RN 23) for aphonia; Yifeng(SJ 17) and Tinggong(SI 19) for loss of hearing; Tiantu(RN 22), Dangzhong(RN 17) and Zusanli(ST 36) for feeling of material choking in the throat; Jianyu (LI 15), Quchi (LI 11), Waiguan (SJ 5) for paralysis, convulsion or trembling in the upper limbs; and Huantiao (GB 30), Yanglingquan (GB 34), Xuanzhong(GB 39) and Kunlun (BL 6) for paralysis, convulsion or trembling in the lower limbs.

Method

Reducing manipulations by twisting, lifting and thrusting the needle are applied during attack of hysteria, and three to five points are selected each treatment session. During the other periods, uniform reinforcing — reducing method is applied and the needles are retained at each point for twenty minutes and twisted once every five minutes during the retention. Three to five points are selected each session and the treatment is given once daily and for ten days as a course.

Introducing An Experiential Technique

Another method for treatment of hysteria is reported in Chinese Convalescent Medicine. Based on psychotherapy, puncture is given. Neiguan (PC 6) is selected for paralysis of upper extremities and Quanzhong(Extra point, 1 cun distal to Yongquan, KI 1)for paralysis of lower extremities. 2 cun long needles are inserted into the points, then, lifted, thrust and twisted, with a gradually increasing stimulation applied. When having the needling sensation, the patient is asked to move his diseased extremities. If recovery of autonomy movement of the diseased extremities is not achieved, electroacuputure is added.

(2) Otopuncture

Selection of Otopoints

Sympathetic, Brain, Heart, Shenmen, Kidney, Occiput.

Method

Three to five otopoints are selected. On puncturing at the points, the needles are retained at each point for twenty to thirty minutes, and strong stimulation is applied. The treatment is given once daily and for ten sessions as a course. Or, in combination, the small needles are inbedded into the points or the vaccaria seeds are stuck on the points.

(3) *Electroacupuncture*

Selection of Points

Neiguan (PC 6), Tongli (HT 5), Shenmen (HT 7), Zusanli (ST 36), Renzhong (DU 26), Taichong (LR 3).

Method

Electroacupuncture is suitable to motor or sensory disturbance. For motor disturbance of upper or lower extremities, eclectroacupuncture is given to the same points as in the filiform needling, with sparse—dense wave and medium strength stimulation applied at each point for five to ten minutes. The treatment is given once daily and for ten sessions as a course.

二十五、精神分裂症

属中医学"癫狂"范畴。狂症起病急,主要表现为两目怒视,狂躁不安,毁物伤人,舌红苔黄,脉弦滑而数;癫症起病缓,表现为表情淡漠,目光呆滞,哭笑无常,忧郁苦闷,幻听、幻视等。

技法运用

1.毫针:取内关、神门、百会、丰隆、三阴交穴。

幻听加听宫,翳风;幻视加攒竹,肝俞,丝竹空,晴明,用平补平泻法,不留针。狂躁不安加行间、劳宫、人中、涌泉,用捻转提插迎随呼吸泻法,不留针,每日1次。

2.耳针:取心、神门、肝、脑、屏间,枕、胃穴。

强刺激,每次针3～5穴,留针30分钟。

3.电针:①,定神(人中沟下1/3与2/3交界处),百会。②头颞(双)(太阳穴后上1寸与耳尖平行,咬牙时颞肌突出处。图5—16)。

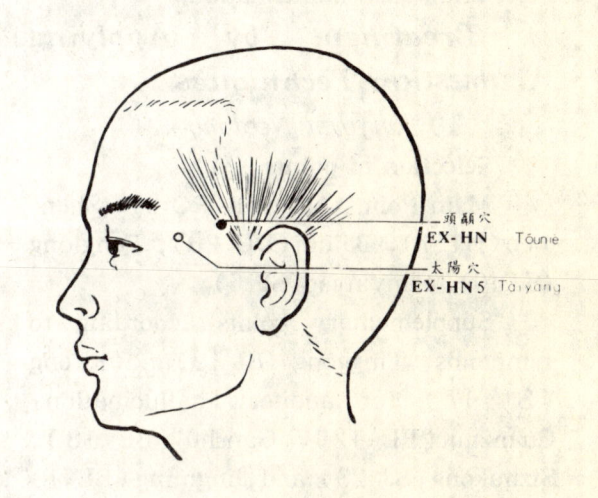

图 5—16 头颞穴
Fig. 5—16 Tounie (Extra point)

每日针2～4次,每次取一组穴针后加脉冲电,电压6伏,用较高频率间断通电,病人局部肌肉抽搐,麻胀感强,施术时严密观察病人情况,调节电流量及通电时间。本法适用于狂躁型精神分裂症。一般2～3天可控制症状,然后减少电针次数(上海中医学院.《针灸学》,1974)。

25. SCHIZOPHRENIA

Manifestations

Schizophrenia belongs to the disease or syndrome categories of Dian (癫), and Kuang (狂) in TCM. Kuang, referring to manic disorders, is manifested mainly by sudden onset, irritability, violent behaviour, red tongue with yellow coating, string—taut, rolling and rapid pulse. Dian, referring to depressive disorders, is manifested mainly by gradual onset, apathy, mental dullness, changing moods, emotional dejection, auditory hallucination, and visual hallucination.

Treatment by Applying Acubustion Techniques

(1) *Filiform Needling*

Selection of points

Main Points: Neiguan(PC 6), Shenmen(HT 7), Baihui(DU 20), Fenglong (ST40), Sanyinjiao(SP 6).

Supplementary points acoording to symptoms: Tinggong (SI 19) and Yifeng (SJ 17) for auditory hallucination; Cuanzhu (BL 12), Ganshu (BL 18), Sizhukong (SJ 23) and Jingming (BL 1) for visual hallucination; Xingjian (LR 2), Laogong (PC 8), Renzhong (DU 20) and Yongquan (KI 1) for excessive motor activity.

Method

Two to four points are employed each treatment session. For auditory and visual hallucination, uniform reinforcing — reducing needling is applied and the needles are not retained. For excessive motor activity, reducing manner by twisting, lifting and thrusting the needle and by manipulatig the needle in cooperation with the patient's respiration is applied, and the neeldes are not retained. The treatment is given once daily and for ten sessions as a course.

(2) *Otopuncture*

Selection of Points

Heart, Shenmen, Liver, Brain, Endocrine, Occiput, Stomach.

Method

Three to five points are selected each treatment session, strong stimulation is chosen, and the needles are retained at each point for thirty minutes. The treatment is given once daily and for ten days as a course.

(3) *Electroacupuncture*

Selection of Points

The following two groups of points are selected. The first group includes Dingshen (extra point, at philtrum, on the junction of lower 1/3 and upper 2/3 of philtrum) and Baihui (DU 20). The second includes bilateral Tounie (extra point, 1 cun superior to Taiyang, EX—HN5), parallel to the apex of the auricle, at the prominence of the temporal muscle when the teeth are clenched. (See Fig. 5—16).

Mehtod

One group of points is employed each treatment session and two groups selected alternately. Following needling, the electric stimulation by intermittent electric pulse at a comparatively high frequency and at a voltage of 6 is applied to the needles inserted in the points, causing local muscular spasm and inducing numbness and distension to the patient. During the electroacupuncture, the patient's response should be observed closely and the intensity of the stimulation adjusted according to the patient's needling sensation and tolerance. The puncture is given two to four times daily. This treatment is suitable to manic type of schizophrenia. Generally speaking, after accepting the electroacupuncture for two or three days, the patient's symptoms and signs will be relieved obviously, and the frequency of giving the electroeacupuncture can be decreased.

二十六、三叉神经痛

三叉神经痛,临床症状为面部突然疼痛发作,阵发性,短暂性烧灼样或刀割样,针刺样疼痛,仅数秒钟至数分钟,间歇有时,一天可发生数次至数十次。一般根据三叉神经的分布部位,区分为眼支(第一支),上颌支(第二支),下颌支(第三支)。常以上、下颌支多见,伴局部抽搐、皮肤潮红、流涎、流泪等。

技法运用

1.毫针:取下关、颊车、地仓、夹承浆(地仓穴直下,承浆旁开1寸),太阳,阳白,四白,攒竹,合谷,中渚,内庭,足临泣,太冲等穴。

针四白时,针尖向外上方刺入(图5—17),使感应传至上唇;针夹承浆时,针尖宜向内下方刺入(图5—17)。使感应传至下唇;针攒竹时,针尖向外下方(图5—17)使感应传至额。用平补平泻法或捻转提插泻法,留针30分钟,每日1~2次,每隔5~10分钟捻转行针1次。血管性头痛亦可取上穴治疗,尤以中渚、足临泣循经取穴为佳。

有人取攒竹穴,用1寸针,呈15°度角,从眉头向眉中缘下方刺眶上裂三叉神经的眼神经支,约0.5~0.8寸,得气后有触电样感传放射到额上,留针1小时。四白穴用1寸针,呈45°角,从鼻翼外侧下方对瞳孔方向刺眶下神经的上颌神经分支,约0.5~0.8寸,得气后有触电样感传放射到鼻及上唇,留针1小时。下关穴用2寸针、呈90°角,从颧弓与下颌切迹形成的凹陷处,直刺三叉神经的下颌神经分支,约1.5~1.8寸。大迎穴用1.5寸针,取15°角,从口角下方下颌骨边缘向外侧横刺颏孔三叉神经的颏神经约0.5~0.8寸,得气后有触电样感传放射到下唇,留针1小时,每日1次(朱天洪,等.中西医结合杂志,6:370;1985)。

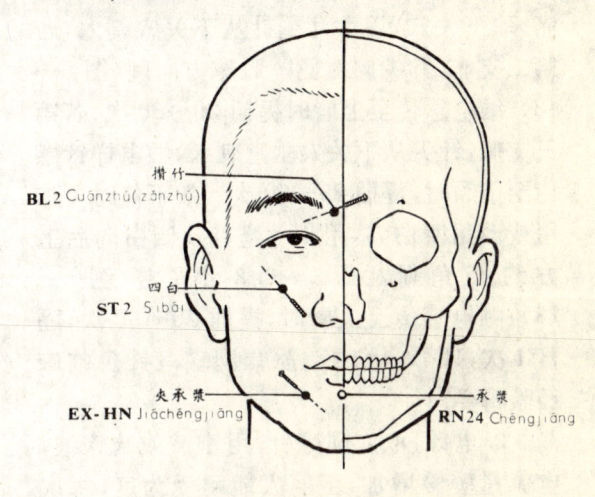

图 5—17 三叉神经痛刺法
Fig. 5—17 The Needling Applied for Trigeminal Neuralgia

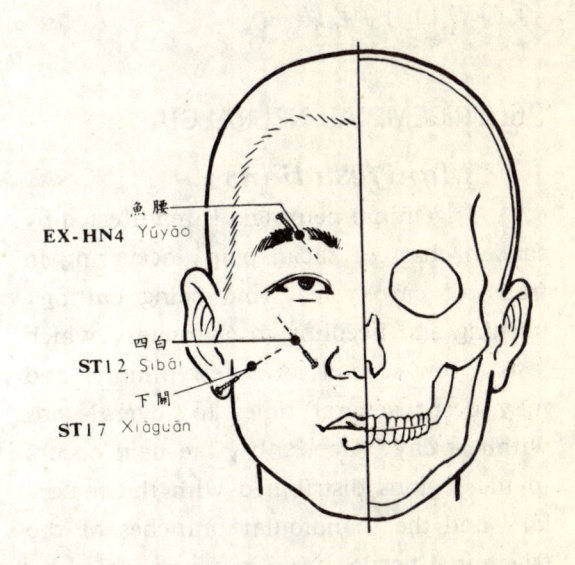

图 5—18 三叉神经痛刺法
Fig. 5—18 The Needling Applied for Trigeminal Neuralgia

还有报道,针治 225 例原发性三叉神经痛,有效率达 98.5%。第一支痛,取眶上孔(相当鱼腰穴),用 1 寸毫针斜向内下方刺入 0.3~0.5 寸(图 5—18),有触电样感传至眼及前额时,提插 20~50 次;第二或第二、三支痛,取下关穴,用 2 寸毫针从下关穴刺入,若第二支痛,针尖向对侧的眼球方向刺(图 5—18),触电感传至上唇时提插 20~50 次;若第三支痛,针尖从下关穴垂直刺入,触电样针感传至下颌时,提插 20~50 次。效不佳时可加用或改用四白穴,用 1 寸毫针从四白向后上方约 45°角刺入 0.7~0.8 寸左右(图 5—18),触电感传至上唇时,提插 20~50 次,隔日 1 次,10 次为 1 疗程(焦国瑞.《针灸临床经验辑要》)。

2. 电针:取穴同毫针,用密波或疏密波,电流量缓慢增加,至病人能耐受为度,每次 20~30 分钟,每日 1 次。

3. 耳针:面颊、上颌、下颌、下脚端、神门、脑。每次取 2~4 穴,强刺激,留针 30~60 分钟,每隔 10 分钟捻转一次。

26. TRIGEMINAL NEURALGIA

Manifestations

Trigeminal neuralgia is manifested by sudden onset of facial pain, occurring in transient paroxysms, and being cutting, burning and needling in character, which lasts a few seconds or a few minutes and may occur several times to several tens within a day. Generally, the pain occurs in the regions distributed with the maxillary and the mandibular branches of the trigeminal nerve, usually accompanied by local spasm and erubescent skin, lacrimation and salivation.

Treatment by Applying Acubustion Techniques

(1) *Filiform Neeling*

Selection of Points

Xiaguan(ST 7), Jiache(ST 6), Dican(ST 4), Jianchengjian(EX., below Dicang, ST4, 1 cun lateral to Chengjian RN 24), Taiyang(EX—HN5), Yangbai(GB 14), Sibai(ST 2), Cuanzhu(BL 2), Hegu(LI 4), Zhongzhu(SJ 3), Neiting(ST 44), Zulinqi(GB 41), Taichong(LR 3).

Method

Three to five points are employed each treatment session. On puncturing at Sibai (ST 2), the needle is inserted upwards and anteriorly (See Fig. 5—17), inducing the needling sensation radiating to the upper lip; on puncturing at Chengjiang(RN 24), the needle is inserted interiorly and downwards (See Fig. 5—17), inducing the needling sensation propagating to the lower lip; and on punctuing at Cuanzhu(BL2), the needle is inserted anteriorly and downwards (See Fig. 5—17), inducing the needling sensation transmiting to the forehead. On puncturing, the uniform reinforcing—reducing manner or reducing manipulations by lifting, thrusting and twisting the needle are chosen, adn the needles are retained in each point for thirty minutes. The puncture treatment is given once daily or twice daily, and for seven sessions as a course.

Besides, the above acupoints can be employed for treatment of vascular headache. Among them, Zhongzhu(SJ 3) and Zulinqi(GB 41) are more effective than the others.

Introducing Some Experiential Tech-

niques

The following technique for treatment of trigeminal neuralgia is reported in Chinese Journal of Integrated Traditional and Western Medicines. A 1 cun long needle is inserted into Cuanzhu (BL 2) at an angle of 15° to the skin and pushed interiorly and downwards to the ophthalmic nerve, a branch of trigeminal nerve, to a depth of 0.5—0.8 cun, inducing electrifying sensation radiating to the forehead. Then, the needle is retained in the point for one hour. Another 1 cun long needle is inserted into Sibai (ST 2) at an angle of 45° to the skin and pushed upwards to the maxillary nerve, a branch of the infraorbital nerve, to a depth of 0.5—0.8 cun, inducing electrifying sensation radiating to the nose and the upper lip. Then, the needle is retained in the point for one hour. A 2 cun long needle is inserted into Xiaguan (ST 7) at an antgle of 90° to the skin and pushed towards the mandibular branch of the trigeminal nerve to a depth of 1.5—1.8 cun. Finally, a 1.5 cun long needle is inserted into Dayin (ST 5) at an angle of 15° to the skin and pushed along the border of the mandible and horizontally towards the mental foramen to the genial branch to a depth of 0.5—0.8 cun, inducing electrifying sensation radiating to the lower lip. Then, the needle is retained in the point for one hour.

In Collection of Outstandings of Clinical Experiences of Acupuncute & Moxibustion another method is recorded, by which a high effective rate of 98.5% in treatment of 225 cases with trigeminal neuralgia was achieved. For neuralgia of the first branch of the trigeminal nerve, Yuyao (EX—HN 4, at the supraorbital foramen) is punctured with a 1 cun long needle inserted obliquely and downwards to a depth of 0.3—0.5 cun (See Fig. 5—18), inducing electrifying sensation radiating to the forehead. Then, the needle is lifted and thrust twenty to fifty times in the point. In treatment of neuralgia of the second branch or the third branch, a 2 cun long needle is inserted into Xiaguan (ST 7). For neuralgia at the second branch, the needle is pushed towards the opposite eyeball (See Fig. 5—18), inducing electrifying sensation radiating to the upper lip, and then, lifted and thrust twenty to fifty times. For neuralgia at the third branch, the needle is pushed perpendicularly, and after the electrifying sensation is induced to the patient and propagated to the mandible, the needle is lifted and thrust twenty to fifty times. If the patient has weak needling sensation, a 1 cun long needle is inserted into Sibai (ST 2) at an angle of 45° to the skin and pushed posteriorly and upwards to a depth of 0.7—0.8 cun (See Fig. 5—18), then, it is lifted and thrust twenty to fifty times after the electrifying sensation is induced to the patient and propagated to the upper lip. The treatment is given once every other day and for ten times as a course.

(2) *Electroacupuncture*

Selection of Points

The same as in the filifrom needling.

Method

Two to four acupoints are employed each treatment session. The intensity of electric stimulation with dense wave or dense-sparse wave is adjusted from weak gradually to maximum that the patient can tolerate without pain. The electric stimulation lasts for twenty to thirty minutes per session and the treatment is given once daily.

（3）*Otopuncture*

Selection of Otopoints

Cheek, Maxilla, Mandible, Sympathetic, Shenmen, Brain.

Method

Two to four otopoints are employed each treatment session, and strong stimulation is applied. The needles are retained in each point for sixty minutes and twisted per ten minutes during the retention. The treatment is given once daily and for ten sessions as a course.

二十七、周围性面神经麻痹

周围性面神经麻痹，属中医学"口眼歪斜"范畴。临床表现为突然口眼歪斜，一侧眼睑不能闭合，不能皱眉、流泪、流涎，不能鼓腮吹气，面肌有麻木感，耳下或乳突常有疼痛，有的病例尚伴患侧舌苔2/3味觉障碍，无肢体瘫痪等。

技法运用

1. 毫针：局部与循经取穴相配合，主要穴位有地仓、颊车、下关、四白、颧髎、迎香、承浆、阳白、翳风、牵正（耳垂前0.5～1寸处），合谷、上巨墟。

每次取4～6穴，用平补平泻法，留针15分钟，每日1次。多数以针刺患侧为主，也有取双侧或单取健侧者。一般主张浅刺轻刺，也有用透刺法者。

有报道治疗周围性面瘫1008例。主要针对病情辨证治疗，早期（一周内）局部有炎症可局部温灸，隔日在口腔患侧颊部锋针泻血，再配合谷、足三里。当炎症缓解后再以面部经穴为主，其中局部经穴多采用两穴对刺，合谷取受病对侧，局部弱刺，远隔部采用强刺，一般留针10～30分钟，并在局部针上通以感应电流。对病程长，局部肌肉萎缩，张力极差者加拔罐。一般1日1次或隔日1次，12次为一疗程（长春中医学院针灸科．《全国针灸针麻学术讨论会论文摘要》．1979年）。

有人取水沟，地仓，瞳子髎，合谷为主穴，配颊车、迎香、承浆、下关、攒竹、四白、风池等。手法：主穴水沟、地仓、瞳子髎三穴用"推位法"，即治疗时先用押手将水沟和患侧的地仓、瞳子髎三穴自歪斜之处推至正常位置，按住后进针。水沟用揣刺法，地仓、瞳子髎用捻转泻法或平补平泻法，合谷穴取健侧或两侧，用捻转补法。对面形恢复正常，但尚感觉面部发麻或板著不舒感的后遗症患者，可用七星针先叩刺患侧面部，使其充血后再针刺（金新海，等．新医药学杂志，5：42；1973）。

2. 拔罐：下关、牵正、太阳、阳白、承浆、颊车，均为患侧。

每次取2～3穴，用小号火罐以闪火法拔罐10分钟，隔日1次。

3. 灸疗：穴位同毫针，适宜于虚寒证或毫针效果不显著者。

用艾卷温和灸，或针上加灸，或隔姜灸。每日1～2次，每次3～5穴，艾炷5～7壮，每穴灸15分钟。

4. 挑治：取患侧腮内膜咬合线，令患者先用盐水漱口，以清洁口腔，并尽量将口张大。医者左手拇、食指用纱布拿住患侧口角，该手余指按压腮部，使其内侧面向口方向翻转，右手持消毒三棱针由内向外点刺咬合线，使其微出血（图5—19）。间隔0.5寸左右挑1针，挑至口角内侧即完毕。挑治后避受风寒，可热敷患部，5～7天挑一次。（孙学全．《针灸临证集验》)。

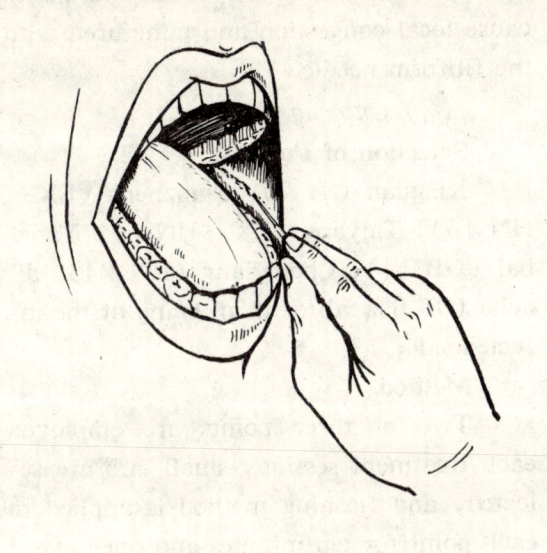

Fig. 5—19 Puncturing at the Line of Occlusion at the Buccal Mucosa

27. PERIPHERAL FACIAL PARALYSIS

Manifestations

Peripheral facial paralysis, belonging to the disease or syndrome category of Kou Yan Wai Xie (口眼歪斜, deviation of eye and mouth) in TCM, is manifested clinically by sudden onset of deviation of eye and mouth, incomplete closure of eye in the affected side, inability to frown, salivation, inability to blow out the cheek, facial numbness, and pain in the mastoid region. In some cases, dysgeusia in the tongue in the affected side may be seen. But no paralysis of extremities is found.

Treatment by Applying Acubustion Techniques

(1) *Filiform Needling*

Selection of Points

Dicang (ST 4), Jiache (ST 6), Xiaguan (ST 7), Sibai (ST 2), Quanliao (SI 18), Yingxiang (LI 20), Ghengjiang (RN 24), Yangbai (GB 14), Yifeng (SJ 17), Qianzheng (EX—HN 16, 0.5—1 cun anterior to ear lobe), Hegu (LI 4), Shangjuxu (ST 37).

Method

Four to six points are employed each treatment session. The points at the affected side are usually taken as the main points. But the points at both sides can be employed, or even the points at the healthy side can be punctured only. Uniform reinforcing—reducing manipulation is applied and the needles are retained at each point for fifteen minutes. Shallow and gentle puncture is more frequently selected and, sometimes, the penetration needling is applied. The treatment is given once daily and for ten sessions as a course.

Introducing Some Experiential Techniques

Another method is reported by acupuncturists in Changchun College of TCM, by which 1008 cases with peripheral facial paralysis were treated. To the operation, at the early stage (i.e., within the first week in disease course) with local inflammation, mild—warming moxibustion is given to the local area. Then, the cheek of the affected side is pricked with a sharp needle to cause bleeding, and Hegu (LI 4) and Zusanli (ST 36) are punctured in coordination. The treatmet is given once daily but except puncture at the affected cheek, which is given once every

• 375 •

other day. To the cases at the stage after relief of the local imflammation, the local points are taken as the main points, and they are punctured in the way that every two points are punctured with the needles inserted towards each other, and with a gentle stimulation administered. Additionally, Hegu (LI 4) at the healthy side is punctured with strong stimulation administered. The needles are retained at each point for ten to thirty minutes. The treatment is given once daily and for ten sessions as a course. To the cases with a prolonged course and local muscular atrophy, cupping may be applied additionally. The treatment is given once daily or once every other day and for twelve times as a course.

In New Medicine the following method is reported. Renzhong (DU 26), Dicang (ST 4), Tongziliao (GB 1) and Hegu (SI 4) are taken as the main points, and Jiache (ST 6), Yingxiang (LI 20), Chengjiang (RN 24), Xiaguan (ST 7), Cuanzhu (BL 2), Sibai (ST 2) and Fengchi (GB 20) taken as the adjuvant. After being pushed to and fixed on the normal position with the pressing hand, Shuigou (DU 26) is punctured with the fathoming manipulation, Dicang (ST 4) and Tongziliao (GB 1) at the affected side punctured with reducing manipulation by twisting the needle or with uniform reinforcing — reducing needling. Then, Hegu (LI 4) at the heathy side or both sides are punctured with reinforcing manner by twirling the needle. To the case who has sequela such as facial numbness and discomfort but whose facial appearance becomes normal, the face at the affected side is tapped with a seven — star needle to cause local congestion and punctured with the filiform needle.

(2) Cupping
Selection of Points

Xiaguan (ST 7), Qianzheng (EX—HN 16), Taiyang (EX—HN 5), Yangbai (GB 14), Chengjiang (RN 24), Jiache (ST 6), all of them being at the affected side.

Method

Two or three points are employed each treatment session, small jars are selected, and flashing method is applied to each point for ten minutes and once every other day.

(3) Moxibustion
Selection of Points

The same as in the filiform needling.

Method

Moxibustion is applicable only to the cold—deficiency type, which is manifested by, besides facial paralysis, cold body and limbs, poor appetite with no thirst, pale complexion, abundant pale urine, pale tongue with whitish coating, deep and small or slow and forceless pulse, and to those acupuncture is not effective. Three to five points are employed each treatment session, mild—warming moxibustion with moxa stick, moxibustion with warming needle, or ginger moxibustion is applied to each point for fifteen minutes or for five to seven cones. The treatment is given once or twice daily.

(4) Pricking Therapy
Selection of Points

The line of occlusion at the buccal

mucosa at the affected side.

Method

Ask the patient to clean his mouth with water and to open it as largely as possible. Take some cloth to hold the angle of mouth at the affected side with the thumb and the index finger of the left hand, press the cheek of the affected side with the other fingers of the hand, and prick the line with a three—edged needle held by another hand from posterior outwards to cause slight bleeding (See Fig. 5—19). Every 0.5 cun portion of the line is pricked from the inside towards the outside until the internal side of the angle of the mouth is reached. The patient is advised to apply hot compress to the affected area and to avoid being attacked by wind—cold evils. The treatment is given once every five to seven days and for three sessions as a course.

二十八、坐骨神经痛

坐骨神经痛,归属于中医学"痹证"范畴。临床常以单侧多见,即沿坐骨神经分布处的腰、臀、大腿后侧,小腿外侧,足背等放散性,烧灼样或刀割样疼痛为主,常因咳嗽、弯腰用力而加重,四、五腰椎旁、臀中点、腘窝中央、外踝后、腓肠肌处有压痛。

针灸对原发性坐骨神经痛效果明显。

技法运用

1.毫针:环跳、阳陵泉、悬钟、委中、秩边、肾俞、殷门、足三里、承山、阿是穴。

腰部压痛明显者加腰阳关,痛久不愈加人中。用捻转提插泻法。针环跳,秩边,殷门等穴,要求针感放射到足;人中施雀啄手法,以眼球充满泪水为度。留针30分钟,每隔10分钟捻转一次,每日1次。亦可配合灸法与拔罐。

有报道,患者取俯卧位,沿髂嵴上缘,在腰三角内下角(背阔肌与髂嵴交点)定上点、髂后上棘内上缘定下点,上点与下点间三等分,上1/3点定中点,共三穴(图5—20)。

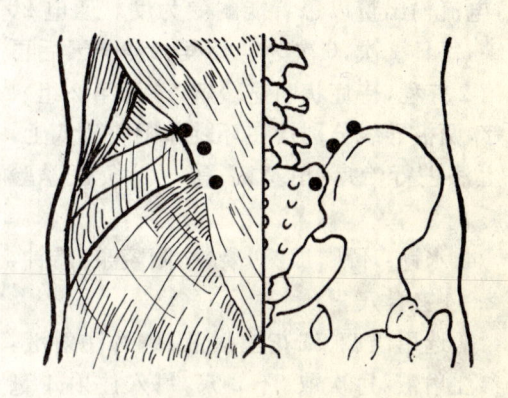

图5—20 坐骨神经痛针刺点
Fig. 5—20 The Needling Points for Sciatica

用28号或30号三寸不锈钢毫针,双手夹持法进针,进针方向与穴位表面垂直,一般采用提插法探索,针深达2.5寸左右,留针20分钟。上点感应至大腿内侧或沿足少阳胆经放射;中点感应沿足阳明胃经与足少阳胆经之间放射;下点感应沿足太阳膀胱经放射至足跟或足底(华延龄,等.上海针灸杂志,2:17;1987)。

2.耳针:坐骨、臀、膝、踝、神门。

腰椎或腰骶椎压痛明显者加腰骶椎,强刺激,留针30分钟,每日一次,行针时活动患肢。

3.电针:取穴同毫针。

每次2～4穴,用疏密波或密波。电流量由中等度到较强度,每次10～20分钟,每日1次。腰部压痛明显者可加刺腰部夹脊穴通电。

有报道,取穴分两组,第一组取四腰穴

（第四腰椎棘突水平旁开2寸处），五腰穴（第五腰椎棘突水平旁开2寸处），次髎，秩边，承扶，条口透承山。电针治疗首先用第一组穴，针刺有针感后，将电针机的两极，一个极接在秩边穴上，另一个极接在条山穴（即条口透承山）。采用快频率（400次以上/分），脉冲间断波，电流输出量以患者能耐受为度。通电20分钟，每日一次，6次为一疗程。停一天后再治第2疗程，待症状明显缓解，改为第2组穴治疗，两极导线分别接在环跳和阳陵泉穴上，按上法进行治疗（田丛豁，等.《针灸医学验集》）。

4. 水针：环跳，殷门，委中，阳陵泉，悬钟，腰2～4夹脊穴。

常选用当归、红花注射液，麝香注射液，丹参注射液，每次取2～3穴，每穴注射1毫升；或用10%葡萄糖注射液10～20毫升，加维生素$B_1$100毫克，或维生素B_{12}100微克混合液注射腰2～4夹脊穴及秩边或环跳穴，每穴5～10毫升。当针刺入一定深度，出现强烈感向下肢放散时，即将针适当上提，再快速推注药液。每天或隔日1次。

5. 皮肤针：取腰骶两侧，臀，下肢足太阳及足少阳循行线。痛点及麻木处重叩，加拔火罐。

28. SCIATICA

Manifestations

Sciatica, belonging to syndrome category of Bi Zheng（痹证, blockage syndrome）in TCM, is manifested clinically by pain distributed through the territory along the course or corresponding to the distribution of the sciatic nerve, characteristically located at the lower back, back of thigh, lateral aspect of calf and dorsum of foot, which is extending, burning or tingling in character, and aggravated by cough or movement. Tender spots may be found at the area lateral to the fourth and fifth lumbar vertebrae, centers of buttock and popliteal fossa, the area posterior to external malleolus, and calf.

Treatment by Applying Acubustion Techniques

(1) *Filiform Needling*

Seletion of Points

Main points: Huantiao (GB 30), Ynaglingquan (GB 34), Xuanzhong (GB 39), Weizhong (BL 40), Zhibian (BL 54), Shenshu (BL 23), Yinmen (BL 37), Zusanli (ST 36), Chengshan (BL 57), Ashi point.

Supplementory points according to symptoms: Yaoyangguan (DU 3) for obviously tender manifestation at lower part of the back, Renzhong (DU 26) for prolonged pain.

Method

Three to five points are employed each treatment session, reducing manipulations by twisting, lifting and thrusting the needle are applied. On puncturing at Huantiao (GB 30), Chibian (BL 54) and Yinmen (BL 37), the needling sensation induced is required to radiate to the foot. On puncturing at Renzhong (DU 26), bird—peck needling is applied until the patient's eyes are filled with tears. The needles are retained at each point for thirty minutes and twisted once every ten minutes during the retention. The puncture treatment is given once daily, or followed by moxibustion or cupping.

Introducing An experiential Technique

In Shanghai Journal of Acupuncture & Moxibustion another method for treating sciatica by puncture is reported. The patient is asked to lie on the abdomen, the crossing point of the platysma of back and the iliac crest at the upper border of the iliac crest is taken as the upper point to be punctured, the internal superior border of the posterior superior iliac spine as the lower point, and the junction of upper 1/3 and lower 2/3 of the line connecting the upper and lower points as the middle point (See Fig. 5—20). No. 28 or No. 30 needles 3 cun long are inserted into the points perpendiculrly to a depth of about 2.5 cun and retained for twenty minutes. The needling sensation caused by puncturing at the upper point radiates to the internal aspect of the thigh or along the course of the Gallbladder Meridian of Foot—Shaoyang; that caused by puncturing at the middle point radiates along the course between the Stomach Meridian of Foot—Yangming and the Gallbladder Meridian of Foor—Shaoyang; and that caused by puncturing at the lower point radiates along the Urinary Bladder Meridian of Foot—Taiyang to the heel or the inferior aspect of foot.

(2) *Otopuncture*

Selection of Otopoints

Ischium, Buttock, Knee, Ankle, Shenmen. Lumbosacral Vertebra is added for severe pain induced by pressure on the lumbar vertebrae or at lumbosacral vertebrae.

Method

two to four points are employed each treatment session, strong stimulation is applied, and the needles are retained in each point for thirty minutes. On manipulating the needles, the patient is asked to move the affected limb in cooperation. The treatment is given once daily and for ten sessions as a course. Next course begins after a week of interval.

(3) *Electroacupuncture*

Selection of Points

The same as in the filiform needling.

Method

Two to four acupoints are employed each treatment session, and the electric stimulation at dense — sparse wave or dense wave is applied to each point for ten to twenty minutes, with medium strength stimulation administered at beginning and comparatively strong stimulation followed. If the lower back is obviously tender, Jiaji (EX—B 2) at the lower back is punctured additionally. The treatment is given once daily and for ten sessions as a course.

Introducing an Experiential Technique

In Collection of Experiences of Acupuncture & Moxcibustion the following method is recorded. Two groups of acupoints are selected, the first group including Siyaoxue (extra point, 2 cun lateral to the spinal process of the fourth lumbar vertebra), Ciliao (BL 32), Zhibian (BL 54), Chengfu (BL 36) and Tiaokou (ST 38), and the second including Huantiao (GB 30) and Yanglingquan (GB 34). At frist, electroacupuncture is given to the first group. After the needling seasation is induced to the patient by puncturing with the filiform needle, one electrode of a pair of the current leads is connected to the needle inserted into Zhibian (BL 54) and the other connected to the needle inserted into Tiaokou (ST 38) which is pushed towards Chengshan (BL 57) with penetration needling, and a high frequency (more than 400 turns/min.) and an electric output tolerable to the patient are administered for twenty minutes. The electroacpuncture is given once daily and for six times as a course. The next course begins after an interval of one day. When a great improvement of the patient's symptoms is achieved, the second group of points is selected in replace of the first one, a pair of leads are connected respectively to the needles inserted into Huantiao (Gb 30) and Ynaglingquan (GB 34), with the same method mentioned above.

(4) *Point Injection*

Selection of Points

Huantiao (GB 30), Yinmen (BL 37), Weizhong (BL 40), Yanglingquan (GB 34), Xuanzhong (GB 39), Jiaji (EX—B 2, L 2—4).

Method

Two or three points are employed each session, and Radix Angelicae Sinesis injection, Safflower injection, musk injection, or Radix Salviae Miltiorrhizae injection is selected. 1 ml of the drug fluid is injected into each point. Or 5—10 ml of mixed solution made of 10—20 ml of 10% glucose solution and vitamin B_1 100 micrograms or vitamin B_{12} 100 micrograms into each point of Jiaji L 2—4 (EX—B 2) and Zhibian (BL 54) or Huantiao (GB 30). Or, 5—10 ml of 1% procaine are injected into the tender spot or Huantiao (GB 30). To the opeartion, a needle is inserted into the point to a certain depth, a strong needling sensation is induced to the patient and propagated downward, the needle is lifted a little, If no blood is found by withdrwaing the piston, then, the drug is injected quickly. The treatment is given once daily or once every other day, and for seven days as a course.

(5) *Tapping*

Selection of Points

Bilateral sides of Lumbosacral spine, Buttock, courses of the Foot — Taiyang Meridian and Foot—Shaoyang Meridian.

Method

Tap at the site with stress on the painful spots and numbness area, followed by cupping.

二十九、肋间神经痛

肋间神经痛属于中医学"胁痛"范畴。临床表现为肋间神经分布区呈阵发性或持续性针刺样,电灼样疼痛,可向同侧肩部,胸背部放散,常因咳嗽,喷嚏或深呼吸时被激发,兼胸脘胀满,嗳气,多随情志变化减轻或加重。

技法运用

1. 毫针:丘墟透照海,支沟,阳陵泉,行间,内关,胸5～10夹脊穴。

用捻转提插泻法。操作丘墟透照海时,可将足背自然蹠屈伸直,右手持2～3寸长28号毫针从丘墟进针,轻捻转用力推进,若碰到阻力则为刺中骨头,即将针后退至皮下再换方向刺入,至无阻力时即为刺中骨缝,可在对侧照海处触到针尖,切忌刺穿对侧皮肤。胸5～10夹脊穴,则斜刺0.5～1寸。一般留针15～20分钟,每5分钟捻转行针一次,每日1次。

2. 耳针：胸、神门、下脚端、脑、肝、相应痛点。每次取3～4穴，强刺激，留针30～60分钟，每日1次。

3. 皮肤针：沿患处肋缘间隙，脊柱两侧、锁骨上窝，叩刺，用中度或重度刺激。

29. INTERCOSTAL NEURALGIA

Manifestations

Intercostal neuralgia, belonging to the disease or syndrome category of Xie Tong（胁痛，hypochondriac pain）in TCM, is manifested clinically by paroxysmal or continuous pain at the area distributed by intercostal nerve, which is stabbing and burning in character and may spread to the shoulder region, chest and back at the affected side, usually induced by cough, sneezing, or deep respiration and aggravated or relieved by emotional change. Distension and fullness in chest and abdomen, and belching are accompanied.

Treatment by Applying Acubustion Techniques

(1) Filiform Needling

Selection of Points

Qiuxu (GB 40), Zhigou (SJ 6), Yanglingquan (GB 34), Xingjian (LR 2), Neiquan (PC 6), Jiaji (EX—B 2, T 5—10).

Method

Select three to five points each treatment session and apply reducing methods by twisting, lifting and thrusting the needle. On puncturing at Qiuxu (GB 40), penetration needling towards Zhaohai (KI 6) is applied. The dorsum of the patient's foot is put at a natural plantar flexion, a 2—3 cun long needle held by the right hand is inserted into Qiuxu (GB 40), and twisted gently and pushed forefully deeper towards Zhaohai (KI 6). If a comparatively strong resistance is felt, indicating the needle is inserted to the bone, the needle should be withrawn to the area beneath the skin and inserted again with the direction somewhat changed and pushed deeper through the interspace of bones until the needle tip can be felt by pressing finger over the Zhaohai (KI 6). On puncturing at Jiaji (EX—B 2, T 5—10), the needles are inserted obliquely 0.5—1 cun deep. Generally, the puncture is given once daily with the needles retained at each point for fifteen to twenty minutes and twisted per five minutes during the retention.

(2) Otopuncture

Selection of Otopoints

Chest, Shenmen, Sympathetic, Brain, Liver, corresponding painful spots.

Method

Select three or four points each treatment session, apply strong stimulation, and retain the needles at each point for sixty minutes. The treatment is given once daily and for ten sessions as a course.

(3) Skin Needling

Tap on the skin over the intercostal space of the affected region, the skin lateral to the spine column of both sides, and the skin over the supraclavicular fossa, and administer medium strength or strong stimulation.

三十、前列腺炎

前列腺炎属中医学"热淋""白浊"、"膏淋"范畴。急性前列腺炎起病急,伴高热寒颤、腰骶部及会阴部胀痛或剧痛,尿频、尿急、尿白浊如泔浆;慢性前列腺炎表现为轻度的尿频、尿急、排尿灼热感,或排尿后有滴尿现象,常有白色分泌物滴出,腰骶部、会阴部及阴囊有坠胀感,常伴性欲减退和神经衰弱。

针灸主要对于慢性前列腺炎有一定疗效。

技法运用

1. 毫针:关元、中极、阴陵泉、膀胱俞、行间、太溪。

急性伴见血尿,加血海、三阴交,用捻转提插配合迎随呼吸泻法;慢性伴见白浊,加用气海俞、肾俞,用捻转提插配合呼吸迎随补法;发热加合谷,曲池,用捻转提泻手法。腹部穴位要求针感传至尿道,腰骶穴位要求针感向前阴传导。留针30分钟,急性每日1次,慢性隔日1次。

有报道以秩边透归来,气海,中极,关元为主,治疗前列腺炎。方法:取屈膝侧卧位,用芒针刺入5~6寸,经秩边透归来,有强烈麻串样感放射至尿道,用平补平泻法,不留针。气海、中极、关元直刺进针3~4寸,针感均达尿道。深刺下腹部穴位时当排空小便,不要大幅度提插捣动(天津中医学院第一附属医院针灸科.《第一届世界针灸学术大会针灸论文摘要选编》)。

2. 挑治:大肠俞,小肠俞,膀胱俞,八髎穴,或腰骶部突出于皮面大头针帽大小(直径1~2毫米)的红褐色反应点。挑治方法同痔疮挑治法,5~7天挑治1次。

3. 耳针:膀胱、肾、枕、下脚端、下屏尖、尿道、输尿管。

强刺激,每次取2~4穴,留针30分钟,每日1次。

4. 磁电疗法:选用表面磁场强度为800~1500高斯的稀土钴合金形磁片,直径为1厘米,厚0.5厘米,选取三阴交,归来,水道,阴陵泉,气海,关元等穴(腹部与下肢穴相配运用),每次2~3个穴位,将G—6805治疗仪导线压在磁片上,以S极接触皮肤,用胶布固定于所选穴位上,采用断续波和疏密波交替,通电量由小逐渐加大,以患者感觉有电流刺激,并向上下传导而无刺激疼痛为准。通电30分钟,每天1次,5次为一疗程(陆明珍.上海针灸杂志,4:43;1987)。

30. PROSTATITIS

Manifestations

Prostatitis, belonging to the disease or syndrome categories of Re Lin (热淋, stranguria due to heat evil), Bei Zhu (白浊, cloudy urine), and Gao Lin (膏淋, stranguria marked by chyluria) in TCM, is classified into the acute type and the chronic type. The acute prostatitis is manifested by acute onset, frequent and urgent urination, white cloudy rice — water — like urine, and distending pain or stabbing pain at lumbosacral region and perineum region, accompanied by high fiver, and chills; the chronic type manifested by mildly frequent and urgent urination, burning sensation in urination, or dropping urination, usually with white cloudy urine, dragging and distending sensation at the lumbosacral region, perineum and scrotum, usually accompanied by sexual hypoesthesia and neurasthenia.

Acupuncture and moxibustion are applicable mainly to chronic prostatitis.

Treatment by Applying Acubustion Techniques

(1) *Filiform Needling*

Selection of Point

Main points: Guanyuan (RN 4), Zhongji (RN 3), Yinlingquan (SP 9), Panggangshu (BL 28), Xingjian (LR 2), Taixi (KI 3).

Supplementary points according to symptoms: Xuehai (SP 10) and Sanyinjiao (SP 6) for cases at acute stage with hematuria; Qihai (RN 6) and Shenshu (BL 23) for chronic type; Hegu (LI 4) and Quchi (LI 11) for fever.

Method

Three to five points are employed each treatment session. For the cases at acute stage with hematuria, reducing manipulations by twisting, lifting and thrusting the needle, taken as the main manner, and reducing manipulation by manipulating the needle in cooperation with the patient's respiration and against the running course of the meridian, taken as the ajuvant, are applied. For chronic type with cloudy urine, reinforcing methods by twirling, lifting and thrusting the needle, which are taken as the main manner, and reinforcing methods by manipulating the needle in cooperation with the patiient's respiration and along the running course of the meridian, which are taken as the adjuvant manner, are applied. For the cases with fever, reducing method by twisting, lifting and thrustiing the needle is applied. On puncturing at the points located on the abdomen, the needling sensation is required to radiate to the urethra, and on puncturing at the points at the lumbosacral region, the needling sensation is required to radiate to the external genitalia. The needles are retained at each point for thirty minutes, and the treatment is given once daily for acute cases and once every other day for chronic cases.

Introducing An Experiential Technique

It is reported by acupuncturists in Tianjin College of TCM the following puncture method is effective in treatment of prostatitis. Zhibian (BL 49), Qihai (RN 6), Zhongji (RN 3) and Guanyuan (RN 4) are selected. On the operation, the patient is asked to lie on one side with the knee flexed. At Zhibian (BL 49) a 5—6 cun long needle is inserted towards Guilai (ST 29) with penetration needling, inducing strong numbness radiating to the urethra, and uniform reinforcing—reducing method is applied without retention of the needle. At Qihai (RN 6), Zhongji (RN 3) and Guanyuan (RN 4), the needles are inserted three or four cun deep, inducing the needling sensation speading to the urethra. On puncturing at the points located at the lower abdomen the patient is asked to evacuate urine and the needle is not lifted or thrust at a large extent.

(2) *Pricking*

Selection of Points

Dachangshu (B 25), Pangguangshu (BL 28), Baliao (a collective term for the eight—liao points, including Shangliao BL 31, Cilao BL 32, Zhongliao BL 33 and Xialiao BL 34). Or the red and brown spots which are above the skin surface at the lumbosacral region and 1—2 mm in diameter are taken as the points to be broken.

Method

The same as in pricking for hemorrhoids. The pricking treatment is given once every five to seven days.

(3) *Otopuncture*

Selection of Otopoints

Urinary Bladder, Kidney, Occiput, Sympathetic, Adrenal Gland, Urethra, Ureter.

Method

Two to four points are employed each treatment session, strong stimulation is applied, and the needles are retained at each point for thirty minutes. The treatment is given once daily and for ten days as a course.

(4) *Magnetoelectric Therapy*

Selection of Points

Sanyinjiao (SP 6), Guilai (ST 29), Shuidao (ST 28), Yinlingquan (SP 9), Qihai (RN 6), Guanyuan (RN 4).

Method

Select a piece of magnete made of rare—earth cobalt, which is 800—1500 abt. in intensity of surface magnetic field and is 1 cm in diameter and 0.5 cm thick, and select two or three points including the points at the abdomen and lower extremites at one treatment session. The magnetic piece is placed over the lead from a G—6805 Electric Stimulator and the electrode is connected to and fixed on the skin of the point selected with adhesive plaster. Intermittent wave or alternate sparse—dense wave is selected, and the intensity of the stimulation is adjusted from weak to the maxium that the pateint feels the electric stimulation radiating upwards and downwards but without pain. The during of the electric stimulation is thirty minutes, and the treatment is given once daily and for five times as a course.

三十一、遗 尿

本病指3岁以上小儿，睡眠中不能自行控制而排尿者，称为遗尿。临床表现为睡中小便自遗，且遗尿后仍能熟睡，轻者数夜一次，重者一夜数次，日久则精神萎靡，智力减退，食欲下降。

技法运用

1. 毫针：取关元、中极、三阴交、肾俞、足三里穴。

用平补平泻法。针腹部穴时要求针感抵达前阴，每次3～5穴，留针15分钟，每日一次。除外尚可配合皮内针埋植命门，长强，次髎，肾俞，三阴交等穴，每次2～3穴，埋植3～5天再于更换穴位。

有报道，用0.5寸毫针在双侧足小趾下的遗尿点（足小趾第一趾横纹中点），用捻转进针法进针，当针尖触到骨面时，加大针的捻转角度，使刺激量加大，此时病人感到局部剧痛，有的病人（尤其是儿童）可感到下腹部发热，发胀时为佳。留针30分钟，中间行针1次，每日或隔日1次（刘继民．新中医，6：46；1974）。

2. 耳针：肾、膀胱、尿道、枕、下脚端、三焦、脑。

中等刺激，留针30分钟，每日1次。亦可配合耳穴贴敷王不留行籽，每日按压2～3次。

3. 灸疗：关元，中极，三阴交，膀胱俞，足三里，神阙，气海。

用艾卷温和灸或艾炷着肤无瘢痕灸（须小儿能合作），每次2～4穴，每穴施灸15～

20分钟或施艾炷3~5壮,每日1次。

4. 皮肤针:背部督脉,膀胱经第一侧线常规叩刺。重点叩刺胸11~21夹脊穴,关元,气海,曲骨,肾俞。用轻度或中度刺激。

5. 腕踝针:双下$_1$。消毒后与皮肤呈30°角,进入皮下后即将针放平,沿皮进针1~1.5寸(约25~40毫米)。病人无酸、麻、胀、痛感觉,留针20~30分钟,隔天针刺1次。

31. ENURESIS

Manifestations

Enuresis refers to involuntary discharge of the urine of a child over the age of three years, occurring during spleep. It is manifested clinically by involuntary micturition during spleep, once in several nights in mild cases and several times a night in severe cases. In the prolonged cases, listlessness, poor intelligence development and poor appetite may be accompanied.

Treatmenr by Applying Acubustion Techniques

(1) *Filiform Needling*

Selection of Points

Guanyuan (RN 4), Zhongji (RN 3), Sanyinjiao (SP 6), Shenshu (BL 23), Zusanli (ST 36).

Method

Select three to five points each treatment session, apply uniform reinforcing—reducing needling, retain the needles at each point for fifteen minutes, and give the puncture treatment once daily and for ten sessions as a course. On needling the point at the abdomen the needling sensation is required to radiate to the external genitalia. Besides, in coordination, intradermal embedding of needle may be given to Mingmen (DU 4), Changqiang (DU 1), Ciliao (BL 232), Shenshu (BL 23) and Sanyinjiao (SP 6), two or three points being employed each session, and the needles being embedded in the points for three to five days. The points are employed alternately.

Introducing An Experiential Technique

Another puncture method for treatment of enuresis is reported in New TCM. The bilateral Enuresis points (extra point, at the midpoint of the first transverse crease of the samll toe) are selected as the puncture points. 0.5 cun long needles are inserted with twisting movements. When the needle tip is pushed to touch the surface of the bone, the needle is twisted at a large amplitude to induce strong stimulation to the patient until the patient complains of severe pain at the local region and distension at the lower abdomen. The needles are retained for thirty minutes and manipulated once during the retention. The treatment is given once daily or once every other day.

(2) *Otopuncture*

Selection of Otopoints

Kidney, Urinary Bladder, Occiput, Sympathetic, Sanjiao, Brain.

Method

Select two to four points each treatment session, apply medium strength stimulation, retain the needles at each point for thirty minutes, and give the treatment once daily. Or stick vaccaria seeds on the otopoints and press them two or three times daily in coordination.

(3) *Moxibustion*

Selection of Points

Guanyuan (RN 4), Zhongji (RN 3), Sanyinjiao (SP 6), Pangguangshu (BL 28), Zusanli (ST 36), Shenque (RN 8), Qihai (RN 6).

Method

Select two to four points each session, give mild — warming moxibustion with the moxa stick or moxibustion with moxa cone on skin to each point for fifteen to twenty minutes or three to five cones, causing no scar left, and give the treatment once daily and for ten sessions as a course. The moxibustion treatment should not be given to the child who is not in cooperation.

(4) *Tapping*

Site to Be Tapped

The Governor Vessel (the Du Meridian) on the back, the first lateral branch of the Urnary Bladder Meridian of the both sides of the spinal column.

Method

Apply the regular tapping on the sites with stress on Jiaji (EX — B 2, T 11 — 21), Guanyuan (RN 4), Qihai (RN 6), Qugu (RN 2), Shenshu (BL 23), and administer mild or medium strength stimulation.

(5) *Wrist — Ankle Puncture*

Selection of Points

Bilateral Lower 1.

Method

After routine sterilization, insert the needle into the point at an angle of 30° to the skin to the subcutaneous tissues. Then, push it horizontally along the skin for 1—1.4 cun, causing soreness, numbness, distension and pain to the patient. Finally, retain the needles at the points for twenty to thirty minutes. The treatment is given once every other day and for seven sessions as a course.

三十二、尿潴留

尿潴留属中医学"癃闭"范畴。临床主要表现为下腹胀满,膀胱充盈小便不能自主排出。虚证主要为小便淋沥不爽,排出无力,甚至点滴不出,小腹膨隆,面色苍白,神疲气短,腰膝酸软,舌淡苔微腻,脉细无力;实证为小便阻塞不通,小腹胀急而痛,烦躁口渴,舌红苔黄腻,脉数。

针灸主要治疗因神经功能障碍所致之尿潴留。

技法运用

1. 针灸:取肾俞、三焦俞、气海、水道、三阴交、中极穴,或由会阳透次髎穴。

实证用捻转提插泻法加阴陵泉,虚证用捻转提插补法配合艾灸,加命门、次髎。针刺中极穴时宜浅刺或向下斜刺或指压按摩,不可垂直深刺,要求感觉抵达尿道。每穴留针20～30分钟,每次取3～4穴,每日1次。

有人用针刺配合穴位指压,治疗骨科,外科,五官科等和泌尿系手术后尿潴留。主穴取气海透曲骨,左归来透右归来。配穴取阴陵泉,三阴交;腹胀明显者加足三里;导尿管停留时间较久或尿道水肿者加太冲,针刺时不宜过深,以免刺入腹腔伤及膀胱。进针后双手快速捻针,持续1分钟,不用提插,留针15～20分钟,中间可捻针1次。阴陵泉,三阴交则用深刺捻转提插泻法。指压法操作时,右手掌心对准脐部,以中指点按关元穴,左手拇指压于右手中指第1节(图5—21),两手由轻渐重地平稳施加压力,着力点在关元穴。同时嘱患者排尿,如有小便流溢、应继续加压,待其排空后,再缓缓将手松开。此法宜用于腹部手术患者(田丛豁,等.《针灸医学验集》)。

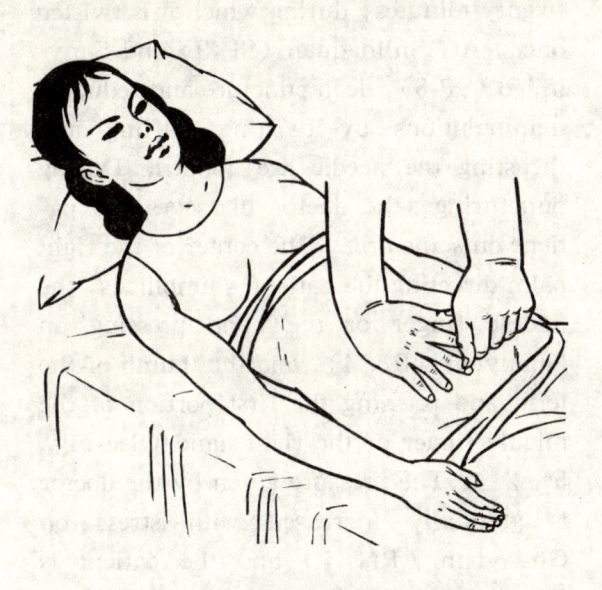

图 5—21 指压关元穴
Fig. 5—21 Pressing Guanyuan (RN 4) with the Finger

2. 耳针:取膀胱、肾、尿道、输尿管、脑、下脚端。

中等刺激,每次 3～4 穴,留针 1 小时,每 10 分钟行针 1 次。

3. 电针:一组为双侧维道穴,针尖沿皮向曲骨(耻骨联合上缘,腹正中线上)透刺约 5.0 厘米;一组为阴陵泉。用断续波通电 15～30 分钟,刺激量可逐渐加强。

有报道,取穴气海,关元,中极,配合水道,三阴交,其中气海沿皮平刺透关元,或关元平透中极。得气后将针接于医用脉冲治疗机正极;水道沿皮向下平刺 1.5～2 寸,或三阴交直刺 1.5～2 寸,得气后接治疗机负极,中等刺激量,频率 140～200 赫,时间 15～30 分钟,治疗术后尿潴留 100 例,获得满意效果。(赵大茵.中国针灸,2:8;1981 年)。

32. RETENTION OF URINE

Manifestations

Retention of urine, belonging to disease category of Long Bi (癃闭) in TCM, is manifested clinically mainly by distension and fullness of the lower abdomen, filling of bladder and difficult urination or even blockage of urine. It may be classified into deficiency and excess types. The deficiency syndrome is characterized by dribbling urination, attenuating in force of the urine discharge, or even retention of urine, fullness of the lower abdomen, pallor, listlessness and shortness of breath, soreness and weakness of the lower back and knee, pale tongue with slightly sticky coating, thready and forceless pulse. The excess type is characterized by blockage of urine, distending pain of the lower abdomen, dysphoria and thirst, red tongue with yellow sticky coating and rapid pulse.

Acupuncture and moxibustion are applicable mainly to the retention of urine due to dysneuria.

Treatment by Applying Acubustion Techniques

(1) *Filiform Needling*
Selection of Points

Main points: Shenshu (BL 23), Sanjiaoshu (BL 22), Qihai (RN 6), Shuidao (ST 28), Sanyinjiao (SP 6), Zhongji (RN 3), Huiyang (BL 35, which is punctured with penetration needling towards Ciliao BL 32).

Supplementary points according to symptoms: Yinlingquan (SP 9) for excess type, and Mingmen (DU 4) for deficiency type.

Method

Three to five points are employed each treatment session. For excess type, reducing method by twisting, lifting and thrusting the needle is applied. For defeficiency type, puncture with reinforcing manipulations by twirling, lifting and thrusting the needle together with moxibustion is applied. On needling Zhongji (RN 3), puncture shallowly or obliquely downwards or with help of massage, causing the needling sensation spreading to the urethra, and avoid perpendicular deep puncture. The needles are retained in each acupoint selected for twenty to thirty minutes each session. The treatment is given once daily and for ten days as a course.

Introducing An Experiential Technique

Another method for treatment of retention of urine after surgical operation is recommended in Collection of Experiences of Acupuncture & Moxibustion. The main points selected include Qihai (RN 6), which is punctured with penetration needling towards Qugu (RN 2), and left Guilai (ST 29), which is punctured with penetration needling towards right Guilai (ST 29). The adjuvant points include Yinlingquan (SP 9) and Sanyinjiao (SP 6). If the patient has severe abdominal distention, Zusanli (ST 36) is added, and if the patient has urethral swelling or prolonged usage of a urinary catheter, Taichong (LR 3) is added. On needling Guilai (ST 29) and Qihai (RN 6), no deep puncture and no lifting or thrusting method are allowed so as not to injure the urinary bladder, and the needle, after being inserted to a depth, is twisted quickly for one minute and retained for fifteen to twenty minutes, during which it is twisted once. At Yinlingquan (SP 9) and Sanyinjiao (SP 6), deep puncture and reducing manipulations by twisting, lifting and thrusting the needle are applied. During puncturing, the doctor massages the patient on some areas, the center of the right palm directing the patient's umbilicus, the middle finger of the hand pressing on Guanyuan (RN 4), and the thumb of the left hand pressing the first portion of the middle finger of the right hand (See Fig. 5−21). The pressure given by the doctor is gradually increased with stress on Guanyuan (RN 4) and the patient is asked to do urination at the same time. If urine is found out of the urethra, the pressure is continuously increased until little urine is in the bladder, then the doctor releases the fingers on the patient slowly.

(2) *Otopuncture*

Seletion of Otopoints

Urinary Bladder, Kidney, Urethra, Ureter, Brain, Sympathetic.

Method

Three or four otopoints are employed each session, medium strength stimulation is applied, and the needles are retained in each point for one hour and manipulated every ten minutes. The treatment is given once daily and for ten sessions as a course.

(3) *Electroacupuncture*

Selection of Points

Two groups of points are selected,

one including bilateral Weidao (GB 28), and the other including Yinlingquan (SP 9).

Method

At first, a needle is inserted into Weidao (GB 28), and pushed towards Qugu (RN 2, at the upper border of the pubic symphysis and at the abdominal median line) for about two cun, then, the electric stimulation is given to the point through the needle for fifteen to thirty minutes, the electric current being at intermittent pulse and the intensity of stimulation gradually increased. Then, a needle is inserted into Yinlingquan (SP 9), and electric stimulation is applied with the same way as above. The treatment is given once daily and for five times as a course.

Introducing An Experiential Technique

A good method is recommended by Chinese Acupunctrue & Moxibustion, by which, it is reported, a satisfactory effect in treating 100 cases with retention of urine was achieved. Firstly, a needle is inserted into Qihai (RN 6) and pushed horizontally beneath the skin towards Guanyuan (RN 4). Or a needle is inserted into Guanyuan (RN 4) and pushed towards Zhongji (RN 3) with penetration needling. After needling sensation is induced to the patient, the needle is connected with the anode of a medical electrostimulator. Then, another needle is inserted into Shuidao (ST 28) and pushed horizontally downwards for 1.5－2 cun, or it is inserted into Sanyinjiao (SP 6) perpendicularly 1.5－2 cun deep. After the needling sensation is induced to the patient, the needle is connected with the cathode of the electrostimulator. Medium strenght stimulation at 140－200 Hz is given for fifteen to thirty minutes. The treatment is given once every other day and for six times as a course.

三十三、男性不育症及性功能障碍

男性不育症，临床常见不射精，精子数量少、死、畸形、活动力低下，或精液中无精子等。多与遗精、早泄、阳萎等性功能障碍（神经系统功能紊乱或器质性病变所引起）并见。

技法运用

1. 毫针：取肾俞，关元，三阴交，命门，足三里，中极，气海，次髎，志室等穴。

用捻转提插补法，如伴见阴囊周围潮湿臊臭，小便黄赤等湿热下注症者，则用泻法或平补平泻法，每次针3～4穴，留针15～30分钟，每日或隔日一次。腹部穴位要求针感到达阴茎。夜梦遗精，口干心烦加大陵，神门；精神不振，耳鸣滑精加复溜，太溪。

有人针治212例男子性功能障碍，主穴：曲骨（针），阴廉（曲骨穴旁2寸，直下2寸）（针），次髎（针），大敦（灸），神阙（灸）。方法：取穴要上下左右按摸触压，选敏感反应强，有间隙或有凹陷感的，牵涉痛的敏感点。针次髎，阴廉穴刺到局部出现酸胀，重感为度。针曲骨以出现电击感向尿道根部放射为止。三穴在针感强者，捻针的手指感到重、紧、滞、用"平补平泻"或轻快的捻转手法；在针感弱者，捻针手指感轻松而滑，则用"飞"或慢搓法运针2分钟，留针10分钟。起针时稍加运针。大敦穴用艾条灸，以雀啄法灸治5分钟，火力要足。治疗前病人应小便，让膀胱排空，用30号2寸半毫针，每隔2～3天针1次，10次为1

个疗程,有些针感弱的病人,最初 3 次可每日针 1 次。治疗期间,每日灸大敦穴和神阙穴 1～2 次,病人在第一疗程内严禁同房。有效率达 86.3%(张钦,等. 上海针灸杂志,3:4。1985)。

有报道治疗射精不能症,每晚临睡前用艾条灸大敦穴 5 分钟或加灸曲泉穴 5 分钟;针大赫(中极穴旁开 0.5 寸)、曲骨(耻骨联合上缘,腹正中线上)、中极、横骨(曲骨穴旁开 0.5 寸),每次 1～2 穴,针刺深度以有电击感放射至尿道根部为佳,然后捻针 1～2 分钟,留针 5～10 分钟;次髎、中髎、关元俞,治阴(骶骨尖端旁开 2 指),每次选 1～2 穴,针刺深度以局部或会阴部有酸胀感为准,然后捻针 1～2 分钟,留针 5～10 分钟;行间、太冲、照海 3 穴中,每次选 1～2 穴,针刺深度以局部有酸胀感为准,然后捻针 1～2 分钟,留针 5～10 分钟,10 次 1 疗程(田丛豁,等.《针灸医学验集》)。

2. 灸疗:穴位同毫针。

用艾卷温和灸或隔姜灸,每次取 3～4 穴,每穴灸 15～30 分钟或 3～5 壮,每日灸治 1 次,亦可针后加温和灸。湿热下注者除外。

3. 耳针:外生殖器,脑,肾,屏间,精宫,肝。

每次取 3～4 穴,中等刺激,留针 20 分钟,隔日 1 次。

33. MALE INFERTILITY AND SEXUAL DISORDERS

Manifestations

Male infertility is manifested by defective ejaculation, oligospermia, dead—sperms, deformity of sperm, lower motility of sperm, or azoospermia. Manifestations of sexual disorders caused by functional disturbance of nervous system or organic disorders such as seminal emission, prospermia and impotence are usually accompanied.

Treatment by Applying Acubustion Techniques

(1) *Filiform Needling*

Selection of Points

Main points: Shenshu (BL 23), Guanyuan (RN 4), Shanyinjiao (SP 6), Mingmen (DU 4), Zusanli (ST 36), Zhongji (RN 3), Qihai (RN 6), Ciliao (BL 32), Zhishi (BL 52).

Supplementary points according to symptoms: Daling (PC 7) and Shenmen (HT 7) for nocturnal emission, thirsty and restlessness, Fuliu (KI 7) and Taixi (KI 3) for listlessness, tinnitus and spermatorrhoea.

Method

Three or four points are employed each treatment session, and reinforcing manipulation by twirling, lifting and thrusting the needle is applied. But for cases due to downward flow of damp—heat, manifested by dampness and faul smell at the surrounding area of the scrotum, reducing method or uniform reinforcing—reducing method is applied. The needles are retained at each point for fifteen to thirty minutes, and the treatment is given once daily or every other day for ten sessions as a course. The next course begins after an interval of five days. Note: the needling sensation induced by needling the point located at the abdomen should be propagated to the penis.

Introducing Some Experiential Techniques

Another method is reported in Shanghai Journal of Acupuncture & Moxibustion, by which a high effective rate of 86.3% in treatment of 212 cases with male sexual disorders was achieved. The points to be selected include Qugu (RN 2), Yinlian (LR 11, 2 cun lateral to and 2 cun below Qugu, RN 2), Ciliao (BL 32), Dadun (LR 1) and Shenque (RN 8). The sensitive spots at the region around the points are taken as needling points too. Ciliao (BL 32) and Yinlian (LR 11) are punctured to cause local soreness, distension and heaviness, and Qugu (RN 2) punctured to induce the local electrifying sensation spreading to the root region of penis. On puncturing these three points, uniform reinforcing—reducing manipulation or swift and gentle twirling manner is applied for the patient who complains of strong needling sensation or when the doctor feels heavy, tight and uneven sensation around the needle by the fingers during twirling the needle. Or flying method or slow twisting manner is applied for two minutes to the patient who complains of weak needling sensation or when the doctor feels soft and smooth sensation around the needle by the fingers. The needles are retained at each point for ten minutes and manipulated a little before withdrawal. On puncturing at Dadun (LR 1), the bird—pecking moxibustion is applied with strong fire force for two minutes. Prior to applying acupuncture and moxibustion the patient is asked to do urination. The treatment is given once per two or three days and for ten sessions as a course, but once daily at the first three times for the patients who complain of weak needling sensation. During the treatment course, moxibustion is given to Dadun (LR 2) and Shenjue (RN 8) once or twice daily. During the first treatment course, no sexual life is allowed to the patient.

In Collection of Experiences of Acupuncture & Moxibustion a good way of treatment of inability of ejaculation with acupuncture and moxibustion is recommended. Before the patient's going to bed, moxibustion with moxa stick is given to Dadun (LR 1) for five minutes or, additionally, to Ququan (LR 8) for five minutes in coordination. Then, the puncture treatment is given. The points to be selected for puncture include three groups. The first group consists of Dahe (KI 12, 0.5 cun lateral to Zhongji, RN 3), Qugu (RN 2, at the upper border of pubic symphysis and at the abdominal medial line), Zhongji (RN 3), Henggu (KI 11, 0.5 cun lateral to Qugu, RN 2), one or two of them being punctured each treatment session. To the operation, a needle is inserted into the point to the depth where the electrifying sensation is induced to the patient and radiates to the root of urethra. Then, the needle is manipulated for one to two minutes and retained for five to ten minutes. The second group consists of Ciliao (BL 32), Zhongliao (BL 33), Guanyuanshu (BL 28) and Zhiyin (extra point, 2 cun lateral to the sacral apex), one or two of them being punctured each treatment session. To the operation, a needle is inserted to the depth where soreness and distension are induced to the patient at the local region or perineum,

Then, it is twisted for one to two minutes and retained for five to ten minutes. The third group includes Xingjian (LR 2), Taichong (LR 3) and Zhaohai (KI 6), one or two of them being punctured each treatment session. To the operation, a needle is inserted to the depth where distension and soreness are induced to the patient at the local area. Then, it is twisted for one or two minutes and retained for five to ten minutes. The puncture treatment is given once daily at the first three sessions and then once every three days, and for ten sessions as a course.

(2) *Moxibustion*
Selection of Points
The same as in the filiform needling.
Method
Three or four points are employed each treatment session, mild warming moxibustion with moxa stick for fifteen to thirty minutes or ginger moxibustion for three to five cones is applied to each point, and the treatment is given once daily and for ten times as a course. Or, mild warming moxibustion is given after puncture. But it should be noted that moxibustion is not applicable to cases due to downward flow of damp—heat, which are manifested by, besides infertility or sexual disorders, fever, heaviness and pain of the body, abdominal distension, loss of appetite, scanty deep — coloured urine, dysentery, yellowish greasy tongue coating, and soft pulse.

(3) *Otopuncture*
Selection of Otopoints
External Genital Organs, Brain, Kidney, Endocrine, Triangular Depression, Liver.
Method
Three or four points are employed each session, medium strength stimulation is applied, and the needles are retained at each point for twenty minutes. The treatment is given once every other day.

三十四、关节炎
〔附〕肩关节周围炎

中医学称本病为"痹证"。临床表现因其病变的性质不同而异,中医辨证分下列类型:

风痹 关节酸痛,上下左右游走不定,兼有寒热。

湿痹 关节酸痛部位固定不移,肢体有重滞感觉,兼有麻木、浮肿。

寒痹 关节疼痛剧烈,遇冷尤其,得热则舒。

热痹 关节局部红肿热痛、拒按、兼身热、咽痛、口干舌燥。

技法运用

1. 针灸:以局部选穴为主,配合循经取穴,用平补平泻法。

脊椎关节—取人中、殷门、大椎、委中穴,脊椎两侧相应节段部位。

肩关节—取肩髃、肩髎、曲池、天宗、臂臑、阿是穴。

肘关节—取曲池、少海、外关、合谷、阿是穴。

腕关节—取阳池、阳溪、腕骨、合谷、养老、阿是穴。

腰骶关节—取腰阳关、委中、昆仑、大肠俞、阿是穴。

髋关节—取环跳、秩边、阳陵泉、阿是穴。

膝关节—内、外膝眼、委中、鹤顶、阴陵泉、阳陵泉。

踝关节—取解溪、丘墟、商丘、太冲、太

溪、昆仑、阿是穴。

痛痹,湿痹针刺加灸,或温针;行痹(风痹),热痹用捻转提插泻法配合点刺出血。每次3～4穴,留针20～30分钟,每日1次。

有人根据疼痛部位,按经络循行,在痛处上或下取1～2个阿是穴,常规消毒后,用皮肤针叩刺出血,随即用闪罐法将罐罩上,5～15分钟后起罐,擦净血污再用艾条温和灸3～7分钟,隔2日治疗1次,5次为1疗程。治疗90例痹症患者,有效率98.9%(阎长赢.中国针灸,3：11;1983)。

有报道,采用"进火补"手法,治疗脊椎关节炎。取穴：大椎、风门、肝俞、大杼、脊中(第十一胸椎棘突下)、命门、关元俞(第五腰椎棘突下旁开1.5寸)、膀胱俞、次髎、秩边、环跳、曲池、委中等。方法：嘱患者呼气一口,随呼气进针1分,找到感觉,将针急插慢提3次,让患者自鼻孔吸气3次(自然呼吸),再进针2分,作同样的急插慢提3～5次,把针摇动,如无酸胀热感,再进针2分,作同样的急插慢提3～5次,即将针慢慢提出,急按其穴(有时不利用呼吸也可),隔日针治1次。(郑魁山。中医杂志,8：426;1956)。

另有人取肩髃透极泉,治疗肩关节周围炎。方法：用双指押手法固定肩髃穴,先用轻刺激手法,垂直刺入0.6～1寸深,待病人产生酸重感后,稍停3息,再用重刺激手法向极泉穴方向垂直刺入3～4寸深,以针尖几将达于极泉穴为止,然后在固定的位置上,施用"烧山火"手法,不断捻转。进针深度应根据病人的胖瘦强弱而定。刺激轻重也要根据病人的耐受程度作标准,但必须使酸胀感达到五指后出针,一般捻转1～2分钟即可,不留针,出针后立即在原位上拔火罐1只,10分钟取下(焦国瑞.《针灸临床经验辑要》)。

2. 耳针：相应区压痛点、神门、脑、肾、屏间。用较强刺激,留针20分钟,每日或隔日1次。适用于以疼痛为主的关节炎。

3. 皮肤针：常用于以肿胀为主的关节炎。叩刺局部肿胀处,或在患病关节作环状叩刺,脊椎两侧自上而下叩刺。

有人用皮肤针治疗肩关节周围炎。取5～7颈椎及1～4胸椎两侧或患部关节周围,患病上肢掌侧面及外侧。重点叩刺压痛点及阳性反应物处。疼痛甚者加刺后颈,骶部;肩部活动障碍加刺肩胛岗,胸椎5～10两侧;肌张力差,肌肉萎缩加刺胸椎7～12两侧,腰以及患肢掌侧和外侧皮区;患肢或指尖有麻木的,可在局部和指尖放血(刘冠军.《中医针法集锦》)。

4. 艾灸：①全身疾病麻木者,可用固定或艾条薰灸器长时间薰灸大椎穴,每次2小时以上,等灸感到达命门穴以下,加薰灸命门穴。②在背部或有不适感处先找到压痛点,再用点燃的艾条在痛区巡回薰灸(蔡耀明.中国针灸,6：3;1986)。

34. ARTHRITIS
(Appendix： Periarthritis of Shoulder Joint)

Manifestations

Arthritis, belonging to syndrome category of Bi Zheng (痹证) in TCM, varies in clinical manifestations due to different pathological natures. There are following types of arthritis according to defferentiation of syndromes with the TCM theories.

Wind — Bi： It is due to attack of wind evil, and mainly characterized by wandering aching pain in the joints, accompanied by fever and chills.

Damp — Bi： It is due to attack of damp evil, and mainly characterized by fixed pain in the joints, heaviness of limbs accompanied by numbness and swelling.

Cold—Bi: It is due to attack of cold evil, and mainly characterized by severe pain in the joints, aggravated by cold and alleviated by warmth.

Heat — Bi: It is due to attack of pathogenic heat, and mainly characterized by local redness, swelling, heat and pain in the joints, aggravated by pressure and accompanied by fever, sore throat, thirst and dry tongue.

Treatment by Applying Acubustion Techniques

(1) *Filiform Needling and Moxibustion*

Selection of Points

The local points are taken as the main points and distal points along the meridian as the adjuvant. The points are selected according to the diseased portion as follows:

Vertebral joints: Renzhong (DU 26), Dazhui (DU 14), weizhong (BL 40), Yinmen (BL 51), bilateral sides of corresponding vertebral joint areas.

Shoulder joints: Jianyu (LI 15), Jianliao (SJ 14), Quchi (LI 11), Tianzong (SI 11), Binao (LI 14), tender spots at the local area.

Elbow joints: Quchi (LI 11), Shaohai (HT 3), Waiguan (SJ 5), Hegu (LI 4), tender spots at the local area.

Wrist joint: Yangchi (SJ 4), Yangxi (LI 5), Wangu (SI 4), Hegu (LI 4), Yanglao (SI 6), tender spots at the local area.

Lumbosacral joints: Yaoyangguan (DU 3), Weizhong (BL 40), Kunlun (BL 6), Dachangshu (BL 25), tender spot at the local area.

Hip joints: Huantiao (GB 30), Zhibian (BL 54), Yanglingquan (GB 34), tender spots at the local area.

Knee joints: Internal and external Xiyan (EX—LE 4,5), Weizhong (BL 40), Heding (EX—LE 2), Yinlingquan (SP 9), Yanglingquan (GB 34).

Ankle joints: Jiexi (ST 41), Qiuxu (GB 40), Shangqiu (SP 5), Taichong (LR 3), Taixi (KI 3), Kunlun (BL 60), tender spots at the local area.

Method

Three to five acupoints or tender spots are employed each treatment session, uniform reinforcing — reducing manipulation is applied, and the needles are retained at each point for twenty to thirty minutes. For cold—bi or damp—bi syndrome, moxibustion is applied additionally, or the needles being inserted into the points are warmed by burning moxa stick on them. For wind—bi or heat—bi syndrome, reducing manipulations by twisting, lifting and thrusting the needle are applied and the points are pricked to cause bleeding. The treatment is given once daily and for ten sessions as a course. The next course begins after an interval of seven days.

Introducing Some Experiential Techniques

Another method is reported in Chinese Acupuncture & Moxibustion, by which an effective rate of 98.9% in treatment of arthritis was achieved. To the operation, one or two tender spots above or below the painful area are selected along the meridian course, and the local and routine sterilization is given. The points selected are tapped with the plum-blossom needle to cause bleeding, and cupping is given there for five to fifteen minutes. After the jars are removed and the skin of the points are cleaned, mild warming moxibustion with stick is given to each point for three to seven minutes. The treatment is given once every three days and for five sessions as a course. The next course begins after an interval of seven days.

The following method for treatment of vertebral arthritis is recommended by Dr. Zheng Koushan, a famous acupuncturist in China. The points to be selected consist of Dazhui (DU 14), Fengmen (BL 12), Ganshu (BL 18), Dashu (BL 11), Jizhong (DU 6, below the spinal process of the 11th thoracic vertebra), Mingmen (DU 4), Guanyuanshu, (BL 26), Pangguangshu (BL 28), Ciliao (BL 32), Zhibian (BL 54), Huantiao (GB 30), Quchi (LI 11), and Weizhong (BL 40), two to four of them being punctured each treatment session. To the operation, "heat — entering reinforcing manner" is applied. The needle is inserted into the point 0.1 cun deep while the patient is breathing out. After the needling sensation is induced, the needle is swiftly thrust and slowly lifted three times. Then, it is pushed 0.2 cun deeper as the patient is breathing in with nose, and at this layer, it is swiftly thrust and slowly lifted three to five times. And then, it is shaked. Through the manipulations, the soreness, distension and heat sensation are induced to the patient. If they aren't, the needle is swiftly thrust and slowly lifted another three to five times. Finally, the needle is withdrawn slowly and the needle hole is pressed immediately. The treatment is given once daily and for ten sessions as a course, and another course begins after an interval of one week.

In Collection of Outstandings of Clinical Experiences of Acupuncture & Moxibustion another method for treatment of periarthritis of shoulder joints is recorded. Jianyu (LI 15) is punctured with penetration needling towards Jiquan (HT 1). To the operation, Jianyu (LI 15) is fixed with the two fingers, and the needle is inserted into the point gently and perpendicularly 0.6 — 1 cun deep, inducing soreness and heaviness to the patient. After the patient breathes in and out three times, the needle is pushed perpendicularly towards Jiquan (HT 1) to a depth of 3 — 4 cun, the needle tip reaching the tissue just beneath the skin of Jiquan (HT 1). Then, at this layer, "heat — producing manipulation" is applied and the needle is twisted continuously. The depth of insertion is adjusted according to the patint's bodily constitution (is he thin or fat, weak or strong), and the intensity of stimulation adjusted according to patient's tolerance. Usually, the needle is twisted one to two minutes and not retained. On puncturing, soreness and distension induced to the patient should be propagated to the fingers. Following withdrawal of the needle, cupping is given for ten minutes. The treatment is given once daily and for ten sessions as a course.

(2) *Otopuncture*

Selection of Otopoints

Corresponding tender spots on the auricle, Shenmen, Brain, Kidney, Endocrine.

Method

Three or four otopoints are employed each treatment session, comparatively strong stimulation is chosen, and the needles are retained at each point for twenty minutes. The otopuncture treatment is suitable to the arthritis to which pain is the main manifestation, and it is given once daily or once every other day.

(3) *Tapping*

It is usually applied to the type of arthritis to which swelling and distension are the main manifestation. Tap on the local swelling and distension area, or tap at the diseased joints in a circle or at the bilateral sides of the spinal vertebra from above downwards.

Introducing An Experiential Technique

Another method is recorded in Collection of Outstandings of the Needling Methods of TCM for treatment of periarthritis of shoulder joint. The bilateral sides of C 5—7 and T 1—4, the surrounding area of the affected joint, and the palmar aspect and lateral aspect of the affected limb are tapped with stress on the tender or sensitive spots. In addition, supplementary areas are tapped according to symptoms. Back of neck and sacral region are added for severe pain, spine of scapula and bilateral sides of the thoracic vertebrae (T 5—10) added for disturbance of shoulder joint in movement, bilateral sides of the thoracic vertebrae T 7—12, lower back, and palmar aspect and lateral aspect of the affected upper limb added for hypomyotonia and muscular atrophy, and the affected area and the finger tips of the affected limb added to cause bleeding for numbness at these areas.

(4) *Moxibustion*

a. To the patient suffering from a general disease with numbness, moxibustion with moxa stick is applied to Dazhui (DU 14) for more than two hours and, when the moxibustion sensation induced to the patient is propagated to the area below Mingmen (DU 4), the moxibustion is given to Mingmen (DU 4) additionally.

b. To the patient who has arthritis, rounding moxibustion with moxa stick is given to the back or to the tender spots at the discomfortable area.

三十五、落 枕

落枕，多表现为睡醒起来后，颈部有牵拉样疼痛，活动时疼痛加剧，以致颈项活动功能明显受限，不能左右转侧或前后俯仰。由于患侧肌群处于紧张、痉挛状态，因而颈项部向一侧歪斜，因此又称为"功能性斜颈"。

技法运用

1. 毫针：落枕、后溪、风池、外关、阳陵泉、中渚、阿是穴。

用平补平泻法，一般先刺四肢远端穴位，行针时嘱患者配合颈项运动，再视情况配合患部穴位针刺。留针15~20分钟，间歇运针1~2次，每日1次。

有报道，按压极泉穴治疗落枕。方法：患者坐位（以右侧为例），把右前臂放在诊断桌上，术者站其右后方，右手拇指放在患者右肩峰上，食指置于腋下极泉穴（图5—22）。由轻到重进行按压。嘱患者做头部左右旋转及屈伸动作,当头转到痛侧时,可用食指弹拨极泉穴一下,患者右手即有触电样感,每次按压5分钟,症状可明显减轻,若局部仍有疼痛时,可作痛点揉按或配合摇颈手法。(杨庆云.《针灸治疗百病荟萃》)。

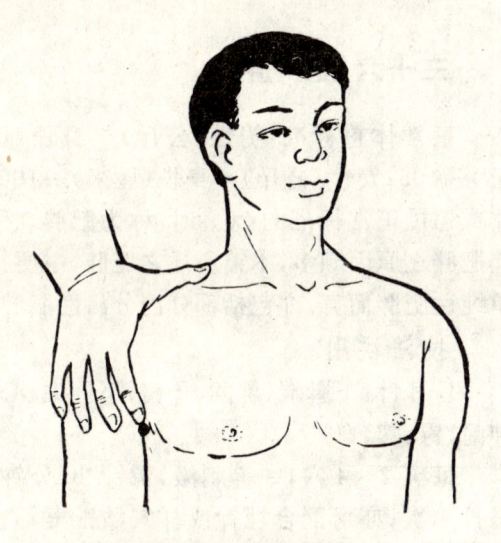

图 5—22 指压极泉穴
Fig. 5—22 Presing Jiquan (HT1) with the Finger

2.耳针:颈、颈椎、肩、枕、神门。

用强刺激手法快速旋转,每日1次,每次留针15～30分钟。亦可耳穴贴压王不留行籽,每次1分钟,按压至有热胀感和疼痛,并同时转动头颈。

3.皮肤针:叩刺颈项强痛部位,使局部皮肤发红,再叩刺肩背压痛点。

4.拔罐:先用皮肤针叩打压痛部位,稍见出血后再拔火罐,亦可针上套拔火罐。

35. STIFF NECK

Manifestations

Stiff neck is usually manifested by dragging pain, occurring after waking up and aggravated by movement, and obvious limitation of movement of the head, inability of the neck to turn left or right, to bend or rise, As the mascular mass of the affected side is at tension and spasm, causing neck to deviate to one side, "functional torticollis" is also termed to it.

Treatment by Applying Acubustion Techntouse

(1) *Filiform Needling*

Selection of Points

Luozhen (EX), Houxi (ST 3), Fengchi (GB 20), waiguan (SJ 5), Yanglingquan (GB 34), Zhongzhu (SJ 3), tender spots.

Method

Three to five points are employed each treatment session, uniform reinforcing — reducing manipulation is applied. Generally, at biginning, the distal points at extremities are punctured in cooperation with the patient's movement of the neck. Then, the points at the affected area are punctured. The needles are retained at each point for fifteen to twenty minutes and manipulated one or two times during the retention. The treatment is given once daily until the disease is cured.

Introducing An Experiential Technique

Another method for treatment of stiff neck is recomemded by Dr. Yang Qingyun, a famous acupuncturist in china. The method is introduced here by taking the disease at the right side as an example. The patient is asked to sit down with the forearm at the diagnostic table, and the doctor stands behind the patient, and places his right thumb on the right acromion of the patient and the index finger at Jiquan (HT 1, See fig. 5 — 22). Then, the acupoint is pressed and the intensity of pressure is gradually increased. At the same time, the patient is asked to turn his head left and right and to bend and to lift the head. As the patient's head turning to the affected side, Jiquan (HT 1) is flicked one time with the index finger, causing electrifying sensation to the patient at the right hand. After five minutes of pressure, the symptoms are relieved obviously. If the local pain is still present, massage is given to the painful spots or the head is shaked additionally in coordination.

(2) *Otopuncture*

Selection of Points

Neck, Cervical Vertebra, Shoulder, Occiput, Shenmen.

Method

Three to five otopoints are employed each treatment session, strong stimulation and swift rotating manner are applied, and the needles are retained at each point for fifteen to thrty minutes. The puncture treatment is given once daily until the symptoms are relieved and eliminated. Or vaccaria seeds are stuck on the otopoints and pressed for one minute, causing heat sensation, distension and pain to the patient, and the patient is asked to move his head while the neck being pressed. The seeds are kept on the points for four or five days and pressed several times daily. Then, some other otopoints are stuck with the vaccaria seeds with the same way.

(3) *Tapping*

The stiff and painful region is tapped until the local skin is reddened. Then, the tender spots at the back are tapped.

(4) *Cupping*

Following tapping at the tender area to cause bleeding slightly, apply cupping on the area. Or apply cupping to the region where a filiform needle is inserted into.

三十六、肥　胖

正常体重标准：男性（公斤）＝身长（厘米）－105；女性（公斤）＝身长（厘米）－100。体重超过正常标准的 20% 时，称为肥胖。引起肥胖之原因颇多，本篇所述之肥胖，主要指单纯性肥胖而言。亦包括部分内分泌性肥胖。

技法运用

1. 耳针：下脚端、屏间、子宫、下屏尖、心、神门、胃、脾、口。

每次 2～4 穴，中等刺激，留针 20 分钟，每日 1 次；亦可配合埋针或耳穴贴压王不留行籽，3～5 天交换一次。

有报道，取耳穴三焦、肺、内分泌（屏间），埋针减肥 253 例。方法：选定穴位后局部常规消毒，以小号止血钳夹持，撳针准确地置入穴位。然后以胶布固定。留针 5 天后取出，再埋下一个穴位。以上穴位每次 1 穴，3 个穴位轮流埋针，6 次为 1 疗程（李士杰. 中国针灸，3：11；1986）。

2. 毫针：梁丘、公孙，每次 1 穴，交替使用，用捻转提插泻法，待患者产生较强烈针感后，再接通电针治疗仪，用连续波，电流量以患者能耐受为度，留针 20 分钟，起针后，用麦粒型皮内针沿皮下刺入 1 厘米左右，用胶布固定。留针期间，嘱病人自行轻按埋针俞穴 2～3 次，每次 1～2 分钟，并在有饥饿感时和进食前 10 分钟，对埋针穴位进行较强刺激的揉按。每 3 天针 1 次，10 次为 1 疗程（雷振萍. 中医杂志，5：52，1987）。

36. OBESITY

Manifestations

The standard of normal body weight is generally taken as follows:

Male: The body weight (Kg) = The body length(cm) − 105

Femal: The body weight (kg) = The body length(cm) − 100

A male person, for example, is 175 cm high, his standard weight is 70 kg. If the body weight is increased by 20% or more to the standard, obesity is considered. There are many facts to cause obesity. But, in this article, only the simple obesity and endogenous obesity are discussed.

Treatment by Applying Acubustion Techniques

(1) *Otopuncture*

Selection of Otopoints

Sympathetic, Endocrine, Uterus, Adrenal Gland, Heart, Shemen, Stomach, Spleen, Mouth.

Method

Two to four points are employed each treatment session, medium strength stimulation is applied, and the needles are retained at each otopoint for twenty minutes. The treatment is given once daily and for ten sessions as a course, the next course beginning after an interval of five days. Or, additionaly, the thumb — tack needles are embedded into the otopoints or the vaccaria seeds are stuck into the otopoints. The needles or the seeds are kept in the otopoints for three to five days, and during the period they are pressed by the patient himself four or five times daily. The otopoints are replaced by some other ones in next session.

Introducing An Experiential Tecnnique

In Chinese Acupuncture and Moxibustion a method is recommended, by which a satisfactory effect was achieved in treatment of 255 cases with obesity. Ot. Sanjiao, Lung, Endocrine are selected. To the operation, following the routine and local sterilization, thumb — tack needle held by a pair of small — sized hemostatic forceps are embedded into the otopoint and then fixed in the skin with adhesive plaster. The needle are kept there for five days and, during the period, the patient is saked to press it three or four tims daily. After removing it, another otopoint is employed for embedment with the same way. The three otopoints are employed alternately, and only one otopoint is employed each treatment session. The embedment is performed once per five days and for six sessions as a course.

(2) *Filiform Needling*

Selection of Points

Lianqiu(ST 34), Gongsun(SP 4).

Method

One point is employed each treatment session, and these two points are employed alternately. On puncturing, reducing manipulations by twisting, lifting and thrusting the needle are applied until comparatively strong needling sensation is induced to the patient. Then, the needle inserted in the point is connected with a lead from an electroacupuncture unit, and electric stimulation at continuous wave is given for twenty minutes. The intensity of the electric stimulation is adjusted to be tolerable to the patient. Following withdrawal of the needle, an wheat — grain — sized intradermal needle is inserted into the point 1 cm deep, and it is fixed in the skin with a piece of adhesive plaster and kept there for three days. The patient is asked to press the point two or three times daily and for one or two minutes each time during the embedment, and additionally, to press the point forcefully whenever the patient himself feels hungry or ten minutes before eating, inducing a strong stimulation to the patient himself. The treatment is given once every three days and for ten times as a course.

第二节 妇产科病症

一、痛 经

本病是指妇女经前，经期或经后发生小腹或腰骶部疼痛，且随着月经周期而反复发作的疾患，严重时可伴有恶心呕吐，甚至昏厥。

技法运用

1. 针灸：取三阴交、中极、气海、关元、归来、足三里。

小腹冷痛，经量少伴血块者加地机，血海，用平补平泻法配合艾灸；小腹胀甚于痛且兼乳胁胀痛者加太冲、内关，阳陵泉，用捻转提插泻法；腹痛绵绵，头晕耳鸣，经色淡者加照海，肾俞，曲泉，用捻转提插补法配合艾灸。

有人取气海、天枢、足三里治痛经。方法：取仰卧位，下肢屈曲。气海用3寸长毫针，先直刺1.5～2寸，上下徐徐提插3～5次后，再将针提至皮下，向中极方向透刺2～2.5寸，按上法上下徐徐提插3～5次，有强烈的沉胀感后留针15～30分钟，天枢针1.5～2寸，刮针手法，留针时间同气海；足三里针1.5～2寸，提插捻转手法，持续行针至腹痛减轻或消失后留针，与上两穴同时起针（孙学全.《针灸临证集验》）

有报道，取关元穴常规消毒后，用28号2寸长毫针垂直刺入1.5寸深，得气后用提插捻转手法，强刺激1分钟。以关元为中心点，上下左右1寸处，各刺1针，深1.5寸，取1.2公分长的艾段，套在针柄上点燃，每日1次，每次在每根针上连用2～3个艾段，3次为1疗程，痊愈后为巩固疗效，分别在下两个月周期治疗1～2次（刘继先.上海针灸杂志，1：13，1987）。

2. 耳针：子宫、屏间、脑、下脚端、肝、肾、腰。

每次取3～4穴，强刺激捻转，留针30分钟，每日1次。亦可配合耳穴贴压王不留行籽。

3. 腕踝针：双侧下$_1$。

采用1.5寸长30号毫针，医者左手拇指食指舒张皮肤，右手持针对准应刺部位，使针体与皮肤呈30°角，刺透皮后，将针放平贴近皮肤皮面，循纵线向上沿皮下平刺入1.4寸左右，留针30分钟。

4. 艾灸：关元、曲骨、三阴交或痛区。

于月经来潮1～2日或月经来潮时，采用隔姜灸或艾条灸，每次每穴3～5壮或10～15分钟。施灸时，以患者感到舒适为度，每日1～2次。

SECTION 2 GYNECOLOGICAL DISEASES

1. DYSMENORRHEA

Manifestations

Dysmenorrhea, a common disease in women, refers to the pain occurring in the lower abdomen or lumbosacral region before, after or during the menstruation, which is proxysmal with the menstrual cycle and is accompanied with nausea, vomiting and even coma in severe cases.

Treatment by Applying Acubustion Techniques

(1) *Filiform Needling*

Selection of Points

Main points: Sanyinjiao (SP 6), Zhongji (RN 3), Qihai (RN 6), Guanyuan (RN 4), Guilai (ST 29), Zusanli (ST 36).

Method & Supplementary Points According to Symptoms

If the patient complains of cold and pain at the lower abdomen, and scanty menses with clots, Xuehai (SP 10) is added, uniform reinofrcing — reducing manipulation is chosen, and moxibustion is applied additionally in coordination. If the patient has distension and pain at the lower abdomen, in which the pain is less severe than the distension, accompanied by distension at the hypochondriac region and breast, Taichong (LR 3), Neiguan (PC 6), and Yanglingquan (GB 34) are added, and reducing manipulations by twisting, lifting and thrusting the needle are applied. If the patient suffers from dull pain in the abdomen, dizziness, tinnitus, and thin menses, Zhaohai (KI 6), Shenshu (BL 23), and Ququan (LR 8) are added, reinforcing manipulations by twirling, lifting and thrusting the needle are applied, and moxibustion is applied additionally in coordination.

Intrdducing Some Experiential Techniques

The following method for treatment of dysmenorrhea is recorded in Collection of Clinical Experiences of Acupuncture & Moxibustion. To this method, Qihai (RN 6), Tianshu (ST 25) and Zusanli (ST 36) are punctured. In the operation, the patient is asked to lie on the back with the lower limbs at flexion. On puncturing at Qihai (RN 6), a 3 cun long needle is inserted into the point perpendicularly to a depth of 1.5~2 cun and, at this layer, the needle is lifted and thrust slowly three to five times. Then, the needle is withdrawn to the area beneath the skin and pushed with penetration needling towards Zhongji (RN 3) for 2~2.5 cun. Then, the needle is lifted and thrust slowly three to five times. After strong heaviness and distension are induced to the patient, the needle is retained for fifteen to thirty minutes. At Tianshu (ST 25), a needle is inserted 1.5—2 cun deep, and shaked. Then, the needle is retained as lomg as in Qihai (RN 6). At Zusanli (ST 36), a needle is inserted 1.5—2 cun deep. Then, it is lifted, thrust and twisted until relief or elimination of abdominal pain. Finally, the needle is retained. The needles at these three points are withdrawn at the same time.

Another method for treatment of dysmenorrhea is reported in Shanghai Journal of Acupuncture & Moxibustion. Following a routine and local sterilization, a No. 28 needle 2 cun long is inserted into Guanyuan (RN 4) perpendicularly to a depth of 1.5 cun. After arrival of qi, a strong stimulation by lifting, thrusting and rotating the needle for one minute is administered. Then, four points 1 cun respectively above, below, left and right to Guanyuan(RN 4) are punctured, with the needles inserted to a depth of 1.5 cun. Finally, five portions of moxa stick, each being 1.2 cun long, are respectively put on the needle handles and ignited for moxibustion. Usually, two or three portions of the moxa stick are burnt at each needle handle in one treatment session. The treatment is given once daily and for three times as a course. After recovery, one to two sessions of the treatment are given respectively in the following two menstrual cycles to consolidate the effect.

(2) *Otopuncture*

Selction of Otopoints

Triangular Fossa, Endocrine, Brain, Sympathetic, Liver, Kidney, Waist.

Method

Three or four otopoints are employed each treatment session, strong stimulation is applied, the needles are retained at each point for thirty minutes, and the treatment is given once daily and for ten sessions as a course. Or the vaccaria seeds are stuck over the otopoints and pressed additionally in coordination.

(3) *Wrist—Ankle Puncture*

Selection of Points

Bilateral Lower I.

Method

Stretch the local skin with the thumb and index finger of the left hand, insert a No. 30 needle 1.5 cun long held with the right hand into the skin at an angle of 30° to the skin. After piercing through the skin, place the needle horizontally and push it beneath the skin upwards for 1.4 cun. Then, it is retained for thirty minutes.

(4) *Moxibustion*

Selection of Points

Guanyuan (RN 4), Qugu (RN 2), Sanyinjiao(SP 6) or painful area.

Method

At the period one or two dyas before the menstruation or on the menstruation, ginger moxibustion to each point for three to five cones or moxibustion with moxa stick to each point for ten to fifteen minutes is applied each treatment session. The intensity of stimulation is adjusted to be tolerable to the patient. The treatment is given once or twice daily.

二、更年期综合征

本病指多发于45～55岁左右的妇女,在月经终止前后,因卵巢性功能减退,或手术摘除卵巢,或放射治疗丧失卵巢功能,而出现的精神和植物神经功能失调为主的症候群。临床表现为月经周期紊乱或突然停止,可出现阵发性面部潮红、出汗、心烦、易怒、抑郁乏力、皮肤麻木、头晕、失眠、心悸、记忆力差等。

技法运用

1. 毫针:内关、足三里、太冲、通里、三阴交。

潮热,汗出,烦怒者加行间,足临泣,用捻转提插泻法;太溪、复溜,用捻转提插补法;心悸、心慌、失眠、健忘者加神门、肝俞、心俞,用平补平泻法。留针15～20分钟,每日或隔日1次。

有人以列缺、照海穴,治疗更年期综合征,也获得了疗效。照海可深刺1.2寸,列缺针0.8寸,用交叉行针法,即左手右足或左足右手,上下轮流,依次捻转提插(陈佑邦,等.《当代中国针灸临证精要》)。

2. 耳针:屏间、下脚端、脑、心、肝、肾、神门。

中等刺激,每次3～5穴,留针20分钟,隔日1次。亦可针刺配合耳穴贴压王不留行籽,每日按压2～3次。

2. MENOPAUSAL SYNDROME

Manifestations

Menopausal Syndrome is usually seen in woman who is 45～55 years old and at the period before or after termination of menstruation. It is characterized mainly by mental and functional maladjustment of vegetative nerve due to hypo—ovaria, decrease of sexual function or ovariectomy, or loss of ovarian function throuhg radiotherapy. It is manifested clinically by menstrual disorder or even sudden termination of menstruation, proxysmal flushed face, lassitude, sweating, listlessness, irritability, mental depression, numbness of the skin, dizziness, insomnea, palpitation, poor memory, etc.

Treatment by Applying Acubustion Techniques

(1) *Filiform Needling*

Selection of Points

Main points: Neiguan (PC 6), Zusanli (ST 36), Taichong (LR 3), Tongli (HT 5), Sanyinjiao(SP 6).

Methods as well as Supplementary Points according to Symptoms

If the patient complains of tidy fever with sweating and irritability, Xingjian (LR 2) and Zulinqi (GB 41) are punctured additionally, with reducing manipulations by twisting, lifting and thrusting the needle, and Taixi(KI 3) and Fuliu (KI 7) Punctured additonally with reinforcing manipulations by twirling, lifting and thrusting the needle. If the patient has palpitation, insomnea and poor memory, Shenmen (HT 7), Ganshu (BL 18) and Xinshu (BL 15) are added, and uniform reinforcing — reducing manipulation is applied. Three to five points are employed each treatment session. Whether reinforcing or reducing mainpulation is applied to the main points is determined according to differentiation of syndromes, i. e. reinforcing manner is selected for deficiency syndrome and vice versa. The needles are retained at each point for fifteen to twenty minutes. The treatment is given once daily or once every other day, and for ten sessions as a course, the next course beginning after an interval of a week.

Introducing An Experiential Technique

An effective method for treatment of menopausal syndrome is recomended in Outstandings of Clinical Experiences of Modern Chinese Acupuncture & Moxidustion. To this method, Lieque (LU 7) and Zhaohai (KI 6) are employed. The depth of insertion of the needle is 1.2 cun at Zhaohai (KI 6) and 0.8 cun at Lieque (LU 7). The left Lieque (LU 7) and right Zhaohai (KI 6) are taken as a group, and left Zhaohai (KI 6) and right Lieque (LU 7) taken as the other group, only one group being punctured each session and these two groups employed alternately, and twirling, rotating, lifting and thrusting manipulations are applied.

(2) *Otopuncture*

Selection of Otopoints

Endocrine, Sympathetic, Brain, Heart, Liver, Kidney, Shemen.

Method

Three to five otopoints are employed each treatment session, medium strength stimulation is applied, and the needles are retained at each otopoint for twenty minutes. The treatment is given once daily and for ten seesions as a course. Or, in coordination, the vaccara seeds are stuck on the otopoints and pressed two or three times daily.

三、带　下

带下,指妇女阴道内流出的一种白色或黄色粘稠液体,现代医学中的阴道炎,宫颈炎,盆腔炎等均可引起。中医学分为脾虚,肾虚,湿热下注三型。

脾虚症见白带量多质稠无臭、纳少、便溏、倦息、体胖、舌淡苔白腻、脉弱;肾虚症见带下色白、量多质稀、淋漓不断、腰部酸痛、小腹发凉、兼头目眩晕、小便清长、舌淡苔薄、脉沉细;湿热下注症见带下粘稠色黄,或夹有血液、量多而气腥秽、阴部作痒、口干口苦、小便短赤、舌红苔黄、脉弦滑数。

技法运用

1. 毫针:带脉、白环俞(第四骶椎棘突下旁开1.5寸)、次髎、关元、归来、三阴交。

脾虚加脾俞、公孙;肾虚加肾俞,太溪均用补法;湿热加阴陵泉、丰隆,用泻法。留针15～20分钟,中间捻转行针1次,每日1次,亦可针后加拔火罐。

有报道,在三阴交穴稍后处,将针尖与皮肤呈30°角向上斜刺1～1.5寸深,留针20～30分钟,10次1疗程。治疗宫颈糜烂1010例,有效率90.1%(梁锐军.《全国针灸针麻学术讨论会论文摘要》;1979)。

有人用针刺加拔火罐治疗白带。主穴:次髎。寒湿配命门,针后加灸;阴痒配蠡沟;湿热配三阴交。方法:嘱患者俯卧,穴位常规消毒,取2～2.5寸毫针,针尖向下肢方向呈45°角斜刺,快速进针,得气后感觉直达小腹及前阴部。寒湿型用平补平泻手法,留针30分钟左右,中间行针2次,湿热型用提插捻转泻法,留针15分钟。针后均留针加拔火罐,留罐15分钟(李欣欣.河南中医,6:13;1985)。

2. 耳针:子宫、脾、肾、三焦、屏间、脑、神门。中等刺激,留针15～20分钟,每日或隔日1次。

3. 灸疗:取穴同毫针。

艾条温和灸或隔姜,隔蒜灸,适宜于脾肾虚证。亦可针后加灸或温针。

有报道,隔姜灸治疗慢性盆腔炎。主穴:气海、中极、归来。方法:用艾绒做成直径1.5厘米,高1.8厘米,重约800毫克的艾炷,置于0.4厘米厚的姜片上(放在所选的穴位上),点燃灸之,每穴灸3壮(张耀华,等.中国针灸,6:36,1986)。

4. 腕踝针:双侧下$_2$。

病人仰卧位。采用30号1.5寸毫针,医者用拇、食、中三指持针柄,针体与皮肤表面呈30°角,用拇指端轻旋针柄,使针尖进入皮肤。过皮后即将针放平,贴近皮肤表面,针尖向上顺直线沿皮下表浅进针。进针速度稍缓慢,如有阻力或出现酸麻胀疼等感觉,则表示针刺太深而已入肌层,应将针退至皮下,重新刺入。进针皮下的长度一般为1.4寸,留针20～30分钟,每日治疗1次,7次为1疗程(田丛豁,等.《针灸医学验集》)。

3. MORBID LEUKORRHEA

Manifestations

Morbid leukorrhea refers to excessive white or yellow mucous vaginal discharge, which may be seen in vaginitis, cervicitis, and pelvic inflammation. It may be classified as three types: the spleen deficiency type, the kidney deficiency type, and the down—flowing of damp—heat type.

The spleen deficiency type is characterized by profuse thick and white vaginal discharge without smell, poor appetite, loose stools, fatty and pale tongue with white and sticky coating, and weak pulse. The kidney deficiency type is characterized by profuse and continuous thin and white vaginal discharge, soreness and pain of the lower back, cold sensation at the lower abdomen, dizziness, excessive urine, pale tongue with thin coating, and deep and thready pulse. The down — flowing of damp-heat type is characterized by profuse yellow and thick mucous viginal discharge with smell or with blood, itching in the vulva, thirst and bitter taste in the mouth, scanty and yellow urine, red tongue with yellow coating, and string — taut, smooth and rapid pulse.

Treateent by Applying Acubustion Techniques

(1) *Filiform Needling*

Selection of Points

Main points: Daimai (GB 26), Baihuanshu (BL 30 1.5 cun lateral to the posterior median line, below the spinal process of the 4th sacral vertebra), Ciliao (BL 32), Guanyuan (RN 4), Guilai (ST 29), Sanyinjiao (SP 6).

Suppelmentary points according to symptoms: Pishu (BL 20) and Gongsun (SP 4) for spleen deficiency; Shenshu (BL 23) and Taixi (KT 3) for deficiency of kidney; and Yinlingquan (SP 9) and Fenglong (ST 40) for down—flowing of damp—heat.

Method

Three to five points are employed each treatment session, reinforcing manipulation is applied to deficiency type and reducing method is chosen for excess type, and the needles are retained at each point for fifteen to twenty minutes and manipulated once during the retention. Following puncture, cupping may be applied. The treatment is given once daily and for ten days as a course, the next course beginning after an interval of a week.

Introducing Some Experiential Techniques

A method, by which an effective rate of 90.1% in treating 1010 cases with erosion of cervix was achieved, is reported by Lian Ruijun, a famous acupuncturist in china. The spot slightly posterior to Sanyinjiao (SP 6) is take as the puncturing point, and a needle is inserted into the spot at an angel of 30° to the skin and pushed obliquely upwards to the depth of 1—1.5 cun, Then, the needle is retained there for twenty to thirty minutes. The treatment is given once daily and for ten sessions as a course.

In Henan Journal of TCM another method for treatment of morbid leukorrhea by acupuncturing and cupping is reported. Ciliao (BL 32) is taken as the main point. The supplementary points according to symptoms include Mingmen (DU 4) for cold—damp type, Ligou (LR 5) for itching in the vulva, and Sanyinjiao (SP 6) for damp—heat type. To the operation, the patient is asked to lie on the stomach, and a routine and local sterilization is given. Then, a 2—2.5 cun long needle is inserted into Ciliao (BL 32) quickly downwards at an angle of 45° to the skin, inducing the needling sensation transmitting to lower abdomen and to the external genitalina. For cold—damp type, unfiorm reinforcing—reducing manipulation is applied, and the needle is retained for about thirty minutes and manipulated two times during the retention. Following the puncture, moxibustion is given additionally in coordination. For heat—damp type, reducing manipulations by lifting, thrusting and twisting the needle are applied, and the needle is retained for fifteen minutes. Additionally, cupping is given for fifteen minutes after the puncture.

(2) *Otopuncture*
Selection of Otopoints
Triangular Fossa, Spleen, Kidney, Sanjiao, Endocrine, Brain, Shenmen.
Method
Three to five otopoints are employed each treatment session, medium strength stimulation is applied, and the needles are retained at each point for fifteen to twenty minutes. The treatment is given once daily or every other day and for ten sessions as a course.

(3) *Moxibustion*
Selection of points
The same as in the filiform needling.
Method
Three to five points are employed each treatment session, and mild—warming moxibustion with moxa stick or ginger moxibustion or garlic moxibustion is applied to each point for approximately fifteen minutes or for three to five cones. Or the moxibustion is given after needling, or the moxibustion with warming needle is applied. But, Moxibustion is only applicable to the types of spleen deficiency and kidney deficiency.

Introduceing An Experiential Technique
A method for treatment of pelvic inflammation is reported in Chinese Acupuncture & Moxibustion. To the method, Qihai (RN 6), Zhongji (RN 3) and Guilai (ST 29) are taken as the main points. Moxa cones 1.5 cm in diameter, 1.8 cm high and 800 mg heavy are made up for usage. In the operation, a moxa cone is placed on a piece of ginger 0.4 cm thick which is on the point selected and ignited for moxibustion. The moxibustion is given to each point for three cones at each treatment session.

(4) *Wrist—Ankel Puncture*
Selection of Points
Bilateral Lower 2.
Method
Ask the patient to lie supine, hold a 1.5 cun long needle with the thumb, index and middle fingers, and insert it through the skin at an angle of 30° to the skin. Then, slowly push it horizontally upwards along the skin. If feeling the resistance around the needle tip or inducing soreness, numbness, distension and pain to the patient, lift the needle to the area beneath the

skin and make antoher try because these phenomena indicate that the needle is inserted too deep to the muscular layer. Generally, insert the needle 1.4 cun deep and retain it for twenty to thirty minutes. The treatment is given once daily and for a week as a course.

四、胎位不正

本症指胎儿30周后,在宫体内位置不正而言。多在产前检查时发现,孕妇并无任何不适。

技法运用

1. 灸疗:至阴穴。

嘱孕妇解松腰带,排空小便仰卧床上,用艾条两根点燃后,同时分别在至阴穴距2~3厘米处悬灸,以局部充血为度,每日1次,每次15~20分钟。

2. 耳穴贴压:有报导用王不留行籽贴压子宫、下脚端、脑、肝、脾、腹等耳穴,每3~4天更换1次,左右两侧轮换,每日早中晚饭后约30分钟,用手指依次压穴15分钟左右,每晚临睡前放松裤带,半卧位再按压1次,治疗169例,成功率81.7%(秦广风.浙江中医杂志,2:83,1988)。

4. MALPOSITION OF FETUS

Mainfestation

Malposition of fetus refers to the abnormal lying of the fetus in the uterus which is found thirty weeks after conception, usually known by prenatal examination and causing no symptoms.

Treatment by Applying Acubustion Techniques

(1) *Moxibustion*

Selection of Points

Zhiyin (BL 67).

Methou

Let the patient loose her girdle and evacuate the urine and lie supine in bed. Then, hold two moxa sticks respectively 2—3cm high to bilateral Zhiyin (B Ⅱ 67) and ignite them for moxibustion for fifteen to twenty minutes, causing local congestion to the patient. The treatment is given once daily until the fetus is at correct position, usually, three to five treatment sessions being needed.

(2) *Otopuncture*

Selection of Points

Triangular Fossa, Sympathetic, Brain, Liver, Spleen, Abdomen.

Method

Two to four otopoints at the same side are employed each treatment session, and two sides are chosen alternately. The vaccaria seed is stuck over each point selected. The patient is aksed to press each seed on her auricle after breakfest, after supper and after dinner, and each time for fiftten minutes, and additionally, to press the seeds another time before going to bed when the patient has losen her girdle. It was reported in Zhejiang Journal of TCM that an effective rate of 81.7% in treatment of 169 cases with malposition of fetus by applying this method was achieved.

第三节 皮肤与外伤科病症

一、急性乳腺炎

乳腺炎,中医学称为"乳痈"。临床主要表

现为乳房红、肿、热、痛,可触及肿块,有明显压痛,并可伴有发热、畏冷、食欲减退等全身反应。炎症进一步发展,可形成脓肿,以致破溃。针灸对该病初起有较好效果。

技法运用

1. 毫针:肩井、乳根、膻中、足三里、内关。

先针足三里,用平补平泻法以防晕针,后针肩井0.5～0.8寸深,用捻转提插并配合呼吸泻法。同时嘱患者自己配合按摩患处肿块。其它穴位,视病情配合运用,取捻转提插泻法。肩井,乳根不宜深刺,乳根向上斜刺或平刺3～5分深。一般留针30～60分钟,留针期间,每隔5～10分钟捻转1次,每日针刺1次,病重者可一日两次。

髎之下骨空处(图5—23),取坐位,体温高者取侧卧法,采用2～2.5寸毫针直刺,用泻法(重刺激),提插到有酸、麻、胀等感觉时,留针,并以艾条灸针柄30～60分钟,每5分钟提插1次。(田丛豁,等.《针灸医学验集》)。

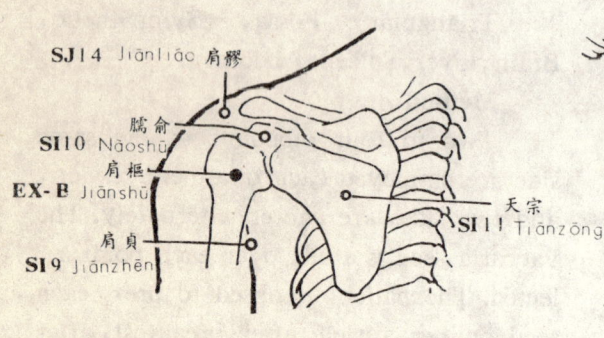

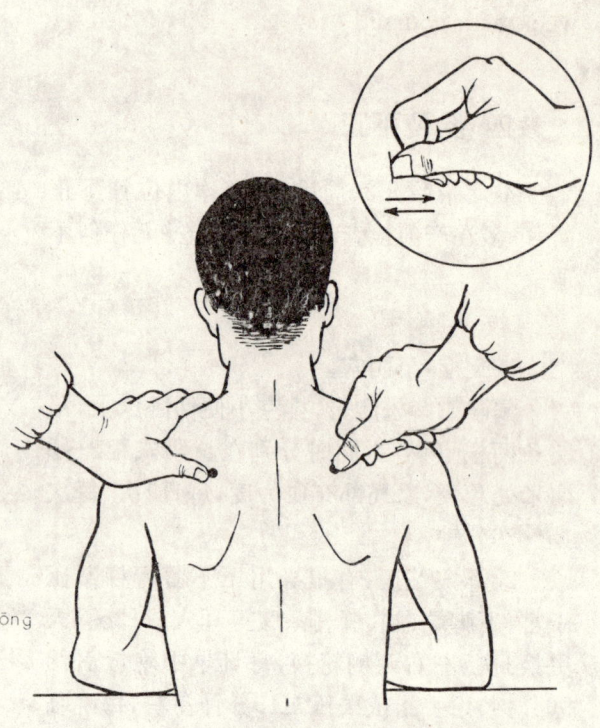

图5—23 肩枢穴
Fig. 5—23 Jianshu (Extra point)

图5—24 天宗穴分筋法
Fig. 5—24 The Tendon—Pushing Method Applied on Tianzong(ST 11)

有报道,用"双穴组"与"单穴组"治疗急性乳腺炎。"双穴组"取患侧的肩贞(上臂内收,腋后纹头上1寸处)、天宗。一般取坐位,体温高者取侧卧位,根据患者身体胖瘦不同,分别采用2～2.5寸毫针直刺,切忌斜刺,用泻法(重刺激)进针后提插到有酸麻胀等感觉时然后留针,并以艾条灸针柄30～40分钟,每灸5分钟提插1次,轻者1次,重者不超过3次,多数均可治愈;"单穴组"取穴肩枢,即肩贞,天宗之上,臑俞(肩贞直上,肩胛岗下缘取之),肩

2. 灸疗:肩井、乳根、曲池、手三里、足三里、阿是穴。

用艾卷温和灸,灸患侧穴位,每穴每次灸5～10分钟,每天灸1～2次。多与针刺,拔火罐配合。

据报道,本病可予膻中穴隔蒜灸5～7壮,至局部潮红,再用右手拇指指尖作分筋,推压,拨动患侧天宗穴(图5—24),手法稍重,反复拨动多次,每天灸、拨2次。结果痊愈43例,显效3例,一例好转。(熊新安.中医杂志,8:

11;1981)。

3. 耳针：取交感、胸、神门、脑、内分泌、下屏尖(肾上腺)。

强刺激，每次取4～5穴，留针20～30分钟，配合局部按摩，每日1次。

4. 刺血疗法：在患者背部第七颈椎以下至第十二胸椎以上的部位，寻找直径为0.5厘米的红疹(指压红疹颜色不褪，稀疏散在，数量不等)。对所有红疹及其周围皮肤进行常规消毒后，再用三棱针刺破红疹，以手挤压，使之出血少许。

有报道，在背部第四胸椎至第十一胸椎间，旁开5寸的范围内进行挑治，右挑左侧，左挑右侧。方法：消毒后，找出皮下出血点，如无可摩擦皮肤，使之红晕，针挑最红处，以出血为度，进针2分深，1次挑1～3处即可。适宜于早期，每天挑治1次，可连续2～3次，(李一卿.赤脚医生杂志,2:30;1977)。

SECTION 3 DISEASES OR SYNDROMES IN DERMATOLOGY, SURGERY AND TRAUMATOLOGY

1. ACUTE MASTITIS

Manifestations

Acute mastitis, belonging to Ru Yong (乳痈, breast abscess) in TCM, is manifested clinically mainly by redness, swelling, heat and pain of the breast, lump in the breast which is tender, accompanied by fever, aversion to cold, poor appetite at early stage. if the inflammation is aggravated the abscess may be formed and even broken. Treatment with acupuncture and moxibustion is comparatively effective to the disease at early stage.

Treatment by Applying Acubustion Techniques

(1) Filiform Needling

Selection of Points

Jianjing (GB 21). Rugen (ST 18), Danzhong (RN 17), Zusanli (ST 36), Neiguan (PC 6).

Methiod

Three to five points are employed each treatment session. With beginning, Zusanli (ST 36) is punctured with uniform reinforcing — reducing manipulation to prevent needling fainting. Then, a needle is inserted into Jianjing (GB 21) to a depth of 0.5 — 0.8 cun, and reducing manipulations by twisting, lifting and thrusting the needle and by manipulating the needle in cooperation with the patient's respiration are applied. On puncturing at Jianjing (GB 21), the patient is asked to massage the affected region in cooperation. According to the patient's condition, some other points may be employed, and reducing manipulations by twisting, lifting and thrusting the needle are applied. At Jianjing (GB 21) and Rugen (ST 18), no deep puncture is allowed, and at Rugen (ST 18), the needle should be pushed obliquely upwards or horizontally upwards for 0.3 — 0.5 cun. Generally, the needles are retained at each point for thirty to sixty minutes and manipulated per five to ten minutes during the retention. The treatment is given once daily or twice daily for severe cases.

Introducing An Experiential Technique

In Collection of Experiences of Acupuncture & Moxibustion another method is recommended. In this method, two groups of points are selected. The first group, i. e. the double points group, includes Jianzhen (SI 19, 1 cun above the posterior end of the axilla transverse crease appearing when the upper arm being at abduct) and Tianzong (SI 11), botn of them being at the affected side. On puncturing at them, the patient is askded to sit down or lie on one side if the patient has high fever, two needles 2 — 2.5 cun long are inserted perpendicularly into these points, and reducing manipulations and strong stimulation by lifting and thrusting the needle are applied until the patient compalins of soreness, numbness and distension. The needles are retained in the points and attached with moxa sticks burning for thirty to forty minutes, during the retention, the needles being lifted and thrust once per five minutes. It is recorded that most patients treated by this method were cured by applying this treatment once for mild cases and no more than three times for severe cases. The second group, i. e. the single point group, includes, Jianshu, an extra point, at the soft space above Jianzhen (SI 9) and Jianzong (ST 11), and below Naoshu (ST 10), which is above Jianzhen (SI 9) and at the lower border of the spine of scapula, and Jianliao (SJ 14) (See Fig. 5 — 23). On puncturing at the point, the patient is asked to sit down or lie on the healthy side if the patient has high fever, and a 2 — 2.5 cun long needle is inserted into the point at the affected side perpendicularly. Then, reducing manipulations by heavily lifting and thrusting the needle are applied until the patient complains of soreness, numbness and distension, Then, the needle is retained there and attached with moxa stick burning on its handle for thirty ot sixty minutes, during the retention, the needle being lifted and thrust per five minutes.

(2) *Moxibustion*

Selection of Points

Jianjiang (GB 21), Rugen (ST 18), Quchi (LI 11), Shousanli (LI 10), Zusanli (ST 36), tender spots.

Method

Three or four points at the affected side are employed each treatment session, mild warming moxibustion with moxa stick is applied to each point for five to ten minutes, and the treatment is given once or twice daily. Usually, Puncturing or cupping is additionally applied in coordination.

Introducing An Experiential Technique

A method of treatment of acute mastitis by combination of moxibustion and massage is reported in Journal of TCM. Following garlic moxibustion at Danzhong (RN 17) for five to seven cones, usually resulting in reddish skin in the local area, massage is applied to TianZong (SI 11) of the affected side by pushing, pressing and poking the point area with the thumb tip of the right hand (See Fig. 5 — 24) forcefully and repeatedly for many times. The treatment by moxibustion and massage is given twice daily and for a week as a course. It was recorded that among 47 cases treated by this method 43 cases were cured, 3 cases markedly improved and one case improved within one course.

(3) *Otopuncture*
Selection of Otopoints
Sympathetic, Shenmen, Brain, Endocrine, Adrenal Gland.

Method
Four or five otopoints are employed each treatment session, strong stimulation is applied, the needles are retained at each point for twenty to thirty minutes, and massage over the local area is applied additionally in coordination. The treatment is given once daily and for ten sessions as a course.

(4) *Pricking to Cause Bleeding*
Selection of Points and Method
Look for red rushes, which are 0.5 cm at diameter, discoloured by pressing with the finger, and on the back below the level of the 7th cervical vertebra and above the level of the 12th thoracic vertebra. Then, give local and routine sterilization to the rush areas, prick the rushes with the three—edged needle and press and squeeze them to cuase slight bleeding.

Introducing An Experiential Technique
Another breaking method for treatment of acute mastitis at the early stage is reported in Journal for Bare—Foot Doctor. The subcutaneous hemorrhage spots at the back below the 4th thoracic vertebra and above the 11th thoracic vertebra, between the posterior median line and the line 5 cun lateral to the posterior median line at the healthy side are looked for and taken as breaking spots. If the spots are not found, the skin at the region is scraped and rubbed until areolae are caused and the reddest point is taken as pricking region. The spots selected are pricked with the three edged needle to cause bleeding. One to three spots are pricked at each treatment session, and the treatment is given once daily and for two or three days.

二、多发性疖肿

多发性疖肿，好发于项背臀部等处，由几个到数十个不等，初起局部皮肤潮红、肿痛、范围局限，有的上面有一黄白色脓头，有的并无脓头，成脓溃破后即自行痊愈。此起彼伏，反复发作，缠绵不愈。

技法运用

1.挑治法：在背部肩胛间部及肩胛下角区寻找红疹，其形如针头大小，初起为充血点，压之褪色；中期压之不褪色，为鲜红色；末期为褐色。用三棱针或圆利针挑破红点，一般1～3个，每周2次。

2.毫针：大椎、曲池、合谷、外关、足三里、风池、身柱、灵台、委中。

用捻转提插泻法，留针15～30分钟，每日1次。其中委中穴以放血为主。

有报道，用直径1.2毫米，长72毫米的粗针，取神道（第五胸椎棘突下）透至阳，配合大椎、命门。患者端坐于板凳上，双手半握拳，屈肘交叉，放在两臂上，肩下垂，头部尽量下低，以便背部皮肤拉紧，充分暴露椎体棘突，以便取穴。方法：皮肤常规消毒，医生左手固定棘突上缘皮肤，右手持针以30°角快速刺入皮下，继而将针压低贴近皮肤，针尖在皮下沿棘突中线缓缓向下刺进（图5—25）。神道进针55毫米，大椎，命门进针40毫米。针的方向和脊柱中线平行，切忌歪向一侧。留针1～6小时，每日1次，10次为1疗程。2099例疔疮，疖肿，痈,治愈率96%(全国高等中医院校函授教材《针灸学》,1987年)。

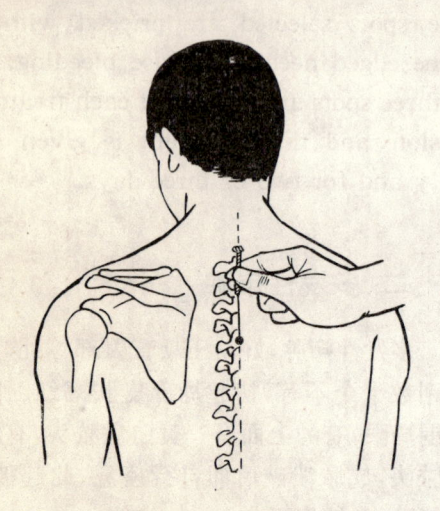

图5—25 神道刺法
Fig. 5—25 Puncturing at Shendao (DU 11)

2. MULTIPLE BOILS

Manifestations

Multiple boils refer to several or several tens of boils occurring frequently in the nape, back, and buttock. At the early stage the boil is manifested by local redness, swelling and pain. The boil may have a yellow and purulent head or not, and may be spontaneously curable throngh diabrosis. The disease is multiple, repeatedly proxysmal and obstinate.

Treatment by Applying Acubustion Techniques

(1) *Pricking*

Selection of Points and Method

Lood for red rushes, whick are like needle head in size, at the upper back. The rush, at the early stage, is a congestion spot and discoloured by pressing. At the middle stage, it becomes bright red and not discoloured by pressing. At the last stage, it becomes brown. prick one to three rushes with the three—edged needle or round—sharp needle at each treatment session, and give the treatment twice per week.

(2) *Filiform Needling*

Selection of Points

Dazhui (DU 14), Quchi (LI 11), Hegu(LI 4), Waiguan (SJ 5), Zusanli(ST 36), Fengchi(GB 20), Shenzhu(DU 12), Lingtai(DU 10), Weizhong(BL 40).

Method

Three to five points are employed each treatment session, reducing manipulations by twisting, lifting, and thrusting the needle are applied, and the needles are retained at each point for fifteen to thirty minutes. Then, Weizhong (BL 40) is pricked to cause bleeding. The treatment is given once daily and for a week as a course.

Introducing An Experiential Technique

A good method is recommended here, by which an effective rate of 96% in treatment of 2099 cases with boil, ulcer and carbuncle was reported to be achieved. Shendao (DU 11, below the spinal process of the 5th thoracic vertebra) is taken as the main point, and Dazhui(DU 14) and Mingman(DU 4) as the adjuvant points. To the operation, the patient is asked to sit with loose fists, to keep the elbows at flexion, to place the left fist on the right shlouder and vice versa, to keep the shoulders at natural position, and to lower the head as far as possible, so as to expose the spinal processes of the vertebrae fully and to make a good condition for selecting the points. After local and routine sterilization is given, the skin at the upper border of the spinal process is fixed with the left hand, a needle 1.2 mm in diameter and 72 mm in length is slowly inserted into Shendao (DU 11) at an angle of 30° to the skin (See Fig. 5—25). Then, the needle is pushed horizontally towarads along the posterior median line for 55 mm, with the penetration needling towards Zhiyang (DU 9), Dazhui (DU 14) and Mingman (DU 4) are punctured with the same way but just with the needles pushed for 40 mm. The treatment is given once daily and for ten sessions as a course.

三、神经性皮炎

神经性皮炎，属中医学"牛皮癣"范畴。临床表现，多好发于颈项部，其次为骶部，四肢内侧等处。初起局部搔痒、后出现扁平圆形或多角形丘疹，肤色呈浅褐色，丘疹密集成群，日久融合成片，呈苔藓样，局部皮肤肥厚干燥，病程缓慢，易于复发。

技法运用

1. 皮肤针

在皮损局部进行经纬形叩刺，每条刺激线相距约0.5厘米（图5—26），每条线反复叩刺3次，或在皮损局部由外向内围刺，以出血为度。另外，在脊柱两侧常规刺激，每日1次或隔日1次。亦可皮肤针重扣患处出血，加拔火罐。

2. 耳针：肺、神门、下屏尖、脑、肝穴。

每次取4～5穴，中等刺激，留针1小时，每日1次。亦可配合耳背静脉，用三棱针刺血。

3. 灸疗：阿是穴（皮损局部）

用艾条温和灸法，每次灸30分钟。

有报道，于皮损处涂以蒜汁，上置小艾炷，点燃施灸，每炷间距15厘米，待艾炷燃尽，除去艾灰，覆盖消毒纱布即可。一般灸1～3次，有明显效果（田丛豁，等.《针灸医学验集》）。

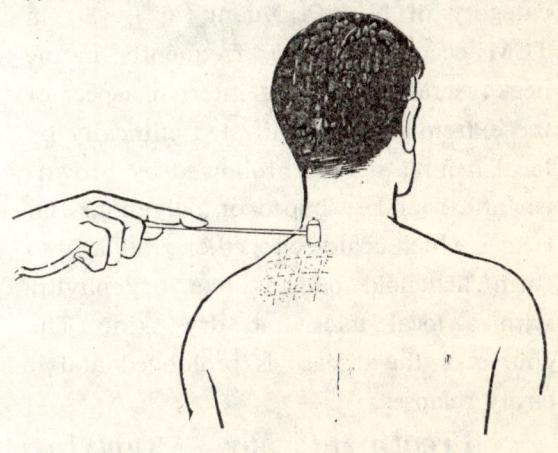

图5—26 经纬叩法
Fig. 5—26 Tapping for Neurodermatitis

4. 毫针：取曲池、血海、三阴交、合谷、阿是穴。

用平补平泻法或捻转提插泻法，留针15分钟，每日1次。局部阿是穴沿病灶基底部皮下，从四方向中心横刺数针。

有人取委中、风门为主，治神经性皮炎。上肢配曲池；面部配合谷、迎香；下肢配风市、三阴交或血海；胸腹及两胁配足三里，阳陵泉。委中用捻转手法，短促行针；针风门时，医者左手拇食两指将风门部位皮肤捏起，右手持针快速刺入皮下后，向肺俞方向沿皮透刺1～1.5寸，留针1～2小时，进针与留针期间均不用其他手法，阳陵泉、足三里均沿皮刺1～1.5寸，曲池向手三里沿皮透刺1.5～2寸，合谷向三间方向沿皮透刺1～1.5寸，迎香向四白方向沿皮透刺0.5～1寸，手法及行针均同风门。留针期间，用艾条灸烤瘙痒重点部位，1日1次，7次1疗程（孙学全.《针灸临证集验》）。

3. NEURODERMATITIS

Manifestations

Neurodermatitis, belonging to disease category of Neu Pi Xuang (牛皮癣) in TCM, occurring mostly frequently in the neck, sacral region, and internal aspect of the extremities, is manifested clinically by local itching at onset, followed by brownish and round — shaped or polygonal flat rushes which coalesce together gradually to form lichenoid patches like bryophyte, with a local thick and dry skin. The course of the disease is prolonged and it easily relapses.

Treatment by Applying Acubustion Techniques

(1) Tapping with the Skin Needle

Selection of Points and Method

Select several lines at the affected region, some of them being perpendicular and some horizontal, the distance between two parallel and near lines being 0.5 cm (See Fig. 5—26). Tap each line for three times at each treatment session. Or give surrounding tapping on the affected region towards its center to cause bleeding. Besides, tap the bilateral sides of the spinal coloum or apply cupping after tapping at the affected region to cause bleeding. The treatment is given once daily or once every other day.

(2) Otopuncture

Selection of Otopoints

Lung, Shenmen, Adrenal Gland, Brain, Liver.

Method

Four or five otopoints are employed each treatment session, medium strength stimulation is applied, and the needles are retained at each point for one hour. Or, in coordination, the veins at the posterior auricle are pricked with the three — edged needle to cause bleeding additionally. The treatment is given once daily and for ten sessions as a course.

(3) Moxibustion

Selection of Points

Affected area (Ashi point).

Method

Mild — warming moxibustion with moxa stick is applied to the affected area for thirty minutes each treatment session. The treatment is given once daily and for ten sessions as a course, the next course beginning after an interval of one week.

Introducing An Experiential Technique

The following method recorded in Collection of Experiences of Acupuncture & Moxibustion is said to be markedly effective to neurodermatitis. The skin at the affected region is smeared with garlic jiuce, and several moxa cones are placed over the skin, each of the cones being 15 cm away from the near one, and ignited for moxibustion. After burning, the skin is cleaned and covered with sterilized cloth. Generally, a markedly effect will be achieved by one to three treatment sessions.

(4) Filiform Needling

Selection of Points

Quchi (LI 11), Xuehai (SP 10), Sanyinjiao (SP 6), Hegu (LI 4), tender spots.

Method

Three or four points are employed

each treatment session, uniform reinforcing—reducing manner or reducing manipulations by lifting, thrusting and twisting the needle are applied, and the needles are retained at each point for fifteen minutes. Additionally, several points at the perifocal area are taken as Ashi points and punctured with the needle tips inserted and pushed horizontally towards the focal center. The treatment is given once daily and for ten sessions as a course, the next course beginning after an interval of a week.

Introducing An Experiential Technique

In Collection of Clinical Experiences of Acupuncture & Moxibustion the following method for treatment of neurodermatitis is recorded. Weizhong(BL 40) and Fengmen(BL 12) are taken as the main points. The supplementary points are selected according to the location of the disease. If the disease is located at the face, Hegu(LI 4) and Yingxiang (LI 20) are added; if it is at the upper limb, Quchi (LI11) is added; if it is at thd lower limb, Fengshi(GB 31) and Sanyinjiao(SP 6) or Xuehai(SP 10) are added; if it is at the chest and abdomen as well as hypochondriac regions, Zusanli(ST 36) and Yanglingquan(GB 34) are punctured additionally. On puncturing at Weizhong(BL 40), twisting and rotating method with quick manner is applied. On puncturing at Fengmen(BL 12), the skin at the point area is pinched by the thumb and index finger of the left hand and a needle held by the right hand is quickly inserted into the point horizontally with the penetration needling towards Feishu(BL 13) for 1.5 cun and retained for one to two hours. On puncturing at Yanglingquan(GB 34) and Zusanli(ST 36), the needles are punctured horizontally for 1.5 cun. On puncturing at Quchi (LI 11), a needle is insertde and pushed horizontally towards Shousanli(LI 10) for 1.5—2 cun. On puncturing at Hegu (LI 4), a needle is pushed with penetration needling towards Ssnjian(LI 3) for 1—1.5 cun. On puncturing at Yingxiang(LI 20), a needle is pushed beneath the skin with penetration needling towards Sibai (ST2) for 0.5—1 cun. The manipulations applied to the points are like that at Fengmen(BL 12). During the retention of the needles, moxibustion is given to the itching area. The treatment is given once daily and for seven days as a course, the next course beginning after an interval of one week rest.

四、湿 疹

湿疹,常发于耳部,阴囊部及肘窝,膝窝。临床表现为局部皮肤奇痒,反复发作,急性多呈红斑,丘疹,水疱,糜烂,渗液,结痂,最后脱屑而愈;慢性多由急性湿疹转变而来,皮肤增厚,皮损局限而边缘清楚,皮纹加深,可呈苔藓样变。常可呈急性发作。

技法运用

1.毫针:取曲池、血海、三阴交、大椎、足三里、合谷穴。

急性者用捻转提插泻法,慢性者用平补平泻法,留针30分钟,每日1次。

有人取主穴曲池、环跳、阳陵泉。面部配合谷,头部配外关;腰背部配委中;胸腹部配足三里,血海。环跳直刺1.5~3寸,用提插手法;委中直刺0.5~0.8,用捻转手法。两穴均短促行针。曲池沿皮向手三里透刺,阳陵泉向下沿皮透刺1~1.5寸,此四穴均留针1~2小时,留针期间用艾条灸曲池,血海,阳陵泉各10~20分钟,1日治疗1次(孙学全.《针灸临证集验》)。

2. 灸疗:取曲池、血海、三阴交、大椎、足三里、阿是穴(即奇痒处)。

用艾卷温和灸或回旋灸,每穴每次灸20分钟,每日1次。亦可用艾炷灸,每穴灸3~5壮,每日1次。

3. 耳针:取肺、肝、神门、下屏尖、脑、屏间、脾穴。

每次取3~4穴,捻转强刺激,留针2小时左右,中间捻针数次,每日1次,10~12次为1疗程。

4. 穴位注射:采用维生素B_{12} 0.1毫克,分注于双侧足三里、曲池,每日1次,10次为1疗程(孙梅倩,等.中国针灸,3:45;1986)。

4. ECZEMA

Manifestations

Eczema, occurring frequently in the auricle, scrotum, cubital fossa and popliteal fossa, is manifested clinically by repeated attack of local severe itching. At the acute stage, erythema, rush, blister, exudate, scar, and desquamation which leads to cure are usually accompanied. At the chronic type, which is usually from the acute one, thick skin, obvious border of the limited lesion, deep skin crease, and lichenois patches may be seen. Acute attack may be seen at the chronic type.

Treatment by Applying Acubustion Techniques

(1) *Filiform Needling*

Selection of points

Quchi (LI 11), Xuehai (SP 10), Sanyinjiao (SP 6), Dazhui (DU 14), Zusanli (ST 36), Hegu (LI 4).

Method

Three to five points are employed each treatment session, reducing manipulations by twisting, rotating, lifting and thrusting the needle are applied to acute cases, and uniform reinforcing — reducing manner is applied for chronic cases. The needles are retained at each point for thirty minutes. The treatment is given once daily and for seven sessions as a course, the next course beginning after an interval of one week rest.

Introducing An Experiential Technique

The following method for treatment of eczema is recorded in Collection of Clinical Experiences of Acupuncture & Moxibustion. Quchi (LI 11), Huantiao (GB 30), and Yanglingquan (GB 34) are taken as the main points. The supplementary points selected according to location of the affected area include Hegu (LI 4) for the disease at the face, Waiguan (SJ 5) for that at the hand, Weizhong (BL 4) for that at the upper and lower back, and Zusanli (ST 36) and Xuehai (SP 10) for that at the chest and abdomen. On puncturing at Huantiao (GB 30), a needle is pushed perpendicularly 1.5—3 cun deep, and lifting and thrusting manipulations are chosen. At Weizhong (BL 40), a needle is pushed perpendicularly 0.5—0.8 cun, and twisting and rotating manner is employed. Short and swift manner is performed at these two points. On puncturing at Quchi (LI 11), a needle is inserted and then penetrating needling towards Shousanli(LI 10) is performed. On puncturing at Ynaglingquan(GB 34) a needle is pushed downwards beneath the skin for 1—1.5 cun. The needles at these four points are retained for one to two hours. During the retention, moxibustion is given to Quchi (LI 11), Xuehai (SP 10) and Yanglingquan (GB 34) respectively for ten to twenty minutes. The treatment is given once daily and for seven days as a course.

(2) *Moxibustion*
Selection of Points
Quchi (LI 11), Xuehai (SP 10), Sanyinjiao(SP 6), Dazhui(DU 4), Zusanli(ST 36), the most itching points.
Method
Three or five points are employed each treatment session, mild—warming or circling moxibustion is applied to each point for twenty minutes, and the treatment is given once daily and for ten sessions as a course. Or, moxibustion with moxa cone is applied to each point for three to five cones, and the treatment is given once daily and for ten times as a course.

(3) *Otopuncture*
Selection of Otopoints
Lung, Liver, Shenmen, Adrenal Gland, Brain, Endocrine, Spleen.
Method
Three or four otopoints are employed each session, twisting and rotating manipulations are appllied, strong stimulation is administered, and the needles are retained at each otopoint for two hours and twisted several times during the retention. The treatment is given once daily and for ten to twenty sessions as a course, the next course beginning after an interval of one week rest.

(4) *Hydro—Puncture*:
Selection of Points
Bilateral Zusanli(ST 36)and Quchi (LI 11).
Method
0.1 mg of vitamin B 12 is injected into each point at one treatment session, and the treatment is given once daily and for ten sessions as a course, the next course beginning after an interval of one week rest.

五、荨麻疹

荨麻疹,中医学称为"瘾疹","风疹块"。临床表现为皮肤上突然出现大小不等、形状不一,高出皮肤,白色或粉红色的片块,界限清楚,剧烈瘙痒,散在出现,此起彼伏,重者可融合成片,遍及全身,可出现发热、恶寒、腹泻、腹痛、恶心等全身症状。慢性者,反复发作,缠绵不断。

技法运用

1. 毫针:曲池、血海、三阴交、风市、足三里、风池、大椎、合谷、阴陵泉。

用捻转提插泻法,每次取4~6穴,留针30分钟,每日1次。

2. 耳针:神门、肺、脾、下屏尖、脑、屏间、下脚端。

强刺激,每次取3~4穴,留针2小时左右,每日1次。亦可耳穴贴压王不留行籽或绿豆,每日按压2~3次,左右两耳交替使用。

有人取耳穴①肺、小肠、内分泌(屏间)②心、大肠、肾上腺(下屏尖)。取单侧耳穴两组交替使用。痒甚加腮腺,即平喘穴(对耳屏边缘的中点)内侧,枕。疗效慢则耳背放血 2～3 滴。用 5 分毫针刺入穴位,留针 30 分钟,每 10 分钟捻针 1 次,隔日 1 次,或用揿针埋入耳穴,胶布固定,每日按压数次,2～5 日取针,间隔 1～2 日再取对侧。(张和嫒.《贵阳中医学院学报》1：41,1987)。

3. 灸疗：取穴同毫针。

用艾条温和灸或回旋灸,每次每穴灸 15 分钟,亦可用艾炷灸,每穴灸 5～8 壮。每日 1 次。

4. 皮肤针：背部夹脊(颈椎至尾骶部)或取风池、血海、风门、委中、肺俞、三阴交穴。使用中度刺激。

5. 拔罐：有报道,采用神阙穴拔罐治疗荨麻疹。用一枚大头针扎入塑料盖,将酒精棉球插到大头针上并点燃,立即将玻璃瓶罩在上面(图 5—27),待吸力不紧后取下,连续拔 3 次,每日 1 次,3 日为 1 疗程(刘天峰.中医杂志,12：43,1986)。

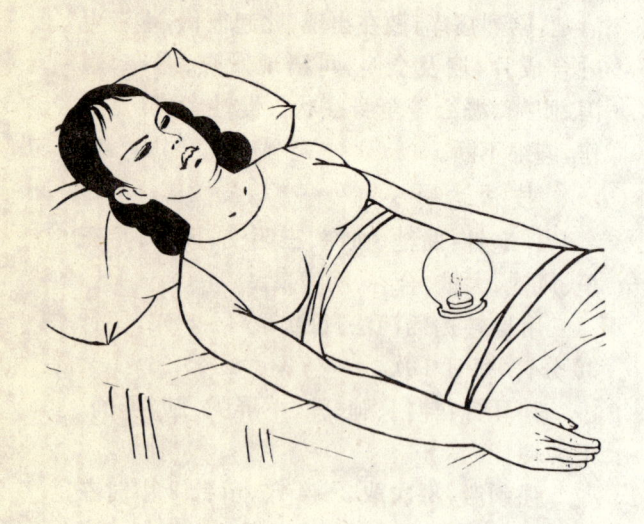

图 5—27 拔罐
Fig. 5—27 Cupping

6. 刺血：大椎、血海。疹发于上肢加曲池；疹发于下肢加风市、委中；疹发于背部加膈俞、风门。方法：先在局部按揉,使其达到红润充血,常规消毒,然后用三棱针点刺,当血溢出,速用闪火法将玻璃火罐吸附在穴位上,并左右旋转,使出血量增加,留罐 15 分钟,隔日 1 次。7 次为 1 疗程(刘志国.上海针灸杂志,3：46；1987)。

5. URTICARIA

Manifestations

Urticaria, termed Yin Zheng, (瘾疹 hidden rush)or Feng Zheng Kuai, (风疹块 wind wheal) in TCM, is manifested clinically by sudden onset with appearance of skin lesions, which are white or pink pitches of varying size or shape with sharply defined edge, raised above the surrounding skin surface, and awful itching. Usually, it occurs simply and rises one after another, but, in severe cases the lesions may coeleace and spread to the whole body, accompanied with general symptoms such as fever, nausea, diarrhea, abdominal pain and aversion to cold. In chronic cases, it may repeatedly occur and have not been cured for a long time.

Treatment by Applying Acubustion Techniques

(1) *Filiform Needling*

Selection of Points

Quchi (LI 11), Xuehai (SP 10), Sanyinjiao (SP 6), Fengshi (GB 31), Zusanli (ST 36), Fengchi (GB 20), Dazhui (DU 14, Hegu (LI 4), Yinlingquan (SP 9).

Method

Four to six points are employed each treatment session, reducing manipulations by twisting, rotating, lifting and thrusting the needle are applied, and the needles are retained at each point for thirty minutes. The treatment is given once daily and for ten times as a course.

(2) *Otopuncture*

Selection of Points

Shenmen, Lung, Spleen, Adrenal Gland, Brain, Endocrine, Sympathetic.

Method

Three or four otopoints are employed each treatment session, strong stimulation is administered, and the needles are retained at each point for two hours. The puncture treatment is given once daily and for ten sessions as a course. Or, the vaccaria seeds or green beans are stuck over the otopoints selected at the one auricle, kept there for three or four days, and pressed two or three times daily. Then, the otopoints at the other aurcle are selected. The two auricle are selected alternately.

Introducing An Experiential Technique

The following method for treatment of urticaria is recommended by Dr. Zhang Heyuan. Two groups of otopoints are selected. The first group includes Lung, Small Intestine, and Endocrine, and the second includes Heart, Large Intestine and Adrenal Gland. The two groups of otopoints at the same side are employed alternately. If the patient complains of awful itching, Ot. Parotid Gland, which is interior to Ot. Soothing Asthma, and Ot. Occiput are added. If the needling effect is achieved slowly, the back of the auricle is pricked additionally to cause two or three drops of bloodletting. The otopoints are punctured with the 0.5 cun long needles, and the needles are retained at each point for thirty minutes and twisted once per ten minutes during the retention. The treatment is given once every other day and for seven sessions as a course. Or, the thumb—tack needles are embedded into the otopoints and fixed with adhesive plaster and pressed several times daily. After embedment for two to five days, the needles are removed, and one or two days later, the otopoints at the opposite side are employed for embedment of the needle.

(3) *Moxibustion*

Selection of Points

The same as in the filiform needling.

Method

Three to five points are employed each treatment session, mild—warming or circling moxibustion with moxa stick is applied to each point for fifteen minutes. Or, moxibustion with moxa cone is performed to each point for five to eight cones. The treatment is given once daily and for seven days as a course.

(4) *Tapping*

Areas and Points to Be Tapped

Jiaji (Ex—B2, the portion of it from the cervical vertebra to the caudal region), Fengchi (GB 20), Xuehai (SP 10), Fengmen (BL 12), Weizhong (BL 40), Feishu (BL 13), Sanyinjiao (SP 6).

Method

Jiaji (E—B2) and some other two to four points are tapped each treatment session, and medium strength stimulation is applied.

(5) *Cupping*

Selection of Points

Shenque (RN 8).
Method

A glass bottle and a plastic lid in which a pin is inserted are selected. The lid is placed on the point, an alcohol cotton ball is attached around the pin and ignited. Immediately, the glass bottle is covered over the lid (See Fig. 5 — 27) for cupping. when the bottle is socked loosely, it is removed. The procedure is repeated three times. The treatment is given once daily and for three days as a course.

(6) *Pricking to Cause Bleeding*
Selection of Points

Main points: Dazhui (DU 14), Xuehai (SP 10).

Supplementary points according to the location of the disaese: Quchi (LI 11) for the disease at upper limb, Fengshi (GB 31) and Weizhong (BL 40) for that at the lower limb, and Geshu (BL 17) and Fengmen (BL 12) for that at the upper back.

Method

At first, massge is performed over the local affected area to cause congestion and routine and local sterilization is given. Then, the points selected are pricked with the three—edged needle. When bleeding is caused by pricking, cupping with the glass bottles to the points is applied, and the bottles are turned left and right to cause bleeding more, and retained at each point for fifteen minutes. The treatment is given once every other day and for seven sessions as a course.

六、带状疱疹

带状疱疹属中医学"蛇丹"范畴。初起皮肤发热灼痛，继则出现密集成簇的绿豆至黄豆大小的丘状疱疹，迅速变成小水疱。三五成群集聚一处或数处，排列成带状，疼痛剧烈，严重时可出现血点、血疱。好发于身体的一侧，以腰肋部、胸部多见，面部次之。

技法运用

1. 毫针：曲池、合谷、血海、三阴交、太冲。

进针得气后，用捻转提插泻法，留针20～30分钟，上穴交替运用，每次2～3穴，每日1次。也可配合局部围刺，即在疱疹连结成块的周围，经皮肤消毒后，用一寸长毫针沿皮刺向成块疱疹的中心，针数的多少，随患处面积大小而定，每针相距1～2寸为宜，留针1～2小时，轻症每日1次，重症每日2次。

有人治右胸带状疱疹，取太冲，阳陵泉，血海，曲池，内关，右胸3～5华陀夹脊穴。方法：先取双侧太冲穴，以提插泻法为主，结合捻转，得气后即出针，再令病人俯卧位，取四肢穴，得气后施行提插捻转法。刺激量以病人适宜为度。留针30分钟。与此同时，取右侧胸挟脊在脊椎棘突旁开0.5寸处进针，深度为1.5寸～1.8寸，力求针感放射至病所，然后在夹脊穴与同侧的曲池穴，接上G6805治疗仪，通电30分钟，电流强度以病人能忍受为度（居贤水. 上海针灸杂志，1：23；1984）。

2. 灸疗：①于皮疹的两端及分叉处，施行艾炷直接灸，灸量为患者灼热感以能忍受为度。此法宜于成人皮疹宜放置艾炷的部位。②沿皮疹之大小，施行艾条旋熨热灸，灸量以皮疹周围正常皮肤红晕为度，时间约20～30分钟。此法宜于小儿或皮疹位置不宜放置艾炷的部位（封爱莲，等. 广西中医药，2：13；1986）。

有人用棉花灸治疗带状疱疹。方法：取微薄一层棉花，越薄越好，不要人为的将厚棉压成薄棉片，薄棉片中切勿有空隙和洞眼，以免影响烧灸疗效。患者要暴露患部，棉片按病损区大小复盖在疱疹上,一切就绪后,令患者闭目,用火柴点燃一端灸之(图258)。患者只感觉有一过性轻微烧灼痛,无须任何处理。每日灸烧1次,最多4次(王松荣.第一届世界针灸学术大会《针灸论文摘要选编》;1987)。

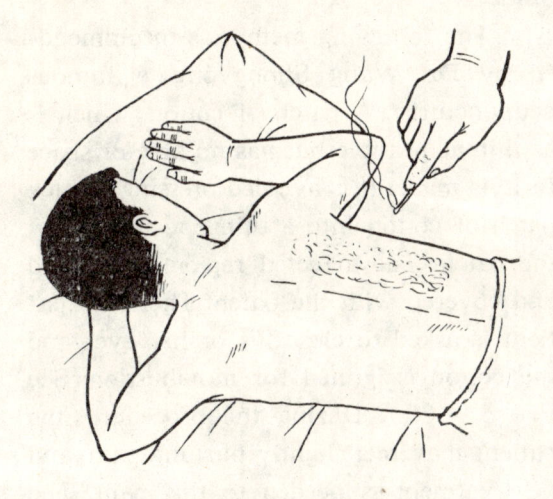

图 5—28 棉花灸
Fig. 5—28 Cotton Attaching Moxibustion

3.梅花针:病变局部常规消毒后,用梅花针叩刺疱疹及周边皮肤,以刺破疱疹,疱内流出液体,病变边缘皮肤变赤为度。部分患者针刺病变区相应节段之华陀夹脊穴。每日1次,重症可每日2次(李淑芹.中国针灸,5:10;1987)。

6. HERPES ZOSTER

Manifestations

Herpes zoster, belonging to disease categorye of She Dang (蛇丹) in TCM, occurs mainly in the lumbar and hypochnodriac regions, and chest. Sometimes, it may occur at the face. At the onset, there are heat and burning pain of the affected skin, on which patches of blisters in the size of mump — bean or soybean are evolved, forming a bandlike distribution with learcut interspace between the patches and causing severe pain. Bleeding spots and bloody bulla may be seen in the affected region at severe cases.

Treatment by Applying Acubustion Technique

(1) *Filiform Needling*

Selection of Points

Quchi (LI 11), Hegu (LI 4), Xuehai (SP 10), Sanyinjaio (SP 6), Taichong (LR 3).

Method

The points are employed alternately and two or three points selected each treatment session. On puncturing, after arrival of qi, reducing manipulations by twisting, rotating, lifting and thrusting the needle are employed, and the needles are retained at each point for twenty to thirty minutes. Or, surrounding puncture at the affected region is applied additionally in coordination. To the operation, following local and routine sterilization, several points around the patches are punctured with the one cun long needle insered horizontally and pushed along the skin towards the center of the patch, the distance between two neighboring points to be inserted being 1—2 cun, and the needles are retained at each point for one to two hours. The treatment is given once daily for mild cases and twice daily for severe cases, and for seven sessions as a course.

Introducing An Experiential Technique

A method for treatment of herpes zoster at the right chest is recommended in Shanghai Journal of Acupuncture & Moxibustion. Taichong (LR. 3), Ynaglingquan (GB 34), Xuehai (SP 10), Quchi (LI 11), Neiguan (PC 6) and Jiaji(EX—B2, T 3—5 at the affected side) are employed. On puncturing, at beginning, bilateral Taichong (LR 3) are punctured with reducing manipulations by lifting, thrusing and twisting the needle, and the needle is removed after arrival of qi. Then, the patient is asked to lie prone and the points at the extremities are punctured. Following arrival of qi, lifting, thrusting and twisting manners and proper strength stimulation which is tolerable to the patient are performed, and the needles are retained at each point for thirty minutes. Meanwhile, the needles are inserted into Jiaji(EX—B2 T3—5) at the right side to a depth of 1.5—1.8 cun to cause the needling sensation radiating to the affected region. Finally, one lead of G6805 type therapeutic instrument is connected to the ceedle in Quchi (LI 11) at the right side and another to the needle in Jiaji(EX—B2). The electric stimulation tolerable to the patient is applied for thirty minutes.

(2) *Moxibustion*

Selection of Points and Method

For adult cases with herpes zoster at the region where moxa cone can be placed, direct moxibustion with moxa cone is applied to the terminal spot and beginning point of the branches of the lesion, with the hot stimulation tolerable to the patient administered.

For child cases or adult cases with the herpes zoster at the region where a moxa cone can not be placed, circling moxibustion with moxa stick is applied to the affected region for twenty to thirty minutes, causing erythema at the normal skin around the lesion. This method is reported in Guanxi Journal of TCM.

Introducing An Experiential Technique

The following method is recommended by Dr. Wang Shongyong, a famous acupuncturist. A patch of cotton, which is as thin as possible but has no hole or space in it, is made. It is avoided pressing a thick patch of cotton into a thin one in making the patch. The affected region is exposed and covered with the patch. Then, the patient is asked to close his or her eyes and the cotton is ignited for moxibustion (See Fig. 5 — 28). During the procedure, the patient may feel slightly burning pain, and no treatment is needed to this pain. The moxibustion is given once daily and four sessions of the treatment is the maximum.

(3) *Tapping with Plum — Blossom Needle*

Selection of Points

Affected region, Jiaji(EX—B2).

Method

Following the routine and local sterilization, tapping with the plum — blossom needle is applied to the plisters and the skin surrounding the lesion until the plisters are broken, the fluid in them flows out and the skin surrounding the affected region is reddened. For some cases, Jiaji(EX — B2) at the corresponding portion is tapped additionally. The treatment is given once daily or twice daily for severe cases.

七、痤　疮

痤疮，好发于青春发育期的男女。临床表

现为黑头粉刺样丘疹,周围色红,用手挤压有小米或米粒样白色脂栓排出,少数为灰白色的小丘疹,以后色红,顶部生有小脓疱,自觉微疼或瘙痒,破溃痊愈,暂时遗留色素沉着或残痕。此起彼伏,缠绵难愈,有的可拖延数年甚至十余年。

技法运用

1. 刺血疗法

(1)耳穴:取内分泌、下屏尖、脑、胃、肺、面颊、额、耳背血管。

(2)体穴:大椎、肺俞、胃俞。

方法:医者以手在应刺部位揉搓数分钟,使其局部充血,皮肤常规消毒后,用三棱针速刺出血,或手术尖刀片割破表皮渗血,用消毒棉球拭去血迹,以后再用消毒棉球或敷料贴盖伤口24小时,以防感染。每次1~3穴,隔日1次。亦可体穴点刺出血后加拔火罐。

2. 毫针:取曲池、合谷、大椎、肺俞、足三里、三阴交。

用平补平泻法,留针20分钟,每日1次。

有人取曲池(双)、合谷(双),捻转进针,中等度刺激,有针感后留针30分钟,行针捻转提插3~4次,每日1次,10次为1疗程。1疗程后,痤疮有收敛者,改隔日1次,一般针3个疗程(李凤波. 中国针灸,4:39;1983)。

3. 耳穴埋针:取内分泌(屏间),用消毒揿针1枚,以针尾在穴位上压深痕作标记,然后在穴区进行常规消毒。待皮肤干后,将揿针紧按在穴区的凹痕上,再用橡皮膏贴在揿针及其周围皮肤上,用手指按压10秒钟加强固定。15天为1疗程,两耳交替进行,埋针期间,每日按揿针3~5次,起针后消毒穴区(史秉才,等. 四川中医,4:53;1986)。

7. ACNE

Manifestations

Acne occurs mainly in persons at adolescence. At the affected region there are rushes with comedo, from which rice—like or millet—like white fat embolus will be excluded by pushing and pressing with the fingers and the skin surrounding the rush is red. But in a few cases there are small rushes with a purulent spot at the head, and mild pain or itching at the affected region, the rushes being greyish and white at beginning and red later. After breaking of the rush, pigmentation or remaining trace is temporarily left. It rises one after another and may not be cured for several years or even more than ten years.

Treatment by Applying Acubustion Techniques

(1) *Pricking to Cause Bleeding*

Selection of Points

Otopoints: Endocrine, Adrenal Gland, Brain, Stomach, Lung, Cheek, Forehead, blood vessels at the posterior auricle.

Acupoints: Dazhui (DU 14), Feishu (BL 13), Weishu (BL 21).

Method

Following twisting the region to be pricked for several minutes to cause local congestion and giving local and routine sterilization, prick the point gently to cause bleeding or break the skin of the point with an operating knife to cause oozing of blood. Then, smear the blood trace with sterilized cotton ball and cover the point with sterilized dress or cotton ball for twenty—four hours to prevent infection. One to three points are employed each treatment session, and the treatment is given once every other day. Or, following pricking the point to cause bleeding, cupping is performed to the pricked point additionally.

(2) *Filiform Needling*

Selection of Points

Quchi(LI 11), Hegu(LI 4), Dazhui (DU 14), Feishu (BL 13), Zusanil (ST 36), Sanyinjiao (SP 6).

Method

Three to five points are employed each treatment session, uniform reinforcing—reducing manipulation is applied, and the needles are retained at each point for twenty minutes. The treatment is given once daily and for seven sessions as a course, the next course beginning after an interval of one week rest.

Introducing An Experiential Technique

The following method is reported in Chinese Acupuncture & Moxibustion. The points to be selected include Quchi(LI 11) and Hegu (LI 4) at the two sides. A needle is inserted into the point with twisting and rotating movements, and medium strength stimulation is administered. After the needling sensation is induced to the patient, the needles are retained at each point for thirty minutes and, during the retention, twisted, rotated, lifted and thrust three or four times. The treatment is given once daily and for ten times as a cours.

(3) *Needle — Embedding in Otopoints*

Selection of Otopoint

Endocrine.

Method

A mark is made with the tail of a sterilized thumb — tack needle on the point, and the routine and local sterilization is given. After the skin is dry, the needle is pressed into the marked spot, and a piece of adhesive plaster is stuck over the needle and the skin surrounding it. Then, the plaster is pressed against skin for ten seconds for consolidation. The needle is kept in the point of one side for fifteen days, during the retention, the needle being pressed three to five times daily, and the point at the other side is employed next time. The points at the two sides are selected alternately. After withdrawal of the needle, the punctured area is sterilized.

八、脱 发

本病分为斑秃和脂溢性脱发两种。斑秃表现为患处头发迅速脱落，呈圆形或椭圆形，斑片大小数目不等，病情进展或发展成全秃；脂溢性脱发为头发稀疏脱落、头皮发痒、皮屑多。

技法运用

1. 梅花针疗法：①局部阿是穴。②第1～7颈椎的两旁与颈椎平行旁开1寸的平行线。③脊椎两侧。

先叩刺颈部及脊柱两侧常规刺激区，还可由耳后通过两侧风池穴向下至后发际横刺2～3排，然后在斑秃局部和头发稀疏脱落部位，由脱发周围向脱发中心区围刺，叩刺至皮肤潮红为度。每日1次，10次为1疗程，间隔一周，再行第二疗程。

2. 毫针：阿是穴、百会、风池、内关、三阴交。

血虚头晕失眠、加足三里、膈俞，用捻转提插补法；血瘀面色晦暗，舌边有瘀点，加血海、合谷，用捻转提插泻法。阿是穴用梅花针叩刺,每日1次。

有报道取风池(针尖斜向下刺入1~1.5寸),后顶(风府穴直上4.5寸,针尖斜向前方刺入0.5~0.8寸)为主穴。前额及两鬓脱发较重,配头维;头部瘙痒较重配大椎;油脂分泌过多配上星(前发际正中直上1寸),留针20分钟。针后均以梅花针雀啄法,斑秃患者在脱发局部以梅花针点刺,每日1次,10次为1疗程。治疗60例,有效率为83.3%(韩之鼎.黑龙江中医药,1:35,1986)。

3.灸疗:阿是穴(脱发周围)。

用艾条温和灸法,在患部上施灸,至皮肤潮红为度。该法一般多在梅花针叩刺后再进行。

8. BALDNESS

Manifestations

Baldness is classified into two types: the alopecia areata and the seborrheic baldness. The former is manifested by alopecia occurring at the affected scalp in a short time and round or elliptic macular patches left with various sizes and number. The latter is manifested by sparse hair and exfoliation of hair, accompanied by itching and many furfures at the scalp.

Treatment by Applying Acubustion Techniques

(1) *Tapping with Plum—Blossom Needle*

Areas to Be Tapped

a. Local Ashi points.

b. Two lines 1 cun lateral to the spinal column from the first to the seventh cervical vertebrae at the two sides.

c. Bilateral sides of the other portion of the spinal column.

Method

At beginning, tap the neck and the regular stimulation area at the back, namely, the bilateral sides of the spinal column. Then, give a surrounding tapping to the affected region from its surrounding area to its center. Apply the tapping method until the local skin and scalp become reddened. The treatment is given once daily and for ten sessions as a course, the next course beginning after an interval of one week.

(2) *Filiform Needling*

Selection of Points

Main points: Ashi points, Baihui (DU 20), Fengchi (GB 20), Neiguan (PC 6), Sanyinjiao (SP 6).

Supplementary points according to symptoms: Zusanli (ST 36) and Geshu (BL 17) for dizziness and insomnea due to blood insufficiency, and Xuehai (SP 10) and Hegu (LI 4) for darkish complexion and ecchymosis at the border of the tongue due to blood stasis.

Method

Three to five points are employed each treatment session. Reinforcing manipulations by twirling, lifting and thrusting the needle are applied for insufficiency of blood, reducing manipulations by twisting, lifting and thrusting the needle are chosen for blood stasis, and tapping with the plum—blossom needle is applied to Ashi points. The treatment is given once daily and for seven days as a course, the next course beginning after an interval of one week.

Introducing An Experiential Technique

In Helongjiang Journal of TCM the

following methods for treatment of baldness are reported. Fengchi (GB 20) and Houding (DU 19) are taken as the main points. The supplementary points according to symptoms include Touwei (ST 8) for comparatively severe baldness at the forehead and bilateral temples, Dazhui (DU 14) for itching at the head, and Shangxing (DU 23) for oleaginous hypersecretion in the scalp. On puncturing at Fengchi (GB 20), the needle is inserted obliquely downward 1—1.5 cun deep, on puncturing at Houding (DU 19, 4.5 cun above Fengfu, DU 12), the needle is inserted obliquely and anteriorly for 0.5—0.8 cun. The needles are retained at each point for twenty minutes. Following the needling, tapping with bird — peck needling with plum — blossom needle is given to the affected area. The treatment is given once daily and for ten times as a course. It is reported an effective rate of 83.3% in treatment of 60 cases with the disease was achieved by applying this method.

(3) *Moxibustion*

Selection of Points

Ashi points, i. e. the surrounding area of baldness.

Method

Mild — warming moxibustion is applied to the affected area until the local scalp is reddened. The moxibustion is given usually after tapping at te affected area with the plum—blossom needle.

九、软组织损伤

本病指皮肤、皮下组织、肌肉、肌腱、筋膜、韧带、关节囊、滑膜囊、神经、血管受外伤后而引起的损伤。属于中医学"筋伤"范畴。临床表现为局部软组织疼痛、活动时加剧,少数局部有肿胀或血肿,一般活动受限,局部有压痛。

技法运用

1. 毫针:以受伤的局部或邻近穴位为主,配合相应的远端循经取穴。用平补平泻法。各部位的软组织损伤取穴,可以"关节炎"各部位的取穴作参考。

要求先针远端穴位并嘱患者配合运动,再针局部穴位。亦可在肿胀周围进行皮下浅刺5～6处,以促进血液循环。

有报道针刺加患部运动治疗急性软组织损伤,其中四肢软组织损伤用左右对称配穴法,即在损伤部位的对侧对称部位取穴;前胸撞伤用前后(背腹)对应取穴;肩腰部、颈部扭伤(落枕)用上下相应配穴,针刺期间嘱患者主动或被动运动。一般在运针后3～20分钟,即出现明显的止痛作用,而且治疗1～3次,即疼痛消失而活动正常(何广新.《全国针灸麻学术讨论会论文摘要》,1979)。

有人针刺天柱穴治腰肌劳损300例。方法:患者取坐位,微垂头,术者用拇指及食指压住双侧穴位,点按片刻,以减轻进针时的疼痛,消毒后迅速进针0.5～0.8寸。针尖斜向椎间孔。因此穴进针后局部针感明显,故不施行针刺手法。留针20～30分钟,嘱患者活动腰部。针天柱穴切不可向内上方深刺,以免损伤延髓(何周智.广西中医药,9:30;1986)。

另有报道皮下针刺治疗扭伤。方法:①于扭伤局部或上下5～10寸的经脉上选1～2点,多经络通过时,可每条经脉取一点。②顺着经过受损部位经络的远端选1点,如腰肌劳损,可在小腿的膀胱经上取1点。③受伤局部及循经远端各取1点配合。操作时,垂直快速进针达皮下后改用平刺,针尖朝病灶,沿经脉走行缓慢进针达1.2～1.5寸,不求酸麻胀重感,留针30分钟,必要时留针24小时,胶布固定。起针快速平拔,每日1次,12次为1疗程(郭佳士,等. 浙江中医杂志,1：43；1984)。

2. 拔罐：于受损局部及邻近部位,针后套拔火罐,或皮肤针叩刺局部后拔火罐,每日1次。

3. 耳针：相应耳穴区、神门、脑。

强刺激配合患部运动,留针30分钟左右,并间歇捻转与运动,每日1次。

4. 灸疗：取穴同毫针,施艾卷温和灸或隔姜灸,每穴每次灸15分钟或每穴施艾炷4~6壮,每日1~2次。亦可温针法或针后配合艾灸。

有人用药饼灸治疗软组织损伤100例。方法：选定软组织损伤处最明显的压痛点,作一标记。根据痛处面积的大小配制药饼(生川乌、生草乌各20克、丁香10克、肉桂10克、樟脑40克,共研细末。用时以米醋,调成饼状)。药饼直径一般为1厘米左右,厚度约0.3厘米。然后将药饼敷于痛处,上盖一层纱布并贴上胶布。再固定薰灸器,艾条火头对准药饼薰灸,一次40分钟,每日1次(李明智. 上海针灸杂志,2：25；1990)。

5. 穴位注射："以痛为腧"为原则,循经邻近取穴为辅。首选醋酸确炎舒松—A注射液2.5毫克或5毫克,维生素B_{12} 0.2毫克,0.9%氯化钠注射液2~5毫升,混合摇匀穴位注射。每次选2~4穴,每穴注药2~3毫升,隔日1次,五次为1疗程。间隔休息一周,再进行第二疗程。一般选用5号短针头、长针头两种规格。穴位常规消毒,应用捏笔式快速进针。病变部肌肉丰厚的穴位,垂直进针；病变部位肌肉浅薄的穴位,提插横刺或斜刺进针。针入穴位后,针下有满意针感,回抽针栓无回血,方可注入药液。体虚者慢推药液；体强者快推药液(郁云亚. 上海针灸杂志,1：20；1990)。

9. SOFT TISSUE INJURY

Manifestations

Soft tissue injury refers to injury of skin, subcutaneous tissue, muscle, tendon, fascia, ligament, joint capsule, synovial bursa, nerve, and blood vessel due to trauma. It is manifested clinically by pain of the local soft tissue, aggravated by movement, local distension and swelling or hematoma at a few cases, motor limitation and local tenderness.

Treatment by Applying Acubustion Techniques

(1) *Filiform Needling*

Selection of Points

The points at the injured area and adjacent area are taken as the main points, and the distal points of the involved meridian as the adjuvant. Selection of points for treatment of soft tissue injury at different areas may be referred to that in the filiform needling for arthritis

Method

Three to five points are employed each treatmen session, and uniform reinforcing — reducing manipulation is applied. At first, the distal points are punctured, and at the same time, the patient is asked to move his affected limb, head, or trunk in cooperation. Then, the local points are punctured. Or, five or six spots around the distension and swelling area are punctured shallowly to promote circulation of blood.

Introducing Some Experiential Techniques

Acute soft tissue injury treated by puncture together with movement of the affected portion of the body is reported. If the injury is at the limbs, the corresponding points at the healthy side are selected, i. e. the corresponging points at the left limb are selected for injury at the right limb and vice versa. The correspoinding points at the back and abdomen are employed for injruy at the chest. The points at the lower extremities are selected for sprain at the lower back, shoulder and neck. On puncturing, the patient is asked to move the affected portion of the body or the patient's relative is asked to help the patient to do the movement in cooperation. Marked relief of the pain is achieved usually by manipulating the needles for three to twenty minutes, and elemination of the pain and recovery of normal movement of the affected portion of the body can be achieved through one to three sessions of the treatment.

The following method is reported, by which a satisfactory effect was achieved in treatment of 300 cases with lumbar muscle strain. The patient is asked to sit down with the head slight bending. Bilateral Tianzhu (BL 8) are pressed with the thumb and index finger for a short time to relieve the possible pain to the patient caused by insertion of the needles. After sterilization, the needles are quickly inserted into bilateral Tianzhu (BL 8) for 0.5 — 0.8 cun, with the needle directig the intervertebral foramen and pushed obliquely. No needling manipuilation is needed because a strong needling sensation is always induced by insertion of the needle at the point. The needles are retained for twenty to thirty minutes, and the patient is asked to move the waist during the retention of the needle. Note: on puncturing at Tianzhu (BL 8), the needle tip should not direct the median—superior area and deep puncture is forbidden, otherwise impairment of bulb may occur.

Another method for treatment of sprain is reported in Zhejiang Journal of TCM. To the method, one or two spots at the local area of sprain or at the portion of the involved meridian which is 5—10 cun above or below the injured region or, if several meridians are involved, one spot at each involved meridian is selected as the first group. A distal point of the involved meridian is taken as the second group. For example, if the patient complains of lumbar muscular sprain, a point at the leg, belonging to the Urinary Bladder Meridian, is selected. Additionally, two points respectively located at the local injured area and at the distal area of the involved meridian are selected as the third group. On puncturing, the needle is inserted through the skin perpendicularly and quickly and then pushed horizontally beneath the skin for 1.2—1.5 cun towards the diseased region along the course of the meridian. The needles are retained at each point for thirty minutes or fixed in the points with adhesive plaster and kept there for 24 hours if negcessary. On withdrwing, the needles are removed quickly. During the needling, no soreness, numbness, distension or heaviness is required. The treatment is given once daily and for twelve sessions as a course.

(2) *Cupping*

Selection of Points and Method

Following needling or tapping with seven—star needle at the affected region, cupping is applied over the region once daily and for ten times as a course.

(3) *Otopuncture*

Selection of Points

Corresponding auricular region, Shenmen, Brian.

Method

Strong needling stimulation is applied in cooperation with the patient's movements of the injured region, and the needles are retained at each otopoint for approximately thirty minutes and manipulated intermittently during the retention. The treatment is given once daily and for ten times as a course.

(4) *Moxibustion*

Selection of Points

See "Filiform Needling".

Method

Three to five points are employed each treatment session, mild — warming moxibustion with moxa stick or moxibustion with moxa cone is applied to each point for fifteen minutes or for four to six cones, and the treatment is given once daily or twice daily and for seven sessions as a course. Or, moxibustion with warming needle or moxibustion performed after puncture is applied.

Introducing An Experiential Technique

In Shanghai Jorunal of Acupuncture & Moxibustion it is reported that 100 cases with soft tissue injury were treated by moxibustion with the moxa cone made of maxa and various herb mediciens. To the method, the most tender spot at the injured region is taken as the area to be given with the moxibustion, and a mark is made on it. 20 g of fresh Radix Aconiti, 20 g of fresh Radix Aconiti Kusnezoffii, 10 g of Flos Caryophylli, 10 g of Cortex Cinnamomi, and 40 g of campnor are ground into powder, and the powder is mixed with rice venegar to make many cakes, each of them being approximately 1 cm in daimeter and 0.3 cm thick. One of the cakes is put on the marked point and covered with a layer of gauze and fixed on the skin with adhesive plaster. Then, a fumigation—moxibustion instrument is placed on the affected region with the burning head of the moxa stck directing the cake, and the moxibustion is applied for forty minutes. The treatment is given once daily and for seven sessions as a course.

(5) *Hydro—Puncture*

Selection of Points

The painful spots at the affected region are taken as the main points, and the corresponding points adjacent to the affected area and belong to the involved meridian as the adjuvant.

Drugs to Be Used

2.5 mg or 5 mg of injection triamcinoione A, 0.2 mg of vetamin B12 and 2—5 mg of 0.9% sodium chloride injection are mixed into the fluid for point injection.

Method

Two to four points are employed each treatment session, and 2—3 ml of the fluid are injected into each point. To the operation, following a routine sterilization given to the local area, a No. 5 needle is inserted into the point perpendicularly if the local muscle is aboundant, or horizontally or obliquely if the local muscle is thin. After inducing the satisfactory needling sensation to the patient and finding no bood in the syringe by withdrawing the piston, inject the fluid quickly into the point if the patient is strong or slowly if the patient is weak. The treatment is given once every other day and for five sessions as a course, the next course beginning after an interval of one week rest.

10. GANGLION

Manifestations

Ganglion, belonging to disease categories of Jing Liu (筋瘤) and Rou Liu (肉瘤) in TCM, occurs usually near joints or tendons, especially at dorsal and palmar aspect of the wrist joint, dorsum of the foot, lateral side of the knee, and popliteal fossa. It is manifested by smooth protuberance with no pain or with soreness and forcelessness at the affected region. A full or undulatory sensation is felt by touching it.

Treatment by Applying Acubustion Techniques

(1) *Centro — Square Needling (Scattering Pricking)*

Selection of Points
The affected region.

Method
No. 28 or No. 26 needles are selected. One needle is inserted into the spot at the center of the affected region, and other four needles are respectively inserted into

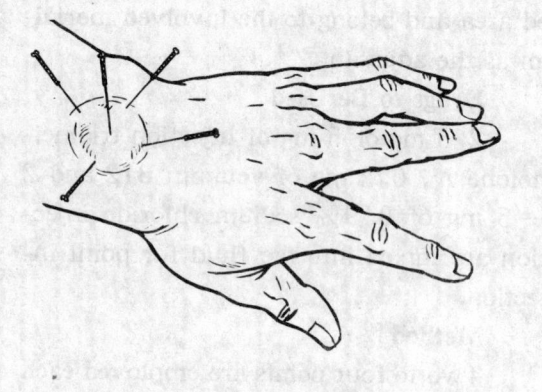

Fig. 5—29 Scattering Pricking for Ganglion

four points which are at the border of the cyst and respectively above, below, left to and right to the center of the cyst (See Fig 5—29). The needles are pushed towards the center of the basis of the cyst and twisted at medium strength. Then, the needles are retained for approximately ten minutes and twisted once during the retention for strengthening the needling sensation. After withdrawal of the needles, the cyst or protuberance is pressed, squeezed or massaged, or moxibustion is applied to it for three cones, cansing local congestion. Or compression bandage is given to it for two or three days. If the protuberance occurs again, the same puncture is applied. Ganglion is usually cured by the treatment for one to five sessions.

Introducing An Experiential Technique

The following method for treatment of ganglion is recommended in Journal of TCM. After local and routine sterilization, the protuberance is punctured with five needles inserted respectively at the center and around it in a square shape as the needles are twisted, and pushed towards the center of the basis of the protuberance until the needle tips reach the cyst wall. Additionally, Waiguan(SJ 5) and Lieque(LY 7) at the affected side are punctured, with the needles inserted obliquely upwards for 0.5—0.7 cun and retained for twenty to thirty minutes and , during the retention, manipulated once per ten minutes. The treatment is given once every other day and for five sessions as a course.

第四节 眼耳鼻咽喉病症

一、鼻 炎

本病主要包括急慢性鼻炎及过敏性鼻炎。急性鼻炎为发热、恶寒、鼻骨作痒、鼻流清涕；慢性鼻炎为鼻塞、鼻流脓涕、鼻粘膜呈慢性充血、肿胀；过敏性鼻炎为阵发性鼻内奇痒、喷嚏、鼻塞、流清水样鼻涕、嗅觉障碍，常在清晨起床时发作。

技法运用

1. 毫针：取迎香、合谷、印堂、上星、风池、足三里、列缺穴。

用平补平泻法，局部与循经取穴相配合。留针20～30分钟，中间捻转行针1～2次，每日1次。

有报道取上迎香穴（鼻翼直上，鼻骨和鼻轮骨结合部图5—30），用"爪切速刺法"，以拇指爪甲紧切其穴，右手持针刺入2分，反复提插3～5次，即将针拔出，使鼻内发痒，打喷嚏，流眼泪。为了巩固疗效，用"透天凉"手法针合谷穴（刘冠军，等.《中国针法集锦》）。

2. 灸疗：取迎香、合谷、印堂、肺俞、足三里、大椎、风池、内关穴。

用艾条温和灸或回旋灸，每次选3～4穴，每穴施灸15～20分钟，每日1次。

3. 耳针：取内鼻、外鼻、肺、下屏尖、额穴。

过敏性鼻炎加屏间。中等刺激，留针20～30分钟，每日一次。并配合耳穴贴压王不留行籽，每日自行按压2～3次。以按至耳部发热或麻胀感或疼痛为度。

4. 指针：①鼻通（又名上迎香）、迎香；②合谷、少商。

①病人取仰卧位，医者位于病人右侧，右手拇指挠侧缘，敷以脱脂棉（防止切伤病人皮肤），切按病人选定的穴位上（鼻通、迎香穴）；拇指伸直，其他手指自然呈半握拳状，逐渐向下用力，病人得气。②用双手拇指指腹敷以脱

脂棉，切按在选定的穴位上（合谷、少商穴），缓慢用力切按，使病人得气。每个穴位切按5分钟，每日1次，两组穴位交替进行，10次1疗程（侯慧先，等．中国针灸 2：42，1990）。

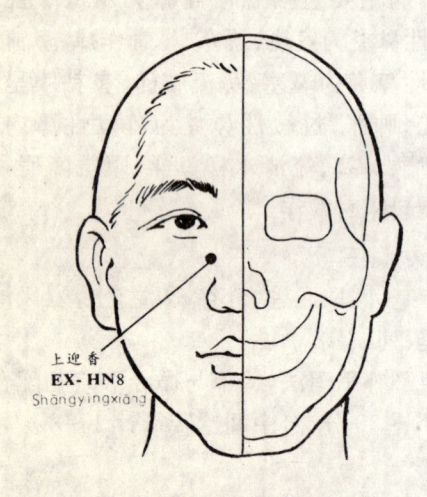

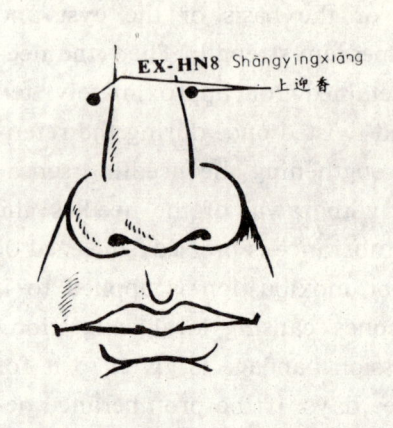

图 5—30 上迎香
Fig. 5—30 Shangyingxiang (EX—HN8)

SECTION 4 DISEASES OF EYES, EARS, NOSE AND THROAT

1. RHINITIS

Manifestations

Rhinitis may be classified into three types: chronic rhinitis, acute rhinitis, and allergic rhinitis. The acute rhinitis is manifested clinically by fever, aversion to cold, itching in the nose, and thin nasal discharge; the chronic rhinitis manifested by nasal obstruction, thick and sticky nasal discharge, and chronic congestion, swelling and distension of the nasal mucosa; and the allergic rhinitis manifested by proxysmal attack, which is ususally at early morning, awful itching in the nose, sneezing, nasal obstruction, watery nasal discharge, and disturbance in smelling.

Treatment by Applying Acubustion Techniques

(1) *Filiform Needling*

Selection of Points

Yingxiang (LI 20), Hegu (LI 4), Yintang (EX — HN3), Shangxing (DU 23), Fengchi (GB 20), Zusanli (ST 36), Lieque (LU 7).

Method

Three to five points are employed each treatment session according to the principle that the local points are selected together with the distal points along the meridian, uniform reinforcing — reducing manner is applied, and the needles are retained at each point for twenty to thirty minutes and twisted one to two times during the retention. The treatment is given once daily and for ten sessions as a course.

Introducing An Experiential Technique

In Collection of Outstandings of the Needling Methods of TCM the following method for treatment of rhinitis is recorded. Shangyingxiang (extra point, above the wing of the nose, at the conjunction of the nasal bone and nasal wheel bone, See Fig. 5—30) is selected. On puncturing, the point is pressed with the nail of the thumb of the left hand, and a needle held by the right hand is inserted into the point to a depth of 0.2 cun. Then, it is repeatedly lifted and thrust for three to five minutes and withdrawh, causing itching of the nose, sneezing, lacrimation to the patient. Additionally, Hegu (LI 4) is punctured with cold — reducing needling to consolidate the needling effect. The treatment is given once daily and for seven days as a cocrse.

(2) *Moxibustion*

Selection of Points

Yingxiang (LI 20), Hegu (LI 4), Yintang (EX—HN2), Feishu (BL 13), Zusanli (ST 36), Dazhui (DU 14), Fengchi (GB 20), Neiguan (FC 6).

Method

Three or four points are employed each treatment session, mild — warming moxibustion or circling moxibustion is applied to each point for fifteen to twenty minutes. The treatment is given once daily and for ten sessions as a course.

(3) *Otopuncture*

Selection of Points

Main points: Interior Nose, Exterior Nose, Lung, Adrenal Gland, Forehead.

Supplementary points according to symptoms: Endocrine for energetic rhinitis.

Method

Three or four otopoints are employed each treatment session, medium strength stimulation is applied and the needles are retained at each otopoint for twenty to thirty minutes. The treatment is given once daily and for ten sessions as a course. Or, additionally, vaccaria seeds are stuck on the otopoints and the patient is asked to press them two or three times daily, inducing distension, numbness, or heat sensation or pain to himself.

(4) *Finger—Pressing Therapy*

Selection of Points

Two groups of points are selected alternately, one including Shangyingxiang (EX—HN8, also termed Bitong), and anoter including Hegu (LI 4) and Shaoshang (LU 11).

Method

One group of points is employed in each treatment session and two groups of the points are selected alternately. To the operation, the patient is asked to lie supine when pressing the points at the face. The point is pressed and pushed by the radial border of the thumb of the right hand, which is covered with sterilized cotton to prevent the patient's local skin form injury during pressing and pushing, and downward pressure with the force being gradually increased is applied to the point when the right thumb is at extension and the othter right fingers at a loose fist, to induce needling sensation to the patient. On pressing the points at the limb, a layer of the sterilized cotton is attached on the abdomens of the thumbs of the left and right hands, and Hegu (LI 4) and Shaoshang (LU 11) are pressed and pushed with the thumbs, with the force acting on the points and gradually increased, inducing the needling sensation to the patient. The pressure with the finger is given to each point selected for five minutes at one treatment session. The treatment is given once daily and for ten sessions as a course.

二、急性扁桃体炎

急性扁桃体炎,中医学称之为"乳蛾"、"喉蛾"、"喉痹"。往往伴有程度不同的急性咽炎。临床表现为突然咽痛,吞咽时加剧,扁桃体充血肿大,表面有淡黄色或白色脓点,有时可融合成片,但不超出扁桃体的范围,易拭去,伴有发热恶寒,头痛等全身症状。

技法运用

1. 毫针:取少商、合谷、颊车、尺泽、商阳。高热加大椎、曲池穴。

用捻转提插泻法,留针15~20分钟,每日1次,少商及商阳点刺放血。

有人治急性扁桃腺炎,取少商速刺出血,合谷用提插泻法(即慢慢将针插入,找到麻胀感觉,急插慢提2~4次),使麻或胀的感觉到手指。翳风用提插泻法(手法同合谷),使麻或胀的感觉至颊部或口腔内(上列穴位不留针)。(刘冠军,等.《中医针法集锦》)。

另有人取天柱穴治急性咽炎。方法:由后外侧斜进针,刺入同身寸1~1.3寸,胀麻针感有时可扩散到头部及肩部,此时施以中等以上的强刺激,提插半分钟至1分钟,每10分钟作同样刺激1次,共留针30分钟(焦国瑞.《针灸临床经验辑要》)。

2. 耳针:扁桃体、咽喉、肺、胃、下屏尖。

强刺激,留针1小时,每隔15分钟间歇捻转行针1次,每天1次;亦可在耳轮上、中、下或耳背静脉用三棱针点刺出血。

3. 拔罐:有人取大椎穴,快速进针2~3毫米深,不留针,再取不易传热大豆片,桔皮等置于大椎部位,上面放一小酒精棉球,点燃后扣上火罐,留罐10~15分钟,反复做2次,结果治疗急性扁桃体炎400例,有效率达98%(金龙洙.中西医结合杂志,8:493;1986)。

2. ACUTE TONSILLITIS

Manifestations

Acute tonsillitis, usually accompanied by acute pharyngitis, is manifested clinically by abrupt onset with sore throat which is aggravated by swallowing, congestion and swelling of the tonsil, yellowish or white purulent spots on the tonsil, which may form a patch but can be wiped away easily, accompanied by fever, aversion to cold, and headache.

Treatment by Applying Acubustion Techniques

(1) *Filiform Needlins*

Selection of Points

Main points: Shaoshang (LU 11), Hegu(LI 4), Jiache(ST 6), Chize(LU 5), Shangyang (LI 1).

Supplementary points according to symptoms: Dazhui(DU 14) and Quchi(lI 11) for high fever.

Method

Three to five points are employed each treatment session, reducing manipulations by twisting, rotating, lifting and thrustig the needle are applied, and the needles are retained at each point for fiftten to twenty minutes. But, at Shaoshang (LU 11) as well as Shangyang (LI 1), pricking is given to cause bleeding. The treatment is given once daily and for five times as a course.

Introducing Some Experiential Techniques

In Collection of Outstandings of the Needling Methods of TCM the following method for treatment of acute tonsillitis is recorded. Shaoshang (LU 11) is pricked to cause bleeding, Hegu (LI 4) is punctured with the needle inserted slowly and, after the patlent complains of distension and numbness, the needle is quickly thrust and slowly lifted two to four times to make the needling sensation propagated to the patient's fingers. Yifeng (SJ 17) is punctured with the same needling metioned above to make the numbness or distension propagated to the cheek or into the mouth. The needles are not retained, and the treatment is given once daily and for five sessions as a course.

Another method for treatment of acute tonsillitis is recorded in Collection of Outstandins of Clinical Experiences of Acupunture & Moxibustion. Tianzhu (BL 10) is selected only, and a needle is inserted into the point obliquely to a depth of 1 — 1.5 cun. When the patient complains of numbness and distension spreading to the head and shoulder region, a medium or more strength stimulation by lifting and thrusting the needle is applied for one minute. Then, the needle is retained for thirty minutes and manipulated in the same way once per ten minutes. The treatment is given once daily and for five times as a course.

(2) *Otopuncture*

Selection of Otopoints

Tonsil, Throat, Lung, Stomach, Adrenal Gland.

Method

Three to five otopoints are employed each treatment session, strong stimulation is chosen, and the needles are retained at each otopoint for one hour and twisted once per fifteen minutes during the retention. The treatment is given once daily and for five sessions as a course. Or, the upper, middle and lower portions of the helix or the veins at the back of the auricle are pricked with the three — edged needle to cause bleeding.

(3) *Cupping*

Selection of Point

Dazhui (DU 14).

A needle is quickly inserted into Dazhui (DU 14) to a depth of 2 — 3 mm and withdrawn immediately. Then, a piece of soybean or tangerine skin on which a small alcohol cotton ball is put s placed on the point, the ball is ignited and covered with a jar for cupping, and the jar is kept on the point for ten to fifteen minutes. This procedure is repeated twice at one treatment session. It is reported in Chinese Journal of Integrated Traditional and Western Mdicine that a high effective rate of 98% in treatment of 400 cases with acute tonsillitis was achieved by applying this method

三、急性眼结膜炎

急性眼结膜炎，中医学称为"天行赤眼"、"火眼"，或俗称"红眼病"。临床表现为发病急骤，球结膜充血、水肿、分泌物多、眼睛红肿、灼热、畏光。

技法运用

1. 毫针：取睛明、太阳、合谷、风池、攒竹、丝竹空、少商、臂臑穴。

少商、太阳点刺出血；攒竹、丝竹空、睛明捻转而不提插；风池行轻微捻转加震颤；合谷用捻转提插泻法；刺臂臑针尖向上方，沿手阳明经脉走向斜刺，与臂成30°角，用捻转提插泻法。口苦、便秘加刺侠溪穴。每次选用3～4穴，留针15～20分钟，每日1次。

有报道用三棱针点刺中冲穴出血，稍加挤压，一眼感染刺一侧，两眼感染刺双侧，治疗红眼病250例，针刺三天以内治愈的，占96%（郭霖.中国针灸，2：47；1989）。

2. 挑治：在肩胛间按压寻找敏感点挑治；或在大椎上下左右各一寸处，沿皮上下左右挑治；或在肺俞，风门等穴挑治。

3. 耳针：肝、眼、目$_1$、目$_2$、耳尖、肺。

强刺激，留针30分钟。亦可耳尖或耳背静脉点刺出血。

4. 刺络拔罐：可于太阳穴处，常规消毒后，医者左手拇、食二指舒张并按压局部皮肤，右手持三棱针快速点刺或梅花针叩刺，出血后拔小火罐。

有报道针罐结合治疗红眼病524例。方法：取大椎、耳尖、少泽为主穴，太阳、肾上腺（下屏尖），攒竹为配穴，治疗时用无菌三棱针在消毒后的耳尖，少泽穴上点刺放血3～5滴；呈梅花样点刺大椎穴（即大椎穴与大椎上下左右各5分处点刺1针），加拔火罐，留罐5分钟左右，出血约3～20毫升；太阳、攒竹、肾上腺等穴出血少许，针刺治疗同时，禁食辛辣、荤腥之物及烟酒。治愈率为100%（李继平，等.上海针灸杂志.1：27；1990）。

5. 灯火灸：取患侧耳背上三角窝处，对光反照，可见一条明显的小血管向耳背部分叉。在血管上部和分叉处各取1点，以圆珠笔作一记号，用75%酒精消毒，取灯芯草蘸上植物油，点燃后迅速灼在记号上，每点各灼一下。灯芯草蘸油时，一般只蘸0.5厘米左右，过长会使灯芯草变软，且火焰过旺易烧伤皮肤，蘸的太短，会使火力不足，未碰到穴位点即减。每点灸一次，可闻及清脆的"啪"音，若无，应重新点灼，但一般不宜超过3次。注意保持皮肤清洁，当天不宜洗擦。若有小水泡不慎擦破，可涂龙胆紫。一般当天获效，若无效，可重新点灼一次（林文谋.四川中医，4：57；1986）。

3. ACUTE CONJUNCTIVITIS

Manifestations

Acute conjunctivitis belonging to the disease category of Tian Xiang Chi Yang (天行赤眼), Huo Yang (火眼), or Hong Yangbing (红眼病) in TCM, is manifested clinically by abrupt onset with congestion and swelling of the bulbar conjunctiva, much discharge, redness, swelling and burning sesnsation of the eye, and photophobia.

Treatment by Applying Acubustion Techniques

(1) *Filifrom Needling*:

Selection of Points

Jingming (BL 1), Taiyang (EX-HN5), Hegu (LI 4), Fengchi (GB 20), Cuanzhu (BL 2), Sizhukong (SJ 23), Shaoshang (LU 11), Binao (LI 14).

Method

Three or four points are employed

each treatment session. At Taiyang(EX—HN5) and Shaoshang(LU 11) pricking is given to cause bleeding, at Cuanznu(BL 2), Sizhukong(SJ 23) and Jingming(BL 1), the needle is inserted and then twisted, and no thrusting or lifting manipulation is allowed. At Fengchi(GB 20), puncture manipulation by twrling the needle plus vibrating the needle is applied, at Hegu(LI 4), reducing needling by twisting, rotating, lifting and thrustng the needle is chosen, and at Binao(LI 14) a needle is inserted obliquely upwards along the course of the Hand—Yangming Meridian at an angle of 30° to the skin and reducing manipulations by twisting, rotating, lifting and thrusting the needle are performed. If the patient has bitter taste in the mouth and constipation, Xiaxi(GB 43) is punctured additionally. The needles are retained at each point selected for fifteen to twenty minutes, and the treatment is given once daily and for five or seven times as a course.

Introducing An Experiential Technique

A simple but good method is recommended, by which a high curative rate of 96% in treatment of 250 cases with the acute conjunctivitis was achieved whthin three days. In this method, Zhongchong (PC 9)at the affected side is pricked with the three—edged needle to cause bleeding, and then the point is squeezed slighgtly. If two eyes being affected, bilateral Zhongchong(PC 9)are employed. The treatment is given once daily.

(2) *Breaking Therapy*
Selection of Areas to Be Broken and

Method

Fibers—pricking method may be applied at sensitive or tender spots at the interscapular region or at four spots 1 cun respectively lateral to, above and below Dazhui(DU 14), or at Feishu(BL13) and Fengmen(BL 12). The treatment is given once daily and for four times.

(3) *Otopuncture*
Selection of Otopoints

Liver, Eye, Frontal Tragic Notch (Eye 1), Back Tragic Notch(Eye 2), Ear Apex, Lung.

Method

Three or four otopoints are employed each treatment session, strong stimulation is chosen, and the needles are retained at each otopoint for thirty minutes. Or, the ear apex or veins at the back of the auricle are pricked to cause bleeding. The treatment is given once daily and for three times as a course.

(4) *Blood—Letting Puncture and Cupping*
Selection of Point

Taiyang(EX—HN5).

Method

Following a local and routine sterilization, the local skin at the point is stretched and pressed with the thumb and index finger of the left hand, and the point is pricked with a three—edged needle held by the right hand or tapped with a plum—blossom needle held by the right hand to cause bleedding. Then, cupping is applied to the point.

Introducing An Experiential Technique

In Shanghai Journal of Acupuncture

&. Moxibustion the following method is recommended, by which a curative rate of 100% in treatment of 524 cases with acute conjunctivitis was achieved. In the method, Dazhui (DU 14), Ot. Ear Apex, and Shaoze (SI 1) are taken as the main points, and Taiyang (EX — HN5), Cuanzhu (BL 2) and Ot. Adrenal Gland as the adjuvant. After a routine and local sterilization, Shaoze (SI 1) and Ot. Ear Apex are pricked with a sterilized three—edged needle to cause bloodletting of 3—5 drops each. Dazhui (DU 14) and four points 0.5 cun respectively lateral, above and below it are pricked and given with cupping for five minutes to cause bloodletting of 3—20 ml. Taiyang (EX—HN5), Cuanzhu (BL 2) and Ot. Adrenal Gland are pricked to cause a little of bloodletting. The patient is advised not to take hot or fat food, and not to smoke or drink during the treatment course.

(5) *Lampwick Moxibustion*

Selection of Point

At the triangular fossa on the back of the auricle of the affected side, a small blood vessel and its branches may be seen obviously under light. Two points respectively superior to the vessel and at the cross are taken as the moxibustion sites.

Method

The two points are marked with a pen, and the local skin is sterilized with 75% of alcohol. Then, a rush soaked with vegetable oil is ignited and dipped accurately onto the marked spot and removed immediately. A clear cracking sound is heard. If not, the procedure is repeated, but the maximum times is three. If the small blister left is broken by pushing, it is smeared with gentian violet to prevent infection. Generally, the disease is cured by one session of treatment. If it is not cured, the treatment may be given once again. During the treatment period the local skin should be kept clean and not washed. Note, the portion of the rush to be soaked in the oil should be approximately 0.5 cm long, because, if the portion of the rush soaked in the oil is more than 0.5 cm long, the rush may become too sofe to apply moxibustion and the fire caused may be so strong that the skin may be burnt, and if the portion soaked in the oil is less than 0.5 cm long, enough fire for moxibustion may not be caused.

四、近 视

近视以视远物模糊不清,视近物清晰为特征,因眼部屈光不正而引起的一种眼病。

技法运用

1. 毫针:取睛明、肝俞、肾俞、承泣、攒竹、风池、丝竹空、翳明、合谷、光明、臂臑等穴。

用平补平泻法,眼区穴宜轻捻缓进,不捣动及大弧度捻转,可留针或不留针,出针时随即用消毒干棉球按压片刻,以防出血。承泣穴垂直进针后,针尖呈30°角,可向睛明斜刺1寸左右,每日1次。

2. 耳针:眼、肝、肾、目$_1$、目$_2$。

中等刺激,留针30分钟,间歇捻转行针,每日1次,两耳交替,亦可耳穴点压王不留行籽,每日自行按压2～3次。

有报道,将中药急性子贴于6毫米见方的小胶布中心备用。取患者耳穴眼、目$_1$、目$_2$、肝、并进行常规消毒后,用北京产 WQ—10B

多用电子穴位测定仪取以上诸穴的敏感点，将急性子胶布块贴压其上。嘱患者每天自行按压3～4穴，每次50～100下，用力大小以有痛感且能忍受为度。每周治疗1次，连续5次为1疗程(黄喜梅.《第一届世界针灸学术大会，针灸论文摘要选编》,1987)。

3.梅花针：叩刺眼周围穴位，脊椎两侧及风池穴，用中等刺激，每日1次。亦可采用电梅花针叩刺。

4.腕踝针：选用上$_1$点(小指侧的尺骨缘前方)，用拇指端按压凹陷处，双眼近视选双侧，单眼近视选患侧，按常规操作法，进针一般应不痛，如痛应将针退至皮下浅表部位，再重新进针。留针1小时，并嘱患者向远处眺望，每日1次，10次为1疗程(江洋.上海针灸杂志，4:11;1987)。

4. MYOPIA

Manifestations

Myopia refers to near sight due to ametropia.

Treatment by Applying Acubustion Techniques

(1) *Filiform Needling*

Selection of Points

Jingming (BL 1), Ganshu (BL 18), Shenshu (BL 23), Chengqi (ST 1), Cuanzhu (BL 1), Fengchi (GB 20), Sizhukong (SJ 23), Yiming (EX—HN14), Hegu (LI 4), Guangming (GB 31), Binao (LI 14).

Method

Three or four points are employed each treatment session, and uniform reinforcing — reducing manipulation is applied. At the points around the eye, the needle is inserted slowly with gentle twirling movement, and shaking or twisting the needle at a large amplitude is forbidden. additionally, after withdrawal of the needle, the needle hole is pressed with sterilized dry cotton ball immediately in order to prevent bleeding. At Chengqi (ST 1), after the needle is inserted through the skin, it is pushed obliquely toward Jingming (BL 1) at an angle of 30° to the skin for 1 cun. The treatment is given once daily and for ten sessions as a course.

(2) *Otopuncture*

Selection of Otopoints

Eye, Liver, Kidney, Frontal Tragic Notch (Eye 1), Back Tragic otch (Eye 2).

Method

Three or four otopoints at the same side are employed each treatment session and the two auricles are selected alternately. On puncturing, medium strength stimulation is applied and the needles are retained at each otopoint for thirty minutes and twisted intermittently during the retention. The treatment is given once daily and for ten sessions as a course, the next course beginning after an interval of one week rest. Or, the vaccaria seeds are stuck over the otopoints and the patient is asked to press them two or three times daily and for seven days.

Introdcuing An Experiential Technique

The following method in treatment of the disease is reported. A garden balsam seed (Semen Impatientis) is put onto the center of a piece of adhesive plaster 6×6 mm in size, and many pieces are made in the same way for use. Ot. Eye, Frontal Tragic Notch, Back Tragic Notch, and Liver are selected, and a local and routine sterilization is given. The sensitive spots on the areas of the otopoints mentioned above are found by using WQ—10 B multi—purpose electronicpoint—probing unit and covered with the plasters. The patient is asked to press each of the point three or four times daily and for fifty to one hundred times at each time, with the force causing painful sensation but being tolerable to himself applied. The treatment is given once daily and for five times as a course.

(3) *Tapping with Plum—Blossom Needle*

Selection of Points

The surrounding areas of the eyes, bilateral sidesof the spinal column and Fengchi(GB2 2).

Method

These areas and points are tapped with the plum—blossom needle once daily, and medium strength stimulation is applied. Or these areas and the points are tapped with the electric plum—blossom needle.

(4) *Wrist—Ankle Puncture*

Seelection of points

Upper 1 at the diseased side, or bilateral Upper 1 if the two eyes are diseased.

Method

Marks are made on the point selected with the thumb, and regular puncture is given. If the patient complains of pain due to insertion of the needle, the needle is withdrawn to the area beneath the skin and pushed deep again. The needle is retained at the point for one hour and the patient is asked to see the place far from

him during the retention. The treatment is given once daily and for ten sessions as a course, the next course beginning after an interval of one week rest.

五、牙 痛

牙痛，为口腔疾患中常见的症状，发病原因很多，一般多因龋齿引起。牙周炎、冠周炎、急性根尖周围炎等亦引起牙痛。其临床表现为突然发作，持续时间长短不一，遇冷，热，酸，甜等刺激时加剧。

技法运用

1. 毫针：取合谷、下关、颊车、太阳穴。

牙痛甚而龈肿，伴形寒身热，为风火牙痛，加外关，风池，曲池；牙痛剧烈，伴有口臭，便秘，为胃火牙痛。加内庭，劳宫，二间，三间；牙痛隐隐，牙齿浮动，腰酸，神疲，口不臭，为虚火牙痛，加太溪，行间。风火牙痛，胃火牙痛用捻转提插泻法，虚火牙痛用捻转提插补法，留针30分钟。

有人取主穴下关(患侧)，颊车(患侧)。上牙痛配合谷；下牙痛配足三里。方法：下关直刺0.5～1寸，提插刮针手法，持续行针至症状减轻或消失后，再留针15～30分钟，5～10分钟行针1次；颊车向地仓透刺1.5～3寸，用捻转刮针手法；合谷针0.5～1寸，足三里直刺1.5～2寸，用提插捻转手法，后三穴均留针15～30分钟，5～10分钟行针1次(孙学全.《针灸临证集验》)。

另有人取昆仑穴，令患者侧卧，患侧在上，进针昆仑穴时，针尖对准内踝前缘。手法：依据"虚则补之"，"实则泻之"原则施针，刺入深度为3～5分深，留针30分钟，每5分钟行针1次(刘致.《中医杂志，2：18；1962》)。

2. 耳针：上颌、下颌、颊、屏尖、神门、肾。

强刺激，捻转留针30～60分钟，或埋揿针

2~3天。

3. 穴位注射疗法：取下关、合谷，用维生素 B_1 100毫克/2毫升，每穴注入0.3~0.5毫升，每日1次。

有报道，用0.5~0.75％盐酸普鲁卡因3~5毫升，进行穴位注射，上牙痛取合谷、太阳、下关；下牙痛用下关、颊车。首先注射合谷，多取健侧，患侧或双侧亦可找到较好感觉。注药0.5~1毫升，然后再注射下关、太阳或颊车，每穴0.5~1毫升，每日1~2次（田丛豁，等．《针灸医学验集》）。

5. TOOTHACHE

Manifestations

Toothache is a common ailment. It is usually due to dental caries. But periodontitis, pericoronitis and acute apical pericementitis may cause it too. In clinic, it may occur suddenly, lasting for a uncertain time, and aggravated by stimulation of cold, heat, sweet or sour material to the tooth.

Treatment by Applying Acubustion Techniques

(1) *Filiform Needling*

Selection of Points

Main points：Hegu (LI 4), Xiaguan (ST 7), Jiache (ST 6), Taiyang (X—HN5).

Supplementary points according to symptoms：Waiguan (SJ 5), Fengchi (GB 20) and Quchi (LI 11) for severe toothache with gingival swelling, accompanied by chills and fever caused by attack by wind-fire evils, Neiting (ST 44), Laogong (PC 8), Erjian (LI 2) and Sanjian (LI 3) for severe toothache accompanied by foul breath and constipation, which is caused by stomach—fire, and Taixi (KL 3) and Xingjian (LR 2) for dull pain, loose tooth, soreness of waist, listlessness, abscence of fo foul breath, caused by asthenic fire.

Mehtod

Three or four points are employed each treatment session. For cases caused by attack by wind—fire evils, reducing manipulations by twisting, lifting and thrusting the needle are applied, and for the cases caused by asthenic fire, reinforcing manipulations by twirling, lifting and thrusting the needle are chosen. The needles are retained at each point for thirty minutes. The treatment is given oncc daily and for three to five treatment sessions as a course. The prolongation or shortening of the course of treatment is made in occordance with the disease condition.

Introducing Some Experiential Techniques

In Collection of Clinical Experiences of Acupuncture &. Moxibustion the following method for treatment of toothache is recorded. Xiaguan (ST 7) and Jiache (ST 6) of the affected side are taken as the main points, and Hegu (LI 4), as the adjuvant for pain of upper tooth, and Zusanli (ST 36) as the adjuvant for pain of the lower tooth. At Xiaguan (ST 7), a needle is inserted perpendicularly 0.5—1 cun deep. Then, it is lifted and thrust and scraped continuously until the symptoms are relieved or eliminated. The needle is retained at the point for fifteen to thirty minutes and manipulated once per five ot ten minutes during the retention. At Jiache

(ST 6), a needle is inserted and pushed beneath the skin with penetration needling towards Dicang(ST 4) for 1.5—3 cun. Then, it is twisted and scraped. At Hegu (LI 4), a needle is pushed and inserted perpendicularly 0.5—1cundeep, and at Zusanli(ST36) a needle is inserted and pushed perpendicularly 1.5—2 cun deep, then, lifting, thrusting and twirling manipulations are applied in these two points. The needles are retained at the last three points for fifteen to thirty minutes and manipulated once per five to ten minutes.

In Journal of TCM another method is recommended. Kunlun (BL 60) is employed. To the operation, the patient is asked to lie on the healthy side, and a needle is inserted into the point and pushed towards the anterior border of the internal malleolus for 0.3—0.5 cun. If the disease is diagnosed as the deficiency type, reinforcing needling is performed, and, if the toothace diagnosed as the excess type, reducing needling employed. The neelde is retained at the point for thirty minutes and manipulated once per five minutes.

(2) Otopuncture

Selection of Otopints

Maxilla, Mandible, Cheek, Tragic Apex, Shenmen, Kidney.

Method

Three or four otopoints are employed each treatment session, strong stimulation is applied, and the needles are retained at each point for thirty to sixty minutes and twisted and rotated several times during the retention. Or the thumb—tack needles are embedded into the otopoints and kept there for two or three days.

(3) Point Injection (Hydro—puncture)

Selection of Points

Xiaguan(ST 7), Hegu(LI 4).

Selection of Drug

Vitamine B_1 100mg [2ml].

Method

Inject 0.3—0.5 ml of the drug fluid into each point. The treatment is given once daily and the points at the two sides are employed alternatley. Three or four treatment sessions constitue a course.

Introducing An Experiential Technique

In Collection of Experiences of Acupuncture & Moxibustion the following method is introduced. Hegu (LI 4) and Taiyang(EX—HN5) and Xiauan (ST 7) are employed for pain at the upper tooth, and Xiaguan(ST 7) and Jiache (ST 6) for pain at the lower tooth. Each point is injected with 0.5—1 ml of 0.5—0.75% procaine hydrochloride. Firstly, Hegu (LI 4), usually at the healthy side, is injected. Then, Xiaguan(ST 7) and Taiyang(EX—HN5) or Jiache(ST 6) are injected. The treatment is given once daily or twice daily and for three to five times as a course.

六、耳鸣、耳聋

耳鸣表现为自觉耳内有各种不同的响声。响声重，伴眩晕易怒为实证；响声低微，伴头晕眼花，腰膝酸软为虚证。耳聋多为听力减退或丧失。针灸治疗多以神经性耳鸣、耳聋为主。

技法运用

1. 毫针：局部与循经取穴相结合。主穴为耳门、听宫、翳风、听会、外关、中渚。

实证加丰隆、侠溪、太冲，用捻转提插泻法；虚证加复溜、太溪，用捻转提插补法。留针30分钟，每日1次。

有报导取翳风、听宫、耳门、听会、瘛脉、百会，治耳聋100例。方法：除百会穴外，各穴针刺深度为3～3.9厘米，用直入直出的"输刺手法"（即垂直刺入较深处候气，得气后慢慢将针退出（奚永江，等.《针尖灸法学》）。不加旋捻，每次留针30分钟，每周针治3次。（焦国瑞.《针灸临床经验辑要》）。

亦有人取耳门、翳风；听会、下关两组穴间日交替使用。耳门张口取之，呈30°角向听宫刺1～1.2寸，听会直刺1～1.2寸，均用捻转手法；翳风直刺1～1.5寸，用刮针手法；下关直刺0.8～1寸，用提插捻转手法，均短促行针，每日针1次，7次1疗程（孙学全.《针灸临证集验》）。

2. 穴位注射疗法：取听宫、翳风、风池、完骨、听会、耳门，采用维生素B_1、维生素B_{12}，10%丹参注射液，5～10%葡萄糖注射液，上药任选一种，每次取3～4穴，每穴注入0.3～0.5毫升，隔日1次。

3. 耳针：耳、下屏尖、肝、肾、屏间。

实证强刺激，虚证弱刺激，留针30分钟，每日1次。亦可针刺配合耳穴贴压王不留行籽，每日按压2～3次。

6. TINNITUS AND DEAFNESE

Manifestations

Tinnitus is manifested by ringing sound in the ears felt by the patient himself. It can be divided into two types according to differentiation of syndromes clinically: the excess type and the deficiency type. The excess type is characterized by strong ringing sound in the ears accompanied by dizziness and irritability. The deficiency type is characterized by low ringing sound in the ears accompanied by dizziness, and soreness and weakness of waist and knee. Deafness is manifested by failing or loss of hearing. Most of tinnitus and deafness which can be treated by acupuncture and moxibustion are neural.

Treatment by Applying Acubustion Techniques

(1) *Filifrom Needling*

Selection of Points

Points at the local area together with the points along the meridian governing the ear are selected.

Main points: Ermen (SJ 21), Tinggong (SI 19), Yifeng (SJ 17). Tinghui (GB 2), Waiguan (SJ 5), Zhongzhu (SJ 3).

Supplementary points according to symptoms: Fenglong (ST 40), Xiaxi (GB 43) and Taichong (LR 3) are selected for excess type, Fuiliu (KI 7) and Taixi (KI 5) for deficiency type.

Method

Three to five points are employed each treatment session, reducing manipulations by twisting, lifting and thrusting the needle are applied for excess type and reinfocring manipulations by twirling, lifting and thrusting the needle applied for the deficiency type, and the needles are retained at each point for thirty minutes. The treatment is given once daily and for ten sessions as a course, the next course beginning after an interval of one week rest.

Introducing Some Experiential Tech-

niques

In Collection of Outstandings of Clinical Experiences of Acupuncture & Moxibustion the following method is recommended, by which a satisfactory effect in treatment of 100 cases with deafness was achieved. The points to be selected include Tinggong (SI 19), Yifeng (SJ 17), Ermen (SJ 21), Tinghui (GB 2), Chimai (SJ 1) and Baihui (DU 20), and three to five points are punctured each treatment session. All points except Baihui (DU 20) are punctured perpendicularly. The needles are inserted and pushed 3-3.9 cm deep to induce the needling sensation. After the needling sensation is induced to the patient, the needles are retained at the points for thirty minutes and then withdrawn slowly. The treatment is given three times per week and for ten times as a course.

Another method for treatment of tinnitus and deafness is recorded in Collection of Clinical Experiences of Acupuncture & Moxibustion. The points to be selected are divided into two groups, one group including Ermen (SJ 21) and Yifeng (SJ 17), and the other including Tinghui (GB 2) and Xiaguan (ST 7), and these two groups are employed alternately. To the operation, the patient is asked to open the mouth and a needle is inserted into Ermen (SJ 21) at an angle of 30° to the skin and pushed towards Tinggong (SI 19) for 1— 1.2 cun. Then, Tinghui (GB 2) is punctured perpendicularly. Twirling and rotating manipulations are applied at these two points. On puncturing at Yifeng (SJ 17), a needle is inserted perpendicularly and pushed 1—1.5 cun deep, and scraping the needle is chosen. On puncturing at Xiaguan (ST 7), a needle is inserted and pushed perpendicularly 0.8—1 cun, and it is lifted, thruste and twisted at a samll extent and with a quck speed. The treatment is given once daily and for seven sessions as a course, the next course beginning after an interval of one week rest.

(2) *Hydro—Puncture*

Selection of Points

Tinggong (SI 19), Yifeng (SJ 17), Fengchi (GB 20), Tinghui (GB 2), Ermen (SJ 21).

Selection of Drugs

Vitamin B 1, B 12, 10% of red sage root (Radix Salviae Miltiorrhizae) injection, 5—10% of glucose injection.

Method

Three or four points and any one kind of drugs mentioned above are selected each treatment session, and 0.3—0.5 ml of the drug fluid is injected into each point. The treatment is given once every other day and for seven treatment sessions as a course.

(3) *Otopuncture*

Selection of Otopoints

Ear, Adrenal Gland, Liver, Kidney, Endocrine.

Method

Three or four otopoints are employed each treatment session, strong stimulation is applied for excess type and gentle stimulation for deficiency type, and the needles are retained at each otopoint for thirty minutes. The treatment is given once daily and for ten sessions as a course, the next course beginning after an interval of five days. Or, the vaccaria seeds are stuck onto the selected otopoints and the patient is asked to press them two or three times daily. The seeds are kept on the otopoints for five to seven days and some other otopoints are plastered with the vaccaria seeds in the same way at the next course. The prolongation or shortening of the times of the treatment course is adjusted accordance with the disease condition.

七、耳源性眩晕

本病是内耳膜迷路积水引起的一种眩晕症。临床表现多为阵发性旋转性眩晕,伴恶心欲呕,耳鸣多在眩晕发生前出现。中医又分为两型,实证(痰浊上蒙)为眩晕头重、耳鸣恶心、胸脘满闷、食少多寐、苔白腻、脉濡滑。虚证(肾阴不足,肝阳上亢)为眩晕、耳鸣、面赤、腰酸、舌红、脉细弦。

技法运用

1. 毫针:印堂、风池、听宫、太冲、百会、内关。实证加丰隆、阴陵泉、中脘;虚证加肾俞、三阴交、太溪、足三里。

实证用捻转提插泻法,虚证用捻转提插补法,留针20~30分钟,每日1次。

有以四神聪、风池(双)、大椎为主穴;丰隆、足三里、三阴交、内关、神门、肾俞为配穴治耳源性眩晕。方法:先采用卧位,穴区皮肤常规消毒,用28号4厘米长的毫针。四神聪用头针刺法,留针20分钟;风池穴以切刺法快速将针刺入皮肤至皮下后缓慢捻针,使酸麻针感放射至前额两侧,留针2分钟后出针;大椎刺法同风池穴,缓慢捻针2分钟后,针上加大号火罐一具,15分钟后取罐起针。一般病人即可缓解。然后再让病人仰卧位,常规针刺以上配穴,用捻转的平补平泻手法,留针20分钟,即可出针(王志秀.中国针灸,5:14;1986)。

另据报道针刺眩晕200例,方法:上星穴透百会。用4寸毫针两枚,一针从上星穴透百会穴,一针从百会穴透达枕外粗隆上,以病人头皮有酸胀及头脑清醒为度;针神门穴,用4寸毫针直刺神门穴0.5~1寸,有针感后将针提至皮下,再向上平刺4寸,以患者肘部有酸胀感为度;针安眠④(在三阴交穴上2寸,胫前内侧缘),用4寸毫针沿皮下向上平刺4寸,以患者自觉足三里处有微热感为度。每日针1次,6~7次为1疗程(李振富.中国针灸,6:11;1988)。

2. 灸疗:百会穴,艾条悬灸或艾炷灸,每日1次,每次15~30分钟或3~7壮。

有报道,艾炷直接灸百会穴治疗耳源性眩晕177例。方法:将百会穴上的头发,从根部剪去约中指甲大,使穴位充分暴露,嘱患者低坐矮凳,医者坐在其正后方的较高位置上,取艾绒少许,做成黄豆大小的上尖下圆的锥形灸炷,首次两壮合并放在百会穴上,用线香点燃,当燃至1/2时,右手持厚纸片迅速将艾炷压熄,留下残绒。以后一壮接一壮加在前次的残绒上,每个艾炷燃至无烟为止。燃完一壮压一壮,压力由轻到重,每次灸25~30壮,使患者自觉有热力,从头皮渗入脑内的舒适感。有效率为98.88%(许美纯.中国针灸,4:14;1984)。

3. 耳针:取肝、肾、神门、内耳、下脚端、下屏尖、脑、缘中、枕穴。

强刺激,每次选3~5穴,留针30分钟,每日1次。亦可配合耳穴撳针或埋置王不留行籽贴压,每日按压2~3次,3~5天更换一次。

7. AURIAL VERTIGO

Manifestations

Aural vertigo, referring to dizziness

due to dropsy in the labyrinth, is manifested clinically by abrupt onset of vertigo, accompanied by nausea, vomiting, and tinnitus occurring before vertigo. It may be divided into excess type and deficiency type according to differentiation of syndromes. The excess type, which, according to TCM theory, is due to retention of phlegm dampness in the head, is characterized by dizziness, nausea, suffocating sensation and fullness in the chest and upper abdomem, anorexia, somnolence, white and sticky tongue coating, and soft and rolling pulse. The deficiency type, which, according to the TCM theory, is due to insufficiency of kidney yin and hyperactivity of the liver yang, is characterized by dizziness, tinnitus, flushed face, soreness of waist, red tongue and thready and string—taut pulse.

Tretment by Applying Acubustion Techniques

(1) Filifrom Needling

Selection of Points

Main points: Yintang (EX—HN 3), Fengchi (GB 20), Tinggong (SI 19), Taichong (LR 3), Baihui (DU 20), Neiguan (PC 6).

Supplementary points according to symptoms: Fenglong (ST 40), Yinlingquan (SP 9) and Zhongwan (RN 12) are selected for excess type, and Shenshu (BL 23), Sanyinjiao (SP 6), Taixi (KI 3), and Zusanli (ST 6) for deficiency type.

Method

Three to five points are employed each treatment session, reducing manipulations by twisting, lifting and thrusting the needle are chosen for excess type, and reinforcing manipulations by twirling, lifting and thrusting the needle chosen for deficiency type, and the needles are retained at each point for twenty to thirty minutes. The treatment is given once daily and for ten sessions of the treatment as a course, the next course beginning after an interval of five days.

Introducing Some Experiential Techniques

In Chinese Acupuncture & Moxibustion the following method is rported. Sishencong (EX — HN 1), Bilateral Fengchi (GB 20) and Dazhui (DU 14) are selected as the main points, and Fenglong (ST 40), Zusanli (ST 36), Sanyinjiao (SP 6), Neiguan (PC 6), Shenmen (HT 7) and Shenshu (BL 23) as the adjuvant. To the operation, the patient is asked to lie prone and the local region is sterilized. On puncturing at Sishencong (EX—HN 1), No 28 4 cm long needles (the other points are punctured with the same size needle) are inseted into the points with a scalp needling method, and retained for twenty minutes. On puncturing at Fengchi (GB 20), the needle is inserted through the skin quickly and then pushed and twisted slowly until the patient complains of soreness and numbness radiating to the two sides of the forehead. Then, the needle is retained for two minutes and withdrawn. On puncturing at Dazhui (DU 14), the same needling as at Fengchi (GB 20) is employed, and the needle is twisted slowly for two minutes. Then, the needle is kept in the point and a large jar is placed on the point for cupping. Fifteen minutes later, the needle and the jar are removed. Most patients will be relieved through the treatment proecedure. Then, the patient is asked to lie supine, some adjuvant points are punctured. On puncturing, uniform reinforcing — reducing manipulation by twirling and rotating the needle is applied, and the needles are retained at each point for twenty minutes before withdrawal of them. The treatment is given once daily and for five times as a course.

Another method for treatment of vertigo is reported in Chinese Acupuncture & Moxibustion, by which a satisfactory effect was achieved in treatment of 200 cases. Shangxing (DU 23) and Baihui (DU 20) are selected. On puncturing, a 4 cun long needle is inserted into Shangxing (DU 23) with penetration needling towards Baihui (DU 20), and another 4 cun long needle is inserted into Baihui (DU 20) and pushed with penetration needling towards the external occipital protuberance. The intensity of needling stimulation is adjusted to optimum by which the patient complains of soreness and distension of the scalp and the patient's mind is clear. Additionally, Shenmen (HT 7) and Anmian (EX—HN 17, 2 cun above Sanyinjiao, Sp 6, at the anterior lateral border of the shin—bone) are employed. On puncturing at Shenmen (HT 7), a 4 cun long needle is inserted and pushed perpendicularly 0.5—1 cun deep at first. Then, it is lifted to the area beneath the skin and pushed deep horizontally upwards for 4 cun, causing soreness and distension of the elbow to the patient. On puncturing at Anmian (EX—HN 17) a 4 cun logn needle is inserted through the skin and pushed upwards along the skin for 4 cun, and the needling intensity is adjusted to optimum by which the patient complains of slight heat sensation at Zusanli (ST 36) area. The treatment is given once daily and for six or seven times as a course.

(2) *Moxibustion*

Selection of Points

Baihui (DU 20).

Method

Suspended moxibustion is applied to the point for fifteen to thirty minutes or moxibustion with moxa cone is applied to the point for five or six cones at one treatment session. The treatment is given once daily and for five or six sessions as a course.

Introducing An Experiential Technique

A good moxibustion method for treatment of aural vertigo is recommended in Chinese Acupuncture & Moxibustion, by which a high effective rate of 98.88% in treatment of 117 cases was achieved. Baihui (DU 20) is selected, and the patient's hair at Baihui (DU 20) area is cut to expose the point fully. The patient is asked to sit down on a low chair, and moxa cones, each of them being as large as a soybean, are prepared. First, two moxa cones are placed on the point and ignited for moxibustion. When the upper half of the cone is burnt out, it is pressed quickly with a piece of thick paper held by the right hand to extinquish the fire, leaving the residual moxa cone on the point. Then another cone is placed on the residual cone and ignited for moxibustion. This course is rpeated until twenty — five to thirty cones are burnt out, with the pressing force gradually increased, causing a comfortable sensation that heat conducts through the scalp into the brain to the patient. The treatment is given once daily and for seven sessions as a course.

(3) *Otopuncture*

Selection of Otopoints

Liver, Kidney, Shenmen, Interior Ear, Sympathetic, Adrenal Gland, Brain, Brain Point, Occiput.

Method

Three to five otopoints are employed each treatment session, strong stimulation is applied, and the needles are retained at each otopoint for thirty minutes. The treatment is given once daily and for seven times as a course. Or, in coordination, the otopoints are embbedded with the thumb — tack needles or stuck with the vaccaria seeds and the patient is asked to press them two or three times daily. The seeds or needles are kept on the otopoints for three to five days and other otopoints are embedded or stuck next time.

第五节 急 症

一、休 克

休克,归属于中医学"厥证"、"脱证"、"亡阴"、"亡阳"等范畴。临床表现以面色苍白,汗出四肢冷、呼吸微弱、脉搏快而微弱、血压急骤下降为特征。

技法运用

1.毫针:取人中、百会、内关、素髎、足三里、涌泉、关元等穴。

先针人中、素髎、内关、足三里,用捻转提插补法,持续运针,待血压回升后,可间歇运针或留针,若血压不升,再加其余穴位。或根据病情,结合西医综合治疗。

2.灸疗:取百会、神阙、气海、关元、涌泉、足三里穴。

用艾条悬灸或艾炷着肤灸,至血压回升为度。

有报道取至阴,百会、足三里、三阴交等穴,大艾炷隔物灸,治失血性休克。方法:隔薄棉各灸5～7壮(先同时灸至阴,气海,百会;后灸足三里、三阴交),艾炷如拇指粗,或艾卷近距离灸灼亦可,每穴灸5～10分钟。如用"太乙神针"药条灸更佳(田丛豁,等.《针灸医学验集》)。

3.耳针:取升压点(耳垂1区上方,图5—31)、肾上腺(下屏尖)、皮质下(脑)、内分泌(屏间)穴。

强刺激,留针1～2小时,间歇运针,效不显时配合其他方法治疗。

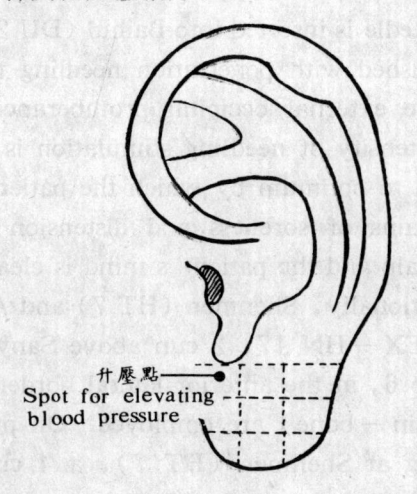

图5—31升压点

Fig. 5—31 The Spot for Elevating Blood Pressure

SECTION 5 EMERGENCY DISEASES

1. SHOCK

Manifestations

Shock, belonging to the disease or syndrome categories of Jue Zheng (厥证), Tuo Zheng (脱证, collapse syndorme), Wang Yin (亡阴, depletion of yin) and Wang Yang (亡阳, depletion of yang) in TCM, is manifested clinically by pallor, cold extremities, sweating, feeble breathing, rapid and faint pulse, as well as quick fall of blood pressure.

Treatment by Applying Acubustion Techniques

(1) Filifrom Needling

Selection of Points

Renzhong (DU 26), Baihui (DU 20), Neiguan (PC 6), Suliao (DU 25), Zusanli (ST 36), Yongquan (KI 1), Guanyuan (RN 4).

Method

At first, Renzhong (DU 26), Suliao (DU 25), Neiguan (PC 6) and Zusanli (ST 36) are punctured, and reinforcing manipulations by twirling, rotating, lifting and thrusting the needles in these points are applied continuously until the blood pressure is elevated to the normal level. Then, the needles are manipulated intermittently or retained in the points. If the blood pressure is not elevated, puncture at the other points is applied additionally or western medical therapy is given in coordination according to the patient's condition.

(2) Moxibustion

Selection of Points

Baihui (DU 20), Shenque (RN 12), Qihai (RN 6), Guanyuan (RN 4), Yongquan (KI 1), Zusanli (ST 36).

Method

Suspended moxibustion or direct moxibustion with moxa cone is applied until the blood pressure is elevated to the normal level.

Introducing An Experiential Technique

In Collection of Experiences of Acupuncture & Moxibustion a method for treatment of hemorrhagic shock is recorded. Zhiyin (BL 67), Baihui (DU 20), Zusanli (ST 36), and Sanyinjiao (SP 6) are selected, and large moxa cones, each of them being as thick as the thumb, are prepared. A thin layer of cotton is placed over the point, and the moxa cone is placed over the cotton. The moxa cone is ignited for moxibustion and five to seven cones are burnt at each point. The moxibustion is given first to Zhiyin (BL 67), Qihai (RN 6) and Baihui (DU 20) and then to Zusanli (ST 36) and Sanyinjiao (SP 6). Or suspended moxibustion is given to each point for five to ten minutes. A better effect will be caused if the moxibustion is performed by applying Taiyi Moxa — Cigar, a special moxa — stick made of chinese medicine.

(3) Otopuncture

Selection of Otopoints

Lower Tragic Notch (Elevating Blood Pressure Point, the upper area of 1st section of lobe, see Fig. (5 — 31, Adrenal Gland, Brain, Endocrine.

Mothod

Three to five otopoints are employed each treatment session, strong stimulation is chosen, and the needles are retained at each otopoint for one to two hours and manipulated intermittently during the retention. If the treatment does not work effectively, other therapies are applied in coordination.

二、中暑

中暑,为发生于夏季的一种急性疾病。中医学称为"暑厥","伤暑","暑风"。临床表现分轻重二类。轻证为发热(38.5°c以上)、头痛、头昏、恶心、胸闷、口渴、汗闭、皮肤灼热、心烦、疲乏无力;重证除上述症状外,尚有高热达40℃以上、昏倒、肢冷或抽搐、腓肠肌痉挛及血压下降,脉细弱而快。

技法运用

1. 毫针:

轻证:取大椎、曲池、合谷、陷谷、内关、足三里穴。用捻转提插泻法,留针15~20分钟。

重证:取百会、人中、十宣、曲池、委中、曲泽、足三里、素髎、涌泉、内关穴。用捻转提插泻法,每次3~5穴。十宣、曲泽、委中,用三棱针点刺放血。

虚脱脉微细欲绝者,急灸神阙、气海、关元,腓肠肌痉挛加针承山。另外,轻证可施刮痧疗法。方法:用光滑平整的陶瓷汤匙、蘸食油或清水,刮脊背两侧,颈部,胸肋间隙,肩、臂、肘窝及腋窝,刮至皮肤紫红为度。

2. 耳针:心、神门、脑、下屏尖、枕、耳尖、下脚端。

强刺激,留针30分钟,耳廓经医师按摩充血后,取耳尖用三棱针点刺放血。

2. SUNSTROKE

Manifestations

Sunstroke is an acute case occurring in summer. It belongs to the disease categories of Shang Shu (伤暑, summer—heat injury), and Shu Feng (暑风, Summer—heat convulsions), and Shu Jue (暑厥, heat exhaustion) in TCM. It may be divided clinically into two types: the mild and the severe. The mild type is manifested by fever (the temperature being above 38.5℃), headache, dizziness, nausea, suffocated sensation in chest, thirst, absence of sweating, hot skin, restlessness, lassitude and forcelessness. The severe type, usually developing from the mild one, is manifested by high fever (the temperature being above 40℃), collapse, cold extremities or convulsion, systremma, fall of blood pressure, thready and faint pulse.

Treatment by Applying Acubustion Techniques

(1) *Filiform Needling*

a. For mild cases:

Selection of Points

Dazhui (DU 14), Quchi (LI 11), Hegu (LI 4), Xiangu (ST 43), Neiguan (PC 6), Zusanli (ST 36).

Method

Three to five points are employed each treatment session, reducing manipulations by twisting, lifting and thrusting the needle are applied, and the needles are retained at each point for fifteen to twenty minutes. Chengshan (BL 57) is punctured additionally if there is systremma.

b. For severe cases:

Selection of Points

Baihui (DU 20), Renzhong (DU 26), Shixuan (EX—UE 11), Quchi (LI

11) Weizhong (BL 40), Quze (PC 3), Zusanli (ST 36), Suliao (DU 25), Yongquan (KI 1), Neiguan (PC 6).

Method

Three to five points are employed each treatment session. Shixuan (EX—UE 11), Quze (PC 3) and Weizhong (BL 40) are pricked to cause bleeding with the three—edged needle. Reducing manipulations by twisting, lifting and thrusting the needle are applied at the other points if they are selected. Chengshan (BL 57) is punctured additionally if there is systremma.

(2) *Moxibustion*

Selection of Points

Shenque (RN 8), Qihai (RN 6), Guanyuan (RN 4).

Method

Moxibustion is only applicable to the cases diagnosed as prostration syndrome with small and indistinct pulse. Moxibustion with the moxa stick is applied to each point until the symptoms are relieved.

(3) *Scraping Therapy*

Selection of Points

Bilateral sides of the spinal column, neck, intercostal spaces, shoulder regions, cubital and axilla fossae.

Method

Scraping therapy is a popular treatment method for mild sunstroke in China. A smooth spoon is dipped into water or vegetable oil, and the regions selected are scraped with the spoon until purplish red colour appears at these region.

(4) *Otopuncture*

Selection of Otopoints

Heart, Shenmen, Brain, Adrenal Gland, Occiput, Ear Apex, Sympathetic.

Method

Three to five otopoints are employed each treatment session, strong stimulation is applied, and the needles are retained at each otopoint for thirty minutes. But to Ear Apex, pricking is performed with the threeedged needle to cause bleeding after the local region is congested by massage.

〔附 1〕　　主要参考书籍

宋.闻人耆年：《备急灸法》，人民卫生出版社仿宋本影印，1955年。
金元.窦汉卿：《针经指南》，回抄本。
元.窦桂芳：《针灸四书》，元至大四年辛亥刊本。
元.王国瑞：《扁鹊神应针灸玉龙经》，四库全书本。
明.陈会：《神应经》，1957年据正保二年翻刻本抄。
明.徐凤：《针灸大全》，人民卫生出版社，1958。
明.汪机：《针灸问对》，江苏科学技术出版社，1985。
明.杨继洲：《针灸大成》，人民卫生出版社，1963。
靳瑞等：《针灸按摩补泻解说》科学普及出版社广州分社，1990。
王雪苔：《中国针灸大全》，河南科学技术出版社，1988。
安徽中医学院等：《针灸学辞典》，上海科学技术出版社，1987。
清.周树冬遗稿，周楣声重订：《金针梅花诗抄》，安徽科学技术出版社，1982。
陆寺康等：《针刺手法一百种》，中国医药科技出版社，1988。
赵缉庵：《针灸要诀与按摩十法》，中医古籍出版社，1986。
马瑞林等：《中国针刺手法汇编》，辽宁中医学院，中华全国中医学会辽宁分会，1982。
刘冠军等：《中医针法集锦》，江西科学技术出版社，1988。
孙学全：《针灸临证集验》，山东科学技术出版社，1982。
陈积祥等：《针术临床实践》，陕西科学技术出版社，1983。
梁庆临等：《针挑疗法》，广东科学技术出版社，1984。
刘万成：《实用毫针刺法手册》，江苏科学技术出版社，1990。
谢锡亮等：《灸法》，山西人民出版社，1984。

方云鹏：《头皮针》，陕西科学技术出版社，1982。
陆瘦燕等：《刺灸法汇编》，上海科学技术出版社，1959。
钟梅泉：《中国梅花针》，人民卫生出版社，1984。
田丛豁等：《针灸医学验集》，科学技术出版社，1985。
安西川等：《实用针灸手册，中英日对照》，吉林科学技术出版社，1989。
章逢润等：《中国灸疗学》，人民卫生出版社，1989。
田丛豁等：《中国灸法集粹》，辽宁科学技术出版社，1987。
焦国瑞等：《针灸临床经验辑要》，人民卫生出版社，1981。
陈佑邦等：《当代中国针灸临证精要》，天津科学技术出版社，1987。
焦顺发：《头针》，山西人民出版社，1982。
宋一同等：《头针与耳针》，中国医药科技出版社，1990。
张心曙：《腕踝针》，上海科学技术出版社，1973。
杨庆云：《针灸治疗百病荟萃》，四川科学技术出版社，1989。
北京中医学院等：《中国针灸学概要》，人民卫生出版社，1979。
程莘农：《中国针灸学》，人民卫生出版社，1982。
李文瑞等：《实用针灸学》，人民卫生出版社，1982。
上海中医学院：《针灸学》，人民卫生出版社，1974。
刘冠军：《针灸学》，湖南科学技术出版社，1987。
江苏新医学院：《针灸学》，上海人民出版社，1975。
奚永红：《针法灸法学》，上海科学技术出版社，1985。
杨甲三：《腧穴学》，上海科学技术出版社，1984。
南京中医学院：《针灸学》，上海科学技术出版社，1979。
邱茂良：《针灸学》，上海科学技术出版社，1985。

邝贺龄等:《内科急诊治疗学》,上海科学技术出版社,1981。

刘冠军:《针灸学》,光明日报出版社,1988。

杨占林:《针刺事故预防》,山西科学技术出版社,1987。

孔介凡等:《实用医生手册》,山东科学技术出版社,1985。

《全国针灸针麻学术讨论会论文摘要》,中国针灸学会,1979。

《第三届全国针灸针麻学术讨论会》论文摘要,中国针灸学会,1984。

第一届世界针灸学术大会《针灸论文摘要选编》,中国针灸学会,1987。

中医研究院医史文献研究室《中西医结合论文选编》,第一分册(针灸),1980。

中山医学院:《内科疾病鉴别诊断学》,人民卫生出版社,1976。

· 453 ·

APPENDIX I BIBLIOGRAPHY

1. **Historical Publications** (the author and the publishing age are given in the bracket for each literature):

Emergency Moxibustion Therapy (Wenren Qinian, 1226)

Handbook of Acupuncture (Dou Hanqing, 1295)

Four Books of Acupuncture and Moxibustion (Dou Guifang, 1311)

Bianque's Acupuncture and Moxibustion Classic of Maraculous Cure (Wang Gourui, the Ming Dynasty, 1368—1644)

The Classic of Miraculous Cure (Chen Hui, the Ming Dynasty, 1368—1644)

A Complete Works in Acupuncture and Moxibustion (Xu Feng, 1439)

The Questions and Answers on Acupuncture and Moxibustion (Wang Ji, 1530)

Great Compendium of Acupuncture and Moxibustion (Yang Jizhou, 1601)

2. **Recent Publications**:

Explanations Concerning Reinforcing and Reducing by Acupuncture, Moxibustion and Massage, edited by Jin Rui, published by Guangzhou Branch of Popular Science Publishing House, 1990.

Complete Works of Chinese Acupuncture and Moxibustion, edited by Wang Xuetai, published by Hunan Science and Technology Publishing House, 1988.

Dictionary of Acupuncture and Moxibustion, edited by Anhui College of TCM, et al, published by Shanghai Science and Technology Publishing House, 1987.

Selection of the Rhymes of Acupuncture and Blossom, edited by Zhou Shudong and Zhou Meisheng, published by Anhui Science and Technology Publishing House, 1982.

One Hundred Techniques of Acupuncture, edited by Lu Shoukang, published by Chinese Medical Science and Technology Publishing House, 1988.

Essence of Acupuncture and Moxibustion and Ten Methods of Massage, edited by Zhao Jian, published by Ancient Traditional Chinese Medical Book Publishing House, 1986.

Collection of Techniques of Chinese Acupuncture, edited by Ma Ruilin, Liaoning Branch of All—china Association of TCM, 1982.

Collection of Outstandings of the Needling Methods of TCM, edited by Liu Guanjun, published by Jiangxi Science and Technology Publishing House, 1988.

Collection of Clinical Experiences of Acupuncture and Moxibustion, edited by Sun Xuequan, published by Shandong Science and Technology Publishing House, 1982.

Clinical Practice of Acupuncture and Moxibustion, edited by Chen Jixiang, published by Shanxi Science and Technology Publishing House, 1983.

Pricking Therapy with the Needle, edited by Liang Qinglin, published by Guangdong Science and Technolgy Publishing House, 1984.

Practical Handbook of Acupuncture Techniques, edited by Liu Wancheng, published by Jiangsu Science and Technology Publishing House, 1990.

Moxibustion Techniques, edited by Xie Xiliang, et al, published by Shanxi People's Publishing House, 1984.

Scalp Acupuncture, edited by Fang Yunpeng, published by Shanxi Science and Technology Publishing House, 1982.

Collection of Acupuncture and Moixbustion Techniques, edited by Lu Shouyan, et al, published by Shanghai Science and Technology Publishing House, 1959.

Chinese Blossom — Needling, edited by Zhong Meiquan, published by People's Medical Publishing House, 1984.

Collection of Experiences of Acupuncture and Moxibustion, edited by Tian Yehou, published by Science and Technology Publishing House, 1985.

Practical Handbook on Acupuncture and Moxibustion, edited by An Xichuan, et al, publshed by Jilin Science and Technology Publishing House, 1989.

Chinese Moxibustion Therapy, edited by Zhang Fengrun, published by People's Medical Publishing House, 1989.

Collection of Outstandings of Chinese Moxibustion Techniques, edited by Tian Yehuo, published by liaoning Science and Technology Publishing House, 1987.

Outstandings of Clinical Experiences of Acupuncture and Moxibustion, edited by Jiao Guorui, published by People's Medical Publishing House, 1981.

Outstandings of Clinical Experiences of Modern Chinese Acupuncture and Moxibustion, edited by Chen Youbang, published by Tianjin Science and Technology Publishing House, 1987.

Scalp Acupuncture, edited by Jiao Shunfa, published by Shanxi People's Publishing House, 1982

Scalp Acupuncture and Ear Acupuncture, edited by Song Yitong, published by Chinese Medical Science and Technology Publishing House, 1990.

Wrist—Ankle Acupuncture, edited by Zhang Xinshu, published by Shanghai Science and Technology Publishing

House, 1973.

Collection of Outstandings of Clinical Experiences in Treatment of Diseases by Acupuncture and Moxibustion, edited by Yang Qingyun, published by Siquan Science and Technology Publishing House, 1989.

Essentials of Chinese Acupuncture, edited by Beijing College of TCM, published by People's Medical Publsing House, 1979.

Chinese Acupuncture and Moxibustion, edited by Cheng Xinnong, published by Foreign Language Press, 1987.

Applied Acupuncture and Moxibustion, edited by Li Wenrui, published by People's Medical Publishing House, 1982.

Science of Acupuncture and Moxibustion, edited by Shanghai College of TCM, published by People's Medical Publishing House, 1974.

Science of Acupuncture and Moxibustion, edited by Liu Guanjun, published by Hunan Science and Technology Publishing House, 1987.

Science of Acupunctute and Moxibustion, edited by Jiangsu College of New Medicne, published by Shanghai People's Publishing House, 1975.

Acupuncture and Moxibustion Techniques, edited by Xi Yongjiang, published by Shanghai Science and Technology Publishing House, 1985.

Science of Acupoints, edited by Yang Jiasan, published by Shanghai Science and Technology Publishing House, 1984.

Science of Acupuncture and Moxibustion, edited by Nanjing College of TCM, pulbished by Shanghai Science and Technology Publishing House, 1979.

Science of Acupuncture and Moxibustion, edited by Qiu Maoliang, pulbished by Shanghai Science and Technology Publishing House, 1985.

Science of Acupuncture and Moxibustion, edited by Liu Guangjun, published by Guanming Daily Publishing House, 1988.

Paper Abstracts of the National Symposia of Acupuncture and Moxibustion and Acupuncture Anaesthesia, Chinese Acupuncture and Moxibustion Association, 1979.

Paper Abstracts of the Second National Symposia of Acupuncture and Moxibustion and Acupuncture Anaesthesia, Chinese Acupuncture and Moxibustion Association, 1984.

Compilation of the Abstracts of Acupuncture and Moxibustion Papers ———— The First World Conference on Acupuncture and Moxibustion, Chinese Acupuncture and Moxibustion Association, 1987.

Therapeutics of Internal Emergency Diseases, edited by Kuang Heling, et al, published by Shanghai Science Publishing House, 1981.

Prevention of Acupuncture Accidents, edited by Yang Zhanlin, Published by Shanxi Science and Education Publishing House, 1987.

Doctor's Applicatory Handbook, edited by Kong Jiefan, published by Shandong Science Publishing House, 1985.

Differential Diagnostics of Internal Diseases, edited by Zhongshan Medical College, published by People's Health Publishing House, 1976.

〔附2〕 图　录

图 1—1	常用骨度分寸
图 1—2	中指同身寸
图 1—3	拇指同身寸
图 1—4	一夫法
图 1—5	简便取穴法
图 1—6	手太阴肺经循行示意图
图 1—7	手太阴肺经穴位图
图 1—8	尺泽、孔最、列缺
图 1—9	列缺穴
图 1—10	手阳明大肠经循行示意图
图 1—11	手阳明大肠经穴位图
图 1—12	二间、三间、合谷、阳溪
图 1—13	合谷穴
图 1—14	臂臑，肩髃
图 1—15	足阳明胃经循行示意图
图 1—16	足阳明胃经穴位图
图 1—17	承泣、四白、地仓
图 1—18	承泣刺法
图 1—19	颊车、下关、头维、人迎
图 1—20	乳根穴
图 1—21	天枢，水道，归来
图 1—22	髀关，伏兔，梁丘
图 1—23	简便取伏兔
图 1—24	足阳明胃经下肢常用穴
图 1—25	足三里穴
图 1—26	足阳明胃经足部常用穴
图 1—27	足太阴脾经循行示意图
图 1—28	足太阴脾经穴位图
图 1—29	足太阴脾经足部常用穴
图 1—30	三阴交、地机、阴陵泉
图 1—31	血海穴
图 1—32	大横穴
图 1—33	手少阴心经循行示意图
图 1—34	手少阴心经穴位图
图 1—35	灵道、通里、阴郄、神门
图 1—36	少府、少冲
图 1—37	手太阳小肠经循行示意图
图 1—38	手太阳小肠经手部常用穴
图 1—40	养老取穴图
图 1—41	支正、小海
图 1—42	肩贞、天宗、肩外俞
图 1—43	颧髎，听宫
图 1—44	足太阳膀胱经循行示意图
图 1—45	足太阳膀胱经穴位图
图 1—46	睛明，攒竹
图 1—47	天柱穴
图 1—48	足太阳膀胱经背腰常用穴
图 1—49	足太阳膀胱经下肢常用穴
图 1—50	足太阳膀胱经足部常用穴
图 1—51	足少阴肾经循行示意图
图 1—52	足少阴肾经穴位图
图 1—53	足少阴肾经下肢常用穴
图 1—54	手厥阴心包经循行示意图
图 1—55	手厥阴心包经穴位图
图 1—56	手厥阴心包经上肢常用穴
图 1—57	劳宫、中冲
图 1—58	手少阳三焦经循行示意图
图 1—59	手少阳三焦经穴位图
图 1—60	关冲、液门、中渚、阳池
图 1—61	阳池穴
图 1—62	手少阳三焦经上肢常用穴
图 1—63	天井、肩髎
图 1—64	翳风、角孙、耳门、丝竹空
图 1—65	角孙穴
图 1—66	足少阳胆经循行示意图
图 1—67	足少阳胆经穴位图
图 1—68	瞳子髎、阳白、听会
图 1—69	听会穴
图 1—70	率谷穴
图 1—71	风池、肩井定位与风池刺法
图 1—72	环跳穴
图 1—73	足少阳胆经下肢常用穴
图 1—74	丘墟、足临泣、侠溪、窍阴
图 1—75	足厥阴肝经循行示意图
图 1—77	大敦、行间、太冲、中封
图 1—78	曲泉穴
图 1—79	章门、期门
图 1—80	任脉循行示意图
图 1—81	任脉穴位图
图 1—82	天突、廉泉
图 1—83	天突穴刺法
图 1—84	督脉循行示意图
图 1—85	督脉穴位图
图 1—86	长强穴
图 1—87	长强穴针刺姿式
图 1—88	哑门、风府
图 1—89	哑门穴刺法
图 1—90	百会，上星，素髎
图 1—91	素髎、水沟（人中）
图 1—92	龈交穴
图 1—93	四神聪穴
图 1—94	印堂、鱼腰、球后
图 1—95	鱼腰、球后
图 1—96	太阳、牵正

图 1—97　翳明、安眠
图 1—98　定喘、夹脊
图 1—99　十宣穴
图 1—100　八邪穴
图 1—101　四缝穴
图 1—102　下肢常用经外奇穴
图 2—1　耳廓表面解剖
图 2—2　耳穴形象分布示意图
图 2—3　常用耳穴分布图
图 2—4　标定线
图 2—5　运动区
图 2—6　侧面刺激区
图 2—7　顶面刺激区
图 2—8　后面刺激区
图 2—9　前面刺激区
图 2—10　前面图
图 2—11　顶面图
图 2—12　侧面图（一）
图 2—13　侧面图（二）
图 2—14　后面图
图 2—15　腕部进针点
图 2—16　踝部进针点
图 3—1　毫针结构
图 3—2　三棱针
图 3—3　麦粒形皮内针
　　　　　环形皮内针
图 3—4　揿针
图 3—5　皮肤针
图 3—6　火针
图 3—7　锟针
图 3—8　G6805电针治疗仪
图 3—9　耳穴探测仪
图 3—10　常用灸材(1)(2)
图 3—11　竹罐
图 3—12　陶罐
图 3—13　玻璃罐
图 3—14　抽气罐
图 3—15　高压灭菌锅消毒
图 3—16　施术部位消毒
图 4—1　两指持针法
图 4—2　三指持针法
图 4—3　四指持针法
图 4—4　指力练习
图 4—5　捻转练习
图 4—6　提插练习
图 4—7　仰卧位
图 4—8　俯卧位
图 4—9　侧卧位
图 4—10　仰靠坐位
图 4—11　俯伏坐位
图 4—12　侧伏坐位
图 4—13　单手进针
图 4—14　指切进针
图 4—15　舒张进针
图 4—16　提捏进针
图 4—17　挟持进针

图 4—18　套管进针
图 4—19　针刺角度
图 4—20　提插法
图 4—21　捻转法
图 4—22　循法
图 4—23　摄法
图 4—24　弹法
图 4—25　刮法
图 4—26　飞法
图 4—27　摇法
图 4—28　盘法
图 4—29　按法
图 4—30　抽法
图 4—31　敲法
图 4—32　推法
图 4—33　捻转补泻
图 4—34　提插补泻
图 4—35　疾徐补泻
图 4—36　迎随补泻
图 4—37　呼吸补泻
图 4—38　开阖补泻
图 4—39　烧山火
图 4—40　透天凉
图 4—41　进火补法
图 4—42　进水泻法
图 4—43　阳中隐阴法
图 4—44　阴中隐阳法
图 4—45　青龙摆尾
图 4—46　白虎摇头
图 4—47　苍龟探穴
图 4—48　赤凤迎源
图 4—49　子午捣白
图 4—50　龙虎交战
图 4—51　龙虎升降
图 4—52　出针
图 4—53　弯针处理
图 4—54　断针处理
图 4—55　点刺法
图 4—56　散刺法
图 4—57　挑刺法
图 4—58　皮内针埋针法
图 4—59　揿针埋针法
图 4—60　皮肤针持针法
图 4—61　皮肤针操作
图 4—62　不正确操作
图 4—63　常规刺激部位
图 4—64　循经条刺
图 4—65　局部叩刺
图 4—66　锟针刺法
图 4—67　电锟针
图 4—68　火针深刺法
图 4—69　火针浅刺法
图 4—70　二穴通电法
图 4—71　一穴通电法
图 4—72　水针技法
图 4—73　肉眼观察法

图 4—74　压按法
图 4—75　耳穴电阻测定法
图 4—76　耳穴刺法
图 4—77　耳穴贴敷法
图 4—78　耳穴皮肤针刺法
图 4—79　头针进针法
图 4—80　头针出针法
图 4—81　腕踝针针刺法
图 4—82　圆柱型艾炷
图 4—83　圆锥型艾炷
图 4—84　直接灸
图 4—85　瘢痕灸
图 4—86　隔姜灸
图 4—87　隔盐灸
图 4—88　温和灸
图 4—89　回旋灸
图 4—90　雀啄灸
图 4—91　温针灸
图 4—92　灯火灸
图 4—93　蒜泥灸
图 4—94　投火法
图 4—95　闪火法
图 4—96　贴棉法
图 4—97　架火法
图 4—98　走罐
图 4—99　针上套罐
图 4—100　抽气拔罐
图 4—101　起罐法
图 5—1　痄腮穴
图 5—2　火柴棒灸
图 5—3　腮腺穴
图 5—4　疟门穴刺法
图 5—5　平喘穴
图 5—6　关闭法刺内关
图 5—7　长针透刺
图 5—8　压按攒竹穴
图 5—9　腹泻特效穴
图 5—10　阑尾压痛点
图 5—11　迎香透四白
图 5—12　腹外穴
图 5—13　二白穴
图 5—14　长强刺法
图 5—15　金津玉液穴
图 5—16　头颞穴
图 5—17　三叉神经痛刺法
图 5—18　三叉神经痛刺法
图 5—19　刺咬合线
图 5—20　坐骨神经痛针刺点
图 5—21　指压关元穴
图 5—22　指压极泉穴
图 5—23　肩枢穴
图 5—24　天宗穴分筋法
图 5—25　神道刺法
图 5—26　经纬叩刺
图 5—27　拔罐
图 5—28　棉花灸
图 5—29　囊肿局部扬刺
图 5—30　上迎香
图 5—31　升压点

APPENDIX Ⅱ CROSS INDEX OF THE FIGURES

Fig. 1—1 Commonly Used Bone—Measurements
Fig. 1—2 Middle Finger Measurement
Fig. 1—3 Thumb Measurement
Fig. 1—4 Four—Finger Measurement
Fig. 1—5 Simple Methods in Locating Points
Fig. 1—6 The Running Course of the Lung Meridian of Hand—Taiyin
Fig. 1—7 Acupoints of the Lung Meridian of Hand—Taiyin
Fig. 1—8 Chize (LU 5), Kongzui (LU 6) and Lieque (LU 7)
Fig. 1—9 Lieque (LU 7)
Fig. 1—10 The Running Course of the Large Intestine Meridian of Hand—Yangming
Fig. 1—11 Acupoints of the Large Intestine Meridian of Hand—Yangming
Fig. 1—12 Erjian (LI 2), Sanjian (LI 3), Hegu (LI 4) and Yangxi (LI 5)
Fig. 1—13 Hegu (LI 4)
Fig. 1—14 Jianyu (LI 15) and Binao (LI 14)
Fig. 1—15 The Running Course of the Stomach Meridian of Foot—Yangming
Fig. 1—16 Acupoints of the Stomach Meridian of Foot—Yangming
Fig. 1—17 Chengqi (ST 1), Sibai (ST 2) and Dicang (ST 4)
Fig. 1—18 Needling at Chengqi (ST 1)
Fig. 1—19 Jiache (ST 6), Xiaguan (ST 7), Touwei (ST 8) and Renying (ST 9)
Fig. 1—20 Rugen (ST18)
Fig. 1—21 Tianshu (ST 25), Shuidao (ST 28) and Guilai (ST 29)
Fig. 1—22 Biguan (ST 31), Futu (ST 32) and Liangqiu (ST 34)
Fig. 1—23 Simple Way for Locating Futu (ST 32)
Fig. 1—24 Acupoints of the Stomach Meridian of Foot—Yangming at the Lower Limb
Fig. 1—25 Zusanli (ST 36)
Fig. 1—26 Commonly Used Acupoints of the Stomach Meridian of Foot—Yangming at the Foot
Fig. 1—27 The Running Course of the Spleen Meridian of Foot—Taiyin
Fig. 1—28 Acupoints of the Spleen Meridian of Foot—Taiyin
Fig. 1—29 Commonly Used Acupoints of the Spleen Meridian at the Foot
Fig. 1—30 Sanyinjiao (SP 6), Diji (SP 8) and Yinlingquan (SP 9)
Fig. 1—31 Xuehai (SP 10)
Fig. 1—32 Daheng (SP 15)
Fig. 1—33 The Running Course of the Heart Meridian of Hand—Shaoyin
Fig. 1—34 Acupoints of the Heart Meridian of Hand—Shaoyin
Fig. 1—35 Lingdao (HT 4), Tongli (HT 5), Yinxi (HT 6) and Shenmen (HT 7)
Fig. 1—36 Shaofu (HT 8) and Shaochong (HT 9)
Fig. 1—37 The Running Course of the Small Intestine Meridian of Hand—Taiyang
Fig. 1—38 The Acupoints of the Small Intestine Meridian of Hand—Taiyang
Fig. 1—39 Commonly Used Acupoints of the Small Intestine meridian at the Hand
Fig. 1—40 The Way of Locating Yanglao (SI 6)
Fig. 1—41 Zhizheng (SI 7) and Xiaohai (SI 8)
Fig. 1—42 Jianzhen (SI 9), Tianzong (SI 11) and Jianwaishu (SI 14)
Fig. 1—43 Quanliao (SI 18) and Tinggong (SI 19)
Fig. 1—44 The Running Course of the Bladder Meridian of Foot—Taiyang
Fig. 1—45 Acupoints of the Bladder Meridian of Foot—Taiyang
Fig. 1—46 Jingming (BL 1) and Cuanzhu (BL 2)
Fig. 1—47 Tianzhu (BL 10)
Fig. 1—48 Commonly Used Acupoints of the Bladder Meridian at the Back
Fig. 1—49 Commonly Used Acupoints of the Bladder Meridian at the Lower Limb
Fig. 1—50 Commonly Used Acupoints of the Bladder Meridian at the Foot
Fig. 1—51 The Running Course of the Kidney Meridian of Foot—Shaoyin
Fig. 1—52 The Acupoints of the Kidney Meridian of Foot—Shaoyin
Fig. 1—53 Commonly Used Acupoints of the Kidney Meridian at the Lower Limb
Fig. 1—54 The Running Course of the Pericardium Meridian of Hand—Jueyin

Fig. 1—55 The Acupoints of the Pericardium Meridian of Hand—Jueyin

Fig. 1—56 Commonly Used Acupoints of the Pericardium Meridian at the Upper Limb

Fig. 1—57 Laogong (PC 8) and Zhongchong (PC 9)

Fig. 1—58 The Running Course of the Sanjiao (Triple Energizer) Meridian of Hand—Shaoyang

Fig. 1—59 Acupoints of the Sanjiao (Triple Energizer) Meridian of Hand—Shaoyang

Fig. 1—60 Guanchong (SJ 1), Yemen (SJ 2), Zhongzhu (SJ 3) and Yangchi (SJ 4)

Fig. 1—61 Yangchi (SJ 4)

Fig. 1—62 Commonly Used Acupoints of the Triple Energizer Meridian at the Upper Limb

Fig. 1—63 Tianjing (SJ 10) and Jianliao (SJ 14)

Fig. 1—64 Yifeng (SJ 17), Jiaosun (SJ 20), Ermen (SJ 21) and Sizhukong (SJ 23)

Fig. 1—65 Jiaosun (SJ 20)

Fig. 1—66 The Running Course of the Gallbladder Meridian of Foot—Shaoyang

Fig. 1—67 Acupoints of the Gallbladder Meridian of Foot—Shaoyang

Fig. 1—68 Yangbai (GB 14), Tongziliao (GB 1) and Tinghui (GB 2)

Fig. 1—69 Tinghui (GB 2)

Fig. 1—70 Shuaigu (GB 8)

Fig. 1—71 Location of Fengchi (GB 20) and Jianjing (GB 21) and Needling of Fengchi (GB 20)

Fig. 1—72 Huantiao (GB 34)

Fig. 1—73 Commonly Used Acupoints of the Gallbladder Meridian at the Lower Limb

Fig. 1—74 Qiuxu (GB 40), Zulinqi (GB 41), Xiaxi (GB 43) and Zuqiaoyin (GB 44)

Fig. 1—75 The Running Course of the Liver Meridian of Foot—Jueyin

Fig. 1—76 Acupoints of the Liver Meridian of Foot—Jueyin

Fig. 1—77 Dadun (LR 1), Xingjian (LR 2), Taichong (LR 3) and Zhongfeng (LR 4)

Fig. 1—78 Ququan (LR 8)

Fig. 1—79 Zhangmen (LR 13) and Qimen (LR 14)

Fig. 1—80 The Running Course of the Conception Vessel (Ren Meridian)

Fig. 1—81 The Acupoints of the Ren Meridian (Conception Vessel)

Fig. 1—82 Tiantu (RN 22) and Lianquan (RN 23)

Fig. 1—83 Needling at Tiantu (RN 22)

Fig. 1—84 The Running Course of the Governor Vessel (Du Meridian)

Fig. 1—85 The Acupoints of the Du Meridian (Governor Vessel)

Fig. 1—86 Changqiang (DU 1)

Fig. 1—87 Patient's Posture in Needling at Changqiang (DU 1)

Fig. 1—88 Yamen (DU 15) and Fengfu (DU 16)

Fig. 1—89 Needling at Yamen (DU 15)

Fig. 1—90 Baihui (DU 20), Shangxin (DU 23) and Suliao (DU 25)

Fig. 1—91 Suliao (DU 25) and Shuigou (DU 26)

Fig. 1—92 Yinjiao (DU 28)

Fig. 1—93 Sishencong (EX—HN 1)

Fig. 1—94 Yintang (EX—HN 3), Yuyao (EX—HN 4) and Qiuhou (EX—HN 7)

Fig. 1—95 Yuyao (EX—HN 4) and Qiuhou (EX—HN 7)

Fig. 1—96 Taiyang (EX—HN 5) and Qianzheng (EX—HN 16)

Fig. 1—97 Yiming (EX—HN 14) and Anmian (EX—HN 17)

Fig. 1—98 Dingchuan (EX—B 1) and Jiaji (EX—B 2)

Fig. 1—99 Shixuan (EX—UE 11)

Fig. 1—100 Baxie (EX—UE 9)

Fig. 1—101 Sifeng (EX—UE 10)

Fig. 1—102 Commonly Used Extra Points at the Lower Limb

Fig. 2—1 Anatomical Structure of the Auricle Surface

Fig. 2—2 Regularity of Distribution of Otopoints

Fig. 2—3 The Commonly Used Otopoints

Fig. 2—4 The Reference Lines on the Scalp

Fig. 2—5 The Motor Area

Fig. 2—6 In lateral View

Fig. 2—7 In Vertex View

Fig. 2—8 In Posterior View

Fig. 2—9 In Anterior View

Fig. 2—10 In Anterior View

Fig. 2—11 In Vertex View

Fig. 2—12 In Lateral View A

Fig. 2—13 In Lateral View B

Fig. 2—14 In Posterior View

Fig. 2—15 Stimulating Points of Wrist—Puncture

Fig. 2—16 Stimulating Points of Ankle—Acupuncture

Fig. 3—1 The Sturcture of the Filiform Needle

Fig. 3—2 The Three—Edged Needle

Fig. 3—3 The Wheat—Granule—Shaped and Circle—Shaped Needle

Fig. 3—4 The Thumb—Pin—Shaped Needle

Fig. 3—5 The Skin Needle

Fig. 3—6 The Hot Needle

Fig. 3—7 The Dull Needle

Fig. 3—8 The G 6805 Electroacupuncture Therapeutic Unit

Fig. 3—9 The Electric Unit for Probing the Otopoint

Fig. 3—10 Materials for Moxibustion

Fig. 3—11 Bamboo Jar

Fig. 3—12 Pottery Jar

Fig. 3—13 Glass Jar
Fig. 3—14 Aspirating Jar
Fig. 3—15 Sterilization by the Autoclave
Fig. 3—16 Sterilization of the Skin to Be Punctured
Fig. 4—1 Holding the Needle with Two Fingers
Fig. 4—2 Holding the Needle with Three Fingers
Fig. 4—3 Holding the Needle with the Four Fingers
Fig. 4—4 Practicing the Finger Force
Fig. 4—5 Twirling and Rotating the Needle
Fig. 4—6 Liting and Thrusting the Needle
Fig. 4—7 The Supine Posture
Fig. 4—8 The Prone Posture
Fig. 4—9 The Lateral Recumbent Posture
Fig. 4—10 The Supine Sitting Posture
Fig. 4—11 The Prone Sitting Posture
Fig. 4—12 The Lateral Sitting Posture
Fig. 4—13 Inserting the Needle with One Hand
Fig. 4—14 Inserting the Needle Aided by the Pressure from the Finger of the Pressing Hand
Fig. 4—15 Inserting the Needle with Fingers Stretching the Skin
Fig. 4—16 Inserting the Needle by Pinching up the Skin
Fig. 4—17 Inserting the Needle by Gripping It
Fig. 4—18 Inserting the Needle with the Help of the Tube
Fig. 4—19 The Angle of the Insertion
Fig. 4—20 Thrusting and Lifting
Fig. 4—21 Twirling and Rotating
Fig. 4—22 Massaging along the Meridian.
Fig. 4—23 Pinching along the Meridian
Fig. 4—24 Flicking Method
Fig. 4—25 Scraping Method
Fig. 4—26 Flying Method
Fig. 4—27 Shaking Method
Fig. 4—28 Circling Method
Fig. 4—29 Pressing Method
Fig. 4—30 Withdrawing Method
Fig. 4—31 Tapping Method
Fig. 4—32 Pushing Method
Fig. 4—33 Reinforcing and Reducing by Twirling and Rotating the Needle
Fig. 4—34 Reinforcing and Reducing by Lifting and Thrusting the Needle
Fig. 4—35 Reinforcing and Reducing Achieved by Rapid and Slow Insertion and Withdrawal of the Needle
Fig. 4—36 Reinforcing and Reducing Achieved by Puncturing along and against the Running Direction of the Meridian
Fig. 4—37 Reinforcing and Reducing Achieved by Manipulating the Needle in Cooperation with the Patient's Respiration
Fig. 4—38 Reinforcing and Reducing Achieved by Keeping the Needle Hole Open or Close
Fig. 4—39 Heat—Producing Needling
Fig. 4—40 Cool—Producing Needling
Fig. 4—41 Reinforcing Method by Fire (Yang)—Producing Needling
Fig. 4—42 Reducing Method by Water (Yin)—Producing Needling
Fig. 4—43 Yin Occluding in Yang
Fig. 4—44 Yang Occluding in Yin
Fig. 4—45 Green Dragon Shaking Tail
Fig. 4—46 White Tiger Shaking Head
Fig. 4—47 Green Tortoise Seeking for Cave
Fig. 4—48 Red Phenix Meeting Resource
Fig. 4—49 Zi Wu Dao Jiu Needling
Fig. 4—50 Dragon—Tiger Fighting
Fig. 4—51 Dragon—Tiger Ascending—Descending Method
Fig. 4—52 Withdrawing the Needle
Fig. 4—53 Withdrawing the Bent Needle
Fig. 4—54 Withdrawing the Broken Needle
Fig. 4—55 Spot Pricking
Fig. 4—56 Scattering Pricking
Fig. 4—57 Fibrous—Tissue—Broken Pricking
Fig. 4—58 The Needle—Embedding Method
Fig. 4—59 Embedment of the Thumb—Tack—Shaped Needle
Fig. 4—60 Holding the Skin Needle
Fig. 4—61 The Correct Way of Manipulating the Skin Needle
Fig. 4—62 The Inccorect Way of Manipulating the Skin Needle
Fig. 4—63 The Routine Stimulating Area in Skin Needling
Fig. 4—64 Tapping along the Meridian with Skin Needle
Fig. 4—65 Tapping at the Affected Area
Fig. 4—66 Pressing with the Dull Needle
Fig. 4—67 The Electrical Dull Needle
Fig. 4—68 Deep Puncture with the Hot Needle
Fig. 4—69 Shallow Puncture with the Hot Needle
Fig. 4—70 The Way of Applying Electroacupuncture to Two Points
Fig. 4—71 The Way of Applying Electroacupuncture to One Point
Fig. 4—72 Manipulating in the Hydro—Acupuncture
Fig. 4—73 Detecting on the Auricle with the Naked Eye
Fig. 4—74 Pressing on the Auricle
Fig. 4—75 Measuring the Electrical Resistance of the Otopoint
Fig. 4—76 Puncturing at the Otopoint with the Filiform Needle
Fig. 4—77 The Otopoint—Mounting Method

Fig. 4—78 Puncturing at the Otopoint with the Plum—Blossom Needle
Fig. 4—79 Inserting the Needle in Scalp Acupuncture
Fig. 4—80 Withdrawing the Needle in Scalp Acupuncture
Fig. 4—81 Wrist—Ankle Needling
Fig. 4—82 The Moxa Cylider
Fig. 4—83 The Moxa Cone
Fig. 4—84 Direct Moxibustion
Fig. 4—85 Scarring Moxibustion
Fig. 4—86 Ginger Moxibustion
Fig. 4—87 Salt Moxibustion
Fig. 4—88 Mild—Warming Moxibustion
Fig. 4—89 Rounding Moxibustion
Fig. 4—90 Sparrow—Pecking Moxibustion
Fig. 4—91 Moxibustion with Warming Needle
Fig. 4—92 Rush—Burning Moxibustion
Fig. 4—93 Mashed Garlic Moxibustion
Fig. 4—94 Fire—Throwing Method
Fig. 4—95 Fire—Twinkling Method
Fig. 4—96 Cotton—Attaching Method
Fig. 4—97 Material—Placing Method
Fig. 4—98 Moving Cupping
Fig. 4—99 Cupping with the Needle inside the Jar
Fig. 4—100 Aspirating Cupping
Fig. 4—101 Removing the Jar
Fig. 5—1 Zhasai (Extra point)
Fig. 5—2 Moxibustion with the Ignited Match
Fig. 5—3 Ot. Parotid Glands
Fig. 5—4 Puncturing at Nuemenxue (Extra point)
Fig. 5—5 Ot. Soothing Asthma
Fig. 5—6 Puncturing at Neiguan (PC 6) for Gastritis
Fig. 5—7 Penetration Needling with the Long Needle
Fig. 5—8 Pressing Cuanzhu (BL 2)
Fig. 5—9 Fuxietexiaoxue (Extra point)
Fig. 5—10 Tender Spots Relating to Appendix
Fig. 5—11 Penetration Needling from Yingxiang (LI 20) to Sibai (ST 2)
Fig. 5—12 Ot. Fuwaixue
Fig. 5—13 Erbai (EX—UE 2)
Fig. 5—14 Puncturing at Changqiang (DU 1)
Fig. 5—15 Jinjin and Yuye (EX—HN 12,13)
Fig. 5—16 Tounie (Extra point)
Fig. 5—17 The Needling Applied for Trigeminal Neuralgia
Fig. 5—18 The Needling Applied for Trigeminal Neuralgia
Fig. 5—19 Puncturing at the Line of Occlusion at the Buccal Mucosa
Fig. 5—20 The Needling Points for Sciatica
Fig. 5—21 Pressing Guanyuan (RN 4) with the Finger
Fig. 5—22 Pressing Jiquan (HT 1) with the Finger
Fig. 5—23 Jianshu (Extra point)
Fig. 5—24 The Tendon—Pushing Method Applied on Tianzong (SI 11)
Fig. 5—25 Puncturing at Shendao (DU 11)
Fig. 5—26 Tapping for Neurodermatitis
Fig. 5—27 Cupping
Fig. 5—28 Cotton Attaching Moxibustion
Fig. 5—29 Scattering Pricking for Ganglion
Fig. 5—30 Shangyingxiang (EX—HN 8)
Fig. 5—31 The Spot for Elevating Blood Pressure

读书札记

读书札记

读书札记

读书札记

NOTE

读书札记

读书札记

读书札记

读书札记

科学出版社
SCIENCE PRESS

科学出版社是中国规模最大的科学书刊出版机构,以出版高水平的自然科学、技术科学读物为基本任务,同时出版法律、医学、文化等方面的图书和画册。目前,年出书约 600 种,学术期刊 150 余种,900 余期。

科学出版社在香港、纽约建有分支机构,并与全球 40 多家出版社和数十家发行商建立了良好的合作关系。近十年来,以各种形式出版了近 200 种优秀英文版图书,并将更积极地促进国际文化、学术交流。

Science Press is the largest publishing house in China in publishing academic works and journals on natural science. It is characterized by publishing scientific and technological works' meanwhile accepts an obligation to publish the publications on law, medicine and culture. Science Press turns out annually about 600 titles of books and more than 900 issues of 150 academic journals.

Science Press has an office in Hong Kong and a branch in New York. It has also established collaborating relations on co-publishing and wholesaling with more than 40 foreign publishing firms and distributors. In the past decade, it has published in various ways nearly 200 titles of excellent scientific books in English edition. As a publisher, We shall exert every effort to actively promote the international cultural and academic exchange in the future.

地　　址：中国·北京　东黄城根北街 16 号
邮政编码：100707
电　　传：210247　SPBJ　CN
电　　话：4019821（国际合作室）
　　　　　4010642（国外发行部）
传　　真：4012180
电　　报：4411

Address: 16 Donghuangchenggen North Street, Beijing 100707
Cable: 4411, Beijing
Telex: 210247 SPBJ CN
Tel: 4019821 (International Cooperation Dept)
　　　441315 (International Sale & Marketing Dept)
Fax: 086-1-4012180

Science Press New York, Ltd.
92—13, 55th Avenue Elmhurst
NY　11373, U.S.A.
Tel: (718) 760—8303

CE—Science Press Ltd. (H. K.)
Block B. 9/F Greatmany Center
109—115
Queen's Road E. Hong Kong
Tel: 5—277689 5—280677
Fax: 5—8654955

湖南科学技术出版社
HUNAN Science & technology Press

湖南科学技术出版社是一家以出版科学技术读物为主的中型出版机构,成立于1979年。(原为湖南人民出版社的一个部门)。拥有年出书200种的出版能力;其中以应用技术读物为主。湖南科技出版社的出版物不仅在中国大陆市场有较高的覆盖面,近年来,还销往港台、北美与欧洲市场。

湖南科技出版社致力于倡导科学精神、推动科技发展。在出版活动中,已形成"精心策划、精编精印、快速高效、奉献一流文化精品"的出版风格。

Hunan Science & Technology Press, which used to be part of Hunan People's Publishing House, was founded in 1979. Being a medium—sized publisher, H. S. T. P. has the ability to publish books as many as 200 kinds yearly, most of which being science and technology readings。The publications by H. S. T. P. not only enjoy a wide coverage in China, but also have entered the book market of Taiwan, Hongkong, North America and Europe in recent years.

With advocating science and promoting, the development of science and technology as its main purpose, H. S. T. P. has evolved a style of "Offering the cream of culture to readers through careful planning , elaborate editing and exquisite printing" in the course of publication.

社址:长沙市展览馆路3号
电话:446777—519(总编室)
　　　446777—516,518(社长)
　　　428446　446742　(发行)
电挂:1516
Address: Echibition Road No 3
　　　　 Changsha 410005
　　　　 P. R. CHINA
Tel: 　　446777-519, 516, 518 (Master)
　　　　 428446, 446742 (Distribution Department)

SKILL WITH ILLUSTRATIONS OF CHINESE ACUPUNCTURE AND MOXIBUSTION

ISBN 7-5357-0931-1/R · 202

All Rights Reserved

© 1992 by Hunan Science & Technology Press and Science Press.

No part of the material protected by this copyright notice may be reproduced or utilized in any form or by any means, electronic or mechanical, including photocopying, recording, or by any information storage and retreval system, without written permission from the copyright owners.

Typesetting: Green Apple Data Center
Printed in Second Xinhua Printing House of Hunan Province
Projector: Wang Yi Fang
Author: Yan Jie
Translator: Yin Ganglin

图解中国针灸技法

严　洁编著　尹钢林译

责任编辑：王一方

湖南科学技术出版社(长沙市展览馆路3号)
科学出版社(北京市东黄城根北街16号)
湖南省科技馆青苹果数据中心排版
湖南省新华印刷二厂印刷

*

1992年2月第1版　1992年3月第1次印刷
开本：850×1168毫米　1/16　印张：31　插页：15
字数：729.2千字
ISBN　7—5357—0931—1
R·202　湘新登记证字004号
02880

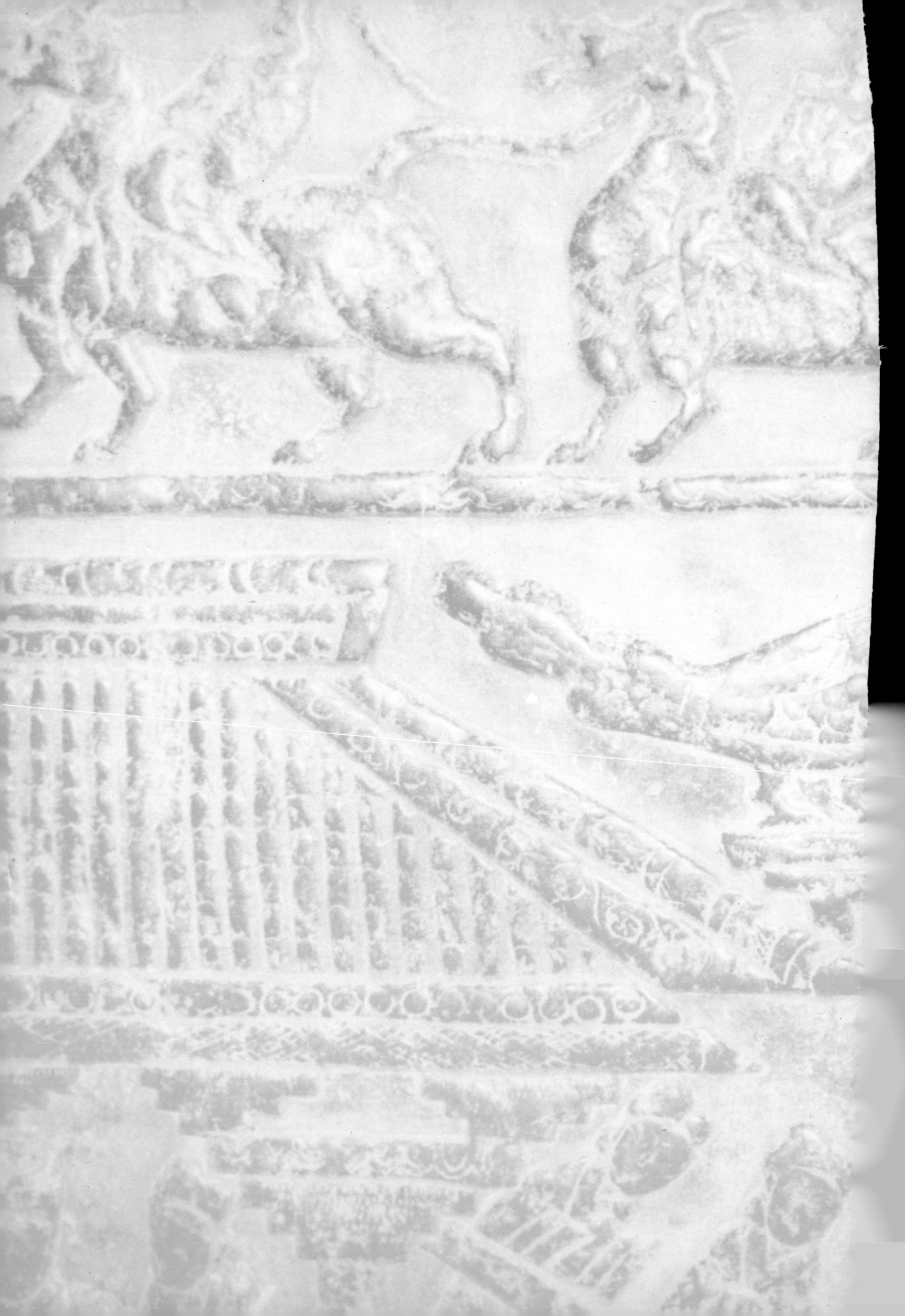